PENGUIN BOOKS

MADNESS EXPLAINED

Born in Sheffield in 1956, Richard P. Bentall was an undergraduate at the University College of North Wales, Bangor. He remained at Bangor to take a Ph.D. in experimental psychology before obtaining a qualification in clinical psychology at the University of Liverpool. He later obtained an MA in philosophy applied to health care from University College Swansea. After a brief period as a National Health Service forensic clinical psychologist, he returned to the University of Liverpool as a lecturer, where he was eventually appointed Professor of Clinical Psychology. In 1989 he received the British Psychological Society's May Davidson Award for his contribution to the field of clinical psychology. In 1999 he moved to a Chair in Experimental Clinical Psychology at the University of Manchester. Apart from his interests in severe mental illness, Richard P. Bentall also studies differences between human and animal learning mechanisms and has carried out research into the treatment of chronic fatigue syndrome. He lives with his partner, Aisling (also a psychologist), and their twin children Fintan and Keeva.

RICHARD BENTALL

Madness Explained
Psychosis and Human Nature

With a Foreword by Aaron T. Beck

PENGUIN BOOKS

PENGUIN BOOKS

Published by the Penguin Group
Penguin Books Ltd, 80 Strand, London WC2R 0RL, England
Penguin Group (USA) Inc., 375 Hudson Street, New York, New York 10014, USA
Penguin Books Australia Ltd, 250 Camberwell Road, Camberwell, Victoria 3124, Australia
Penguin Books Canada Ltd, 10 Alcorn Avenue, Toronto, Ontario, Canada M4V 3B2
Penguin Books India (P) Ltd, 11 Community Centre, Panchsheel Park, New Delhi – 110 017, India
Penguin Books (NZ) Ltd, Cnr Rosedale and Airborne Roads, Albany, Auckland, New Zealand
Penguin Books (South Africa) (Pty) Ltd, 24 Sturdee Avenue, Rosebank 2196, South Africa

Penguin Books Ltd, Registered Offices: 80 Strand, London WC2R 0RL, England

www.penguin.com

Published by Allen Lane 2003
Published in Penguin Books 2004
1

Copyright © Richard Bentall, 2003
Foreword copyright © Aaron T. Beck, 2003
All rights reserved

The moral right of the author has been asserted

The Acknowledgements on page x constitute an extension of this copyright page

Set by Rowland Phototypesetting Ltd, Bury St Edmunds, Suffolk
Printed in England by Clays Ltd, St Ives plc

For my family

Aisling
Keeva and Fintan

Everyone is much more simply human than otherwise.

Harry Stack Sullivan,
The Interpersonal Theory of Psychiatry

Contents

Part Four
Causes and their Effects

Acknowledgements

Verse

p. 118: Extract from 'We and They' by Rudyard Kipling reproduced by permission of A. P. Watt Ltd on behalf of the National Trust for Places of Historical Interest or Natural Beauty. p. 465: Extract from 'This be the Verse' by Philip Larkin reproduced by permission of Faber & Faber Ltd, on behalf of the estate of Philip Larkin.

Figures and tables

Table 3.1: Reprinted by permission of Oxford University Press. Table 3.4: Reprinted with permission from the *Diagnostic and Statistical Manual of Mental Disorders*, Third Edition. American Psychiatric Association. Table 3.5: Reprinted by permission of Cambridge University Press. Figure 4.1: From *Manic-Depressive Illness* by Fredrick K. Goodwin and Kay R. Jamison © 1990 by Oxford University Press, Inc. Used by permission of Oxford University Press Inc. Figure 4.2: Reprinted by permission of Cambridge University Press. Figure 6.1: Reprinted by permission of Cambridge University Press. Figure 7.1: Reprinted by permission of Elsevier Science. Figure 7.2: Copyright © 2001 by Oxford University Press, Inc. Used by permission of Oxford University Press, Inc. Figure 7.3: From *In Search of Madness: Schizophrenia and Neuroscience* by R. W. Heinrichs, copyright © 2001 by Oxford University Press, Inc. Used by permission of Oxford University Press, Inc. Figure 9.1: Copyright © Addison Wesley Longman Limited 1996, reprinted by permission of Pearson Education Limited. Figure 10.1: Copyright © 1999 by American Psychological Association. Adapted with permission. Figure 11.1: From *Manic-Depressive Illness* by Fredrick K. Goodwin and Kay R. Jamison, copyright © 1990 by Oxford University Press, Inc. Used by permission of Oxford University Press, Inc. Figure 11.3: Copyright © 1999 by American Psychological Association. Adapted with permission. Figure 12.3 : Reproduced by permission of Taylor & Francis. Figure 13.1: Reproduced with permission from the *British Journal of Medical Psychology*, copyright © The British Psychological Society. Figure 14.1: Reproduced with permission from the *British Journal of Medical Psychology*, copyright © The British Psychological Society. Figure 14.2: Reprinted by permission of Carol Donner. Figure 14.3: Copyright © 2000 by American Psychological Association. Reprinted with permission. Figure 14.4: Copyright © 2000 by American Psychological Association. Reprinted with permission. Figure 15.1: Reprinted by permission of Loris Lesynski. Figure 18.1: Copyright © Sage. Reprinted by permission of Sage Publications.

While every effort has been made to contact copyright holders, the author and publisher are happy to rectify any errors or omissions in subsequent editions.

Foreword by Professor Aaron Beck

As we move into the twenty-first century, a radical shift in the way many of us look at severe mental disorders has been taking place. Irrespective of the label – whether schizophrenia, psychosis or severe mental disease – a new humanizing trend is observable. In contrast to the more mechanistic framing of schizophrenia in terms of abnormal brain chemistry or anatomical lesions, the new approach views the patient as a whole person troubled by apparently baffling problems, but also having the resources for ameliorating these problems. This New Look can be contrasted with the prevailing biological paradigm with its emphasis on the disordered neurochemistry and anatomical defects and especially the perception of the patient as a passive recipient of the treatment. Although the laboratory tests, brain scans, and post-mortem studies have advanced our understanding of the neurological substrate and provided a variety of new medications, the distancing of the mental patient from the rest of humanity has persisted.

The more recent work spearheaded by Richard Bentall has brought the patient back into the mainstream of humanity. He and his co-workers have been able to demonstrate that the apparently mysterious, incomprehensible symptoms of the mentally ill are actually extensions of what many of us experience every day. The rather arcane extreme beliefs manifested by the patients can be seen to be on a continuum with ideas of the population at large. Beliefs in mind-reading, clairvoyance and alien possession are especially common in young people and a surprisingly large percentage of the population believe that they have received communications from God, the Devil and aliens. The 'bizarre' thinking of the severely disturbed patient represents an extract of these common notions. These beliefs, however, become a problem when they come to dominate the patients' thinking and especially their interpretations of their experiences. By analysing these beliefs within the framework of human nature and mainstream psychology, we can begin to make sense out of them. Further, the so-called 'negative symptoms' can be understood as a natural detachment from a stressful environment. By disengaging, the patients attempt to shut out those stimuli that activate their delusions and hallucinations. Part of the withdrawal also represents a 'giving up' produced by the profound demoralization over others' having given up on them.

Concurrent with the ground-breaking work of Bentall and his team, there has been an upsurge of interest in cognitive therapy of schizophrenia, with a number of successful attempts to ameliorate the patients' psychotic symptoms already published. The new approach, inspired in part by Bentall's work, views patients as agents in their own change, rather than passive recipients of the treatments that are administered to them. Further, the 'normalizing rationale' derived from Bentall's formulations provides a basic construct by which patients can understand and cope with their distressing, unusual experiences.

As the leader in the investigations of the psychology of psychosis, Bentall is uniquely qualified to explain this new approach and make it available not only to readers of scholarly journals, but also to a much broader audience. His approach demystifies psychosis and restores the patient to a proper place with the rest of humankind. By reversing the dehumanizing trend, he makes it possible to relate to the afflicted individuals as though they are just like the rest of us, although ostensibly quite different. The book is of particular interest to anybody who is curious about human nature and its vicissitudes. It will be of a special interest to those individuals who suffer from these mental disturbances or are related to such individuals or are professionals who treat them.

Like the legendary Theseus winding his way through the Labyrinth, Bentall has in his personal and private life encountered many obstacles and taken many twists and turns. As he faced and solved one problem, he was confronted with another, then another, which he proceeded to resolve. Like Theseus, he has endeavoured to slay the monster – mental illness – and in this volume he shows how he has trapped it, if not finished it off.

Author's Preface

In this book have I tried to tell three stories. First, I have tried to trace the history of our current understandings of serious mental illness and to show that these understandings are fatally flawed. Second, I have attempted to draw together recent research to suggest a radically different way of thinking about the most severe types of mental disorder, known as the psychoses. Finally, I have tried to tell a fraction of my personal story, about how I came to conduct research on delusions and hallucinations, and how the ideas outlined in these pages have come together in my mind. I have tried to write these stories in a straightforward way that will be accessible to non-specialists and lay people, because I believe that the way we think about psychiatric problems should be important to everybody, given that most people have some acquaintance with these problems, either through direct experience or by observing the suffering of a close relative or friend. At the same time, I have tried to be thorough enough in my treatment of the various issues to satisfy both my sympathetic colleagues and my critics from within psychiatry and clinical psychology. Inevitably, balancing the needs of these two quite different audiences has been difficult. The extent to which I have succeeded can only be judged by my readers.

The most important of the three stories is undoubtedly the second. I believe that many psychologists and psychiatrists can sense that a new way of thinking about psychiatric disorders is emerging, but few will have had the opportunity to try to gather together the many different strands of research that are contributing to this shift in thinking. Over the four years that it has taken me to assemble the relevant evidence I have found myself exploring surprising avenues, such as, for example, developmental psychology, medical anthropology, the new molecular genetics, developmental neurobiology and ideas from the branch of mathematics known as non-linear dynamics. These explorations have confirmed a view I have held for many years: that psychosis shines a particularly penetrating light on ordinary human functioning. Indeed, I do not think it is an exaggeration to say that the study of psychosis amounts to the study of human nature.

Of course, in many of the areas that I have explored I remain an amateur. Inevitably, there are gaps. One virtue of writing a book rather than an academic paper is that it is possible to speculate. However, the price of speculation may well be that I have got some things wrong. This is very much an unfinished project. For example, for completeness it would have been good to have included something about anxiety and obsessional thinking, thereby bringing the psychoses and the neuroses within a single framework. I think it is quite easy to see how this could be accomplished. However, to do so would take fifty extra pages and at least another year, so this part of the project will have to wait until another time.

I have said something about my personal story because I believe that it is important to recognize that science, and especially the scientific study of abnormal mental states, is a human activity. Scientists, like ordinary folk and psychiatric patients, are flawed, emotional and excitable human beings who are sometimes wise and sometimes stupid, sometimes lovable and sometimes bloody irritating. By talking about my own experiences, both positive and negative, I have attempted to highlight an important theme of this book, which is the vanishingly small difference between the 'us' who are sane and the 'them' who are not. At a recent conference I was introduced as 'Someone who has done more than most to move the dividing line between sanity and madness', which I think was a compliment. In any case, in these pages I have tried to demonstrate that the differences between those who are diagnosed as suffering from a psychiatric disorder and those who are not amounts to not very much. This is an important insight because of its implications for psychiatric care. As I hope to demonstrate in a later publication, the dreadful state of our psychiatric services is not only a consequence of muddled thinking about the nature of psychiatric disorders, but also a consequence of the way in which psychiatric patients have been denied a voice by being treated as irrational and dangerous, like wild animals in a zoo.

A word to my critics from within the mental health professions. Commentators on my work (you know who you are) have very occasionally dismissed my ideas as 'angry', anti-biological, a rehash of old ideas from the sixties, 'a politically motivated anti-psychiatric rant' (to quote an extremely unhappy member of the audience at a conference where I spoke) or Szaszian (readers who are unfamiliar with long-running arguments about the nature of madness will know, by the seventh chapter of the book, what this latter epithet means, and that its application to me is inaccurate). Perhaps I have been angry on occasions; certainly this seems to be an appropriate response to the way in which psychiatric patients are often dehumanized by a system that purports to care for them. However, the rest is false. Because I believe that these impressions arise from a superficial acquaintance with my work I will give unsympathetic readers of this volume an important clue: *you will not be able to understand the approach I am advocating without reading the fourth part of the book*, in which I attempt to show how an approach which is based on symptoms, and which therefore appears to be fragmented, can be welded together into a coherent whole.

Writing this book has been an interesting journey, during which there have been several important distractions, including my migration along the M62 from the University of Liverpool to the University of Manchester and, much more importantly, the birth of my two children Keeva and Fintan. In developing the ideas herein, I have been influenced by many people, but above all by the talented Ph.D. and D. Clin.Psychol. students it has been my privilege to supervise over the last fifteen years. One of the best-kept secrets in science is that most successful academic reputations are built on the backs of hard-working postgraduates, and my career is no exception to this rule. For their contributions to my thinking about the psychoses, I single out (in alphabetical order): Kim Bowen-Jones, Jennie Day, Gill Haddock, Sue Kaney, Peter Kinderman, Peter Rankin, Rebecca Swarbrick, Sara Tai and Heather Young, all of whom have since moved on to greater things. Current postgraduates who continue to keep me on my toes, and who constantly feed me ideas, include Paul French, Paul Hammersley, Becca Knowles, Peter Simpson, Joanna Teuton and Justin Thomas. Numerous collaborators who have supported and encouraged me, while tolerating my dreadful time-keeping and other idiosyncrasies, include David Healy, David Kingdon, Shôn Lewis, Tony Morrison, Richard Morriss, David Pilgrim, Anne Rogers, Jan Scott, Nick Tarrier and Doug Turkington. I would also like to thank Tim Beck, whose recent interest in the work carried out by myself and colleagues in Britain has been an important source of encouragement. Despite his abrupt departure from the British clinical psychology community a few years ago, it would be wrong not to mention Peter Slade, who strongly supported me during the early years of my career. I should also mention Don Evans and Martin Evans who ran the famous MA course in philosophy applied to health care at Swansea in the late 1980s; I hope that parts of this book show that their efforts were not entirely wasted.

Thanks for reading early drafts of various chapters and making encouraging noises go to my partner Aisling O'Kane, to the father (psychologist) and son (biologist) team of David and Ben Dickins (who checked my genetics), to Paul French, to John Read and finally to Tim Beck (who reminded me that it takes much less time to write a good chapter than a very, very good chapter). I would also like to offer special thanks to Stefan McGrath of Penguin Books, who first asked me to write this volume, tolerated my complete inability to stick to deadlines, and whose helpful feedback ensured that the final product was not so large that a wheelbarrow would be required to move it from one place to another.

No doubt I have left important people out of this list, and will find myself apologizing to them at a later date. Of course, my memory is less than perfect. In any case, it is time to reclaim my life and move on to projects new.

Richard Bentall
August, 2002

Part One

The Origins of our Misunderstandings about Madness

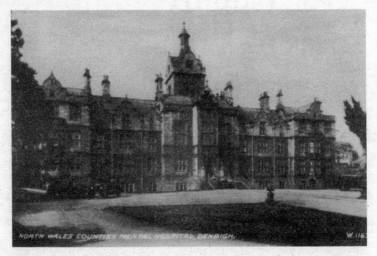

Figure 1.1 The North Wales Hospital, Denbigh, photographed in 1930 (reproduced from C. Wynne (1995) *The North Wales Hospital Denbigh, 1842–1995*. Denbigh: Gee & Son). The hospital was opened in 1848 on twenty acres of land donated for the purpose by a local landowner, Joseph Ablett, of Llanbedr Hall. At its peak, during the 1950s, the hospital was home to some 1500 patients. Its closure, first announced in 1960, was not completed until 1995.

1

Emil Kraepelin's Big Idea

What a curious attitude scientists have – 'We still don't know that;
but it is knowable and it is only a matter of time before we get to
know it!' As if that went without saying.   Ludwig Wittgenstein[1]

It is nearly twenty years since I first walked on to a psychiatric ward. At
the time I was an undergraduate psychology student at the University
College of North Wales, naive about the harsh realities of psychiatric
care, but determined to prove myself in the hope of securing a career
in clinical psychology.* Like most students in the 1970s, I wore faded
blue jeans and a sweatshirt for all occasions. This caused at least one
nurse to mistake me for a patient. (She attempted to overcome her
embarrassment by explaining that she had assumed I was a psychopath
rather than a schizophrenic. Apparently the patients attending the
hospital's drug rehabilitation unit nearly all wore jeans and nearly all

---

* Rob Buckman, doctor and humorist, has characterized the difference between
psychologists and psychiatrists in the following way: 'According to psychologists,
a psychologist is a scientist who has trained in various aspects of experimental
psychology, neurophysiology, operant conditioning and interpersonal dynamics,
whereas a psychiatrist is a doctor who couldn't keep up the payments on his
stethoscope. Psychiatrists, on the other hand, tend to view the schism in a more
allegorical style. Thus, according to a very senior psychiatrist, "neurotics are
people who build castles in the air, psychotics are people who live in them, while
psychiatrists are people who charge the rent, and psychologists are like Men from
the Council who come round once in a blue moon, talk incomprehensible crap,
and do damn all" (*Medicineballs II*. London: Papermac, 1988, pp. 78–9).

As this quotation suggests, the training of clinical psychologists and psychiatrists is quite different. For short accounts of these differences, see the Appendix, (pp. 513–26), which also contains brief definitions of many of the technical
terms included in the text.

were thought to show evidence of a 'psychopathic' or anti-social personality.)

The North Wales Hospital was located just outside the quiet market town of Denbigh. I was visiting in order to carry out a small research project with some of the hospital's long-term patients. I commuted the forty-two miles between Bangor and Denbigh in a disintegrating Austin mini, purchased with £300 I had earned by labouring in a Sheffield tool factory during my summer vacation. Descending the winding A543 into the centre of the town, I had to proceed cautiously because my brakes were not reliable. Unable to afford repairs, I was no exception to the delusion of immortality that is peculiarly strong in the ambitious young.

From the centre of Denbigh, a narrow road led up a hill and past a ruined thirteenth-century castle. Beyond the summit, the hospital came into view – a stone-grey Victorian fortress, standing in spacious and neatly maintained gardens, behind which stood the Clwyd hills. On a sunny day, it looked like an 'asylum' in the true sense of the word: a refuge, a place isolated from the troubles of the world. This illusion would be broken only after stepping through the imposing entrance, into the dark, antiseptic-smelling corridors that led to the psychiatric wards.

The ward on which I attempted to carry out my research was a large dormitory divided by wooden partitions into sleeping, sitting and dining areas. The paint was yellowing and the furniture had seen better times. The ward always reeked of cigarettes and sometimes also smelt of urine. It was home to about ten women, mostly elderly, who had spent most of their lives in psychiatric hospitals, and all of whom had been diagnosed as suffering from schizophrenia. They were cared for by uniformed nurses who, like generations of their predecessors, had been drawn from the population of the nearby town. In order to improve the women's self-care skills, a form of behaviour-modification programme (known as a 'token economy') had been introduced under the supervision of one of the hospital's few psychologists. The women were rewarded with plastic tokens if they completed various routine tasks (for example, getting up by a particular time, washing and dressing appropriately) and they could exchange their accumulated tokens for various forms of 'reinforcement' (usually cigarettes or sweets). It was a mechanistic form of rehabilitation (and one that has largely fallen out of favour) but its effects were occasionally dramatic. Before its introduction, one patient had been so determined to mutilate herself that the nurses had taken to tying her arms to her bed to prevent her from harming herself during the night. A year after the programme had been introduced, she was sleeping normally and was able to work as a nursing assistant on one of the other wards.

Despite these kinds of benefits, most of the women continued to exhibit a bewildering range of symptoms. Some appeared to talk to imaginary voices. Others expressed bizarre ideas. One believed that she had written a famous Russian novel. Another kept insisting that 'Peter Pickering has plucked my brain', a delusion which became more intelligible when inspection of her case notes revealed that she had been given a prefrontal leucotomy (a crude brain operation) many years earlier. (The notes recorded that the operation had been given under local anaesthetic and that she had become highly distressed at the precise moment that the knife had been inserted into her brain.)

One of the women had been mute for many years. Another spoke in a chaotic jumble of invented words and half-finished sentences. Most exhibited emotional or disorganized behaviour of one sort or another. (I recall that one lady of about 70 would periodically announce 'I'm going up the pole' before running from one end of the ward to the other, screaming loudly.) They were all vulnerable to maltreatment and exploitation. For example, one had been sexually abused in a toilet by a hospital visitor, who had attempted to buy her silence with a cigarette. How the women had come to be at the North Wales Hospital was something of a mystery. Most of the medical notes were too old and too vague to give any useful information about their early lives.[2]

The experiment I conducted under the supervision of the psychologist who was running the token system was designed to test the effectiveness of a simple form of psychological treatment, known as *self-instructional training*. The aim of the treatment was to improve the patients' ability to focus their attention when attempting daily tasks, on the assumption that this would facilitate their rehabilitation. The study called for each of the women to be given a short battery of memory and reasoning tests before and after several sessions of treatment, each lasting for perhaps half an hour. In each session, I would encourage the women to talk out aloud to themselves while solving various puzzles – to literally instruct themselves about what they were doing. In this way, the psychologist and I hoped that they would regain the capacity for focused verbal thought that we assumed they had lost as a consequence of their many years of living in an institution.

Some years later, I formulated what I now refer to as my 'first law of research', with which I entertain students who are about to embark on their first scientific projects. The law states that, by the time an experiment has been completed, the researcher will know how it should have been done properly. My own first adventure in experimental clinical psychology was no exception to this rule. I worked with each of the women for several hours, trying to teach them the relatively simple strategies that I believed would help them, becoming increasingly frustrated at their indifference to my efforts which, in retrospect, had little relevance to their needs. They, in turn, sometimes became frustrated with me, but more often struggled to be nice to the scruffy young man in jeans who energetically cajoled them to speak out loud while assembling simple jigsaws, or while matching groups of similar patterns. There was not a single aspect of my relationship with the women that I would now describe as therapeutic for either party.

Life has been kind to me in the years following the completion of the study. Some months later, I wrote up my results, said goodbye to the North Wales Hospital and collected my degree.[3] Although I failed to secure a place on a clinical psychology training course, I was not particularly disappointed – competition for training places was very strong. Plan B was to study for a doctorate in experimental psychology, so I gratefully accepted an offer to stay on at Bangor. Four years later, after completing my Ph.D., I secured a place on the clinical psychology course at the University of Liverpool. Sixteen years later still, I head up a small research team at the nearby University of Manchester, studying the kinds of problems that I had observed but poorly understood at Denbigh.

I suspect that life has been less kind to the women who suffered from those problems. Even a self-absorbed and ambitious young student could sense that the best they might experience in their declining years was humane custodial care. I imagine that most have now died. The North Wales Hospital now lies silent and empty, closed down like many similar institutions in the effort to move psychiatric services into the community. From the vantage point of the hospital bowling green, once immaculate but now overgrown, the building still looks peaceful in a ghostly sort of way. Because of its fine architectural features it is protected from demolition. Perhaps it will find a new lease of life as company offices or a large hotel.

With few exceptions, the psychiatric wards of today are located in general hospitals alongside surgical, medical and other types of services. Long-stay patients, unless they are judged to pose a significant danger to themselves or other people, live in small apartments or hostels hidden in the suburbs of towns and cities. Admissions to hospital are restricted to those who are floridly disturbed. Discharge back into the community is usually after a matter of weeks by which time, hopefully, the patient's worst symptoms have been controlled by medication. Visiting such a ward, one sees patients with a variety of diagnoses wandering aimlessly around. Some talk out loud to their voices, or charge around in a manic frenzy. However, on closer scrutiny, the overwhelming impression is one of inactivity and loneliness. Many patients sit in the ward lounge, silently smoking cigarettes, their faces glued to daytime television shows. The nurses, who now wear casual clothes instead of uniforms, spend most of their time in the nursing office, talking only to those patients who are most obviously distressed. The psychiatrists and psychologists are even less in evidence – patients on many wards see their psychiatrists for only a few minutes every week and the psychologists are almost entirely absent, confined by their own choice to outpatient clinics. There seems to be a lack of therapeutic contact between the patients and the staff. The patients are simply being 'warehoused' in the hope that their medication will do the trick.

I do not believe that this reflects much improvement compared to the standard of care that I encountered twenty years ago. Indeed, the psychiatrist and anthropologist Richard Warner, who has studied changes in psychiatric practice over many years, has argued that the success of psychiatric treatment today is little improved on that achieved in the first decades of the twentieth century, before the development of modern psychiatric drugs.[4] It would be tempting to blame this depressing state of affairs on the quality of the staff who work in our psychiatric services. Certainly, I have met some nurses, psychiatrists and psychologists who appear to be indifferent to the needs of their patients, and who would be much better employed in some other line of work. However, they are the exceptions. Most mental health professionals are hard-working, caring and thoroughly frustrated at their inability to do better for their patients.

In this book I will argue that the main problem faced by modern psychiatric services is not one of personnel or resources (although these may be important) but one of *ideas*. I will suggest that we have been labouring under serious misunderstandings about the nature of madness for more than a century, and that many contemporary approaches to the problem, although cloaked with the appearance of scientific rigour, have more in common with astrology than rational science. Only by abolishing these misunderstandings can we hope to improve the lot of the most impoverished, neglected and vulnerable of our citizens.

The orthodox approach which I will show must be rejected is based on two false assumptions: first, that madness can be divided into a small number of diseases (for example, schizophrenia and manic depression) and, second, that the manifestations or 'symptoms' of madness cannot be understood in terms of the psychology of the person who suffers from them. These assumptions were spelt out explicitly by the early psychiatrists whose writings have most influenced modern psychiatric thinking, and whose ideas remain unquestioned by many psychiatrists today. By tracing the history of these apparently innocuous assumptions, we will be able to see why they proved so disastrous to the well-being of patients.

Who was Emil Kraepelin?

> Trusting in the wings of my will
> I swore to dispatch the misery of my people,
> To drive us through peril and danger
> And fulfil the promise of their prosperity

Arduous and long the journey. In bloody victories
And with an ardent heart did I execute my mission
To but one *enemy was I to succumb:*
The thanklessness and delusion of my own people.

Emil Kraepelin, *c.* 1920[5]

Despite important developments elsewhere, the world centre of psychiatry and most other medical specialities in the nineteenth century was Germany, partly because more researchers pursued higher degrees there than anywhere else. It was a German, Johann Christian Reil, who first coined the term 'psychiatry' from the Greek 'psyche' (soul) and 'iatros' (doctor).[6] Teaching in psychiatry began in Leipzig in 1811, and professors of the new discipline began to appear at other German universities soon afterwards. In 1865 Wilhelm Griesinger established the first modern-style university psychiatry department in Berlin, where teaching and research were pursued alongside clinical work. Two years later, he founded one of the first academic journals in psychiatry, the *Archives for Psychiatry and Nervous Disease*.

Researchers of the period spent much of their time staring down microscopes at post-mortem brain tissue in the hope of discovering the biological basis of mental illness. In the process, they made many important discoveries about the structure of the human nervous system. The historian Edward Shorter has dubbed this era 'the age of the first biological psychiatry' to contrast it with our own times, in which a biological approach is also dominant.

As Shorter has observed, it is the German psychiatrist Emil Kraepelin rather than Freud who should be seen as the central figure in the history of psychiatry.[7] Kraepelin was born in 1856 (the same year as Freud) in Neustrelitz, a village near the Baltic Sea. It is said that he learned early to respect authority, a disposition that in later life would manifest itself in his unwavering admiration of Bismarck and in his authorship of nationalistic poems, the quality of which can be judged from that quoted at the beginning of this section. He was much influenced by his older brother Karl, a respected biologist who made contributions to the classification of plant species. Studying medicine at Würzburg, Kraepelin graduated in 1878, having earlier won a prize for an essay entitled 'The influence of acute diseases on the origin of mental diseases'.

His enthusiasm for psychiatry was reinforced by a period of further study in Leipzig, where he had planned to work under the supervision of the noted psychiatrist and brain anatomist Paul Flechsig.[8] However, Flechsig had little interest in the psychological issues that interested Kraepelin. (It is said that Flechsig only once recorded the life circumstances of a patient, a depressed young man whom he wrote up for his doctoral dissertation.) The two men did not get on and, after a couple of months, Kraepelin was sacked, allegedly because Flechsig did not consider him able enough to deputize in his absence. (This dispute was apparently quite personal. Flechsig later formally accused Kraepelin of making derogatory remarks about his official oath, briefly stalling Kraepelin's promotion, until friends persuaded the Ministry of Culture to intervene on his behalf.) It was in these difficult circumstances that Kraepelin was rescued by Wilhelm Wundt, a philosopher who is widely credited with being the first experimental psychologist. Working in Wundt's laboratory, he immersed himself in simple psychological experiments. His new master was to remain an important influence on Kraepelin's life and work, and encouraged him to write the first, fairly insubstantial edition of his *Compendium of Psychiatry*. After a series of revisions, this book would have near-revolutionary impact on the theory of psychiatry.

In 1883, the year in which the first edition of the *Compendium* appeared, Kraepelin became a lecturer at the District Mental Hospital in Munich. He was appointed professor of psychiatry in Dorpat in Russia (now Tartu in Estonia) in 1886, and it was there that he first began to develop his ideas on psychiatric classification. It was not until 1891, however, when he moved to the psychiatric hospital of the University of Heidelberg in the German state of Baden, that he was able to put these ideas to the test by amassing data from a large number of patients. By 1896 he had collected over 1000 case studies. This effort brought him into some conflict with the local authorities responsible for the administration of psychiatric services.[9] At that time, the care of the insane in Baden was organized into three districts, each served by a hospital, one of which was the University clinic at Heidelberg. From there, patients could be transferred to the two other institutions at Emmendingen and Pforzheim, the former specializing in the care of patients who were capable of productive work and the latter in the care of patients whose illnesses were chronic and unremitting.

Kraepelin's complaint was, first, that records transferred with the patients became difficult to access for the purposes of scientific investigation and, second, that transfers were not happening speedily enough, limiting the number of new patients that were available for him to study. The dispute escalated into an argument about Kraepelin's clinical autonomy and it was partly for this reason that he accepted a position at the University clinic in Munich in 1902, where he opened the German Psychiatric Research Institute (now the Max Planck Institute of Psychiatry) in 1917.

Although those who recorded their meetings with Kraepelin usually wrote about him with some affection, it is doubtful whether he was fun to be with. Perhaps the closest he came to his colleagues in his later years was during annual walks in the countryside (nicknamed 'catatonic walks' by the junior staff), which it was his custom to take with his assistants. At other times he would browbeat his colleagues with his strongly held views about the dangers of alcohol, having decided in 1895 to live a life of uncompromising abstinence in order to set an example to others.[10] An American psychiatrist who knew him remarked on the relationship between Kraepelin's personality and his approach to his work:

Kraepelin's personal nature was guarded by a wall of reserve. He held himself sternly to his goals; he devoted himself unremittingly to his work, uncompromisingly following what he believed to be the path of investigation – exact, demonstrable and well established by the assembling of all possible testimony step by step. It was consistent with this nature that only the precision of experimental psychology should seem applicable, that the more elastic boundaries of a subjective psychology of mental disease, like psychoanalysis, should seem forbidden and untrustworthy territory.[11]

Apparently, Kraepelin's reserve could cross the boundary into complete insensitivity. One of his assistants, who became seriously ill while accompanying him on a visit to the United States, remarked on his return that: 'If I had died on the trip, Kraepelin would probably have collected my ashes in a cigar box and brought them home to my wife with the words, "He was a real disappointment to me".'[12]

Although Kraepelin is usually remembered for his diagnostic concepts, his research interests were broad ranging. For example, influenced by Wundt he advocated the use of psychological tests in psychiatric research, and carried out simple studies of memory and reaction times with his patients. He wrote an interesting study of the role of speech in dreams based on his own dream diary, although, unlike Freud, he believed dreams to be meaningless phenomena caused by transient neuropathological conditions.[13] He was also a pioneer of psychopharmacology (the study of the psychological effects of drugs) and carried out experiments on the mental effects of tea, alcohol and various sedatives. In 1903 he travelled to Java with his brother in order to determine whether the forms of mental illness observed there in both Europeans and natives would correspond to those observed in Germany. He concluded that they did,[14] and returned convinced of the importance of the human will, although, as a recent commentator has remarked, 'He was in no manner consistent in conceiving it as being either free or biologically determined and preferred instead to empha- size the former in describing his own condition and the latter in diagnosing that of his patients.'[15]

Kraepelin wrote about every major type of psychiatric disorder recognized in his time. However, he was particularly interested in the more severe forms of madness in which the individual appears to lose touch with reality. Today, these disorders are known as the *psychoses* (although the term was used somewhat differently in Kraepelin's day). Despite the wide range of information that he was prepared to draw upon, his approach was uncompromisingly medical:

Judging from our experience in internal medicine it is a fair assumption that similar disease processes will produce identical symptom pictures, identical pathological anatomy and an identical aetiology. If, therefore, we possessed a comprehensive knowledge of any of these three fields – pathological anatomy, symptomatology, or aetiology – we would at once have a uniform and standard classification of mental diseases. A similar comprehensive knowledge of either of the other two fields would give us not just as uniform and standard classifications, but *all of these classifications would exactly coincide.*[16]

This was Kraepelin's big idea (see Figure 1.2), announced tentatively in the second edition of the *Compendium* (renamed the *Textbook of Psychiatry*), which appeared in 1887, and which he elaborated until just before his death in 1926, soon after which the ninth and last edition was published. Mental illnesses fell into a small number of

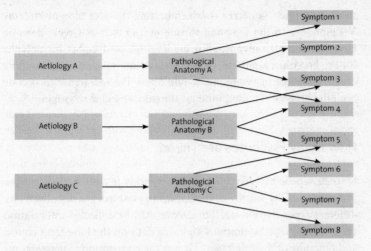

Figure 1.2 Emil Kraepelin's big idea. Kraepelin assumed that there was a discrete and discoverable number of psychiatric disorders. Although he recognized that some symptoms could occur in more than one disorder, he argued that each disorder has a typical symptom-picture. He also believed that the different disorders were associated with different types of brain pathology and with different aetiologies. On this view, the first step towards discovering the causes of mental illness was to identify the different disorders on the basis of their symptoms.

discoverable types, and these could be independently identified by studying symptoms, by direct observation of brain diseases, or by discovering the aetiologies of the illnesses (for example, by finding out whether they ran in families and were therefore determined by heredity). Of course, the only practical method of classification available at the time was by symptoms, as very little was known about the neuropathology or aetiology of psychiatric disorders. However, precisely because individuals with the same illness, defined by symptoms, were assumed to have the same brain disease, it could confidently be assumed that the identification of the illness would lead directly to an understanding of aetiology. On Kraepelin's analysis, therefore, the correct classification of mental illnesses according to symptoms would provide a kind of Rosetta stone, which would point directly to the biological origins of madness. The Rosetta stone, discovered in 1799 by Napoleon's soldiers during their invasion of Egypt, contained the same inscription (a decree commemorating the accession of Ptolemy V Epiphanes to the Egyptian throne in 197 BC) in Greek, demotic Egyptian and hieroglyphs, allowing linguists to decipher hieroglyphs for the first time. Similarly, on Kraepelin's analysis, an understanding of the language of symptoms would allow the researcher to decode both the biological underpinnings of madness and their origins.

How Many Psychoses are There?

Once Kraepelin had decided that the psychoses fell into a small number of discoverable types, the next step was to establish exactly how many different types there were. To achieve this, he collected information about his patients' symptoms and also data on the long-term course and outcome of their illnesses.[17] It was the recognition that symptoms changed with time, and therefore that patients should be observed throughout their lifetimes, that led Kraepelin to collect the thousand and more case studies which, in 1896, still seemed inadequate for his purposes. And it was on the basis of these case studies that he began to conclude that different groups of symptoms followed characteristically different courses.

Between 1893, when he published the fourth edition of the *Textbook*, and 1915, when the eighth edition was published, Kraepelin began to group together illnesses described by other researchers that apparently had a poor outcome. He included *catatonia*, a disorder characterized by stupor and abnormal postures. Also included was *hebephrenia*, a disease that struck during adolescence and which led to a rapid deterioration of mental functions. Finally, there was *dementia paranoides*, a disease which again led to rapid deterioration, but which was characterized by bizarre fears of persecution. This focus on illnesses with poor outcome reflected a preoccupation with psychological degeneration that was common among psychiatrists of his time, and that had been stimulated by the writings of Augustin Morel, a French psychiatrist who had died in 1873. Morel had suggested that mental illness (like sin) is passed on and exacerbated by heredity, weakening successive generations. (Many years later, this theory would have disastrous implications for the practice of psychiatry in the Third Reich.) It was therefore striking that Kraepelin, on deciding that catatonia, hebephrenia and dementia paranoides were manifestations of the same illness, chose to name the illness *dementia praecox*, a term originally proposed by Morel as an alternative name for hebephrenia.

The Latin term 'dementia praecox' means senility of the young, and that was exactly how Kraepelin saw the disorder. Its various subtypes – ten according to the eighth edition of the *Textbook* – were reflected in a variety of symptoms which usually first appeared in adolescence or early adulthood. Patients might experience an absence of emotion, or their emotional responses might be highly inappropriate (for example, a patient might laugh at a funeral). They might display stereotyped behaviour (for example, clapping five times before entering a room) or adopt catatonic postures. Problems of attention were also common, so that patients became distractible and easily confused. They might suffer from strange perceptions, particularly auditory (hearing imaginary voices) and tactile (feeling something touching them in the absence of an actual stimulus) hallucinations. Irrational beliefs were also frequently observed, particularly delusions of persecution (for example, patients might believe that they were being persecuted by the German royal family) or of grandiosity (believing that they had improbable powers). However, the common underlying feature that was always present was an irreversible deterioration of the intellectual functions. Dementia praecox patients became mentally disabled, unable to lead productive lives, and they never recovered. It was for this reason that Kraepelin could confidently assert that:

Although there still are in many details far reaching differences of opinion, the conviction is gaining ground more and more, that dementia praecox is by and large a distinct disease entity; and that we are justified in regarding at least the main group of often very diverse clinical pictures brought here together as the expression of a uniform morbid process.[18]

During the years in which he was developing the concept of dementia praecox, Kraepelin came to believe that he could recognize a second major type of mental illness, characterized by a periodic course and a good prognosis. As was the case for dementia praecox, this second type emerged gradually over successive editions of the *Textbook*, in which he collapsed a number of previously described disorders into a single category. The common feature of these disorders was a recurrent or 'circular' disorder of mood in which episodes of illness were followed by periods of normal functioning. By the eighth edition of the *Textbook*, Kraepelin had grouped all mood disorders into the single category of *manic depressive illness*.[19] His use of this term was broad by modern standards. He included disorders in which there are episodes of depression but no episodes of mania, which would now be described as *unipolar depression*. He also included illnesses in which the individual experienced only one episode followed by a complete recovery.[20]

A final category of illness described by Kraepelin, but given less attention by later historians of psychiatry, was *paranoia*. From the fifth edition of the *Textbook* onwards, this term was used to refer to a chronic illness characterized by delusional beliefs in the absence of significant changes to the patient's personality. It was differentiated from dementia praecox – in which delusions were also observed – because more general deficits of thinking or will were absent. Until the eighth edition of the *Textbook*, Kraepelin believed that paranoia had a similar unremitting course to dementia praecox. However, he eventually came to the view that paranoia included cases of low severity, in which at least a partial recovery was possible.

Kraepelin's Legacy

In the final decade of his life, Kraepelin wrote a number of papers that attempted to draw together his conclusions about mental disorders and the methods by which they could be studied. The most important, published in 1920, was entitled 'Clinical manifestations of mental illness',[21] and has sometimes been mistaken for a retraction of his previous ideas. To be sure, the tone adopted in the paper was less certain than in many of his earlier publications. Indeed, he began by conceding that progress in understanding the aetiology of most disorders had been painfully slow:

In the past, when tissue was first examined microscopically, new discoveries were made daily. Today we can only make significant progress by using very refined methods. In the case of some diseases many questions have already been answered. It is difficult to broaden our knowledge in such instances. The more we scratch below the surface, the more obvious the problems become and the more refined our tools must be. In spite of all this our successes are becoming more modest. We shall have to resign ourselves to this state of affairs, which after all corresponds to that found in other branches of scientific inquiry.

In passages that anticipated debates that would haunt psychiatry for the remaining years of the twentieth century, he acknowledged the difficulty of distinguishing between disease entities:

No experienced physician would deny that cases occur with unwelcome frequency in which, despite the most assiduous observation, it is impossible to reach a diagnosis. The experience that we cannot significantly reduce the number of misdiagnoses has a crippling effect on one's job satisfaction.

And:

We shall have to get accustomed to the fact that our much used clinical checklist does not permit us to differentiate reliably manic depressive insanity from [dementia praecox] in all circumstances; and that there is an overlap between the two, which depends on the fact that the clinical signs have arisen from certain antecedent conditions.

However, this did not mean that manic depression and dementia praecox were no longer to be regarded as separate diseases. On the contrary:

We cannot help but maintain that the two disease processes themselves are distinct. On the one hand we find those patients with irreversible dementia and severe cortical lesions. On the other are those patients whose personality remains intact. This distinction is too overwhelming for us to accept much overlap between the two groups, particularly as we can often predict the course of the two from the clinical signs.

The problem, as Kraepelin now saw it, was that the patient's symptoms are not uniquely determined by the disease process. Rather, the symptoms brought out by the disease depend on the individual nature of the patient. Therefore:

It seems absurd to propose that neurosyphilis [damage to the brain that occurs in the final stages of a syphilitic infection] causes patients to believe that they are the proud possessors of cars,* mansions or millions of pounds,

---

* Of course, in Kraepelin's time, cars were owned only by the very rich.

and that cocaine causes visual hallucinations of mites and lice. Rather, the general desires of such people are reflected in their delusions of grandeur.

These kinds of influences, Kraepelin believed, could be revealed by the methods of comparative psychiatry, which allowed the varying manifestations of a disorder to be studied in different people and different circumstances. Studies of this kind revealed that symptoms were affected by personal and social factors such as sex ('women show a greater propensity to erotic delusions and are less flamboyant in the presentation of delusions of grandeur'), age ('the clinical form of juvenile dementia praecox is . . . characterized by occasional excitement on a background of apathy and obtuseness') and culture ('it goes without saying that [in Java] no one suffered from delusions of guilt because these have their origins in religion').

These subtle qualifications were all but ignored by the majority of Kraepelin's followers. To many readers of the successive editions of the *Textbook*, his work appeared to bring order to a field that had previously lacked an agreed language. However, his system was not adopted immediately or uncritically, partly because alternative models of psychiatric classification were available from his academic rivals. In France, Kraepelin was attacked because of the 'woolliness of his suggested clinical pictures',[22] and the concept of dementia praecox was accepted only grudgingly. In Germany, Great Britain and the United States his system of diagnosis was vigorously debated before finally being embraced by most clinicians. This ultimate triumph partly reflected the simplifying effect that Kraepelin's ideas had on the theory and practice of psychiatry. He had asked himself how many different types of psychosis there actually were and had come up with a surprising answer: only three.

After Kraepelin

Every great man nowadays has his disciples, and it is always Judas who writes the biography.   Oscar Wilde[1]

Unlike Freud, Kraepelin never encouraged the formation of a group of disciples who would revere his case studies and proselytize his theories for the benefit of later generations of clinicians. Nevertheless, those who have followed him have by and large regarded his diagnostic system as the foundation stone around which a scientific psychiatry could be built. Indeed, Kraepelin's success is evident from the fact that his diagnostic concepts have survived until the present time. Two of the names he selected to describe major classes of mental illness – manic depression and paranoia – are in use today. The third – dementia praecox – was discarded in the first important revision of his system, which was brought about by a Swiss psychiatrist, Eugen Bleuler.

The Evolution of Schizophrenia

Bleuler was born in 1857 in the village of Zollikon, approximately one hour's walk from the centre of Zurich, and now a suburb of the city.[2] According to an account of his life written by his son Manfred (also a psychiatrist), his decision to become a doctor was partly inspired by observing local dissatisfaction with the German-speaking medical professors who had been appointed to positions at the nearby Burg-hölzli Mental Hospital, which had opened its doors for the first time in 1870.

After graduating in medicine at the University of Zurich in 1881, Bleuler studied in Paris, London and Munich, before joining the staff at the Burghölzli. There, he worked under the director, August Forel, a biological psychiatrist who had developed an appreciation for the more psychological aspects of psychiatric care after discovering that laymen were sometimes better able to cure alcoholics than physicians. (Consulting one successful lay therapist, Forel was told, 'No wonder, Herr Professor, I am an abstainer while you are not.')[3]

In 1886, at the age of 29, Bleuler became director of a psychiatric clinic at Rheinau, a small farming village. The clinic was located in an eighth-century monastery on an island in the Rhine, which had been turned into a hospital in 1867 and which, at the time of Bleuler's arrival, was reputed to be one of the most backward psychiatric institutions in Switzerland. He set about reforming the hospital and improving the quality of life of its patients. In Manfred's account:

Bleuler was not yet married, and lived there alone, in contact with his patients. He worked with them (mostly in agriculture), organized their free time (for instance, hiked with them, played in the theatre with them, and danced with them). He was also the general physician of the patients of the Clinic and the inhabitants of the village. During his life with the patients, Bleuler had always a memo-pad at hand, where he noted what touched and interested him in his patients' behaviour. He frequently noted in shorthand what the patients actually said.[4]

When a typhoid epidemic broke out, Bleuler was able to recruit some of his patients as nurses. They performed well, prompting him to observe that mental illness, far from dominating the life of patients, could retreat into the background when a crisis loomed. Because he had formed such close relationships with the inhabitants of the hospital, it was with regret that he returned to the Burghölzli, where, in 1898, he was appointed Forel's successor. Two years later, he appointed Carl Gustav Jung to a junior post in the hospital. Jung, who was to become Sigmund Freud's most famous disciple, and later the first rebel of the psychoanalytic movement, was to have an important impact on Bleuler's thinking about the causes of mental illness. However, it seems that the two men never really liked each other, although the fact that most observers commented on Bleuler's warmth and openness suggests that the fault was Jung's. Certainly, Jung adapted with difficulty to the workaholic regime established by Bleuler at the hospital, which required doctors to make their rounds before breakfast.

At the time, Freud's theory of *psychoanalysis* was just beginning to attract the attention of psychiatrists and psychologists outside his home city of Vienna. According to the theory, mental illness was caused by unconscious mental forces or repressed ideas, which intruded into consciousness in a distorted form, and thereby generated the patient's symptoms. This discovery seemed to promise a new kind of psychological treatment for the mentally ill. During the period that he worked in the Burghölzli between 1900 and 1910, Jung therefore formed a small discussion group dedicated to examining the claims of psychoanalysis. He also undertook a series of studies of dementia praecox that, although initially developed with his colleagues in Zurich, drew him progressively closer to Freud's ideas. Most important of these were studies in which word associations were used to probe the unconscious 'feeling-toned-complexes' which Jung believed lay at the root of the patient's dreamlike thoughts and speech.[5]

Encouraged by the successful work of his junior colleague, Bleuler participated in the discussion group and became convinced that psychoanalysis represented an important breakthrough in the theory and practice of psychiatry. This enthusiasm became very important to Freud, as Bleuler was the first respected academic psychiatrist to take the new theory seriously. Unfortunately for Freud, Bleuler's enthusiasm did not blunt his critical faculties. By the time of the first international meeting of psychoanalysts, organized by Jung and held in the Hotel Bristol in Salzburg in April 1908, tensions had begun to develop between the two great men. These tensions, which eventually led to Bleuler's resignation from the newly formed International Psychoanalytic Association, reveal much of Bleuler's character and his approach to his work.

According to a letter written by Bleuler to Freud in October 1910:

There is a difference between us, which I decided I shall point out to you, although I am afraid it will make it emotionally more difficult for you to come to an agreement. For you evidently it became the aim and interest of your whole life to establish firmly your theory and to secure its acceptance. I certainly do not underestimate your work. One compares it with that of Darwin, Copernicus and Semmelweis. I believe too that for psychology your discoveries are equally as fundamental as the theories of those men for other branches of science, no matter whether or not one evaluates advancements in psychology as highly as those in other sciences. The latter is a matter of subjective opinion. For me, the theory is only one new truth among other truths. I stand up for it because I consider it valid and because I feel I am able to judge it since I am working in a related field. But for me this is not a major issue, whether the validity of these views will be recognized a few years sooner or later. I am therefore less tempted than you to sacrifice my whole personality for the advancement of the cause.[6]

In March 1911 Bleuler wrote to Freud in defence of a psychiatrist who had been asked to resign from the Association because of a difference of opinion:

'Who is not with us is against us,' the principle 'all or nothing' is necessary for religious sects and for political parties. I can understand such a policy, but for science I consider it harmful. There is no ultimate truth. From a complex of notions one person will accept one detail, another person another detail. The partial notions, A and B, do not necessarily determine each other. I do not see that in science if someone accepts A, he must necessarily swear also for B. I recognise in science neither open nor closed doors, but no doors, no barriers at all.[7]

This kind of eclecticism is clearly evident in Bleuler's most famous work, *Dementia Praecox or the Group of Schizophrenias*, which drew heavily on his observations of patients at Rheinau, and which was rich in clinical detail. It began with acknowledgements to Kraepelin (for grouping together and describing the separate symptoms of dementia praecox) and to Freud (for enlarging the concepts available to psycho-pathologists). However, just as Bleuler found it difficult to swallow the entire body of Freudian theory without reservation, so too he found it difficult to agree completely with Kraepelin's characterization of the most severe type of mental illness.

The first and most obvious difference between Kraepelin and Bleuler concerned the name that should be given to the illness. Bleuler believed that the term 'dementia praecox' was misleading for two reasons. First, the illness did not always result in an extreme form of mental deterioration (it was not a dementia). Second, although it usually began in late adolescence, the illness sometimes first appeared in later life (it was not always praecox). To the confusion of lay people ever since, Bleuler proposed the new term *schizophrenia* to describe the disorder. In doing so, he did not mean to imply that the illness caused a split personality of the kind sometimes portrayed in paperback novels and Hollywood films.* Rather, Bleuler was suggesting that, at the core of the illness, there was a separation between the different psychic functions of personality, thinking, memory and perception.

Bleuler, like Kraepelin, believed that schizophrenia was the product of some kind of biological disorder, and toyed with the idea that it was caused by an accumulation of abnormal metabolites in the blood. However, unlike the early Kraepelin, he was also interested in the psychology of his patients' symptoms, and was impressed by the extent to which they could vary from one individual to another. In order to make sense of this variation, he made use of ideas borrowed from Freud and psychoanalysis, and combined them with his own notions about the mental mechanisms responsible for normal thinking and reasoning. This approach led him to suppose that, underneath the most obvious but varied symptoms of schizophrenia, there was a less obvious inner unity. In an attempt to characterize this unity, he identified four subtle symptoms which he believed to be fundamental to the illness, and which have since been known to English-speaking psychiatrists as Bleuler's four 'As'.

First, and most importantly, there was a loosening of the *associations* that linked together the stream of thought, so that the patient could no longer reason coherently. In extreme cases, this could cause the sufferer to speak in a jumbled word salad, as exemplified by a modern patient's attempt to answer the question 'Why do you think people believe in God?'

Uh, let's, I don't know why, let's see, balloon travel. He holds it up for you, the balloon. He don't let you fall out, your little legs sticking out down through the clouds. He's down to the smoke stack, looking through the smoke trying to get the balloon gassed up you know. Way they're flyin' on top that way, legs sticking out, I don't know, looking down on the ground, heck, that'd make you so dizzy you just stay and sleep you know, hold down

---

* For a brief but interesting account of this lay misunderstanding of the concept of schizophrenia see T. Turner (1995) 'Schizophrenia', in G. E. Berrios and R. Porter (eds.), *A History of Clinical Psychiatry*. London: Athlone Press. According to Turner, the earliest recorded misrepresentation of this sort occurs in an essay on literary criticism written by T. S. Eliot in 1933.

and sleep there. The balloon's His home you know up there. I used to be sleep out doors, you know, sleep out doors instead of going home.[8]

(Since Bleuler, this kind of speech has commonly been described as *thought disorder*. However, in a later chapter we will see that this term is quite misleading.)

The second of Bleuler's four 'As' was *ambivalence* – the holding of conflicting emotions and attitudes towards others. Third, schizophrenia patients were said to suffer from *autism*, a withdrawal from the social world resulting from a preference for living in an inner world of fantasy. Finally, there was inappropriate *affect*, the display of emotions that are incongruent with the patient's circumstances.

Bleuler held that, in contrast to these fundamental symptoms, the most obvious features of schizophrenia described by Kraepelin, namely hallucinations and delusions, were mere accessory symptoms – psychological reactions to the illness rather than direct products of the disorder. Indeed, he argued that a substantial subgroup of patients, who were said to suffer from *simple schizophrenia*, did not experience these symptoms at all. Such people might include individuals who 'vegetate as day labourers, peddlers, even as servants', or 'the wife . . . who is unbearable, constantly scolding, nagging, always making demands but never recognising duties'.[9]

Enlarging the category of schizophrenia even further, Bleuler argued that:

There is also a latent schizophrenia and I am convinced that it is the most frequent form, although admittedly these people hardly ever come for treatment. It is not necessary to give a detailed description of the various manifestations of latent schizophrenia . . . Irritable, odd, moody, withdrawn or exaggeratedly punctual people arouse, among other things, the suspicion of being schizophrenic.[10]

In his less well known *Textbook of Psychiatry*, the fourth edition of which was published in 1924, Bleuler extended this analysis to reconsider the relationship between schizophrenia and manic depression. Unlike Kraepelin, he came to the view that these were not separate disease entities after all, but that there was a continuum running between them, without a clear line of demarcation.[11] On this view, patients could be regarded as predominantly schizophrenic or predominantly manic depressive according to the extent to which they experienced or did not experience schizophrenia symptoms (the affective symptoms normally attributed to manic depression being regarded as non-specific).

Bleuler's contribution, then, was not only to provide an account of the psychology of dementia praecox, but also to widen the concept substantially. Indeed, on his account there seemed to be no precise dividing line between normality and illness, or between one type of madness and another. This analysis was entirely consistent with Bleuler's clinical attitude which, as we have seen, was markedly different from Kraepelin's. Whereas for Kraepelin the mad were subjects of scientific interest and scrutiny, for Bleuler they were fellow human beings engaged in the same existential struggles as the rest of humanity, struggles that were made more difficult by their illness.

Defining the boundaries of madness: the philosophical approach of Karl Jaspers

Broad conceptions of schizophrenia, such as Bleuler's, highlighted the difficulty of determining exactly who suffered from the illness and who did not. This important problem was addressed, in different ways, by a group of psychiatrists who were Kraepelin's successors at Heidelberg, whose ideas brought about further shifts in the way that researchers thought about the illness. Foremost among them was Karl Jaspers, who became better known as a philosopher than as a psychiatrist, and who worked as a doctor for only seven years, between 1908 and 1915.[12]

Jaspers was born in 1883 in Oldenburg, close to the North Sea. His father was a jurist and his mother came from a local farming family. According to Jaspers' own account, his father actively encouraged him to question authority at an early age which, unfortunately, led him into conflict with his teachers and isolated him from potential friends. Seeking solace by exploring the nearby coast and countryside, Jaspers' mind turned to matters philosophical. He read Spinoza at the age of 17 but decided to study law rather than philosophy at university. Almost immediately it became evident to him that this decision had been a great mistake: 'The abstractions which were used to refer to social life – a life still entirely unknown to me – proved so disappointing that I occupied myself instead with poetry, art, graphology and the theatre, always turning to something else.'[13]

In 1902, Jaspers decided to abandon his legal studies and study medicine. In order to explain this decision to his parents, he wrote them a memorandum:

My plan is the following: I shall take my medical state examination after the prescribed number of semesters. If then I still believe – as I do now – to possess the necessary talent for it, I shall transfer to psychiatry or psychology. After that I shall first of all start practicing as a physician in a mental hospital. Eventually I might enter upon an academic career as a psychologist, as for example Kraepelin in Heidelberg – something which I would not, however, care to express because of the uncertainty and of its being dependent upon my capabilities . . . Therefore, I had best state it this way: I am going to study medicine in order to become a physician in a health resort or a specialist, for example, a doctor for the mentally ill. To myself I add: the rest will come if and when.

The memorandum proved to be remarkably prescient. Despite health problems that were to affect him throughout his later life, he received his MD in 1909. By this time he had already started voluntary work at the psychiatric hospital in Heidelberg, seven years after Kraepelin had left for Munich. Kraepelin's successor at the hospital was Franz Nissl, whose main research interest was neuropathology, but who encouraged his junior staff to develop projects across the spectrum of disciplines relevant to psychiatry. Jaspers experimented with intelligence tests, and with a new apparatus for measuring blood pressure. Describing the intellectual environment in which he began to assemble his ideas about the very nature of madness, Jaspers later recorded that:

The common conceptual framework of the hospital was Kraepelin's psychiatry together with deviations from it, resulting in points of view and ideas for which no one person could claim individual authorship. Thus, for example, the polarity of the two broad spheres of dementia praecox (later called schizophrenia) and of the manic-depressive illnesses was considered valid.

However, Jaspers doubted whether this broad acceptance of Kraepelin's doctrine provided a secure basis for progress in the understanding of madness. On the contrary:

The realization that scientific investigation and therapy were in a state of stagnation was widespread in German psychiatric clinics at that time. The large institutions for the mentally ill were built constantly more hygienic and more magnificent. The lives of the unfortunate inmates, which could not be changed essentially, were controlled. The best that was possible consisted of shaping their lives as naturally as possible as, for example, by successful work therapy as long as such therapy remained a humane and reasonable link in the entire organization of the patient's life. In view of the exceedingly small amount of knowledge and technical know-how, intelligent, yet unproductive psychiatrists, such as Hoche, took recourse to a sceptical attitude and to elegant sounding phrases of gentlemanly superiority.

Jaspers therefore set himself the task of rethinking the way in which he and his colleagues studied mental illness. The originality of his approach first became evident to his colleagues in 1910, when he published a paper in which he considered whether paranoia should be regarded as an abnormal form of personality development or as an illness.[14] Jaspers' distinction between these two possibilities was novel in itself. If paranoia was a form of personality development it should reflect the understandable evolution of the patient's inner life. If, on the other hand, paranoia was an illness it must inevitably be considered a product of the biological changes that were presumed to accompany the onset of psychosis. Even more original, however, was Jaspers' method of addressing this distinction. In his paper he described several cases of paranoia in unusual detail, paying attention to his patients' accounts of their lives before they entered hospital, and also their subjective experience of their symptoms. 'With this mode of presentation, Jaspers introduced the *biographical method* into psychiatry: a summons to regard a patient's illness always as part of his life history.'[15]

The paper on paranoia was soon followed by others on a variety of topics, including a review of the role of intelligence testing in psychiatry, and further case studies, the last of which was published in 1913. During this period Jaspers was working on his only book on psychiatry, which was also published in 1913, two years before he became a professional philosopher.

General Psychopathology, completed when he was 30 years of age, attempted a grand sweep, bringing together the biological and the psychological. In it, Jaspers made a distinction between two apparently irreconcilable methods of comprehending mental symptoms: *understanding* and *explaining*. According to Jaspers, a patient's experiences can be understood if they are seen to arise meaningfully from the person's personality and life history. The key to a psychological analysis of a patient's abnormal experiences is therefore the clinician's empathetic understanding of the patient's subjective world and life story. In some cases, however, symptoms arise in such a way that no amount of empathy can link them understandably to the patient's background. Such symptoms, Jaspers asserted, cannot be understood but can only be explained as caused by an underlying biological disorder.[16] *Ununderstandability* was, of course, the hallmark of the psychoses, and allowed them to be distinguished from the less severe psychiatric disorders, which later became known as the neuroses.*

Nowhere is this distinction clearer than in Jaspers' account of abnormal beliefs. Such beliefs (which are discussed in more detail in later chapters) are often expressed by psychotic patients and usually follow particular themes, the most common of which are persecution (for example, 'The Royal Family and the British Home Office are conspiring to kill me') and grandiosity (for example, 'I am Christ reborn'). Jaspers identified three key features of such beliefs. First, they are held with extraordinary conviction. Second, they are resistant to counter-arguments or contradictory evidence. Third, they have bizarre or impossible content. However, according to Jaspers, these criteria are not sufficient to determine whether a belief is a true delusion. True delusions are ununderstandable because they arise suddenly without any context. The clearest case of this phenomenon is the delusional perception, in which the individual interprets a particular stimulus in a bizarre way. An example (described by Kurt Schneider) is of a young man who considers the position of a salt-cellar on his table and suddenly concludes that he will become the Pope.

The problem with this distinction is that, far from making the borderline between normality and madness more objective, it introduces an alarming degree of subjectivity. For Jaspers, the empathetic

---

* This theory anticipated recent philosophical discussions, for example by Dan Dennett, about the relationship between 'folk' psychology and scientific explanations of human behaviour. See note 16, p. 51.

attitude of the psychiatrist towards the patient functions as a kind of diagnostic test. If the empathy scanner returns the reading 'ununderstandable' the patient is psychotic and suffering from a biological disease. However, behaviours and experiences may vary in degree according to how amenable they are to empathy. By not empathizing hard enough, we may fail to recognize the intelligible aspects of the other person's experiences. Moreover, once we have decided that the patient's experiences are unintelligible, we are given an apparent licence to treat the patient as a disordered organism, a malfunctioning body that we do not have to relate to in a human way.

A real-life example illustrates this danger. Some years ago, my research assistant, Sue Kaney, was administering a battery of psychological tests to patients suffering from delusions. One patient's delusional belief, 'Professor B has turned me into a portfolio', had been dismissed by her doctors and nurses as meaningless. As Professor B was a well-known gynaecologist it seemed to us a good idea to check whether the lady had any unusual medical complaints. Investigation of her medical notes revealed that she suffered from a rare condition that the Professor was researching. 'Professor B has turned me into a portfolio' seemed an odd way for the woman to declare that she felt uncared for and an object of scientific scrutiny. Nonetheless this is what she appeared to be asserting.

This brief anecdote illustrates the central irony of Jaspers' work. In his great book he tried to identify a role for psychological explanations in psychiatry. In the process, he gave madness to the biologists and inadvertently discouraged the psychological investigation of the psychoses.

Schneider and the 'First-Rank Symptoms'

In 1913 Jaspers became a teacher of psychology in the Department of Philosophy at the University of Heidelberg. At first, he assumed the move would be temporary but in 1922 he was appointed to a full chair in philosophy, and he never returned to psychiatric practice.

Kurt Schneider's career overlapped with Jaspers' and was greatly influenced by it.[17] Like Jaspers, he studied both medicine and philosophy and addressed the problem of deciding who was mad and who was not. Yet, unlike his predecessor, his approach was pragmatic rather than philosophical.

Born in 1887 in Crailsheim in the state of Württemberg, Schneider trained in medicine in Berlin and Tübingen. After military service in the First World War, he obtained his academic qualification in psychiatry in Cologne in 1919. In 1931 he was appointed director of the Psychiatric Research Institute in Munich, which had been founded by Kraepelin.

In the following years, Nazi policies were gradually embraced by the German psychiatric establishment, championed in particular by Ernst Rüdin, who had been recruited to the Institute by Kraepelin in order to develop the new field of psychiatric genetics. The eugenic theories that Rüdin proposed led, first, to the enforced sterilization and then, later, the killing of mentally ill patients.[18] These developments horrified Schneider, who eventually left the Institute to serve as an army doctor during the Second World War.*

In 1945, the invading US army decided to reopen the famous university at Heidelberg and appointed a group of anti-Nazi academics to advise them. The group, led by Jaspers, attempted to identify fellow academics who could be safely entrusted with the rebuilding of the University. Schneider was sufficiently free of the taint of Nazism to be appointed Dean of the Medical School, a position he retained until his retirement in 1955. He died, aged 80 years, in 1967.

Although Schneider's work was to have a profound impact on the way in which English-speaking researchers thought about schizophrenia, his approach became known to the English academic world largely via accounts provided by British and American psychiatrists who had studied him in German. Indeed, the English translation of his famous textbook on *Psychopathology*, published in 1959, was allowed to go out of print after one edition, and has never been reissued. It is doubtful whether Schneider himself felt his analysis of schizophrenia

---

* The role of German psychiatry in promoting Nazi eugenic policies is not widely known but has been well documented. Foremost among those who played a role was Alfred Hoche (the man criticized by Jaspers as 'intelligent, yet unproductive' and prone to 'elegant sounding phrases of gentlemanly superiority'), who, together with the philosopher and jurist Karl Binding, in 1920 published a pamphlet entitled 'Permission to destroy life unworthy of living', advocating compulsory euthanasia for the inmates of 'idiot institutes'. It was supporters of the National Socialist Movement, notably Rüdin, who pioneered genetic studies of schizophrenia while at the same time advocating the most extreme eugenic measures. Their work is considered in more detail in Chapter 4.

to be his most important contribution; he also wrote extensively about disorders of personality, and about forensic problems that lay at the boundary between legal and psychiatric practice.

According to Canadian psychiatrist J. Hoenig, 'Schneider's work ... was not in the area of system design, but it was firmly planted at the bedside' (a curious description, as psychiatrists almost never see their patients when they are lying in bed). Applying Jaspers' phenomenological approach, he addressed himself to the problem of diagnosing schizophrenia and differentiating it from more general problems of personality. He hit on the strategy of identifying those characteristics that were peculiar to schizophrenia, and which would therefore provide the best guide for the practising clinician. In this way, he identified what he believed to be the *first-rank symptoms* of the disorder, which are listed in Table 2.1. These symptoms, which were to be distinguished from other symptoms of the second rank, were all forms of hallucination, delusion, or passivity experience. For example, the patient might hear an auditory hallucination in the form of a voice speaking about him in the third person and commenting on his actions, or he might feel that his will was being controlled by some external force or agency.

When trying to determine whether patients suffered from any of these symptoms, Schneider believed that it was more important to pay attention to the *form* rather than the *content* of the patient's experience:

Diagnosis looks for the 'How?' (form) not the 'What?' (the theme or content). When I find thought withdrawal, then this is important to me as a mode of inner experience and as a diagnostic hint, but it is not of diagnostic significance whether it is the devil, the girlfriend or a political leader who withdraws the thoughts. Wherever one focuses on such contents, diagnostics recedes; one sees then only the biographical aspects or the existence open to interpretation.[19]

For Schneider therefore, the meaning of first-rank symptoms was irrelevant to the diagnostician. Moreover, he was careful to deny that these symptoms were crucially important features of schizophrenia. They were chosen purely for convenience, because they were easy to recognize. Accordingly, any patient who showed any of these symptoms would, more likely than not, be suffering from schizophrenia,

Table 2.1 Schneider's first-rank symptoms of schizophrenia (adapted from K. Schneider (1959) *Clinical Psychopathology*. New York: Grune & Stratton)

Symptom as described by Schneider	Example given by Schneider
1 Audible thoughts	A schizophrenic woman, for instance, replied to the question about hearing voices with the answer, 'I hear my own thoughts. I can hear them when everything is quiet.'
2 Voices heard arguing	Another schizophrenic heard his own voice night and day, like a dialogue, one voice always arguing against another.
3 Voices heard commenting on one's actions	A schizophrenic woman heard a voice say, whenever she wanted to eat, 'Now she is eating, here she is munching again', or when she patted the dog, she heard, 'What is she up to now, fondling the dog?'
4 Experience of influences playing on the body	A schizophrenic woman speaking of electrical influences said, 'The electricity works of the whole world are directed on to me.'
5 Thought withdrawal	A definite schizophrenic disturbance may only be supposed when it is recounted that 'other people' are taking the thoughts away . . . A schizophrenic man stated that his thoughts were 'taken from me years ago by the parish council'.

Symptom as described by Schneider	Example given by Schneider
6 Thoughts are ascribed to other people who intrude their thoughts upon the patient	A skilled shirtmaker knew exactly how large the collars should be, but when she proceeded to make them, there were times when she could not calculate at all. This was not ordinary forgetting; she had to think thoughts she did not want to think, evil thoughts. She attributed all this to being hypnotized by a priest.
7 Thought diffusion	The diffusion of thoughts is illustrated by a schizophrenic shopkeeper who said, 'People see what I am thinking; you could not prove it but I just know it is so. I see it in their faces; it would not be so bad if I did not think such unsuitable things – swine or some other rude word. If I think of anything, at once those opposite know it and it is embarrassing.'
8 Delusional perception	Another schizophrenic woman said: 'The people next door were strange and offhand; they did not want me; perhaps I was too quiet for them. The previous Sunday my employers had a visitor who embarrassed me. I thought it was my father. Later on, I thought it was only the son of the house in disguise. I don't know if they wanted to find out about me.'
9–11 Feelings, impulses (drives) and volitional acts that are experienced by the patient as the work or influence of others	A schizophrenic student said, 'I cannot respond to any suggestion; thousands and thousands of wills work against me.'

but 'We often have to base our diagnosis of schizophrenia on the second rank symptoms, in exceptional cases now and then even merely on expressional [behavioural] symptoms, provided they are adequately distinct and present in large numbers.'[20]

Despite these qualifications, many English-speaking researchers assumed that Schneider had found a more precise way of identifying 'real cases' of schizophrenia. The term 'Schneider-positive schizophrenia' – to refer to a group of patients suffering from his first-rank symptoms – was first used in 1965 by a group of investigators searching for metabolic abnormalities in psychotic patients.[21] Somewhat later, Schneider's account was used to define a core group of schizophrenia symptoms by a British team, led by John Wing, which was attempting to find more reliable ways of defining and diagnosing psychiatric disorders.[22] As we will see in the next chapter, subsequent definitions of schizophrenia developed in Britain and the United States, and now employed throughout the world, have all emphasized hallucinations and delusions rather than the intellectual deficits described by Kraepelin or the so-called fundamental symptoms described by Bleuler.

It is likely that Schneider himself would have been shocked by these developments. As we have seen, his goal in defining the first-rank symptoms was merely to make the task of the clinician more straightforward. Indeed, Schneider the pragmatist denied that psychiatric diagnosis identified cases with a common aetiology as supposed by Kraepelin. In an essay celebrating Kraepelin's influence on psychiatry published in 1956 he remarked that:

Today no one will any longer attempt a sharp differential diagnosis between cyclothymia [manic depression] and schizophrenia (as they are now called). There is only a differential typology, that means there are transitions . . . One should really no longer argue about such cases: 'this is a cyclothymia, no, this is a schizophrenia'. One can argue this about GPI versus a cerebral tumour. Here the 'is' can be verified. With the endogenous psychoses, which are purely psychological forms, one can make assessments only according to one's own concepts. One can only say: this is for me, or I call this a cyclothymia or a schizophrenia. The crucial point in such an argument is merely to make it clear that in a descriptive psychopathology of this kind Kraepelin's forms are still basically accepted.[23]

The sceptical reader may be forgiven for wondering whether the two main assertions in this quotation (that 'one can make assessments only according to one's own concepts' and that 'Kraepelin's forms are still basically accepted') are entirely consistent with each other.

The Evolution of Manic Depression

Just as the concept of dementia praecox evolved, and even changed dramatically in the years following Kraepelin's original formulation, so too the concept of manic depression underwent a series of transformations. These transformations followed the growing perception among psychiatrists in Europe and North America that Kraepelin's account created problems of two kinds. The first problem was the embarrassment for psychiatric classification presented by patients who suffered from a mixture of schizophrenic and manic-depressive symptoms. The second problem was the apparent over-inclusiveness of the manic-depression concept, which demanded that it be broken down into several subtypes.

As we have seen, Bleuler believed that psychotic patients could be more or less schizophrenic or manic depressive depending on the extent to which schizophrenia symptoms were more evident than abnormal mood. Extending this idea to its logical conclusion, in 1933 the American psychiatrist Jacob Kasanin proposed the concept of *schizoaffective disorder* to describe a kind of illness which combined symptoms of both disorders, but which was distinct from both.[24] According to Kasanin, schizoaffective patients usually suffered from 'marked emotional turmoil' and 'false sensory impressions' (hallucinations) but rarely experienced the passivity symptoms (delusions of control) usually seen in cases of schizophrenia. These symptoms most often appeared suddenly after a stressful experience, and there was usually evidence of good premorbid adjustment (in other words, patients showed little evidence of social or personality difficulties prior to their illness). Recovery was often rapid, although many patients went on to suffer further episodes.

A similar but not identical concept of *cycloid psychosis* was proposed in 1926 by Karl Kliest, professor of psychiatry at Frankfurt University. His student Karl Leonhard, who, in 1936, became head of the Frankfurt University Mental Hospital, later elaborated this concept.[25] In a series of papers published in the 1950s, Kliest and Leonhard grouped together under this term all those disorders that appeared to have such a variable course that patients appeared schizophrenic at one point in time and manic depressive at another.[26] Despite the apparent similarities with Kasanin's account, Leonhard denied that the two proposals were the same. The essential feature of cycloid psychosis was the change in symptomatology observed over time. In contrast, the schizoaffective patients described by Kasanin appeared to experience symptoms of schizophrenia and manic depression simultaneously.

It was Leonhard who introduced a final modification to Kraepelin's system that appeared to solve the second problem of over-inclusiveness. Leonhard undertook an analysis of the varying symptoms of a large group of manic-depressive patients, which he summarized in his book on *The Classification of the Endogenous Psychoses*, which was published in 1957. He observed that some patients experienced both episodes of mania (characterized by euphoria, excitement and irritability) and episodes of depression, whereas others appeared to suffer only from episodes of depression.[27] He therefore proposed the term *bipolar disorder* to describe the first type of illness, because patients appeared to experience at different times two opposite types of extreme mood. (The term 'manic depression' is now often used exclusively to describe this bipolar type of illness.) The term *unipolar depression* was suggested for the second type of illness, in which episodes of mania never occurred. Importantly, Leonhard and subsequent investigators observed that mania in the absence of a history of depression is extremely rare. For this reason, it is usually assumed that apparently 'unipolar manic' patients either have experienced episodes of depression which they have forgotten about, or will go on to develop depression in the future.[28]

Prior to the 1970s, researchers studying mood disorders rarely distinguished between patients suffering from bipolar and unipolar illnesses. Following the publication of an English translation of *The Classification of the Endogenous Psychoses* in the 1970s, it became commonplace to do so. By the last quarter of the twentieth century, therefore, Kraepelin's model had been substantially elaborated and yet remained, in most respects, intact. A consensus model of psychiatric classification, outlined in Figure 2.1, was widely embraced. It began with the distinction between the psychoses and the minor psychiatric disorders or neuroses, as outlined by Jaspers. The psychoses, in turn, were divided into two major categories, schizophrenia and manic depression as proposed by Kraepelin, and two perhaps more contentious categories, paranoia and schizoaffective disorder. Finally, manic depression was deemed to consist of two subtypes, unipolar depression and bipolar disorder.

Will the Real Concept of Schizophrenia Please Stand up?

In these first two chapters we have examined the development of the Kraepelinian approach to psychiatry from its beginnings in the last half of the nineteenth century through to the last quarter of the twentieth. Although I have presented no more than an outline sketch of this process, focusing narrowly on the work of four giants of psychiatry, the astute reader will already have recognized that Kraepelin's ideas underwent a series of radical transformations as they progressed through the hands of Bleuler, Jaspers, Schneider and onwards. This was most obviously the case for the concept of dementia praecox. For Kraepelin the cardinal features of the disorder were intellectual, for Bleuler they were cognitive and emotional, whereas Schneider emphasized hallucinations and delusions. Indeed, we may be forgiven for wondering whether these explorers of the mind and its disorders were writing about the same illness. Writing in 1980, the psychiatric geneticist Seymour Kety had little doubt about this question, and argued that Schneider's account of schizophrenia amounted to nothing less than a perversion of Kraepelin's original concept:

Schneider, 50 years later ... [after Bleuler] gave renewed support to those who preferred to think of schizophrenia as a benign process by simply redefining schizophrenia to make it so. Features regarded by Kraepelin and Bleuler as fundamental and characteristic (impoverishment of affect, disturbances of personal contact and rapport, ambivalence, lack of motivation, depersonalisation and stereotypes) were significantly rejected and the new criteria were restricted to particular kinds of hallucinations and delusions which Bleuler had regarded as accessory symptoms. Schneider

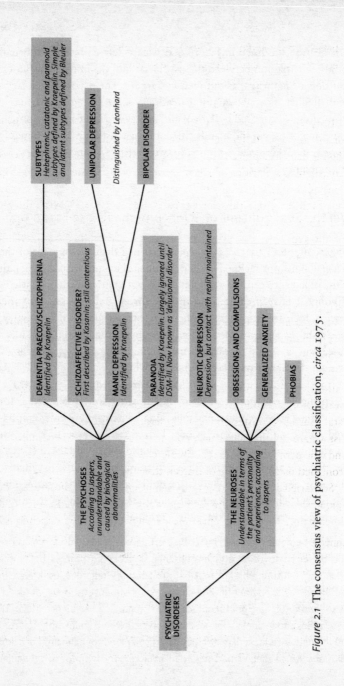

Figure 2.1 The consensus view of psychiatric classification, *circa* 1975.

PSYCHIATRIC DISORDERS

THE PSYCHOSES
According to Jaspers, ununderstandable and caused by biological abnormalities

THE NEUROSES
Understandable in terms of the patient's personality and experiences according to Jaspers

DEMENTIA PRAECOX/SCHIZOPHRENIA
Identified by Kraepelin

SCHIZOAFFECTIVE DISORDER?
First described by Kasanin; still contentious

MANIC DEPRESSION
Identified by Kraepelin

PARANOIA
Identified by Kraepelin. Largely ignored until DSM-III. Now known as delusional disorder'

NEUROTIC DEPRESSION
Depression, but contact with reality maintained

OBSESSIONS AND COMPULSIONS

GENERALIZED ANXIETY

PHOBIAS

SUBTYPES
Hebephrenic, catatonic and paranoid subtypes defined by Kraepelin. Simple and latent subtypes defined by Bleuler

UNIPOLAR DEPRESSION

Distinguished by Leonhard

BIPOLAR DISORDER

established a new syndrome with features which are economically put into check lists and fed into computers. That syndrome may be more prevalent, have a more favourable outcome, and be more responsive to a wide variety of treatments, but it is not schizophrenia.[29]

British psychologist Mary Boyle has offered a different explanation for the apparent differences between modern schizophrenia patients and the dementia praecox patients of Kraepelin's time.[30] She has noted remarkable similarities between Kraepelin's case studies and descriptions of people suffering from *encephalitis lethargica*, a viral disease that swept through Italy during the 1890s, and then through the rest of Europe between 1916 and 1927. In the epidemic of 1916–27, five million people were affected, about one third of whom died or fell into a coma after a period of intense sleeplessness. Many of those who survived went on to develop a form of post-encephalitic Parkinson's disease (named after a London physician James Parkinson who, in 1817, first described the non-viral manifestations of this condition; symptoms include uncontrollable tremor, sudden accelerated movements interspersed with periods of stiffness or rigidity, and other crippling disorders of will and action). Sometimes, survivors would remain conscious but unable to move for years, frozen in their chairs without obvious motive, emotion or desire, apparently indifferent to the world around them.[31] The biological basis of the illness was established by Constantin von Economo, a Greek-born neuropathologist who found characteristic lesions in the brains of victims at autopsy, and who demonstrated that a submicroscopic, filterable virus obtained from victims was capable of transmitting the disease to monkeys.[32]

So varied were the long-term symptoms observed following the epidemic, that encephalitis lethargica originally received a variety of other names, including 'epidemic delirium', 'epidemic disseminated sclerosis', 'atypical poliomyelitis' and 'epidemic schizophrenia'. The last of these terms was sometimes used because the movement disorders of patients were similar to those recorded in patients thought to suffer from catatonic schizophrenia.

The important lesson of Boyle's argument is not that Kraepelin was sometimes mistaken when assigning diagnoses (we will never know for certain whether some of his patients were suffering from a brain infection) but that the concept of dementia praecox was less certain than either he or his followers supposed. As we will see, this is not the only problem that has threatened to undermine the Kraepelinian system.

3

The Great Classification Crisis

If any man were bold enough to write a history of psychiatric classifications he would find when he had completed his task that in the process he had written a history of psychiatry as well.

Robert Kendell[1]

The philosopher Thomas Kuhn[2] has observed that sciences do not develop by the mere accumulation of knowledge (although the accumulation of knowledge is important). Rather, scientific progress sometimes occurs in abrupt leaps or shifts, for example when Newton justified a Copernican model of the solar system by proposing his law of gravitation, or when Einstein abolished the concept of absolute motion by introducing his theory of special relativity. In each of these examples (and many others from the physical and biological sciences that can be easily invoked) one theoretical framework was eventually abandoned in favour of another, incompatible, framework. During this process, according to Kuhn, researchers are usually reluctant to accept the evidence in favour of the new approach until limitations of the old approach become so obvious that they can no longer be avoided.

Kuhn argued that these sudden theoretical leaps could be understood, at least in part, in sociological terms. According to his account, each science begins in fits and starts until researchers eventually accept a common *paradigm* (framework or set of assumptions about the nature of their subject matter). During the subsequent phase of *normal science*, researchers work within the paradigm, even though they may be hardly aware that they are doing so (for example, after Newton physicists assumed that space was best described by the principles of Euclidean geometry, until Einstein showed that non-Euclidean geometries were required to describe the curvature of space under the influence of gravity). Over time they begin to accumulate observations that cannot be understood within the existing framework and this leads, eventually, to a *scientific revolution* in which a replacement paradigm is accepted. Afterwards there follows another period of normal science.

Although Kuhn's model has sometimes been criticized for oversimplifying the processes involved in the growth of scientific knowledge,[3] it allows us to understand Emil Kraepelin's position within the history of psychiatry. It is a position that bears some resemblance to that of Newton within the history of physics. Like Newton, he established a paradigm or a set of assumptions that would guide the activities of successive generations of researchers, but which were so ingrained that they have been difficult to question. According to this paradigm, psychiatric disorders fall into a finite number of types or categories (dementia praecox, manic depression, paranoia, etc.), each with a different pathophysiology and aetiology. Of course, modern psychiatrists and psychologists have sometimes quibbled with details of the system (for example, arguing whether the true number of psychotic illnesses is three or more than three). Often they have also acknowledged the multifactorial origins of particular illnesses ('schizophrenia is caused by an interaction of biology and the environment . . .'). Nonetheless, the practice of most psychiatrists and clinical psychologists – the way that they assign diagnoses and decide treatments for their patients, the way that they conduct their research into the causes of madness – reveals that the Kraepelinian paradigm remains almost unchallenged within the mental health professions as a whole. That this is so is evident from four observations.

First, modern textbooks of psychopathology, whether written by psychiatrists or psychologists, almost without exception, are organized according to some variant of Kraepelin's system, with chapter headings on 'schizophrenia', 'manic depression' and so on. Second, as we will see later in this chapter, the official diagnostic systems currently advocated by influential bodies such as the World Health Organization (WHO)[4] and the American Psychiatric Association (APA),[5] are similarly organized in a way that reflects Kraepelin's assumptions about the nature of madness. Third, most research in psychiatry (whether conducted by psychiatrists or psychologists) is based on Kraepelin's paradigm. Usually, patients with a particular diagnosis are compared with other people, on the assumption that those with the diagnosis have something in common that makes them different. And finally, clinicians throughout the world typically employ Kraepelin's diagnostic concepts during their routine work, for example when explaining to patients what is wrong with them ('I'm afraid you suffer from manic depression, Mr Smith') and when deciding what treatment should be offered ('so you should therefore take lithium carbonate').

Because Kraepelin's paradigm remains the main organizing principle for psychiatric practice and research, any evidence that draws it into question has revolutionary implications for both the understanding and treatment of madness. Evidence of this kind would undermine most of the research into psychiatric disorders conducted since Kraepelin's death. (After all, the attempt to find the cause or causes of schizophrenia is doomed to failure if the diagnosis does not pick out a group of people who suffer from the same disorder.) It would also undermine any routine clinical decisions – for example, advice about whether patients are likely to recover, or to benefit from particular kinds of medication – that are based on Kraepelinian diagnoses.

These disastrous consequences of a poorly founded method of classification point to the necessity of evaluating Kraepelin's system. There are many different ways of approaching this problem. However, in this chapter we will be concerned only with the first and most obvious test that a diagnostic system must pass in order to be deemed useful. This test is known as *reliability*, and concerns the consistency with which diagnoses are employed by different clinicians or on different occasions. If two psychiatrists met the same patient, we would expect both to make the same diagnosis. Similarly, we would expect a patient to be assigned the same diagnosis on two different occasions (unless the patient recovered and later developed a separate illness altogether). Without this kind of diagnostic consistency, there would be no way of agreeing about who suffers from a particular disorder and who does not.

The Problem of Reliability

In order to achieve reliable psychiatric diagnoses it is first necessary to reach a consensus about the main features of each disorder. Although early attempts to create the required standard definitions were made elsewhere (the first being a list of eleven mental diseases agreed at a Congress of Mental Science in Paris in 1889),[6] it is fair to say that this process of mass-producing psychiatric diagnoses has been mostly an American enterprise. From our vantage point at the beginning of the twenty-first century, it therefore seems almost paradoxical that American psychiatrists working in the middle years of the last century were mostly sceptical about the value of diagnoses. This scepticism reflected the influence of Adolf Meyer, a Swiss-born psychiatrist who played a leading role in shaping American thinking about madness during the first decades of the twentieth century.

Meyer was born in 1866 in Niederweingen, near Zurich, and studied medicine in Switzerland before undertaking postgraduate work in Paris, London, Edinburgh and Berlin. In 1892, he migrated to the United States where, after working in a series of neurology posts, he eventually became director of the Pathological Institute of the New York State Hospitals. In 1909 he received an honorary doctorate from Clark University at the same time as did Sigmund Freud and Carl Jung, who were mid-way through a lecture tour of the United States.

During this early period of his career, Meyer was a firm advocate of Kraepelin's approach and has been credited, along with a few other émigrés, for introducing the concept of dementia praecox to the United States. Indeed, the only book he published in his lifetime was entitled *Dementia Praecox*. It attempted (with somewhat less success than Bleuler's book of the same title) to integrate Kraepelin's ideas with those of Freud. On being appointed to a chair in the Department of Psychiatry at Johns Hopkins University in Baltimore in 1910, where he was to remain until retiring in 1941, Meyer intended to model the new University clinic on Kraepelin's Institute in Munich. The Henry Phipps Psychiatric Clinic, as it became known, was housed in an elegant building, with a roof garden and unbarred windows. Like the Munich Institute, the clinic was run along medical lines, so that patients usually arrived in ambulances, physical restraints were employed as rarely as possible, and few patients were compulsorily detained. It is therefore all the more remarkable that Meyer's subsequent reputation was as an *anti*-Kraepelinian.

Historian Edward Shorter was probably unfair when he described Meyer as, 'a second-rate thinker and verbose writer, [who] was never, in his own mind, able to disentangle schools that were absolutely incompatible, and ended up embracing whatever new came along'.[7] However, Meyer was certainly enthusiastic about Freud's theories, and therefore shares some responsibility for the success of psychoanalytic ideas in the United States. He also supported the psychologist J. B. Watson's first attempts to apply the theory of Pavlovian conditioning in a psychiatric setting, and therefore can also be credited with encouraging the psychological doctrine of *behaviourism** (an approach to psychology that is usually regarded as the antithesis of psychoanalysis). Meyer's later writings, mostly published after his death in 1950, advocated a holistic approach to psychiatry in which biological, psychological and sociological approaches were considered to be equally important. Despite his earlier enthusiasm for Kraepelin's system, he became pessimistic about the value of psychiatric classification, arguing that 'We should give up the idea of classifying people as we do plants.' He felt that psychiatric categories did little justice to the complexity of patients' problems, their individual histories, and the social circumstances in which their problems arose. He also objected to the superstition that a diagnosis led automatically to a choice of treatment and suggested that, rather than grouping different behaviours under one name, clinicians should base their treatment decisions on a concrete specification of the various problems from which the patient suffered.

Despite Meyer's influence, the American Psychiatric Association contributed a section on psychiatric disorders to a nationally accepted *Standard Classified Nomenclature of Disease* organized by the New York Academy of Medicine, which was published in 1933. It was the attempt to use this classification during the Second World War that led both military and civilian psychiatrists to reconsider their attitudes

---

* In 1913 Watson coined the term 'behaviourism' (roughly, the idea that human behaviour should be studied objectively, using the same techniques that had been successfully used to study animal behaviour). Behaviourism became the most influential approach in psychology between the 1930s and the 1960s.

towards the whole process of diagnosis. During the war, nearly 10 per cent of all discharges from the armed forces were for psychiatric reasons. However, the range of disorders contained within the *Nomenclature*, based largely on clinical experience within asylums, was inadequate to describe many of the problems suffered by the returning men. In particular, stress reactions, psychosomatic problems and problems of personality were inadequately described. To make matters worse, the US army, the US navy and the Veterans Administration (responsible for providing medical care to ex-service personnel and their families) all employed their own idiosyncratic systems of classification alongside the *Nomenclature*.[8] It was in order to bring an end to this chaos that the American Psychiatric Association in 1948 formed a task force to create a new standardized diagnostic system. The result, published in 1952, was the first edition of the APA's *Diagnostic and Statistical Manual of Mental Disorders*.

DSM-I (as it became known) was a triumph of the doctrine of truth by agreement. Great care was taken to represent the broad spectrum of contemporary psychiatric opinion in the USA. One tenth of the Association's members were sent a questionnaire, which elicited their opinions about an early draft of the manual, allowing revisions to be made before it was officially adopted by a vote of the entire membership. The final version came as a handy-sized book with a grey cover. Within its pages, each diagnosis was given a simple definition, usually accompanied by a thumbnail description of the disorder. The impact of this simple and practical system proved to be as great outside the United States as within, shaping attempts to produce an international consensus about psychiatric classification.

The attempt to achieve such a consensus was led by the World Health Organization. On its creation in 1948, WHO had assumed responsibility for an *International List of Causes of Death*, which had been first compiled in 1853, and which had undergone four major revisions sponsored by the French government. Expanding the manual to include non-fatal diseases, WHO published a sixth edition (now renamed the *International Classification of Diseases*, or ICD-6 for short) in 1951, but was disappointed by its impact. The mental disorders section of the manual was adopted for official use only in Finland, Great Britain, New Zealand, Peru and Thailand and, even in these countries, its use by practising psychiatrists was fairly haphazard.

A committee chaired by Erwin Stengel, a British psychiatrist, was therefore mandated to consider how the section on psychiatric disorders might be improved in future editions. Stengel became convinced that aetiological prejudices were largely responsible for the difficulty in achieving agreement. Some diagnostic concepts then in wide use seemed to imply that disorders had particular causes. For example, many psychiatrists believed that the term 'schizophrenia' implied an endogenous disorder (that is, a disorder caused by some biological dysfunction within the individual), whereas other widely used terms, such as 'reactive depression', seemed to imply that disorders were largely caused by environmental factors. For these reasons, Stengel embraced an idea originally suggested by the American philosopher Carl Hempel, and proposed that future classifications of psychiatric diseases should include only *operational definitions*, which is to say definitions that precisely specified the rules to be followed when making each diagnosis. DSM-I, with its relatively clear definitions and its thumbnail descriptions, was the closest he could find to this ideal approach.

Stengel's advice that diagnoses should make no reference to aetiology was followed for the eighth edition of the *International Classification of Disease*, which was published in 1965 and officially adopted by WHO in 1969. ICD-8 was the product of an unusual degree of co-operation between psychiatrists in different countries. Scandinavian and German psychiatric societies supported the new taxonomy, and the American Psychiatric Association agreed to base a revision of their *Diagnostic and Statistical Manual* on the ICD-8 system. Accordingly, in 1965 the APA appointed a small committee of eight experts and two consultants, and DSM-II was published three years later as a spiral-bound notebook, 150 pages in length, available to clinicians for $3.50.

Troublesome data

By the middle decades of the twentieth century, it was becoming obvious to many psychiatrists that the achievement of a consensus about the main features of each psychiatric disorder would not be enough to ensure that diagnoses were reliable, let alone scientifically meaningful. Empirical research was required. Unfortunately, the earliest studies of diagnostic reliability proved to be discomfiting to those who wished to believe that Kraepelin had at last discovered the correct taxonomy of psychiatric disorders.

Jules Masserman and H. Carmichael, two American psychiatrists, published the first study of the reliability of psychiatric diagnoses, in 1938.[9] These researchers followed up 100 patients one year after they had been admitted to a university psychiatric clinic in Chicago, in order to see whether their diagnoses had changed during that period. They noted that the majority of patients had symptoms that seemed to fit more than one diagnostic category. By the end of the follow-up interval, 40 per cent of the patients had been assigned diagnoses different from those they had been given on admission. Although it might be argued that these disappointing findings were merely a reflection of the poor diagnostic skills of particular clinicians in a particular city at a particular time, later studies established that this was not the case. For example, similar results were obtained in a much larger investigation conducted by three US navy psychiatrists, William Hunt, Cecil Wittson and Edna Hunt, published in 1953.[10] Nearly 800 enlisted men discharged from naval boot camps for psychiatric reasons were followed up in the hospitals to which they were discharged and their diagnoses there were compared with those they had been given by the navy psychiatrists. There was agreement about specific diagnoses in only 32.6 per cent of cases.

Of course, diagnoses may change over time for genuine reasons (because patients' symptoms change), so unstable diagnoses are not incontrovertible evidence of diagnostic destitution. Of much greater importance is the extent to which different clinicians assign the same diagnoses to the same patients when conducting assessments at the same point in time. This question was first addressed in a pioneering investigation conducted by an American postgraduate student of industrial psychology, Philip Ash, which was published in 1949.[11] Three psychiatrists interviewed fifty-two male patients attending an outpatient clinic and the results, at least on first sight, were even less impressive than those obtained by Masserman and Carmichael. All three psychiatrists agreed on diagnoses in only 20 per cent of cases, whereas two out of three agreed about 48.6 per cent of cases. These figures improved to 45.7 per cent and 51.4 per cent respectively when only major diagnostic categories (for example, psychosis) were considered, but even then fell well short of the desired level of agreement. Unfortunately, as later commentators pointed out, Ash's study suffered from a defect that made interpretation of his findings difficult. Three quarters of the major diagnoses given were 'normal with a predominant personality characteristic'. On the one hand, it might therefore be argued that the psychiatrists were being asked to make judgements of personality rather than illness. On the other hand, with such a high *base rate* for a single category, relatively high rates of agreement were bound to occur by chance. (To see that this is the case, imagine what would happen if only one diagnosis was employed. In these circumstances there would inevitably be 100 per cent agreement between different clinicians. Now imagine that there is a choice between only two diagnoses. Even under these circumstances two psychiatrists deciding diagnoses by a toss of a coin would agree on 50 per cent of occasions. The chance level of agreement therefore decreases as the base rate of each diagnosis decreases, and as the number of available diagnoses increases.) It is for this reason that simple percentage agreement figures usually give an *inflated* impression of diagnostic agreement.

Several other early studies of diagnostic agreement were less affected by these limitations, and yet produced results that were little better.[12] For example, a new standard in the field was set in a report published by Myron Sandifer, Charles Pettus and Dana Quade in 1964. Sandifer and his colleagues studied the diagnoses assigned to first-time psychiatric patients admitted to three hospitals in North Carolina.[13] Ninety-one patients were interviewed by a psychiatrist in front of a team of experienced clinicians, also mostly psychiatrists. Levels of agreement between the interviewing psychiatrists and their colleagues varied substantially across the different diagnoses. Some diagnoses fared reasonably well. For example, 74 per cent of the observers agreed when the interviewer assigned a diagnosis of schizophrenia. Others performed very badly. For example, only 36 per cent of the observers agreed when a diagnosis of manic depression was assigned. (Of course, these figures do not correct for the base rate problem.)

Worlds apart

At about the same time that these studies were drawing attention to difficulties in ensuring agreement between clinicians, other studies were pointing to substantial differences in diagnostic practices in different countries. The first detailed study of this phenomenon was published by Morton Kramer in 1961.[14] Kramer compared the diagnoses given to patients when first admitted to hospitals in England, Wales and the United States, finding that the diagnosis of schizophrenia was used much more frequently in the United States than in Great Britain. The opposite appeared to be true for manic depression.

These observations stimulated a substantial study of transatlantic differences in diagnostic practices, which became known as the US–UK Diagnostic Project, and which was conducted by a team of British and American psychiatrists. In a significant advance on Kramer's approach, the team examined patients in the two countries using a structured interview schedule (to ensure that all patients were asked the same questions) and assigned them ICD-8 diagnoses.[15] This procedure largely eliminated the transatlantic differences in the rates at which various diagnoses were given. For example, when local diagnoses were examined, 61.5 per cent of New York patients but only 33.9 per cent of London patients were given a diagnosis of schizophrenia. However, when ICD-8 diagnoses were assigned, 29.2 per cent of New York patients and 35.1 of London patients were given the diagnosis. These findings were important because they implied that different diagnostic practices (rather than actual differences between the patient populations) were responsible for the transatlantic differences that had previously been observed.

This conclusion was supported by a further study conducted by the team, in which large groups of British and American psychiatrists were shown videotaped interviews with patients. When the diagnoses given by the participating psychiatrists were studied, it was again found that the Americans in comparison with the British were much more willing to make a diagnosis of schizophrenia and much less willing to make diagnoses of mania, depression or neurosis. These differences were summarized by the project team in the form of a Venn diagram, reproduced in Figure 3.1, which shows how the American concept of

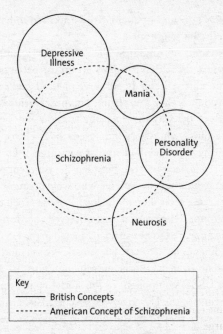

Figure 3.1 Venn diagram showing relationships between US and UK diagnostic concepts as revealed in the US–UK Diagnostic Project (from R. E. Kendell, J. E. Cooper, A. J. Gourlay, J. R. M. Copeland, L. Sharpe and B. J. Gurland (1971) 'Diagnostic criteria of American and British psychiatrists', *Archives of General Psychiatry*, 25: 123–30).

schizophrenia overlapped the other diagnostic categories used more frequently in Britain.

The World Health Organization subsequently conducted a much broader investigation of international discrepancies in diagnostic practices, which became known as the International Pilot Study of Schizophrenia (IPSS).[16] A total of 1202 recently ill patients were recruited from Columbia, Czechoslovakia (now divided into the Czech Republic and Slovakia), China, Denmark, India, Nigeria, the then Soviet Union, the UK and the USA. Three different approaches were made to assigning diagnoses. First, patients were diagnosed according to the customs and practices of the local psychiatrists. Second, they were given an ICD-8 diagnosis on the basis of their responses to a standardized psychiatric interview. Third, a computer program was used to identify a core group of patients who appeared to have a common set of schizophrenia symptoms.

When presenting its findings, the WHO drew attention to the unsurprising fact that a 'concordant group' of patients identified as suffering from schizophrenia by all three methods were very alike, no matter which country they came from. This observation was, of course, a consequence of the way in which the study was designed (as these patients were those who everyone agreed had schizophrenia it was hardly surprising that they had similar symptoms). Of more interest were the discrepancies observed between the different approaches to diagnosis. Large numbers of patients who were diagnosed as suffering from schizophrenia according to the local criteria failed to fall into the concordant group. Moreover, it was observed that local concepts of schizophrenia appeared to be especially broad in the USA (confirming the earlier findings of the US–UK Diagnostic Project) and in the USSR.

The apparent over-diagnosis of schizophrenia in Moscow (the centre for the USSR component of the study) merits further examination. At the time of the IPSS, Soviet psychiatrists' attitudes towards schizophrenia were shaped by the views of Andrei Snezebryakova, an ambitious Communist Party member who had advocated a politically favoured Pavlovian approach to mental illness. Snezebryakova had been appointed a full member of the prestigious Academy of Medical Sciences in 1962. At the same time, he had become Director of the Academy's Institute of Psychiatry, a position of considerable power in the Soviet system, as it made him chief adviser in psychiatry to the Ministry of Health. He had therefore been able to determine the training given to junior psychiatrists, their progress in the profession, and the policies that they would pursue when working in hospitals.

Snezebryakova had an extremely broad conception of schizophrenia, and suppressed views that differed from his own. He believed that the disorder appeared in a spectrum of guises ranging from idiosyncratic thinking through to full-blown psychosis, and that it could develop gradually rather than suddenly, so that its onset was often indistinguishable from eccentric behaviour. Moreover, for Snezebryakova, dissatisfaction with the Soviet political and economic system, or with communism in general, was itself evidence of mental instability. The consequence of this line of reasoning was a unique classification of schizophrenia according to both course (whether the illness was continuous, periodic or intermittent) and severity, as shown in Table 3.1. Symptoms of the mildest forms of schizophrenia were said to include 'neurotic self-consciousness', 'conflicts with parental and other authorities', 'reformism', 'social contentiousness' and 'philosophical concerns'. Small wonder that, by the late 1960s, individuals who were regarded as political dissidents in the West were being forcibly treated for schizophrenia in the USSR, notably in the notorious Serbsky Institute of Forensic Psychiatry in Moscow.[17] In a commentary on this apparent abuse of psychiatry, American psychiatrist Walter Reich noted that Soviet psychiatrists, far from acting as conscious agents of the state, were often acting in good faith:

Those Soviet psychiatrists really *saw* the patients as schizophrenic; or, to put it another way, *the system created a category, first on paper and then, with training, in the minds of Soviet psychiatrists, which was eventually assumed to represent a real class of patients and which was inevitably filled by real persons* ... Had those psychiatrists been sensitive to the capacity of diagnostic systems to shape the way psychiatrists understand, categorise, and perceive psychopathology, they might have been able, one hopes, to avert this result.[18]

Rethinking agreement

To many psychiatrists working in the mid-1970s, the findings from these international comparisons, together with the discouraging results from the earlier reliability studies, signalled nothing less than a crisis in the theory and practice of psychiatry. Some clinicians of this era advocated abandoning the practice of assigning diagnoses, on the grounds that they were meaningless and dehumanizing to patients (we will examine some of these arguments later). Others, however, believed that the crisis was caused by an unrigorous and insufficiently medical approach to mental illness and that the problems of classification might still be solved. A leading exponent of this conservative position was Robert Spitzer, a psychiatrist who would influence American attitudes towards diagnosis in the second half of the twentieth century as much as Adolf Meyer had done in the first.

Spitzer was an unlikely candidate for this role. Born in White Plains, New York, in 1932, he studied psychology at Cornell University before

Table 3.1 The Moscow school criteria for schizophrenia employed in the Soviet Union in the early 1970s (adapted from W. Reich (1984) 'Psychiatric diagnosis as an ethical problem', in S. Bloch and P. Chodoff (eds.), *Psychiatric Ethics*. Oxford: Oxford University Press).

Types	Continuous			Periodic	Shift-like		
Life course of the illness	Steady deterioration			Intermittent episodes	Intermittent episodes, superimposed on a steady deterioration		
Subtypes	*Sluggish* (mild)	*Paranoid* (moderate)	*Malignant* (severe)		*Mild*	*Moderate*	*Severe*
Some characteristics	Neurotic self-consciousness; introspectiveness; obsessive doubts; conflicts with parental and other authorities	Paranoid delusions; hallucinations; parasitic life-style	Early onset; unremitting; overwhelming	Acute attacks; fluctuations in mood; confusions	Neurotic, with affective colouring; social contentiousness; philosophical concerns; self-absorption	Acute paranoid	Catatonia; delusions; prominent mood changes

Course Forms

completing his MD at New York University in 1957.[19] While training at the New York State Psychiatric Institute, he attended the Columbia University Psychoanalytic Clinic for Training and Research, and qualified as a psychoanalyst. It was after completing this training that he was appointed to a research fellowship, which brought him into contact with epidemiologically sophisticated researchers at the New York State Psychiatric Institute, most notably Joseph Fliess, a statistician, and Joseph Zubin and Jean Endicott, both psychologists. His experience in this position led him to become one of the consultants to the APA's Task Force on Nomenclature and Statistics, which introduced DSM-II. Indeed, Spitzer co-authored the article in the *American Journal of Psychiatry* which introduced and defended the new manual.[20]

In a paper published with Joseph Fliess in 1974, Spitzer attempted an empirical summary of the art of psychiatric diagnosis at that point in time.[21] A novel aspect of their treatment of the reliability problem was their use of a relatively simple mathematical procedure to compensate for the base rate problem (that is, to allow for the extent to which randomly assigned diagnoses would be in agreement by chance, especially for frequently used diagnoses). The measure of reliability that they advocated, known as Cohen's kappa, gave a value between 0 for chance agreement and 1 for perfect agreement, with values above 0.7 being regarded as acceptable.* Using this statistic, Spitzer and Fliess were able to reanalyse data from the six best reliability studies then available, including the US–UK Diagnostic Project (for which they reported separate analyses of the New York and London data). Their findings are summarized in Table 3.2.

Their reanalysis suggested more modest levels of agreement than those claimed by the authors of the original studies. For example, in the study by Sandifer, Pettus and Quade, levels of agreement calculated using kappa (for example, schizophrenia = 0.68; psychotic depression = 0.19; manic depression = 0.33) appeared consistently lower than those calculated as percentages (schizophrenia = 74 per cent; psychotic depression = 22 per cent; manic depression = 36 per cent).[22]

---

* For the statistically unafraid, the formula for kappa is as follows:

$$k = \frac{P_O - P_C}{1 - P_C}$$

where P_O is the proportion of observed agreement between clinicians and P_C is the level of agreement expected by chance.

Table 3.2 Kappa measures computed for six studies (adapted from R. L. Spitzer and J. L. Fliess (1974) 'A reanalysis of the reliability of psychiatric diagnosis', *British Journal of Psychiatry*, 123: 341–7).

Specific diagnoses (e.g. schizophrenia) are listed under the major diagnostic categories (e.g. psychosis). A kappa value of 1 indicates perfect agreement between raters whereas a value of 0 indicates agreement at chance level. This statistic corrects for the 'base rate problem' (see text) and is a better measure of agreement than raw percentages. The studies from which the data were derived were (I) Schmidt and Fonda (1956); (II) Krietman (1961); (III) Beck et al. (1962); (IV) Sandifer et al. (1964); (V) Cooper et al. (1972); (VI) Spitzer et al. (1974). The data from (V) (the US–UK Diagnostic Project) are analysed separately for the New York and London samples.

| | | | | | STUDY V | | | |
Diagnosis	I	II	III	IV	US	UK	VI	Mean
Mental deficiency				.72				.72
Organic brain syndrome	.82	.90					.59	.77
Acute brain syndrome				.44				.44
Chronic brain syndrome				.64				.64
Alcoholism					.74	.68		.71
Psychosis	.73	.62		.56	.42	.43	.54	.55
Schizophrenia	.77		.42	.68	.32	.60	.65	.57
Mood disorder					.19	.44	.59	.41
Neurotic depression			.47		.20	.10		.26
Psychotic depression				.19	.24	.30		.24
Manic depression				.33				.33
Involutional depression			.38	.21				.30
Personality disorder			.33	.56	.19	.22	.29	.32
Neurosis		.52		.42	.26	.30	.48	.40
Anxiety reaction			.45					.45
Psychophysiologic reaction				.38				.38

DSM-III and the Industrialization of Psychiatry

The unsolved problem of reliability was one factor among many that led the APA to embark on the production of the third and most influential edition of its *Diagnostic and Statistical Manual*. Also important were political and economic concerns, together with changes in the scientific Zeitgeist.

The political concerns mainly centred on homosexuality, which was listed as a disorder in DSM-II. Following the emergence of the gay rights movement in the late 1960s, activists lobbied APA meetings – at first angrily protesting outside but later taking part in debates supported by sympathetic psychiatrists – in order to have homosexuality removed from the manual. Robert Spitzer played an important role in these discussions, shifting his support from those who saw homosexuality as a disease to those who saw it as part of normal human variation. Although these developments were peripheral to the classification of the psychoses, they drew problems of psychiatric classification to the attention of the American public for the first time, and established Spitzer as an authority on diagnostic issues in the eyes of many of his peers.[23]

The economic issues sprang from attempts to regulate the availability of psychological and medical treatments for psychiatric conditions. Health insurance companies in North America required a diagnosis before they would make reimbursement available to claimants, and looked to the APA for criteria to discriminate between those who really needed psychotherapy and those who did not. The US Food and Drugs Administration's demand that drug companies specify the disorders that their new compounds were to treat created similar pressures for a comprehensive and standardized approach to psychiatric diagnosis.[24]

However, more important than any of these factors was a shift in the way in which many American psychiatrists thought about psychiatric disorders. During the decades following the Second World War, Freudian theory had dominated American psychiatry, and the terminology of DSM-I had reflected this. For example, psychotic disorders were grouped under the heading 'disorders of psychogenic origin or without clearly defined physical cause or structural change in the brain' and, in deference to the ideas of Adolf Meyer, were individually listed as 'reaction types' (for example, 'manic-depressive reaction', 'schizophrenic reaction'). By the end of the 1960s, many American psychiatrists had become disenchanted with psychoanalysis, partly because it had failed to deliver effective treatments but also because it threatened to sever for ever the ties between psychiatry and medicine. It was mainly in reaction to this threat that Spitzer and others placed their hopes in a thoroughly biological approach to mental illness.

American psychiatrist Gerald Klerman coined the term *neoKraepelinian* to describe this new attitude to mental illness. In a 1978 article, which came close to being a manifesto, Klerman identified the nine propositions that he believed united the movement (see Table 3.3).[25] These recapitulated the approach to mental disorder taken by the movement's forefather nearly a century before and emphasized psychiatry's roots in physical medicine. According to Klerman, the neo-Kraepelinians assumed that a line could be drawn between mental illness and normal behaviour (proposition 4), and that there was a discrete and discoverable number of psychiatric disorders (proposition 5). There was an emphasis on the biological causes of mental illness and the psychiatrist's expertise in biological matters (proposition 6). Finally, emphasis was also placed on the importance of developing a reliable and valid system of psychiatric classification (propositions 7, 8 and 9).

One of the most important early achievements of the movement was a new, unofficial diagnostic system. In a landmark paper published in 1972, a group of neoKraepelinians from Washington University noted that the unsolved reliability problem made it difficult to ensure that the patients studied by one research group were comparable to those studied by another.[26] They therefore proposed what came to be known as *Feighner criteria* (after John Feighner, the first author of the paper) for sixteen commonly researched disorders. The paper became one of the most highly cited publications in the field of psychiatry. It was successful because the authors had finally adopted the suggestion made more than a decade earlier by the philosopher Carl Hempel. For each disorder, a precise list of symptoms was given, together with rules that specified exactly how many of the symptoms were required before the diagnosis could be made. This level of precision promised to abolish entirely the ambiguity and doubt which had previously affected the

Table 3.3 The main points of Gerald Klerman's neoKraepelinian manifesto (from G. L. Klerman (1978) 'The evolution of a scientific nosology', in J. C. Shershow (ed.), *Schizophrenia: Science and Practice*. Cambridge, MA: Harvard University Press).

1 Psychiatry is a branch of medicine.

2 Psychiatry should use modern scientific methodologies and base its practice on scientific knowledge.

3 Psychiatry treats people who are sick and who require treatment for mental illness.

4 There is a boundary between the normal and the sick.

5 There are discrete mental illnesses. Mental illnesses are not myths. There is not one, but many mental illnesses. It is the task of scientific psychiatry, as of other medical specialties, to investigate the causes, diagnosis and treatment of mental illnesses.

6 The focus of psychiatric physicians should be particularly on the biological aspects of mental illness.

7 There should be an explicit and intentional concern with diagnosis and classification.

8 Diagnostic criteria should be codified, and a legitimate and valued area of research should be to validate such criteria by various techniques. Further, departments of psychiatry in medical schools should teach these criteria and not depreciate them, as has been the case for many years.

9 In research efforts directed at improving the reliability and validity of diagnosis and classification, statistical techniques should be utilized.

selection of patients for inclusion in research. The thirst for certainty in diagnosis had at last been quenched.

The Feighner criteria became the model for DSM-III. The precise strategy for developing the new edition of the manual was decided at a day-long meeting in 1974 attended by Spitzer, Melvin Sabshin, then President of the APA, and Theodore Millon, a psychologist at the Illinois Medical Center. The production of the manual was to be a major undertaking. The task force set up to execute this project – chaired, of course, by Spitzer – decided to undertake field trials to determine whether various draft criteria were usable in practice. By the time the task had been completed, no fewer than 600 clinicians had become involved.

The DSM-III definitions of schizophrenia and manic episode, which illustrate the clarity of the manual, are given in Table 3.4. DSM-III definitions have what some have called a 'Chinese menu' structure. For example, in the definition of a manic episode there are three main elements. First of all, the patient must meet criterion A (one or more distinct periods of elevated, irritable or expansive mood). Second,

---

Table 3.4 DSM-III definitions of schizophrenia and manic episode (American Psychiatric Association (1980) *Diagnostic and Statistical Manual of Mental Disorders* (3rd edn). Washington, DC: APA).

SCHIZOPHRENIA

A   At least one of the following during a phase of the illness:

1 bizarre delusions (content is patently absurd and has *no* possible basis in fact), such as delusions of being controlled, thought broadcasting, thought insertion, or thought withdrawal

2 somatic, grandiose, religious, nihilistic or other delusions without persecutory or jealous content

3 delusions with persecutory or jealous content, if accompanied by hallucinations of any type

4 auditory hallucinations in which either a voice keeps a running commentary on the individual's behaviour or thoughts, or two or more voices converse with each other

5 auditory hallucinations on several occasions with content of more than one or two words, having no apparent relation to depression or elation

6 incoherence, marked loosening of associations, markedly illogical thinking, or marked poverty of content of speech if associated with at least one of the following:
   (a) blunted, flat, or inappropriate affect
   (b) delusions or hallucinations
   (c) catatonic or other grossly disorganized behaviour

B   Deterioration from a previous level of functioning in such areas as work, social relations and self care.

C   Duration: Continuous signs of the illness for at least six months at some time during the person's life, with some signs of the illness at present. The six-month period must include an active phase during which there were symptoms from A, with or without a prodromal or residual phase.

MANIC EPISODE

A   One or more distinct periods with a predominantly elevated, expansive, or irritable mood. The elevated or irritable mood must be a prominent part of the illness and relatively persistent, although it may alternate or intermingle with depressive mood.

B   Duration of at least one week (or any duration if hospitalization is necessary) during which, for most of the time, at least three of the following symptoms have persisted (four if the mood is only irritable) and have been present to a significant degree:

   1 increase in activity (either socially, at work, or sexually) or physical restlessness
   2 more talkative than usual or pressure to keep talking
   3 flight of ideas or subjective experience that thoughts are racing
   4 inflated self-esteem (grandiosity, which may be delusional)
   5 decreased need for sleep
   6 distractability, i.e. attention is too easily drawn to unimportant or irrelevant external stimuli
   7 excessive involvement in activities that have a high potential for painful consequences which is not recognized, e.g. buying sprees, sexual indiscretion, foolish business investments, reckless driving

C   Neither of the following dominates the clinical picture when an affective syndrome is absent (i.e. symptoms in criteria A and B above):

   1 preoccupation with a mood-incongruent delusion or hallucination
   2 bizarre behaviour

D   Not superimposed on either schizophrenia, schizophreniform disorder or a paranoid disorder.

E   Not due to any organic mental disorder, such as substance abuse.

criterion B requires that the patient has suffered from at least three out of a list of seven symptoms over a period of at least a week. Finally, criterion C indicates some exclusion criteria, for example symptoms that, if present, would indicate an alternative diagnosis.

The final manual, at 500 pages, was more than three times longer than DSM-II.[27] During a period when the American publishing industry was experiencing serious difficulties, it became an unlikely bestseller. Nearly half a million copies were bought, generating estimated revenue for the APA of over $9.8 million (a sum that does not include earnings from the numerous pocket guides to DSM-III which were later published). In the USA, the manual was widely embraced both by psychiatrists and psychologists fearful that, without a DSM-III diagnosis for each of their patients, payment from health insurance companies would not be forthcoming. Many journals would not accept papers for publication unless investigators could reassure their readers that the patients studied had been diagnosed according to the DSM-III system, thus ensuring that the criteria became a standard among researchers, not only in America but also elsewhere in the world.

Astonishingly, DSM-III has been revised twice since its publication in 1980. Within three years, a new task force, again chaired by Robert Spitzer, set to work on the changes that would be required for the revised third edition, known as DSM-III-R, which was published in 1987.[28] Despite Spitzer's assurances that only minor adjustments were necessary, twenty-five committees involving over 200 consultants worked on the project. The criteria for half of the diagnostic categories were altered, and thirty new diagnoses were added. Not surprisingly, the appointment of a DSM-IV task force within four months of the publication of DSM-III-R led some psychiatrists to protest. British psychiatrist Robert Kendell suggested that the exercise was little more than a cynical attempt to repeat the huge profits the APA had made from selling the earlier editions.[29] Despite these objections, the APA decided to proceed with the new edition, partly to ensure that the official classification would be consistent with the mental disorders section of the tenth edition of the International Classification of Diseases (ICD-10), scheduled for publication in 1992. When it appeared in 1994, DSM-IV weighed in at 900 pages, and credited over 1000 consultants.[30] By the end of 2000, over 960,000 copies had been sold, a remarkable volume of sales given that there were just 42,000 psychiatrists and about 300,000 other mental health care professionals in the USA.[31] At about the same time, the lead character of the hit television comedy show *Frasier* read out spoof DSM criteria for 'phase of life problem' without explaining what the letters stood for, thereby indicating the extent to which the manual had become part of American culture.

At the time of writing, the American Psychiatric Association has just released a provisional timetable for the publication of the fifth edition of the *Diagnostic and Statistical Manual*, which is tentatively scheduled for 2010. Although the structure of the manual is yet to be determined, some observers have already speculated about its contents. For example, the American psychologist Roger Blashfield, in a paper ridiculing the entire approach, used statistical techniques to analyse trends in DSMs I–IV.[32] Based on his calculations, he predicted that DSM-V will have 1256 pages, will contain 1800 diagnostic criteria and eleven appendices, and will generate $80 million in revenue for the APA. As the only basic colour that has yet to be used on the cover of a DSM is brown, Blashfield has predicted that this colour will be used for DSM-V.

By now the reader may be wondering whether the enormous effort and expenditure required to complete these successive revisions of the DSM has yielded the promised improvements in reliability. The neoKraepelinians clearly believed that they had succeeded in this respect. Reviewing the results of the DSM-III field trials, Spitzer described the reliability of the manual as extremely good.[33] Similarly, Gerald Klerman (the psychiatrist who had given the name to the neoKraepelinian movement) felt able to declare that, in principle, the reliability problem had at last been solved.[34]

In a detailed review of the evidence from the field trials, psychologists Herb Kutchins and Stuart Kirk reached a starkly different conclusion, arguing that, 'The DSM revolution in reliability has been a revolution in rhetoric, not in reality.'[35] They noted that the trials were beset with numerous methodological problems. For example, little control was exercised over the way in which the studies were conducted at different sites, so that estimates of reliability were often calculated on the basis of agreements between close colleagues about small numbers of patients. Even so, the results for many diagnoses were hardly impressive, and often failed to reach the kappa value of 0.7 defined in advance as acceptable by Spitzer and his colleagues.

Following the publication of DSM-III, ever more ambitious reliability studies were conducted, but most obtained comparable results. For example, a seven-centre study carried out in the USA and Germany was reported by a team that included Spitzer.[36] Nearly 400 patients and just over 200 ordinary people were examined by pairs of specially trained psychiatrists. The psychiatrists used an interview schedule specifically designed to yield the information required for assigning DSM-III-R diagnoses. Even under these ideal circumstances, levels of agreement for patients averaged at a kappa of 0.61.

Of course, the diagnoses obtained in these kinds of studies are often obtained in ideal conditions. The diagnosticians taking part usually receive special training and employ standardized interview schedules that define precisely the questions they may ask their patients. Australian psychiatrist Patrick McGorry and his colleagues have argued that the levels of agreement observed therefore give a spuriously positive impression of what can be achieved in routine clinical practice.[37] To investigate the effects of varying interview procedures, they asked psychiatrists to assign DSM-III-R diagnoses using four different methods. Three of the methods involved the use of special interview schedules or checklists to assess patients' symptoms. The fourth involved each patient being interviewed by a team, which then arrived at a consensus diagnosis by discussion. When any two methods were compared, kappa values varied between 0.53 and 0.67. Full agreement between all four procedures was achieved for only twenty-seven out of the fifty patients who participated in the study.

The Vanishing Consensus Effect

The development of the DSM system has so mesmerized recent thinking about psychiatric disorders that it is easy to forget that rival sets of criteria have also been proposed, such as the eighth and subsequent editions of the *International Classification of Disease*, and the Feighner system. In addition to these major challengers to the diagnostic hegemony of the American Psychiatric Association, there are also a number of idiosyncratic definitions of specific disorders proposed by various researchers (for example, definitions of schizophrenia suggested by Taylor and Abrams[38] and by Carpenter and his colleagues[39] in the United States). When these different criteria are compared there is little to indicate which, if any, embodies the most meaningful taxonomy of mental disorders. What is clear is that the apparent consensus created by the DSM system is illusory.

A dramatic demonstration of this vanishing consensus effect was reported by Ian Brockington of the University of Birmingham, who applied various definitions of schizophrenia to symptom data collected from patients studied in the US–UK Diagnostic Project.[40] Eighty-five patients from Netherne Hospital in London had received a hospital diagnosis of schizophrenia at the time of the study. Brockington estimated that 163 would have received the diagnosis according to the then existing American criteria. When the project team applied the ICD-8 definition, only 65 were found to suffer from schizophrenia. This number fell to 55 when a computer-generated diagnosis based on Schneider's first-rank symptoms was employed. When the Research Diagnostic Criteria (a variant of the Feighner system) were used, the number of schizophrenia patients was 28, and the use of the DSM-III criteria saw this number fall even further to 19. Thus, the number of schizophrenia patients in the sample varied between 163 and 19, according to the definition chosen.

These troubles have not been restricted to the diagnosis of schizophrenia. In a study recently published by Jim van Os and his colleagues in Britain and Holland, over 700 patients with chronic psychosis were classified according to the RDC, DSM-III-R and ICD-10 systems.[41] The numbers of patients meeting various definitions of schizophrenia, depression, mania and other diagnoses are shown in Table 3.5. For example, it can be seen that the number of patients in the sample suffering from mania varied from 18 (according to the RDC definition) to 87 (according to the DSM-III-R definition), a staggering nearly fivefold difference.

As a remedy for the vanishing consensus effect, some researchers have advocated a 'polydiagnostic' approach, in which several diagnostic systems are used simultaneously. A leading exponent of this approach is Peter McGuffin, Professor of Psychiatry at the Institute of Psychiatry in London, who has developed a computer program known as OPCRIT, which generates diagnoses according to the

Table 3.5 Distribution of diagnoses in 706 psychotic patients according to three different diagnostic criteria (from J. van Os et al. (1999) 'A comparison of the utility of dimensional and categorical representations of psychosis', *Psychological Medicine*, 29: 595–606).

Diagnosis	RDC		DSM-III-R		ICD-10	
	N	%	N	%	N	%
Schizophreniform disorder	–		20	2.8	–	
Schizophrenia	268	38.0	371	52.6	387	54.8
Schizoaffective manic	98	13.9			41	5.8
Schizoaffective bipolar	129	18.3	13	1.8	23	3.3
Schizoaffective depressed	118	16.7			40	5.7
Major depression	16	2.3	71	10.1	19	2.7
Mania	18	2.6	87	12.3	61	8.6
Bipolar disorder	16	2.3	66	9.4	6	0.9
Unspecified functional psychosis	43	6.1	68	9.6	95	13.5
Delusional disorder	–		10	1.4	18	2.6
Not classified	–		–		16	2.3

DSM-III, DSM-III-R, DSM-IV, ICD-9 and ICD-10 systems.[42] Whether this approach clarifies or obscures the business of conducting psychiatric research is open to debate. Certainly, it offers no guidance to the practising clinician.

4

Fool's Gold

In his fantastic essay 'John Wilkins' analytical language', the Argentinian writer Jorge Luis Borges remarks on a classification of animals described in a certain Chinese encyclopaedia, *The Celestial Emporium of Benevolent Knowledge*:

In those remote pages it is stated that animals can be divided into the following classes: (a) belonging to the Emperor; (b) embalmed; (c) trained; (d) sucking pigs; (e) mermaids; (f) fabulous; (g) stray dogs; (h) included in this classification; (i) with the vigorous movements of madmen; (j) innumerable; (k) drawn with a very fine camel hair brush; (l) etcetera; (m) having just broken a large vase; (n) looking from a distance like flies.[1]

Borges thereby reminds us that not all taxonomies are meaningful. If his joke seems far removed from reality, consider the real-life example of astrology, a system of classification that provides a fool's-gold standard against which to evaluate modern psychiatric diagnoses. Like diagnoses, star signs are supposed to describe human characteristics and to predict what will happen to people in the future. Although there is no evidence to support these claims, astrology is a system of classification that continues to capture the imagination of large numbers of otherwise intelligent people. Indeed, a recent poll revealed that almost one quarter of American adults believe in astrological theories.[2]

In the last chapter, we saw that one way of assessing the usefulness of a diagnostic system is to measure its reliability. However, the example of astrology illustrates the limitation of this approach. Star signs are highly reliable (we can all agree about who is born under Taurus), so reliability alone cannot ensure that a diagnostic system is scientific. Further tests of the *validity* of the system are necessary to determine whether it fulfils the functions for which it has been designed. We can test the validity of astrological theories by seeing whether people born under the sign of Libra really are well-balanced, or whether most Scorpios really do meet the beautiful stranger of their dreams in the first quarter of the year. Similarly, we can evaluate the validity of diagnostic categories by seeing whether they lead us to useful scientific insights or helpful clinical predictions.

Of course, although reliability does not guarantee validity, it is obvious that *a diagnostic system cannot be valid without first being reliable*. Unless psychiatrists and psychologists can agree about which patients suffer from which disorders there is no possibility that the process of diagnosis will fulfil any useful function. In the last chapter I established that, for the most part, modern psychiatric diagnoses fail to meet adequate standards of reliability. Some readers might therefore be forgiven for wondering whether there is any point in proceeding to examine validity evidence in detail. However, there are two good reasons for doing so. First, some readers, particularly those who have trained in the mental health professions, may require further per-suasion before abandoning long-held assumptions about the nature of madness. Second, as we study the validity of psychiatric diagnoses we will encounter evidence that will be useful when attempting to construct a scientific alternative to the Kraepelinian system.

Diagnoses as Descriptions

One function of a diagnosis is to provide a shorthand description of a patient's complaints. On the basis of a diagnosis recorded in the medical notes, a clinician about to meet a patient for the first time should be able to anticipate the range of symptoms that the patient will be suffering. However, diagnoses can only achieve this function if they accurately reflect the way that symptoms cluster together. Determining whether they do or do not is quite difficult, and requires the use of complex statistical procedures. Fortunately, the principles behind these procedures can be readily understood without knowledge of the relevant mathematical equations.

How many psychoses are there?

For a categorial system of diagnosis to work, diagnoses must be jointly exhaustive (there should be no psychiatric patients who fail to meet the criteria for a diagnosis) and mutually exclusive (patients, unless they are very unlucky, should not suffer from more than one disorder).[3] In Kraepelin's original system, there were only two or three major categories of psychosis. However, in order to make the DSM exhaustive, its authors have dramatically increased the number of definitions included in successive editions of the manual, and have also included catch-all 'not otherwise specified' diagnoses in order to sweep up anyone who does not fit the criteria for a specific disorder. At the same time, in order to ensure that diagnoses are mutually exclusive, the authors have had to include special exclusion rules to limit the possibility that patients will fall into more than one category.

Including subtypes as well as major diagnoses, 94 categories of disorder were included in DSM-I. This number rose to 137 in DSM-II, to 163 in DSM-III, to 174 in DSM-III-R and finally to 201 in DSM-IV. This expansion has been accompanied by an increasingly fine-grained subdivision of the major categories. For example, DSM-IV describes five subtypes of schizophrenia; two milder forms of psychosis (schizophreniform disorder and brief psychotic disorder); schizoaffective disorder; delusional disorder (formerly paranoia); shared psychotic disorder (*folie à deux*); psychotic disorder due to a medical condition; substance-induced psychotic disorder; and, finally, the catch-all 'psychotic disorder not otherwise specified'. Bipolar disorder appears as two different subtypes (Type I and Type II, distinguished by the severity of manic episodes) in a separate section on mood disorders, along with seven other types of mood disorder, 'mood disorder not otherwise specified', and four types of mood 'episodes'.

The arbitrary exclusion rules designed to limit the risk that patients will be judged to suffer from more than one type of illness – a phenomenon known as *comorbidity*[4] – are listed at the end of each set of diagnostic criteria. For example, DSM-IV states that patients may not be diagnosed as suffering from schizophrenia if they also meet the criteria for schizoaffective disorder, major depression or mania. Similarly, the criteria for bipolar disorder specify that the patient's symptoms should, 'Not be better accounted for by schizoaffective disorder and are not superimposed on schizophrenia, schizophreniform disorder, delusional disorder, or psychotic disorder not otherwise specified.'

That the exclusion rules hide, rather than eliminate, the problem of comorbidity became evident in one of the most impressive surveys of psychiatric symptoms ever conducted. Funded by the US National Institute of Mental Health and carried out during the 1980s, it was known as the Epidemiological Catchment Area (ECA) Study, and its overall purpose was to determine the prevalence of various types of psychiatric disorder in the general population. A total of 18,500 people over 18 years of age were randomly selected from five US cities, and interviewed about their experiences of psychiatric symptoms and emotional distress. Over 15,000 agreed to a further interview one year later. The interview data were then used to assign diagnoses according to DSM-III criteria.

When the researchers suspended the arbitrary exclusion rules built into the DSM system, they found that 60 per cent of those who had met the criteria for one disorder during their lifetime had also met the criteria for at least one other.[5] In order to quantify the extent of *current comorbidity* – the presence of two or more DSM-III disorders at the same point in time – they calculated a statistic known as the *odds ratio*, which indicates the chance of having a second diagnosis if a first one is present. (An odds ratio of 1 indicates no increased chance of a second diagnosis, an odds ratio of 2 indicates that the presence of one diagnosis doubles the chance of another, and so on. The researchers decided in advance that an odds ratio of 10 implied a strong association between diagnoses.)

On average, the odds that any two diagnoses would occur together turned out to be 2 (that is, twice what would be expected by chance). The odds ratio for depression and mania was 36, which was perhaps unsurprising as both are regarded as phases of a single disorder. However, the odds ratio for schizophrenia and mania was 46, and for schizophrenia and depression it was 14. Project leader Lee Robins and his colleagues concluded that 'The most likely explanation for co-occurrence is that having one disorder puts the affected person at risk of developing other disorders.'[6] Presumably, they had in mind the possibility that patients suffering from, say, schizophrenia, might be so distressed by the experience that they would become depressed as well. Strangely, they did not discuss the possibility that their findings might instead reflect the inadequacies of the neoKraepelinian system. Clearly, the most likely explanation for the strong associations observed between schizophrenia, depression and mania is that these diagnoses do not describe separate disorders.

We can test this suspicion by looking at symptoms in a different way. Suppose that, instead of diagnosing patients as schizophrenic or manic-depressive, we instead assign them scores indicating the extent to which their symptoms correspond to one diagnosis or the other. If we then place patients along this dimension of schizophrenic versus manic-depressive, we should be able to observe whether they fall into two separate groups with clearly different scores, or whether many patients have intermediate scores indicating a mixture of the two types of symptoms. I have just described, in a very simple way, the rationale for a statistical technique known as *discriminant function analysis*. The actual methods used to calculate the scores of individual patients are fairly complex and can be ignored for present purposes.[7]

In a pioneering study using this method, Robert Kendell and Jane Gourlay studied the symptoms of nearly 300 patients.[8] They used a computer to assign negative scores to schizophrenia symptoms such as delusions and hallucinations and positive scores to mood symptoms such as abnormal gregariousness, manic speech and depressed behaviour. When the scores for each patient's symptoms were added together, it was found that most patients fell in the middle range, close to zero, indicating that there is a continuum between schizophrenia and manic depression, rather than two separate illnesses. Subsequent studies using variations on the technique,[9] although producing results that have varied in some respects from those obtained by Kendell and Gourlay, have all failed to find the neat dividing line between schizophrenic and bipolar symptoms that was the one of main assumptions of the Kraepelinian paradigm, and which, for this reason, was described by Kendell and Gourlay as one of the 'cornerstones of modern psychiatry'.

Which symptoms go together?

Although psychotic symptoms do not fall into two main categories as supposed by Kraepelin, this does not mean that the relationships between them have no structure. Symptoms may cluster together in ways that were never envisaged by the father of modern psychiatry, perhaps in ways that cut across the major categories described in modern diagnostic systems. To discover whether this is the case, researchers have resorted to another statistical procedure, known as *factor analysis*. In the initial phase of this kind of analysis, information about symptoms is collected from a large number of patients and a matrix (table) of correlations is calculated showing the relationships between all possible pairs. (If two symptoms are highly correlated this means that they typically occur together.) Further analysis of the matrix then leads to the discovery of different clusters or groups of symptoms, known as *factors*. One of the main goals of factor analysis is to discover the minimum number of factors required to describe the data. If only one factor is discovered, there is only one cluster of symptoms, and patients can be placed on a single dimension running from well (no or very few symptoms) to very ill (many symptoms). If two or more factors are discovered, it is likely that there are two or more symptom clusters and that patients vary according to their severity on each.

Factor analysis was developed in the 1920s by psychologists who were interested in the relationships between different measures of human intelligence. They wanted to know whether there is just one type of general intelligence, or several different intellectual faculties. As the invention of the computer lay some way in the future, the necessary calculations were carried out by teams of clerks, who would often take several weeks to complete each analysis.[10]

The technique was first applied to the problem of psychiatric classification by an American psychologist, Thomas Moore, who published his findings in 1930.[11] From data on the symptoms of a group of 367 seriously ill patients, Moore was able to extract no less than eight symptom clusters. Hallucinations and delusions seemed to occur together (a finding that has been consistently repeated in later research). However, Moore found two types of depression, two types

of mania, a syndrome of uninhibited behaviour, a syndrome of catatonic behaviour, and a syndrome of cognitive deficits.

Following Moore's work, interest in the use of factor analysis in
psychiatry has waxed and waned as the technique has been progressively refined.[12] However, the method has been used extensively in the
past ten years, partly in response to an influential theory proposed by
the British psychiatrist Tim Crow. In a paper published in 1980, Crow
broke away from the Kraepelinian paradigm and suggested that there
are two different types of schizophrenia.[13] According to the theory,
the main symptoms of Type I schizophrenia are hallucinations and
delusions, which are caused by a biochemical imbalance in the brain.
Borrowing from the literature on neurological illnesses, Crow referred
to these as *positive symptoms* (because they consist of experiences and
behaviours that we would prefer to be absent).* The symptoms of
Crow's Type II schizophrenia consist of apathy, emotional flatness
and social withdrawal. Crow called these *negative symptoms* (because
they involve the absence of desirable behaviour) and argued that they
are caused by a progressive atrophy of certain areas in the brain.
Although this theory made bold use of evidence from biological studies
of brain structure and function, it was essentially speculative and was
not based on analyses of symptom data. However, the theory leads to
some fairly obvious predictions about what should emerge from a
factor analysis of psychotic symptoms.

In fact, the first study that attempted to test Crow's theory obtained
not two symptom clusters but three. Analysing data from a group of
chronically ill schizophrenia patients, British psychiatrist Peter Liddle
obtained one factor consisting of positive symptoms and one consisting

---

* The concept of positive and negative symptoms can be traced to the British
neurologist Hughlings Jackson. Writing at the end of the nineteenth century,
Jackson assumed a hierarchical-evolutionary model of the nervous system, in
which the most evolved regions of the brain were not only responsible for the
highest forms of mental functioning, but also regulated the expression of more
primitive functions. On this view, negative symptoms were the consequence of the
loss of higher functions whereas the release of lower functions was responsible for
positive symptoms. Jackson's use of metaphor reveals the cultural origins of this
theory: 'If the governing body of this country were destroyed suddenly, we should
have two causes of lamentation: 1. The loss of services of eminent men; 2. the
anarchy of the now uncontrolled people' (quoted in J. Miller (1978) *The Body in
Question*. London: Jonathan Cape).

of negative symptoms. The unexpected third factor consisted of symptoms of cognitive disorganization, for example disturbed speech and problems of attention.[14] These findings have since been replicated by many other researchers,[15] although, to complicate matters further, some have argued that the three clusters can be further subdivided.[16]

Of course, it is impossible to conclude much about psychosis in general from these findings, as they were obtained from groups of patients who had already been selected for a diagnosis of schizophrenia. What we would like to know, therefore, is whether the same three dimensions can be used to describe the symptoms of psychotic patients with other diagnoses. There is at least some evidence that they can. For example, in a recent study published by researchers at Harvard Medical School, factor analysis was used to investigate the symptoms of psychotic patients diagnosed as suffering from schizophrenia, major depression and bipolar disorder according to DSM criteria. Although there was some variation in the results when the analyses were restricted to the individual diagnostic groups, the overall picture that emerged was consistent with the three-factor model.[17]

In this account, I have simplified the steps involved in carrying out a factor analysis, and underplayed the difficulties involved. The number of factors revealed can be affected by decisions about which symptoms to include in the analysis (if important symptoms are not recorded the results are likely to be misleading) or about which patients to study (the broader the sample, the more likely that the results will be meaningful). Moreover, a number of different methods of carrying out the analysis employ different rules to determine the number of factors, so that researchers, finding that a particular analysis is uninterpretable, are sometimes tempted to experiment with other methods before selecting the one that yields the most credible results. Despite these opportunities for subjectivity, and similar limitations affecting discriminant function analysis, it is striking that analyses of patients' symptoms have *never* provided clear support for Kraepelin's theory. Indeed, at first sight, the results obtained from the two statistical approaches we have considered appear to deviate from Kraepelin's system in opposite directions. The findings from discriminant function analysis imply that we should collapse all the psychotic disorders into one, whereas the findings from factor analysis seem to suggest that we need to subdivide the psychoses into many more components than those proposed by Kraepelin. This apparent paradox is resolved when we remember that the symptom dimensions revealed by factor analysis seem to describe efficiently the symptoms of both schizophrenia and bipolar patients. Therefore, although the distinction between schizophrenia and bipolar disorder does not seem to survive examination with these techniques, we can be fairly confident that all psychotic symptoms cannot be explained in terms of a single underlying disease process.

What Families Can Teach us about Psychiatric Diagnoses

A second function of a diagnosis is to group together people whose problems are likely to have a common aetiology. Indeed, as we have already seen, the most common strategy employed in psychiatric research – comparing those with a particular diagnosis with people who are psychologically healthy – assumes that those with the diagnosis have something in common that is of aetiological significance. Although discussion of many of the factors thought to influence the development of psychosis must wait until later chapters, there is one aetiological factor that has been thought to have special significance for psychiatric classification, and which we will therefore consider here. This will require a short digression into the difficult world of genetics, an effort that will save us time later in the book.

On the assumption that psychiatric problems are, at least in part, inherited, some researchers have attempted to address the validity of diagnoses by observing whether they breed true in families. If this is so, people who suffer from a particular disorder are likely to have many relatives who suffer from the same disorder, but few relatives who suffer from any other kind of mental illness. Some researchers conducting this kind of work have argued that genetic studies provide an unassailable riposte to those who question the Kraepelinian paradigm. For example, the American psychiatrist Seymour Kety once commented that, 'If schizophrenia is a myth, it is a myth with a strong genetic component.'[18]

As we have already seen, genetic research into psychiatric disorders has suffered from an unhappy history. Many of the German pioneers in the field held political views that were in sympathy with the Nazi movement. The first genetic studies of schizophrenia were carried out by Ernst Rüdin, who later served with Heinrich Himmler on a committee that, in 1933, drafted legislation enabling the compulsory sterilization of psychiatric patients.[19] His student Franz Kallman advocated the sterilization, not only of mentally ill people, but also of their relatives.* Ironically, Kallman was forced to move from Germany to the United States in the 1930s because he was half-Jewish. Given these unpromising beginnings, it is understandable that some critics have viewed all genetic research into madness with suspicion.[20]

Before proceeding further, it will be useful to consider the three main research strategies that psychiatric geneticists have followed when attempting to determine the contribution of heredity to mental illness. All exploit the fact that we share alleles (particular versions of genes) with other individuals according to how closely we are related to them. For example, we obtain half of our alleles from each of our two parents who, in turn, obtained half of theirs from each of their two parents. Half of our alleles are therefore shared with each parent and a quarter are shared with each grandparent. As ordinary brothers and sisters are each a product of the random combination of alleles from the same two parents, it turns out that sibs, on average, also have half their alleles in common.

Matters become slightly more complicated when it comes to twins. *Dizygotic* (sometimes called non-identical or fraternal) twins are born after two eggs, appearing at the same time in the uterus, are fertilized by two sperm. They are therefore sibs who happen to be born at the same time and, on average, have half their alleles in common. About 50 per cent of dizygotic twin pairs consist of a boy and a girl, about a quarter consist of two boys and about a quarter consist of two girls. Even when the twins are of the same sex, they often look quite different

---

* Kallman, who became one of the most influential of the early psychiatric geneticists, believed that the gene for schizophrenia was recessive and therefore would be carried by many of the healthy relatives of schizophrenia patients. He therefore held that the spread of schizophrenia genes into successive generations could only be checked if both patients and their healthy relatives were prevented from breeding. In their book *Not in Our Genes*, Steven Rose, Leon Kamin and Richard Lewontin (Harmondsworth: Penguin, 1985) have noted a curious rewriting of history by some contemporary American writers, who have argued that Kallman was motivated to believe that schizophrenia was a recessive disorder precisely because he knew that this would make eugenic measures impractical.

from each other, although this is not invariably the case. *Monozygotic* or identical twins, on the other hand, are born after a single zygote (fertilized egg) splits in two and both halves develop separately in the uterus. These twins are genetically identical and are always the same sex, although they may still be differentially affected by factors in the inter-uterine environment.*

The simplest method of exploiting these differences in genetic similarity is the *family study*. In this kind of research, cases of an illness are traced within large families. If the illness is mostly inherited, close relatives of an affected member should be more likely to suffer from the illness than distant relatives. The second widely used strategy is the *twin study*. If genes make a major contribution to an illness, the probability that an identical twin of an affected individual will also suffer from the illness should be very high and the concordance rate for fraternal twins should be lower. Of course, twins belonging to the same family may be raised similarly and this may also affect concordance rates. To control for this possibility, geneticists sometimes carry out *adoption studies*. For example, children of affected parents who have been adopted away at birth and raised by normal families can be compared with the adopted-away children of unaffected parents. If

---

* Identical twins are not always identical in the uterus. Very rarely, genetic mutations may affect one foetus and not the other. More commonly, one foetus receives a better blood supply than the other, and is born heavier as a consequence. Also, infectious or toxic agents may have differential effects on twins. One twin may be affected by a virus whereas the other is not (a study of six pairs of twins born to HIV-positive mothers found that only one of the twins was affected in three of the pairs). Similarly, drugs taken by the mother may have a greater effect on one twin than on the other.

One way of estimating the influence of such factors on the development of twins is by the study of congenital abnormalities that are present at birth. Identical twins are often discordant for such abnormalities, and the degree of concordance or discordance varies according to the organ system affected. For example, concordance rates for clubfoot have been estimated at approximately 75 per cent whereas those for brain abnormalities are much lower, leading some researchers to conclude that non-genetic factors are the main cause of the latter. (For discussions of these and other factors complicating twin studies, see E. F. Torrey, A. E. Bowler, E. H. Taylor and I. I. Gottesman (1994) *Schizophrenia and Manic-Depressive Disorder*. New York: Basic Books, and also L. Wright (1997) *Twins: Genes, Environment and the Mystery of Identity*. London: Weidenfeld & Nicolson.)

genetic factors play a role in the aetiology of the illness, the children of the affected parents should show higher rates of illness than the children of the unaffected parents, even though both groups have been raised apart from their biological families. An alternative adoption study strategy starts with the adoptees but follows the same logic. In this case, the researcher attempts to trace the biological parents of adoptees who have become ill, in order to compare them with the biological parents of adoptees who show no evidence of psychiatric illness.

It is fair to say that each of these strategies has proved to be fraught with difficulties. For example, the poor reliability of psychiatric diagnoses means that there must be some uncertainty about the diagnoses assigned by genetic researchers. (This problem was most evident in a famous series of adoption studies carried out in Denmark by Seymour Kety and his colleagues, who used such a broad definition of 'schizophrenia' that almost anyone who was slightly eccentric was regarded as mentally ill.[21] Inevitably, some commentators have dismissed the results from these studies as almost worthless, although they are still cited in textbooks of psychiatry.)[22] Surprisingly, it can also be difficult to decide whether twins are identical or fraternal without genetic testing, which has only become available in recent years.

When the individuals who are examined in a genetic study are relatively young, geneticists make mathematical corrections to their data to allow for the possibility that some unaffected individuals will become ill later in life (in effect, they guess how many of the well individuals will become ill as they get older). Confusingly, there are also several ways of estimating concordance in twin studies, some of which give higher values than others. The commonsense approach is the *pairwise* method. For a group of twins in which at least one member of each pair is affected, the pairwise concordance rate is the percentage of pairs in which both are affected. For example, if in three out of ten twin pairs both are affected, but in the remaining seven only one is affected, the pairwise concordance rate is $^3/_{10}$ or 30 per cent. The less commonsensical *probandwise* method gives higher values and is therefore preferred by geneticists. This is calculated as the proportion of twins who have the illness who have an affected twin. In the above example, six twins have an affected twin (i.e. both members of each concordant pair are counted as having a twin who is also ill) whereas only seven do not, leading to a concordance rate of $^6/_{13}$ or 46 per cent (an increase in concordance of more than a half).*

A further difficulty with twin studies is that twin status itself is associated with slightly abnormal development. Twins (whether fraternal or identical) have a higher risk of congenital difficulties and, on average, reach developmental milestones slightly later than singletons.[23] It is also possible that they are treated differently from singletons by their parents, who will certainly face more than the usual difficulties when struggling to provide them with adequate attention. Whether these subtle influences might, in extreme circumstances, culminate in a higher risk of psychosis remains unclear. In an analysis of twin data from schizophrenia studies, Steven Rose, Leon Kamin and Richard Lewontin (distinguished neuroscientist, psychologist and geneticist, respectively) calculated that concordance rates for fraternal twins were significantly greater than those for non-twin sibs, an observation that clearly points to the adverse effect of being a twin.[24] However, attempts to find out whether twins have an increased liability to psychosis compared to the general population have reported inconsistent results.[25]

Given these problems, it is remarkable that genetic researchers have been almost blind to obvious environmental influences on the people they have studied. The case of the Genain quadruplets, four genetically identical women believed to be suffering from schizophrenia, provides an astonishing example of this kind of myopia. American psychologist David Rosenthal and his colleagues estimated that the probability that identical quadruplets would be affected by the illness was one per one and a half billion births.[26] The pseudonyms given to the quadruplets to maintain their anonymity give some indication of where the researchers were coming from. *Genain* was derived from the Greek for 'dreadful

---

* In an essay that is highly critical of the quality of genetic research in psychiatry, the late J. Richard Marshall showed that the same logic could be used to inflate estimates of *dis*cordance. For example, in the above example the pairwise discordance rate is 70 per cent. However, if we calculate a probandwise discordance rate for the sample by counting separately each member of the discordant pairs, we arrive at a discordance rate of 82 per cent, so that, 'It could then be argued that the *concordance* rate is negligible' ('The genetics of schizophrenia: axiom or hypothesis?' in R. P. Bentall (ed.) (1990) *Reconstructing Schizophrenia*. London: Routledge).

gene' and the first names selected for the unfortunate women, Nora, Iris, Myra and Hester, when written in their birth order, spelt out the initials of the US National Institute for Mental Health.

Despite his obvious bias, Rosenthal's publications provide compelling reasons for questioning his exclusively genetic account of their difficulties. First, there were considerable differences in the psychiatric problems experienced by the women. Myra, who had married, suffered from much milder symptoms than the others, and preferred minimal contact with the investigators. Follow-up studies carried out in 1981 when the quadruplets were 51 years old[27] and in 1996 when they were 66[28] showed that Myra and Iris performed much better than Nora and Hester on a range of psychological tests, with Myra's performance falling mostly in the normal range. Moreover, Myra and Iris showed much less deterioration than Nora and Hester when their medication was stopped.

More importantly, there was considerable evidence that the quadruplets had suffered unfortunate experiences during childhood, which may have contributed to their difficulties as adults. Their father, who often drank excessively, was described as unstable and paranoid. It is likely that he sexually abused some of his daughters. The investigators report that 'He chose Nora as his favourite, at times fondling her breasts and being intrusive when she was in the bathroom.' A less than ideal family environment can also be inferred from the following observations:

Iris and Hester engaged in mutual masturbation and the parents, horrified, agreed with an attending physician to have both girls circumcised and their hands tied to their beds for thirty nights. Nora and Myra were not allowed to visit their sisters and 'couldn't understand the whole situation'. Three of the girls completed high school; Hester did not. Her parents kept her at home in her senior year and she cried a great deal.[29]

Rosenthal and his colleagues never seriously considered that these kinds of experiences might have contributed to the women's problems. Nor did they consider the impact of the study on the women's lives. Visiting them at home for several days every six months or so, the researchers would take the three co-operating Genains out to dinners and lunches, and talk with them about their current circumstances, activities and problems, creating a powerful incentive for the women to describe their experiences in a way that was consistent with the researchers' expectations.

In the light of the limitations of much of the genetic research, it is impossible at present to reach definitive conclusions about the contribution of heredity to madness. However, even the hardiest sceptic must concede it unlikely that genes play no role whatsoever. In a review of twin study evidence, American psychiatrist E. F. Torrey estimated the pairwise concordance rate for monozygotic twins to be 28 per cent in the case of schizophrenia, and 6 per cent for fraternal twins. For bipolar disorder it was estimated at 56 per cent for identical twins and 14 per cent for fraternal twins.[30] Although these figures indicate that genes play a more substantial role in bipolar disorder than in schizophrenia, they should not lead us to suppose that there is a simple causal arrow pointing from genes to mental illness. Assuming that these figures are correct, about half of those who inherit genes for bipolar disorder do not become ill, and only one in seven of those closely related to an affected person are also affected. On similar reasoning, only about a quarter of those who inherit genes for schizophrenia actually become schizophrenic, and the risk to close relatives of schizophrenia patients is only one in seventeen. These figures therefore provide very strong evidence that non-genetic factors influence the development of mental illness.

The implications of genetic research for Kraepelin's paradigm have been examined by British psychiatrist Tim Crow[31] and by American psychiatrist Michael Taylor.[32] Although the findings from family studies have not always been consistent, Crow and Taylor were able to point to studies in which the observed risk of a diagnosis of affective disorder in the relatives of schizophrenia patients was greater than chance,[33] or in which there was an increased risk of a diagnosis of schizophrenia in the relatives of bipolar patients.[34]

Crow has also noted that many of the studies which appear to show that schizophrenia and manic depression breed true have been compromised by what he has termed 'the fallacy of the excluded middle' – researchers' tendency to exclude or ignore individuals whose symptoms do not fit the classic pictures of schizophrenia and bipolar disorder. In studies that have included patients with mixed states, their close relatives have been found to be at increased risk for both schizophrenia and affective disorders. Angst and Scharfetter, for example, have analysed data from the families of patients suffering from unipolar depression, bipolar disorder, schizoaffective illness with predominantly affective symptoms, schizoaffective illness with predominantly schizophrenic symptoms, and 'pure' schizophrenia. The proportion of first-degree relatives who were found to suffer from affective disorders or schizophrenia varied systematically across this spectrum. The more 'schizophrenic' the patient, the more likely it was that their relatives would suffer from schizophrenia. The more 'mood disordered' the patient, the more likely it was that their relatives would suffer from mood disorder (see Table 4.1).[35] Crow has interpreted these findings as suggesting that schizophrenia and bipolar disorder lie at two ends of a spectrum of psychosis.

Table 4.1 Data from Angst and Scharfetter (1990) showing the risk that first-degree relatives of psychotic patients will meet criteria for schizophrenia or affective disorder (from T. Crow, 'The failure of the binary concept and the psychosis gene', in A. Kerr and H. McClelland (eds.) (1991) *Concepts of Mental Disorder: A Continuing Debate.* London: Gaskell).

Patients are grouped into five diagnostic categories reflecting the extent to which they suffered from mainly affective symptoms, mainly schizophrenia symptoms, or a mixture of symptoms. The last row shows the ratio of relatives who meet the criteria for schizophrenia vs affective disorder. Ratios less than 1 indicate that most ill relatives meet the criteria for affective disorder whereas ratios greater than 1 indicate that most meet the criteria for schizophrenia.

Diagnosis of patients

	Unipolar depression	Bipolar disorder	Schizoaffective (predominantly affective)	Schizoaffective (predominantly schizophrenic)	Schizophrenia
No. of patients	58	31	34	35	105
No. of relatives with schizophrenia	10	4	19	18	31
No. of relatives with affective disorder	24	6	14	4	5
Ratio of schizophrenic to affective relatives (age-corrected)	0.30	0.47	0.92	2.99	5.05

Twin studies have also undermined the Kraepelinian distinction between schizophrenia and manic depression. Several cases of twins have been reported in which one appears to suffer from schizophrenia and the other seems to suffer from an affective illness.[36] In a study of schizophrenia conducted by British psychiatrists Ann Farmer and Peter McGuffin in collaboration with US psychologist Irvine Gottesman, seven out of twenty-four identical twin pairs had one member diagnosed as suffering from schizophrenia and the other diagnosed as suffering from a mood disorder according to DSM-III criteria. Of the remaining seventeen pairs, six were concordant for schizophrenia whereas, for the other eleven, only one member of each pair suffered from schizophrenia. Farmer and her colleagues attribute these findings to deficiencies of the DSM-III definition of schizophrenia, but they obviously point to a close relationship between schizophrenia and affective disorder.[37]

Better than Astrology?

From the point of view of the clinician, one of the most important functions of a diagnosis is prediction. When a doctor interprets your chest pain as evidence of angina, you know that she is predicting a different future for you than if she had interpreted your pain as evidence of indigestion. Similarly, if Kraepelin was correct, a diagnosis of schizophrenia should predict a more unremitting course of illness than a diagnosis of manic depression.

In practice, this claim has proved difficult to test. One reason for this is that the course and outcomes of psychiatric disorders are hard to quantify. American psychiatrists John Strauss and William Carpenter have noted that outcome can be measured across several domains that are only loosely correlated. Whereas *clinical outcome* is determined by assessing the persistence of symptoms, *occupational outcome* is defined according to how well the individual maintains a steady job, and *social outcome* reflects the individual's ability to maintain an adequate network of social relationships.[38]

In their studies of schizophrenia patients, Strauss and Carpenter came across patients whose functioning could not be classified as simply good or poor, but varied across these three domains. For example, one woman they interviewed was very delusional but was successfully taking care of her child and holding down a job. Her clinical outcome was therefore poor, but her occupational and social outcomes were excellent. Another, whose symptoms had almost disappeared, had not worked for two years, had lost touch with most of her friends, and spent most of her days sitting in a darkened room.[39] Similar dissociations between different kinds of outcomes have been observed in bipolar patients.[40]

Despite these difficulties, three consistent findings have emerged from outcome studies. The first is that *the course of psychosis is very unpredictable*. For example, the time between the mood episodes experienced by bipolar patients may be as short as several weeks or as long as many years.[41] Some patients experience episodes of depression followed by mania followed by normal functioning, others experience mania followed by depression and eventually remission, whereas the majority follow no particular discernible sequence of episodes.[42] However, underneath this variability a pattern can be perceived. Towards the end of his life, Kraepelin's own data led him to believe that the average time between bipolar episodes decreased as the number of episodes increased. This finding has been replicated by more recent investigators (see Figure 4.1), leading some biological psychiatrists to suppose that each episode leaves the brain more sensitive to future episodes, a process sometimes described as 'kindling'.[43]

Similar findings have been obtained in studies of schizophrenia patients, who have sometimes been followed up for decades. For example, in a classic study, Luc Ciompi, a Swiss psychiatrist, observed the fate of a group of patients followed up for more than thirty years. The majority spent less than one tenth of this time as inpatients but a quarter spent more than twenty years in hospital. Some patients suffered a sudden breakdown followed by complete recovery. Others had many episodes of illness that began abruptly. Still others experienced a slow onset of illness and, if periods of remission occurred, recovery would be only partial. Some remained ill continuously.[44] A similar study carried out by Manfred Bleuler, the son of Eugen, yielded almost identical results.[45] Reflecting on the heterogeneity of the outcomes they observed, both Ciompi and the younger Bleuler were moved to reject the idea that schizophrenia is a simple brain disease. This conclusion is particularly striking in the case of Bleuler,

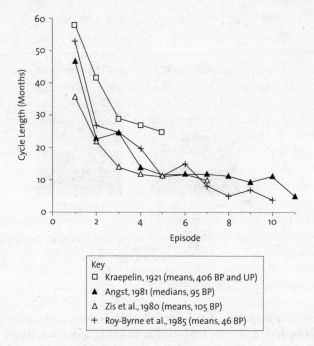

Figure 4.1 Average cycle length in bipolar (BP) patients from four studies (from F. K. Goodwin and K. R. Jamison (1990) *Manic-Depressive Illness*. Oxford: Oxford University Press). Note that Kraepelin's data included unipolar (UP) patients.

given his relationship to the man who coined the term 'schizophrenia'.

A second conclusion that can be drawn from research data on the course of psychosis is that *outcome is enormously variable between individuals with the same diagnosis*. For example, although Kraepelin held that schizophrenia patients inevitably remain ill for the majority of their lives, the long-term studies of Luc Ciompi and Manfred Bleuler both revealed that this was the case for only a minority of patients (see Figure 4.2). About a third of patients completely recovered over the long term, the remaining patients having intermediate outcomes.

Extreme variability has also been observed in the outcome of patients diagnosed as suffering from bipolar disorder. Kraepelin, it will be recalled, believed that manic depression was a relatively benign illness. Indeed, he estimated that the majority of his manic-depressive

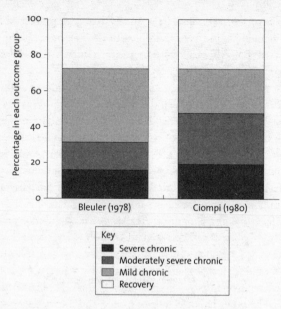

Figure 4.2 Bleuler and Ciompi data on long-term outcome of schizophrenia (redrawn from J. Zubin, J. Magaziner and S. R. Steinhauer (1983) 'The metamorphosis of Schizophrenia', *Psychological Medicine*, 13: 551–71).

patients (many of whom would be diagnosed as suffering from uni-polar depression by modern standards) experienced only one episode. Modern studies, by comparison, indicate that a much broader range of outcomes is experienced by bipolar patients.[46] For example, in a thirty-five-year follow-up of patients who had been diagnosed as suffering from mania on first admission to hospital, American psychiatrist Michael Tsuang and his colleagues found that 64 per cent had recovered completely, whereas 22 per cent remained seriously ill.[47] This outcome was better, on average, than the outcome for a group of patients diagnosed as suffering from schizophrenia, but not strikingly so.

Tsuang's study leads to the third general conclusion that can be drawn from the data on the long-term course of psychiatric disorders. Despite the unpredictable course and extremely variable outcome of psychotic illnesses, *patients who receive a diagnosis of manic depression have a better outcome on average than patients who receive a diagnosis of schizophrenia.* This finding has been reported in many studies, including a five-year follow-up of the first-admission patients recruited to the World Health Organization's International Pilot Study of Schizophrenia.[48]

At first sight, this difference seems to be strong evidence in favour of Kraepelin's distinction between the two main categories of psychosis. However, as British psychiatrist Tim Crow has pointed out, this conclusion is based on the error of reasoning that he has described as 'the fallacy of the excluded middle', namely the tendency to focus on 'textbook' patients who appear to be clearly schizophrenic or clearly manic-depressive, while ignoring the large number of patients who have both types of symptoms.[49]

The effects of controlling for this fallacy were explored in an important study conducted by Robert Kendell and Ian Brockington.[50] They argued that, if schizophrenia and manic depression are separate entities, we should see a clear 'gap' or discontinuity between the outcomes associated with one disorder and the outcomes associated with the other. On the other hand, if schizophrenia and manic depression are variants of the same disorder, outcome might well be affected by the exact mix of symptoms experienced by the patient. On this latter view, schizoaffective patients should have an average outcome that lies somewhere in between those observed for patients suffering from 'pure' schizophrenia and those suffering from bipolar disorder.

Kendell and Brockington studied the progress of a large number of patients who had been classified into ten groups along a continuum of symptomatology ranging from mostly manic-depressive, through mixed, to mostly schizophrenic. Outcome was measured after two years using six different methods, and the findings are shown in Figure 4.3. There is no evidence of a sharp discontinuity of outcomes according to any of the measures. On the contrary, the average outcomes seem to form a gradient that depends on the extent to which patients are suffering from schizophrenia or affective symptoms.

At the beginning of this chapter I suggested that astrological predictions provide a fool's-gold standard against which to evaluate the predictions achieved by psychiatric diagnoses. We are now in a position to apply this standard. While diagnoses clearly are superior to star signs, this superiority is not striking and is only evident when large groups are studied. When the focus is on the individual, the clinician

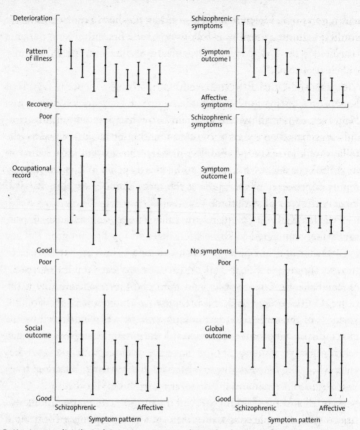

Patients are distributed into ten groups along the horizontal axes according to the extent to which they suffered mainly schizophrenia symptoms, a mixture of schizophrenia and affective symptoms, or mainly affective symptoms. There are six different measures of outcome on the vertical axes: overall pattern of illness (ranging from recovery to deterioration); occupational record (based on work records); social outcome (based on the quality of social relations); two measures of symptoms (one grading the symptoms on a spectrum from schizophrenia to affective symptoms, the other indicating the overall severity of schizophrenia symptoms alone) and finally a composite or global measure. Note that worse outcomes are associated with schizophrenia symptoms. However, note also that there is no clear evidence of separate groups of schizophrenia and mood-disorder patients.

Figure 4.3 Relationships between symptoms and outcome in patients with psychosis, from R. E. Kendell and I. F. Brockington (1980) 'The identification of disease entities and the relationship between schizophrenic and affective psychoses', *British Journal of Psychiatry*, 137: 324–31.

wanting to predict what will happen to her patients in the years ahead would do almost as well by resorting to horoscopes.

The Specificity of Psychiatric Drugs

Diagnoses should allow the clinician to predict not only the course and long-term outcome of a disorder, but also what kind of treatment is likely to be effective. For example, different drugs should be effective for different conditions. Oddly, with the exception of one study, this important clinical property of psychiatric diagnoses has not been systematically investigated. This omission is remarkable, as drugs have been the mainstay of psychiatric treatment for at least fifty years, and were widely used even in Kraepelin's time.

Today, four main types of medication are available to psychiatrists. The less severe psychiatric disorders are usually treated with *anxiolytics* (the benzodiazapines such as Valium and Librium, normally used to treat anxiety but sometimes useful in the treatment of mild depression) or *anti-depressants* (mainly tricyclic drugs such as imipramine and the new selective serotonin re-uptake inhibitors such as Prozac, usually employed in the treatment of depression but also effective in the treatment of anxiety). Although the development of these drugs is certainly of historical interest, I will say no more about them in this book.[51] *Anti-psychotic* (also called *neuroleptic*) medications (for example, phenothiazines such as chlorpromazine – also known as Largactil*) are the most commonly prescribed drugs for schizophrenia patients. Patients with a diagnosis of bipolar disorder, on the other hand, are usually offered various *mood-stabilizing* medications (for example, lithium carbonate or carbamazapine).

Readers without a background in medicine or pharmacology may assume that the development of new drugs usually follows from advances in our understanding of the biological bases of disease. For example, it might be expected that some breakthrough in understanding the biochemistry of the brain would lead to the identification of

---

* Confusingly, drugs are given two names. The generic name (for example, chlorpromazine) refers to the active compound, whereas the trade name (for example, Largactil) is used by the drug company when marketing the compound. I will follow convention and begin generic names in lower case and trade names in upper case.

abnormalities in the brains of schizophrenia patients, and from there to the design of novel drugs. In fact, progress in psychopharmacology has nearly always been in the opposite direction – the accidental discovery of an apparently effective drug has led to speculation about its mode of action, and from there to research on the biological origins of mental illness.

In the fifty years before the discovery of chlorpromazine, described by historian of psychiatry Edward Shorter as 'the first drug that worked',[52] there had been few or no genuine advances in the drug treatment of mental illness. Writing in 1899, Kraepelin had listed the drugs available to him as narcotics (for example, opium and morphine), soporifics (for example, chloral hydrate), chloroform, ether, ethyl bromide, bromides, amyl nitrate and digitalis.[53] Many of these compounds were still in use at the outbreak of the Second World War.

The effects of chlorpromazine (later known by the trade name Largactil) were first observed by a French naval surgeon named Henri Laborit, who was something of an eccentric. According to the obituary published in the *Guardian* newspaper when Laborit died in 1995, 'The world has just lost the chance of awarding an Oscar, a Pulitzer and a Nobel Prize to the same person.'[54] Many years after achieving fame for his pharmacological discovery, he appeared in Alain Renais' film *Mon Oncle d'Amerique*, which won the Palme d'Or at the Cannes film festival. He also won several literary awards for his best-selling books on popular science, and campaigned for the abolition of the Paris–Dakar rally because, 'In our world, competition is disgusting, a most stupid triviality.'

As a consequence of his war experience, Laborit developed an interest in physical shock, a condition that had many manifestations (low temperature, faint pulse and low blood pressure, accompanied by apathy and anxiety), and that affected his patients' ability to recover from surgery. Believing that this condition resulted from an excessively strong biological emergency reaction involving the chemicals adrenaline, acetylcholine and histamine, Laborit began experimenting with various compounds that were known to have inhibitory effects on these substances. As luck would have it, at this time the Rhône-Poulenc pharmaceutical company was synthesizing novel anti-histamine compounds, some of which were made available to Laborit.

In 1951, aged 37, Laborit was transferred from a marine hospital in Tunisia to the Val-de-Grâce military hospital in Paris, where he continued his experiments. One of the compounds sent to him by Rhône-Poulenc was labelled 4560 RP, and had already been identified as having useful sedative effects. Finding that the drug lessened the anxiety felt by his patients prior to surgery but left them with a curious disinterest in their surroundings, Laborit wondered about its potential value in psychiatry. Perhaps disturbed psychiatric patients would benefit from this kind of psychic indifference. After disastrously testing its tolerability on a volunteer psychiatrist at a nearby hospital (immediately after receiving an intravenous injection of 4560 RP she stood up to go to the toilet and fainted) he finally managed to persuade three colleagues at Val-de-Grâce to try the drug on a manic patient. The results were impressive. Within a few weeks the patient was much calmer and able to lead a relatively normal life.

In 1952, Laborit's experiments came to the attention of Jean Delay, who worked at the Ste-Anne mental hospital in Paris, and who was one of the best-known French psychiatrists of the day. Delay asked for samples of 4560 RP from Rhône-Poulenc and, together with his colleague Pierre Deniker, conducted the first clinical trial of the new medicine with psychotic patients. Delay and Deniker were able to report the positive results of their experiment just three months later at a meeting of the Société Médico-Psychologique. Their subsequent publications prompted further successful trials elsewhere. By the mid-1950s, the new drug – by now known as chlorpromazine – had become the treatment of choice for schizophrenia, and was in use throughout the developed world. Other similar compounds were rapidly tested, mainly because other pharmaceutical companies wanted to profit from this therapeutic breakthrough, so that by the early 1960s a range of anti-psychotic drugs was available to practising psychiatrists.

Curiously, the mood-stabilizing effects of lithium carbonate, the most widely used drug in the long-term treatment of mania, were also discovered accidentally by a relative outsider, and at almost exactly the same time that Laborit began his experiments with synthetic antihistamines. John Cade, the medical superintendent of the Repatriation Mental Hospital in Bundoora, Australia, wanted to test his theory that mania was caused by an endogenous toxin, and began injecting guinea pigs with urine from his manic patients. Although these ill-thought-out experiments inevitably ended in the death of the guinea pigs, Cade proceeded to devise a series of studies to investigate the effects of the various chemical constituents of urine. He first used lithium as a solvent for uric acid and then, on impulse, tried injecting lithium alone. Observing that the guinea pigs became lethargic and resistant to startle, Cade injected himself with lithium compounds to discover his ability to tolerate them, and rapidly progressed to a small-scale trial in which the drug was administered to patients diagnosed as suffering from schizophrenia, mania and depression. His results, which showed that lithium calmed schizophrenia patients but had even more dramatic therapeutic effects on those suffering from mania, were published in the *Medical Journal of Australia* in 1949, where they lay almost unnoticed for years. Despite the success of a more carefully conducted study undertaken by Mogens Schou in Denmark, published in 1952, the first trials of lithium carbonate in North America were not conducted until the 1960s, and the drug was only licensed for use in the USA in 1970. Although a licence was granted earlier in Great Britain, the drug's impact was similarly negligible at first. Edward Shorter has suggested that these delays partly reflected a lack of enthusiasm by drug companies, who were reluctant to support a compound that was abundant in nature, and therefore difficult to turn into profit.

In the half century since the discovery of the therapeutic effects of chlorpromazine and lithium, the idea that these drugs are diagnostically specific has driven a prodigious volume of biochemical research. This has been especially true for the neuroleptics; analysis of their biological effects led rapidly to the hypothesis that schizophrenia was caused by a disorder of those parts of the brain that contain the neurotransmitter substance dopamine. At one time, this hypothesis was so widely held that it almost acquired the status of an established truth, which only a raving heretic would question. (When I gave a talk about the concept of schizophrenia at Sheffield University only a few years ago, a neurobiologist in the audience angrily challenged me to draw a circuit diagram of the pathways in the brain that utilized dopamine.) I will discuss this theory in more detail in a later chapter; for the moment I am only concerned with one of the principal assumptions behind this kind of research – that the therapeutic effects of neuroleptics and lithium are specific to the two groups of patients who normally receive them. Clearly, evidence of treatment specificity would be strong evidence that schizophrenia and bipolar disorder are separate and distinct conditions.

Of course, the only way of adequately testing the specificity of psychiatric drugs is by randomly assigning them to patients regardless of diagnosis. To my knowledge, only one adequate experiment of this sort has ever been conducted. It was carried out by Eve Johnstone, Tim Crow and their colleagues at the Northwick Park Hospital in Middlesex, England, and their findings were reported in the medical journal the *Lancet* in 1988.[55]

One hundred and twenty psychotic patients were carefully assessed for delusions, hallucinations and abnormal mood before being randomly assigned to different drug treatments. Some received pimozide (a neuroleptic) alone, some received lithium carbonate alone, and others received either both drugs in combination or neither. The study was a double-bind trial, which is to say that neither the patients nor the assessing psychiatrists were aware which treatments the patients were assigned. This was achieved by giving all patients two drugs, one or both of which were sometimes placebos (inert substances). At the end of three weeks, it was found that pimozide had an effect on hallucinations and delusions, regardless of the patients' DSM-III diagnoses. Lithium carbonate similarly had a specific effect on elevated mood; although its non-specificity for diagnosis was less clear-cut than was the case for pimozide, this was because nearly all the patients who exhibited elevated mood were diagnosed as manic. Drug response, it seemed, was specific to particular symptoms, but not to particular diagnoses.

Biological psychiatrists who were aware of the history of their calling should not have been astonished by these findings. Evidence that the effects of neuroleptic drugs were diagnostically non-specific was available from the very beginning of modern psychopharmacology. Although most clinical trials of neuroleptics have been carried out with schizophrenia patients, the first successful trial – that carried out by Delay and Deniker in 1952 – was conducted on patients suffering from mania.

Categories or Dimensions?

In this chapter I have drawn on a wide range of research. None of the findings we have considered supports Kraepelin's diagnostic system. Studies of patients' symptoms, of the role of genes, of the course and outcome of illnesses over time, and of the response of symptoms to treatment, all point to similarities between schizophrenia and bipolar patients, rather than to differences.

Clearly people who suffer from psychiatric problems vary in their experiences. The taxonomists have attempted to accommodate this fact by dividing the geography of psychological distress into separate territories, but their efforts have been neither successful nor consistent. In the face of these difficulties, psychiatrists and psychologists have occasionally suggested alternatives to Kraepelin's system. Some, like Adolf Meyer, have argued that we should give up the idea of classifying people like plants. Others have argued that there is but one type of psychosis, or *einheitspsychose*, an idea that was championed by Kraepelin's rival Hoche.[56] This approach is currently favoured by Tim Crow,[57] among others.

Still others, mostly psychologists, have advocated the development of dimensional systems of classification, in which an individual is regarded as suffering more or less from different kinds of disorder.[58] (This suggestion is given some credence by the editors of DSM-IV. However, as they note, the present lack of consensus about the best way of constructing a dimensional classification means that a workable system may be a long way off.)[59] A recent study by Jim van Os and his colleagues provides some empirical support for this approach. Using his sample of over 700 psychotic patients, van Os assessed the power of categories (DSM-III-R diagnoses) and symptom dimensions to predict illness course, employment history, suicidal behaviour, the patients' perceived quality of life, and a number of other variables. For nearly all of these, the dimensions were more powerful predictors than the categories.[60]

None of these strategies has received support from the majority of clinicians, perhaps because they have found it difficult to see how these alternatives would work in practice.

The Boundaries of Madness

Madness need not be regarded as an illness. Why shouldn't it be seen as a sudden – more or less sudden – change of character?

Ludwig Wittgenstein[1]

In 1799 a German bookseller named Nicola read a paper to the Royal Society of Berlin, in which he described a series of hallucinations that he had experienced some nine years earlier.[2] They had been provoked by a period of stress, and he first became aware of them when he saw the figure of someone he knew to be dead. The figure, which was unobservable to his wife, disappeared after a few minutes but reappeared later in the day. Over the following months other hallucinatory figures came and went and sometimes spoke to Nicola, who became proficient at differentiating them from living people. Anticipating modern debates about the nature of psychosis, he claimed that his story demonstrated that hallucinations could be experienced by the sane.

Kraepelin's paradigm, articulated almost 100 years after Nicola's paper, assumed a non-arbitrary division between sanity and madness, an assumption that was explicitly embraced by the designers of DSM-III (see proposition 4 of Gerald Klerman's neoKraepelinian manifesto, given in Table 3.3, p. 59). According to Kraepelin, people either suffer from mental illness or they do not, and we are not free to choose whether to regard some kind of unusual behaviour as evidence of madness or mere eccentricity. This attitude was also evident in the theories of most of the other giants of psychiatry whose work we have considered. For Karl Jaspers, the psychiatrist's inability to form an empathetic appreciation of a patient's experiences was a sure sign of the patient's madness. For Kurt Schneider, the observation of certain behaviours and experiences (the first-rank symptoms) carried a similar implication. Only Eugen Bleuler was more flexible, conceiving of a continuum that ran from normality to the extreme experiences of people suffering from psychosis.

In the last chapter I examined Kraepelin's division of the psychoses into various types. In this chapter and the next, I will focus on this more fundamental division between madness and sanity. In particular, I will address the suggestion (succinctly expressed in the above quotation from the philosopher Ludwig Wittgenstein) that psychosis should be seen as just part and parcel of human variation, rather than as an illness. This claim, in its strongest form, suggests that the attribution of mental illness, either to individuals or to particular types of behaviour, is arbitrary rather than scientific, and that psychotic people are eccentrics who are misunderstood and victimized by society.

How Common are Psychotic Experiences?

Let us begin by considering whether Nicola's experiences were extraordinary or whether, on the contrary, ordinary people experience psychotic symptoms more commonly than is usually supposed. According to the Kraepelinian model, symptoms should be confined to those who are severely ill. Of course, we can accept that mentally ill people sometimes fail to receive appropriate treatment and consequently are left undetected in the community. However, this should happen only rarely. Evidence that large numbers of otherwise well-adjusted people report psychotic experiences on questioning would therefore further undermine the Kraepelinian paradigm.

Hallucinations

The first systematic study of hallucinations in ordinary people was conducted in Britain at the end of the nineteenth century by the Society for Psychical Research.[3] The Society assumed that their findings would have implications for the understanding of apparently supernatural phenomena. A large team of interviewers questioned over 14,000 men and women. Although no attempt was made to obtain a truly random sample, anyone suffering from obvious signs of mental or physical illness was excluded. Of those questioned, nearly 8 per cent of men and 12 per cent of women reported at least one vivid hallucinatory experience, the most common being a vision of a living person who was not present at the time. Hallucinations with a religious or supernatural content were also reported, and auditory hallucinations were recorded less often than visual hallucinations. Fifty years later, the Society attempted to check these findings by conducting a much less extensive survey, obtaining very similar results.[4]

Modern surveys have continued to provide evidence that hallucinations are experienced by people who appear to be otherwise normal, who do not regard themselves as mentally ill, and who have not felt the need to seek psychiatric treatment. For example, in the United States, psychologists Thomas Posey and Mary Losch[5] questioned 375 college students and found that 39 per cent had heard a voice speaking their thoughts aloud – a first-rank symptom of schizophrenia according to Kurt Schneider. Perhaps even more surprisingly, 5 per cent reported holding conversations with their hallucinations. Subsequent surveys of students in Britain (carried out by myself and others)[6] and in the United States (carried out by Tim Barrett and his colleagues)[7] have obtained comparable results.

Of course, college students are hardly representative of the population as a whole, so it may be wrong to generalize from student samples. However, this limitation does not apply to the most comprehensive survey of hallucinations in the general population so far conducted, which was reported in 1991 by American psychiatrist Allen Tien.[8] Tien's data were collected as part of the Epidemiological Catchment Area (ECA) Study, the large US population survey of psychiatric symptoms described in the previous chapter. Although the definition of hallucinations used by Tien was taken from DSM-III-R, his findings were remarkably similar to those obtained almost a century earlier by the Society for Psychical Research. He estimated that the proportion of the 18,000 ECA participants who had experienced hallucinations at some time in their lives was between 11 and 13 per cent.* Hallucinations were reported approximately twice as often by women as by men. Tien noted only two differences between his findings and the

* The 13.0 per cent figure was based on data from the first interview, whereas the 11.1 per cent figure was based on data collected at the follow-up interviews one year later.

much earlier findings from Britain. First, the Society for Psychical Research reported that people between 20 and 29 years of age were most likely to experience hallucinations, whereas the ECA data suggested that hallucinations occur across the age spectrum but most often in the elderly. Second, visual hallucinations were recorded less often in the ECA survey in comparison with the Society's data.*

Two subsequent studies have provided broad support for Tien's findings. Jim van Os and his colleagues conducted psychiatric interviews with over 7000 people randomly selected from the general population of Holland.[9] When abnormal experiences secondary to drug-taking or physical illness were excluded, 1.7 per cent were found to have experienced 'true' hallucinations, but a further 6.2 per cent had experienced hallucinations that were judged not clinically relevant because they were not associated with distress. Comparable results were obtained in a survey of 761 residents of Dunedin, New Zealand, recently reported by Richie Poulton and others.[10]

To appreciate the significance of these findings it may help to compare them with the available epidemiological data on schizophrenia. Recent estimates suggest that, in most countries, fewer than 1 per cent of the general population receive a diagnosis of schizophrenia at some point in their lives.[11] It now appears that about ten times as many people have experienced hallucinations.

Delusional beliefs

There has been much less research on the prevalence of delusional beliefs, a symptom usually attributed either to schizophrenia, manic depression or paranoia. This is probably because researchers have recognized that distinguishing between delusions and beliefs that are just bizarre or unusual is an inherently uncertain enterprise. A Gallup poll of 1236 American adults revealed that approximately one quarter believed in ghosts.[12] A similar proportion reported telepathic experi-

---

* There is evidence of both cross-cultural and historical variation in the extent to which visual hallucinations are reported by psychiatric patients, which I review in later chapters. Modern psychiatric patients in the West appear to report fewer visual hallucinations than patients in Kraepelin's time. This difference between Tien's findings and the earlier British findings may therefore reflect a genuine historical trend.

ences, about one in ten claimed to have been in the presence of a ghost, and about one in seven thought they had seen a UFO. In a similar interview study of 502 people from the general population of Winnipeg, Canada, it was found that over 15 per cent claimed to have experienced telepathy and that nearly 18 per cent reported experiencing dreams that predicted future events. In this study, belief in the paranormal was associated with various indices of psychiatric problems, including Schneider's first-rank symptoms.[13] However, other researchers have observed that those reporting paranormal experiences often experience high levels of subjective well-being.[14]

Psychiatrists have sometimes suggested that spiritual experiences should be regarded as evidence of mental illness[15] (an idea that has been supported by the government of the People's Republic of China, where members of the Falun Gong religious movement have recently been subjected to compulsory psychiatric treatment).[16] Although this argument cannot be taken seriously by anyone capable of respecting religious sentiments shared by a large proportion of the world's population, this does not mean that we should not consider similarities between religious beliefs and the delusional beliefs of patients. That these similarities can be marked is evident from a study reported by Mike Jackson, a psychologist at the University College Bangor in Wales, and Bill Fulford, an Oxford-based psychiatrist and philosopher.[17] Jackson and Fulford carried out a detailed study of three people whose experiences were recorded by the Alistair Hardy Research Centre at Oxford University, which investigates religious experiences. All three reported beliefs that met standard psychiatric definitions of delusions (two also experienced auditory hallucinations). For example, 'Simon', a 40-year-old man, was raised as a Baptist and enjoyed a successful career until he fell into a legal dispute with his colleagues. After praying for guidance late at night, he noticed that wax from a candle had dripped on to his Bible, obscuring certain words. Interpreting this event as a message from God, he realized that he was 'The living son of David . . . also a relative of Ishmael, and . . . captain of the guard of Israel'.

British psychiatrist Glen Roberts conducted a study comparing deluded patients, patients who had recovered from delusions, trainee Anglican priests (chosen because of their presumed religious convictions) and ordinary people, finding that both the currently deluded patients and the trainee priests, but not the recovered patients or the ordinary people, expressed an extremely strong need to find meaning in their lives.[18] In a more recent study, Emmanuelle Peters and her colleagues at the Institute of Psychiatry in London compared psychotic inpatients and ordinary people to members of new religious movements (Druids and members of the Hare Krishna religion). Although the members of the new religious movements were not 'ill' in the sense of wanting or appearing to need treatment, the two groups could not be distinguished on a measure of delusional beliefs.[19]

A similar controversy has concerned the relationship between psychosis and beliefs about visits to Earth by extraterrestrials. In the United States in recent years, a surprising number of people have reported being kidnapped by aliens. Typically, 'abductees' describe being taken from their beds at night. Later they find themselves in a UFO, being inspected by aliens (usually described as 'greys' – small humanoid creatures with thin faces and slanting eyes). They are forced to lie helpless as their bodies are probed and penetrated by alien devices, presumably as part of some kind of interplanetary zoology experiment. Eventually, they are returned to their beds unharmed. Estimates of the number of people in the USA who have had 'abduction experiences' have been as high as 3.7 million.[20] One prominent psychiatrist has concluded that they are honest accounts of real events,[21] provoking harsh criticism from his colleagues. Some features of abduction accounts are strikingly reminiscent of the passivity delusions included in Schneider's list of first-rank symptoms, but whether these kinds of experiences are associated with psychopathology remains a matter of dispute.[22] Although an American study failed to find evidence of psychopathology in abductees,[23] a recent British study found that belief in UFOs was associated with high scores on questionnaire measures of psychotic thinking.[24]

It is only very recently that attempts have been made to assess the prevalence in the general population of delusional beliefs defined by psychiatric criteria. In the recent survey of more than 7000 Dutch people conducted by Jim van Os and his colleagues, 3.3 per cent of the sample were found to have 'true' delusions and 8.7 per cent had delusions that were not clinically relevant (that is, which were not associated with distress and did not require treatment).[25] Higher estimates were obtained in Poulton's developmental study of the residents of Dunedin, New Zealand, in which 20.1 per cent of the sample were recorded as having delusions by the end point of the study, and 12.6 per cent were judged to be paranoid.[26]

I am aware of only one study in which an attempt has been made to assess the prevalence of different kinds of delusions. In June 1996, thirty-one family doctors in the Aquitaine region of southwest France asked over 1000 patients attending their clinics to complete a questionnaire measuring twenty-one commonly reported delusional beliefs. Only 11.5 per cent of those approached had attended their doctor because of psychiatric problems. The most common delusional ideas reported were that people were not who they seemed to be (69.3 per cent of those with no history of psychiatric disorder); that the individual had experienced telepathic communication (46.9 per cent); that seemingly innocuous events had double meanings (42.2 per cent); that the individual was being persecuted in some way (25.5 per cent); and that occult forces were at work (23.4 per cent).[27]

Language and communication disorders

Incoherent speech has often been regarded as an important symptom of psychosis. As we saw in Chapter 2, Bleuler believed that this kind of speech reflected the loosening of associations that he held to be a fundamental feature of schizophrenia. The American psychiatrist Nancy Andreasen has developed a formal method of assessing psychotic speech that has been extensively used in recent research. Anticipating our more detailed discussion of this symptom in a later chapter, for present purposes we need only note that her method requires investigators to score segments of speech for twenty different kinds of abnormality. In a validation study, Andreasen reported ratings of abnormal speech from schizophrenia patients, bipolar patients, patients suffering from unipolar depression and ordinary people. The most surprising discovery was that incoherent speech was more often observed in manic patients than in schizophrenia patients (further evidence that the distinction between these diagnoses is not meaningful). Andreasen also observed that incoherence was, to a lesser degree, a feature of the speech of some depressed patients and even of some of the normal people she examined.[28] This finding raises the possibility that incoherent speech, like other symptoms of psychosis, is more frequently observed in non-psychotic individuals than has previously been supposed.

This inference receives some support from an unusual study conducted by David Weeks, a clinical psychologist based in Edinburgh, Scotland. Weeks conducted an investigation of self-styled eccentrics (people who believed that their manner and behaviour made them different from ordinary folk) who responded to advertisements he placed in newspapers.[29] Many of those who volunteered to participate had very odd attitudes and behaviour. For example, Norma, a woman who lived in Connecticut, played in a kazoo band, wore a fireman's outfit in the winter, and held parties in the summer in which she served only canned food and dressed as a member of the British royal family. She believed that it was immoral to throw anything away and had to buy an abandoned opera house to hold all of her possessions. Al, another member of Weeks' sample, rode around his hometown in Virginia on a device that was half bicycle and half rocking horse, behind which he towed a milk crate mounted on a golf cart.

Weeks used Andreasen's scale to analyse recorded speech samples collected from his eccentrics. As might be expected of a group that had been so loosely defined, the quality of their speech was highly variable. Over half of the eccentrics showed no evidence of speech disorder whatsoever, whereas others showed evidence of severe communication difficulties. The following is an example:

I have since resolved to actually Sherlock Holmes a manuscript, anticipatory, of many practicing psychiatry, this conjectural profession, none to date have concentrated their probes into the mind's cognitive faculties, which ... I suspect ... is ... as it were, a high-octane, rather than the typically average petrol ... that circumstances, IQ and health, is responsible for neurosis. Is it a key to the wonderful fulfilment of this gift of life? Whiter light needs darker shadow. The greyest gap in psychiatry is that it must accept creative individuals are left to stew in their own portentous juices to work out their eccentricity unaided.[30]

Weeks was careful *not* to claim that his eccentrics were psychotic. Indeed, in the case of two categories of abnormal speech – *derailment* (a pattern of speech in which ideas seem to slip off one track on to another, obliquely related track) and *loss of goal* (failure to follow a chain of thought to its logical conclusion) – the eccentrics showed less evidence of abnormality than ordinary people. However, for most of the other types of speech disorder, and particularly for *pressure of speech* (rapid talking that is difficult to interrupt), *tangentiality* (responding to questions in an oblique or irrelevant manner), and *circumstantiality* (speech that is delayed in reaching its goal because of the intrusion of many tenuously related ideas), the eccentrics showed more evidence of abnormality than ordinary people.

Of course, just as some kinds of peculiar beliefs may not be related to delusions, so too some kinds of abnormal speech should not be regarded as forms of language and communication disorder. For example, glossolalia, the speaking in unknown tongues practised by some Christian sects, has sometimes been described as similar to the speech of schizophrenia patients,[31] but is, in fact, linguistically quite different[32] and, unlike the disordered speech of patients, is usually brought on wilfully in specific religious settings.[33]

So far as I am aware, only one study has reported a population estimate for psychotic speech. In Poulton's study of people in Dunedin, the speech of the participants was rated by a social worker as they arrived to be assessed, and 17.9 per cent of the sample were rated as having disorganized speech.[34]

Hypomania

Mood swings, like the other symptoms we have considered, appear to be much more commonly experienced than would be anticipated on the basis of Kraepelin's paradigm. For example, American psychologist Ronald Depue and his colleagues have estimated from questionnaire studies that 6 per cent of college students show evidence of abnormal variations in mood.[35]

In the Zurich canton of Switzerland, a team led by psychiatrist Jules Angst interviewed a representative sample of the general population and estimated that 4 per cent had experienced mild episodes of mania (known as *hypomania*).[36] In a later study, in which the sample was followed up over a fourteen-year period, 5.5 per cent had experienced an episode meeting the DSM-IV criteria for hypomania and a further 11.3 per cent had experienced 'subdiagnostic' hypomanic symptoms.[37]

Reviewing similar investigations conducted in several different countries, Hagop Akiskal, a psychiatrist at the University of California at San Diego, concluded that, 'Softer bipolar expressions are at least 4–6 times more common than the usual prevalence of 1 per cent given for classic manic-depressive illness.'[38]

From Sanity to Madness

It seems that there is some truth in Bleuler's view that the differences between sanity and madness are matters of degree. In the 1920s, Ernst Kretschmer, a professor of psychiatry at the University of Tübingen, elaborated Bleuler's theory, arguing that both schizophrenia and manic depression were related to variations in normal personality.[39] According to Kretschmer, there is a type of 'schizothymic' personality characterized by a combination of coldness and hypersensitivity. Similarly, he argued that there is a 'cyclothymic' personality type that resembles manic depression, in which the individual is prone to extreme moods. Kretschmer believed that these personality types, and the clinical states related to them, were associated with particular bodily constitutions. The schizophrenia patient, on his view, was most likely to be of *asthenic* build, that is, frail with a narrow physique. The manic-depressive patient, on the other hand, was most likely to have the *pyknic* build, being middle in height, and rounded, with a tendency towards fat around the trunk. (Although some early studies reported data consistent with Kretschmer's theory,[40] so far as I am aware, these relationships between psychopathology and physical stature have never been verified by modern research.)

The concept of schizotypy

Unfortunately, Kretschmer's ideas had no immediate impact on psychiatric research (although they did influence some psychologists studying normal variations in personality)[41] and it was nearly half a century before the hypothesized continuum between sanity and madness was investigated properly. Modern studies in this area were stimulated by the ideas of American psychologist Paul Meehl, expressed in a 1962 speech he made as president of the American Psychological Association.[42] Focusing on schizophrenia, Meehl argued that inconsistent findings from genetic research could be accounted for by supposing that individuals inherit a vulnerability to the disorder rather than the disorder itself. He proposed the term 'schizotaxia' to describe this predisposition, and suggested that it might lead the individual to experience 'cognitive slippage' (his term for the loosening of associations) and 'anhedonia' (an inability to experience pleasure). Meehl argued that the majority of people who suffered from schizotaxia would not develop full-blown schizophrenia, but would instead have *schizotypal personality* characteristics – for example eccentric beliefs and magical thinking. Such people would only become schizophrenic if exposed to some kind of stress.

Meehl's arguments later gained some support from the adoption studies carried out in Denmark by Seymour Kety, David Rosenthal and their colleagues (see pp. 77–8 for a brief discussion of these investigations). In these studies very little evidence of full-blown psychotic illness was observed in the biological relatives of adoptees who had been diagnosed as suffering from schizophrenia, a finding which, at first sight, seemed to undermine the genetic theory of schizophrenia. However, Kety and Rosenthal argued that many of these biological relatives showed eccentric personality characteristics, for example unusual beliefs about the supernatural, constricted emotions, suspiciousness and social anxiety. Assuming that such people were suffering from a subclinical variant of schizophrenia, they proposed the new diagnostic category of 'schizophrenia spectrum disorder' in order to describe these characteristics.[43]

The work of Kety, Rosenthal and their colleagues preceded the publication of DSM-III. Partly influenced by their observations, the authors of the manual decided to include a multi-axial system in which information in addition to diagnoses would be classified. Whereas clinicians were invited to describe their patients' psychiatric illnesses using axis 1, axis 2 was to be used to classify disorders of personality. These were defined as 'enduring patterns of perceiving, relating to, and thinking about the environment and oneself' and were considered to be distinct from illnesses because they were present throughout adulthood, whereas the illnesses were episodic.

The definitions of the axis-2 disorders were drawn from various sources, including psychoanalysts and theories of normal personality. After some debate, eleven were included. Among these were criteria for 'schizotypal personality disorder' devised by Robert Spitzer on the basis of Kety and Rosenthal's concept of 'schizophrenia spectrum disorder'. Spitzer also constructed a definition of 'borderline personality disorder' from earlier formulations suggested by psychoanalytic authors. This term was used to describe a type of personality characterized by extreme emotional instability, severe problems of self-esteem, self-destructive behaviours and intense and unstable relationships with others.[44] The confusing name 'borderline' was used because some psychoanalysts had theorized that such people lay on the borderline between psychosis and neurosis. However, it was assumed that borderline patients would not show active psychotic symptoms.

Axis 2 of DSM-III and its successors attempted to accommodate dimensions of disorder within a categorial system. However, as might be expected of such an attempt, the division of abnormal personalities into separate categories proved problematic from the outset. Research showed that the reliability of these categories was very low (one study found an average kappa value of 0.41)[45] and the authors of DSM-III were forced to acknowledge that many patients would meet the criteria for more than one type of personality disorder.

A psychological approach to psychosis-proneness

Meehl's ideas prompted psychologists to search for personality 'markers' or indicators of schizotaxia in the hope that these could be used to detect people at risk of schizophrenic breakdowns. As it was believed that the features of schizotaxia were quite subtle, many investigators believed they might be detected by examining unusual responses to conventional personality questionnaires. A common research strategy involved asking the mentally well (but presumably schizotaxic) relatives of schizophrenia patients to complete standard personality tests. Unfortunately, this line of research led nowhere and had been all but abandoned by the end of the 1970s.[46]

At about this time it became obvious to some psychologists that a better way of approaching this problem might be to question people directly about psychotic experiences. In the United States, Loren and Jean Chapman at the University of Wisconsin devised a series of questionnaires for this purpose, each of which focused on a different symptom. Their early questionnaires measured physical and social anhedonia (items included 'I have had very little desire to buy new kinds of foods', and 'It's fun to sing with other people', to be marked as either 'true' or 'false') and perceptual aberrations ('Occasionally I have felt as if my body did not exist'). Later questionnaires measured magical thinking ('Some people can make me aware of them just by thinking about me') and hypomania ('I am so good at controlling others that it sometimes scares me').[47] In Britain, at the Department of Experimental Psychology at Oxford University, Gordon Claridge took a slightly different approach, and devised a single questionnaire based on Robert Spitzer's DSM-III definition of schizotypal personality disorder.[48] These questionnaires have been followed by many others, so that scales of schizotypy or psychosis-proneness, if not quite a dime a dozen, have now become commonplace instruments of psychological research.

Gordon Claridge has recognized that the apparent continuum from sanity to madness, confirmed by studies that have employed these questionnaires, necessitates a revision of the Kraepelinian model of psychosis.[49] However, he does not believe that it is necessary to abandon a biomedical model of madness altogether. He has pointed out that there are widely recognized physical diseases that are extremes of normal variation. An example is hypertension, an abnormal elevation of blood pressure, which leads to an increased risk of strokes and heart attacks. Blood pressures are distributed normally* in the population. Some people have very low pressure, some have very high pressure, but the majority of the population lies somewhere in between these two extremes. The cut-off point between low and high blood pressure is arbitrary, and is determined pragmatically by doctors, who balance the need to identify those most at risk of vascular disease with the hazards of unnecessarily treating a large proportion of the population. Nonetheless, as high blood pressure has disastrous (and sometimes fatal) consequences, few people would doubt that it is a cause for medical concern.

On this analogy, psychosis might be thought of as the extreme end of a normally distributed spectrum of personality traits on which we

---

* A normal distribution, as defined by statisticians and epidemiologists, is characterized by the familiar 'bell curve' when values of a trait are plotted on the x-axis of a graph, and the proportion of the population having different values of the trait are plotted on the y-axis (see Figure 5.1).

impose an arbitrary cut-off point to separate those who are mentally ill from those who are not. Claridge's approach is slightly more complex than this, in that he assumes that there is a discontinuity between madness and sanity, which, using the blood pressure analogy, might be thought of as equivalent to a stroke. He argues that a person who has psychotic traits may lead a normal life, much as a person with high blood pressure can lead a normal life, unless some kind of adverse environmental event precipitates a breakdown. Claridge suggests that there are many different kinds of events that might lead to such a crisis, including both psychological and physical traumas (see Figure 5.1). This model is similar to Meehl's, and assumes that individuals differ in their vulnerability to mental illness, so that a relatively minor life event can precipitate a breakdown in someone who is especially at risk, whereas a major crisis is required to precipitate a breakdown in someone who is less vulnerable.

There is insufficient space here to review the very large volume of research that has been conducted with questionnaire measures of psychosis-proneness. However, two general findings are worth noting. First, there is some evidence that scores on these questionnaires predict future psychotic breakdown, although not with the kind of precision that would be useful to clinicians. In a study carried out by Loren and Jean Chapman, several hundred Wisconsin students were tested on a battery of schizotypy questionnaires and were then divided into high scoring and normally scoring groups. After ten years, fourteen of the high scorers and only one of the low scorers had been admitted to hospital with a psychotic illness.[50] While this finding would not justify the mass testing of young adults in the hope of preventing mental illness, it does suggest that there is a real link between schizotypal personality characteristics and outright madness, as supposed by Meehl, Claridge and the Chapmans.

Second, the same kinds of arguments that have been made about the continuum between normal personality and schizophrenia have also been made about mood disorders. Hagop Akiskal of the University of California at San Diego has suggested that many patients treated by psychiatrists or psychologists for 'borderline personality disorder' in fact suffer from subclinical bipolar disorder.[51] This type of personality, it will be recalled, has been characterized in terms of extreme emotional reactions, unstable self-esteem, self-destructive behaviour and intense

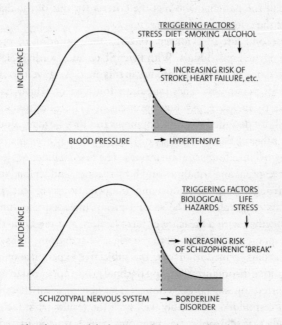

Figure 5.1 Claridge's model showing the relationship between schizotypal personality and schizophrenia, and showing the parallel with systemic diseases such as hypertension (from G. S. Claridge (1990) 'Can a disease model of schizophrenia survive?', in R. P. Bentall (ed.), *Reconstructing Schizophrenia*. London: Routledge). Note the familiar bell-shaped normal distributions for both blood pressure and schizotypal traits.

and unstable relationships with others. In addition to the obvious clinical similarities between prototypically bipolar and borderline patients, Akiskal was able to point to evidence of high levels of mood disorder in the close relatives of borderline patients.

Given the evidence against Kraepelin's division between dementia praecox and manic depression, which we considered in the previous chapter, it would obviously be interesting to know whether borderline mood states overlap with measures of psychosis-proneness derived from the concept of schizophrenia. Two lines of research suggest that they do. First, in a study by Robert Spitzer, psychiatrists were asked to evaluate their patients on the proposed DSM-III definitions of schizotypal and borderline personality disorder. It was found that about half the patients who met the criteria for one of the diagnoses also met the criteria for the other.[52]

The second line of evidence concerns the clustering of psychotic traits in normal individuals. With Peter Slade and Gordon Claridge, I conducted one of the earliest studies in this area. We gave 180 students a range of personality questionnaires, fourteen of which had been designed to measure psychosis-proneness. (The questionnaires included those designed by the Chapmans and by Claridge, along with various others.) Factor analysis of the questionnaire scores revealed that they fell into four separate groups. The first included scales measuring perceptual abnormalities and bizarre ideas, and seemed to correspond (roughly) to delusions and hallucinations, or the positive symptoms of psychosis. The second group included the anhedonia scales together with a measure of introversion, and might be thought to correspond (again roughly) to the negative symptoms of psychosis. A third group seemed to involve the subjective experience of anxiety and cognitive disorganization, and the final group appeared to measure self-reported anti-social behaviour.[53] The first three of these dimensions corresponded reasonably well with the results from factor analytic studies of schizophrenia symptoms, which we considered in the previous chapter.

Although it would be risky to base a theory entirely on the questionnaire responses of a relatively small number of British university students, these findings have now been repeated by other investigators who have carried out studies with much larger and more representative samples.[54] (Indeed, we eventually replicated our original findings with a sample of 1095 people drawn from various walks of life.)[55] The findings also seem to have some cross-cultural validity, as a study of over 1200 people living in Mauritius has shown that this pattern of scores on schizotypy measures seems to be unaffected by culture, gender or religious affiliation.[56] In general, these studies have found that hypomanic traits (presumably related to mania) correlate very highly with odd beliefs and perceptual aberrations (traditionally thought of as a characteristic of schizophrenia). This finding suggests that schizophrenia and bipolar personality characteristics overlap, and therefore further undermines Kraepelin's assumption that there are two separate types of psychosis.

Madness, Creativity and Evolution

In her biography of Nobel-prize-winning mathematician John Nash Jr, Sylvia Nasar describes the following encounter:

It was late on a weekday afternoon in the spring of 1959, and, though it was only May, uncomfortably warm. Nash was slumped in an armchair in one corner of the hospital lounge, carelessly dressed in a nylon shirt that hung limply over his unbelted trousers. His powerful frame was slack as a rag doll's, his finely moulded features expressionless. He had been staring dully at a spot immediately in front of the left foot of Harvard professor George Mackey, hardly moving except to brush his long dark hair away from his forehead in a fitful, repetitive motion. His visitor sat upright, oppressed by the silence, acutely conscious that the doors to the room were locked. Mackey finally could contain himself no longer. His voice was slightly querulous, but he strained to be gentle. 'How could you,' began Mackey, 'how could you, a mathematician, a man devoted to reason and logical proof . . . how could you believe that extraterrestrials are sending you messages? How could you believe that you are being recruited by aliens from outer space to save the world? How could you?'

Nash looked up at last and fixed Mackey with an unblinking stare as cool and dispassionate of that of any bird or snake. 'Because,' Nash said slowly in his soft, reasonable southern drawl, as if talking to himself, 'the ideas I had about supernatural beings came to me the same way that my mathematical ideas did. So I took them seriously.'[57]

Some authors have argued that the discovery of a continuum (or several continua) linking psychosis and normal functioning may help to explain a feature of madness that has puzzled evolutionary thinkers, namely its persistence within populations over many generations. On the face of it, madness has grim implications for survival and reproduction. People suffering from severe psychotic symptoms often find it difficult to work, are relatively poor, are often socially isolated, and face a high risk of early death from suicide.[58] Not surprisingly, research has shown that they enjoy less reproductive success (that is, they have fewer children on average) than their fellow human beings.[59]

A paper co-authored by the evolutionary biologists Julian Huxley and Ernst Mayr and psychiatrists Humphrey Osmond and Abram

Hoffer, published in *Nature* in 1964, first pointed out that genes causing vulnerability to psychosis should be selected out over successive generations unless these social and reproductive disadvantages are balanced by advantages. They suggested that some kind of physiological benefit to non-affected relatives, for example enhanced resistance to infection, might compensate for the selective disadvantage of lower survival and reduced fertility experienced by the severely ill.[60] However, over thirty years later there is still no evidence to support this theory, and more recent researchers have argued that the benefits associated with psychosis lie in the social rather than the physical domain. Various kinds of social benefits have been postulated. For example, it has been suggested that genes for paranoia encourage a healthy defensiveness in threatening environments,[61] or that schizophrenia genes cause just the right degree of social strife to facilitate the splitting of overlarge groups in primitive societies.[62] Most of these hypotheses are evolutionary 'just so' stories of little merit, and the only substantial research exploring the positive consequences of madness has focused on creativity.

The idea that madness and creative genius are related predates modern psychiatry, and can certainly be traced back to Aristotle.[63] The evolutionary arguments of Huxley and others have given new life to this idea, provoking several lines of investigation. Some researchers have conducted biographical surveys of historically important people in the hope of finding evidence of high rates of psychiatric disorder. Table 5.1 gives a list of historical figures thought to suffer from serious mental illness, compiled from various sources by the American psychologist Dean Simonton.[64]

The problems faced by studies of this sort should not be underestimated. It is difficult to decide who should be included in this kind of survey, and even more difficult to make inferences about mental health from biographical data. Inevitably, psychiatric symptoms are inaccurately attributed to some people, and others who were clearly mentally ill are overlooked. (Simonton's table misses out two of my own favourite examples of disturbed genius, the mathematicians Kurt Gödel and John Nash. Gödel suffered from paranoid delusions and died from malnutrition after refusing to eat.[65] As we have already seen, Nash, a Nobel prize-winner and creator of a mathematical theory of rational behaviour, spent much of his life in psychiatric hospitals,

Table 5.1 Eminent persons with supposed mental illness (adapted from D. K. Simonton (1994) *Greatness: Who Makes History and Why.* New York: Guilford).

Schizophrenia

Scientists: T. Brahe, Cantor, Copernicus, Descartes, Faraday, W. R. Hamilton, Kepler, Lagrange, Linnaeus, Newton, Pascal, Semmelweiss, Weierstrass, H. Wells

Thinkers: Kant, Nietzsche, Swedenborg

Writers: Baudelaire, Lewis Carroll, Hawthorne, Hölderlin, S. Johnson, Pound, Rimbaud, Strindberg, Swift

Artists: Bosch, Cellini, Dürer, Goya, El Greco, Kandinsky, Leonardo da Vinci, Rembrandt, Toulouse-Lautrec.

Composers: Donizetti, MacDowell, F. Mendelssohn, Rimsky-Korsakov, Saint-Saëns

Others: de Sade, Goebbels, Herod the Great, Joan of Arc, Nero, Nijinsky, Skaha

Affective disorders (depression or bipolar disorder)

Scientists: Boltwood, Boltzmann, Carothers, C. Darwin, L. de Forest, J. F. W. Herschel, Julian Huxley, T. H. Huxley, Jung, Kammerer, J. R. von Mayer, V. Meyer, H. J. Müller, J. P. Müller, B. V. Schmidt, J. B. Watson

Thinkers: W. James, J. S. Mill, Rousseau, Sabbatai Z'vi, Schopenhauer

Writers: Balzac, Barrie, Berryman, Blake, Boswell, V. W. Brooks, Byron, Chatterton, J. Clare, Coleridge, William Collins, Conrad, Cowper, H. Crane, Dickens, T. Dreiser, R. Fergusson, F. S. Fitzgerald, Frost, Goethe, G. Greene, Hemingway, Jarrell, Kafka, C. Lamb, J. London, R. Lowell, de Maupassant, E. O'Neill, Plath, Poe, Quroga, Roethke, D. G. Rossetti, Saroyan, Schiller, Sexton, P. B. Shelley, C. Smart, T. Tasso, V. Woolf

Artists: Michelangelo, Modigliani, Pollock, Raphael, Rothko, R. Soyer, Van Gogh

Composers: Berlioz, Chopin, Elgar, Gershwin, Handel, Mahler, Rachmaninoff, Rossini, R. Schumann, Scriabin, Smetana, Tchaikovsky, Wolf

Others: C. Borgia, Clive, O. Cromwell, A. Davis, J. Garland

Note: Because almost all of these diagnoses are not based on objective clinical assessments, most are highly tentative.

believing that he was receiving messages from extraterrestrials.)[66] These problems notwithstanding, the most carefully conducted biographical surveys have consistently pointed to unusual levels of psychiatric disturbance in creative and influential people.[67]

Other investigators have attempted to avoid the uncertainties of historical research by studying living people. For example, Nancy Andreasen interviewed a group of creative writers living in Iowa, and found abnormally high levels of mood disorder in both the writers and their relatives.[68] American psychologist Kay Redfield Jamison similarly interviewed a group of eminent British writers and artists (chosen on the basis of having won at least one top award in their field) and also found high levels of mood disturbance. Although very few in Jamison's sample had been treated for bipolar disorder (most having been treated for depression) many described creative episodes in which they had experienced mood and energy changes consistent with hypomania.[69]

If psychosis and creativity have common genetic roots, the relatives of mentally ill patients should show evidence of unusual creativity. This prediction was tested in a study conducted in Iceland by psychiatrist John Karlsson, who investigated the occupations of the relatives of schizophrenia patients and found evidence of high levels of creativity.[70] In a more recent study carried out in Denmark by Ruth Richards and her colleagues, manic-depressive patients and their relatives were interviewed about their lives, and their responses were evaluated using a standard measure of lifetime creative achievement. The patients and their relatives scored higher than a mentally well control group.[71]

The account I have given by no means exhausts the ways in which the relationship between psychosis and creativity has been explored.[72] Suffice it to say that, overall, the research is surprisingly consistent, and the long-held association between madness and creativity seems to be a real one. One unresolved issue concerns whether creativity is related to any particular type of psychosis. Writers such as Nancy Andreasen and Kay Jamison have favoured a link between creativity and mania whereas others, notably John Karlsson, have argued for a link with schizophrenia.

This question was addressed directly by Gordon Claridge, who studied in depth ten authors who had written at length about their mental troubles. The writers were Margery Kempe, Thomas Hoccleve, Christopher Smart, William Cowper, John Clare, John Ruskin, Arthur Benson, Virginia Woolf, Antonia White and Sylvia Plath. When their self-reported symptoms were coded using the OPCRIT computer diagnostic program, many diagnoses fell in the schizophrenia spectrum, but some diagnoses of bipolar disorder were also made. Interestingly, several of the writers received both types of diagnosis, depending on the precise criteria employed. For example, William Cowper was diagnosed as suffering from depression according to Taylor and Abrams' criteria, bipolar disorder according to DSM-III and DSM-III-R, schizoaffective disorder according to the RDC, and schizophrenia according to five less widely used diagnostic systems.[73] Once again, it seems, we are confronted with the limitations of Kraepelin's distinction between dementia praecox and manic depression.

A Matter of Perspective?

Everywhere we look, it seems that the boundaries between sanity and madness are indistinct and permeable. Contrary to the neoKraepelinian assumption that a clear line can be drawn between mental illness and normal functioning, it seems reasonable to assume, as a general principle, that abnormal behaviours and experiences exist on continua with normal behaviours and experiences. This *principle of continuity* might be formally stated as follows:

Abnormal behaviours and experiences are related to normal behaviours and experiences by continua of frequency (the same behaviours and experiences occur less frequently in non-psychiatric populations), severity (less severe forms of the behaviours and experiences can be identified in non-psychiatric populations), and phenomenology (non-clinical analogues of the behaviours and experiences can be identified as part of normal life).

Some of the evidence we have considered poses problems even for sophisticated accounts of madness. For example, Gordon Claridge's revised biomedical model – in which madness is regarded as the dysfunctional manifestation of an extreme variant of normal personality – seems threatened by the apparent association between madness and genius. It might be argued that these observations undermine *any* approach that automatically assumes madness to be a medical condition.

Challenges to the medical approach to madness have a long history. Freud, for example, although a doctor by training, came to believe that medicine provides a poor framework for either understanding or treating mental disorders, and defended the right of 'lay analysts' to practise psychotherapy.[74] Popular concerns about the value of the medical approach reached something of a crescendo during the 1960s and 1970s. At this time, those who opposed conventional psychiatry (mainly because they regarded it as dehumanizing) often styled themselves as 'anti-psychiatrists'. Some historians of psychiatry have argued that the neoKraepelinians emerged as a group partly in reaction to the anti-psychiatry movement.[75] Certainly, it can be no accident that anti-psychiatry was a popular intellectual position at the same time that Robert Spitzer and his colleagues were fashioning DSM-III.

Many of those who proposed anti-psychiatric arguments were psychiatrists themselves. In Britain, R. D. Laing became one of the most celebrated contributors to the anti-psychiatry debate following the publication of his books *The Divided Self* and *The Self and Others*.[76] These built on Laing's training in psychoanalysis and his experiences with a group of Scottish psychiatrists who had argued that schizophrenia patients should be treated with psychotherapy. Laing's main claim was that psychotic symptoms are meaningful and therefore cannot be understood as medical phenomena. In his later books, *Sanity, Madness and the Family* and *The Politics of Experience*, he suggested, first, that schizophrenia patients were driven insane by persecutory family systems and, later, that madness could be seen as a creative, mystical experience.[77] Although these ideas were passionately expressed and resonated well with the Zeitgeist (for me, reading Laing as an undergraduate psychology student who had not long escaped from the grip of parental authority was an almost intoxicating experience) it is probably fair to say that their expression was often muddled and inconsistent. This was partly because Laing flirted with various poorly thought out, New Age ideas, and partly because his own creative powers were unable to survive his almost legendary predilection for alcohol.[78] This is a pity because his early work revealed an uncanny empathy with psychotic patients, and appeared to offer intriguing insights into the psychology of their experiences.

Other influential critics of conventional psychiatry have put forward different arguments against the medical approach to psychosis. In the United States, for example, the Hungarian-born psychiatrist Thomas Szasz (who has been highly critical of Laing, and who denies that he is an anti-psychiatrist) has claimed that schizophrenia cannot be an illness, because no evidence of pathology has ever been found in the brains of psychotic patients. Indeed, he has gone as far as to assert that mental illness is a myth.[79] We will examine these arguments (which I will ultimately reject, although in a way that will offer little comfort to the neoKraepelinians) in a later chapter. For the moment, we need only note that the research on the continuum or continua between psychosis and normal functioning suggests a startling conclusion that is in some ways consistent with Laing's loosely expressed philosophy. Perhaps the line between sanity and madness must be drawn relative to the place at which we stand. Perhaps it is possible to be, at the same time, mad when viewed from one perspective and sane when viewed from another.

6

Them and Us*

> *Father, Mother, and Me,*
> *Sister and Auntie say*
> *All the people like us are We,*
> *And everyone else is They,*
> *And They live over the sea,*
> *While We live over the way,*
> *But – would you believe it? – They look upon We*
> *As only a sort of They.*
>
> Rudyard Kipling[1]

During my career, I have met mental health experts in many different parts of the world. Perhaps the most unusual meeting of this kind that I have so far experienced took place in a small village, high in the hills above the town of Mbarara in southern Uganda. I had travelled to the country in support of a British Council-sponsored link between my own university and the Psychology Department at Makarere University in Kampala, where plans were afoot to establish a clinical psychology training course. The trip southwards from the capital had been arranged by Joanna Teuton, a British clinical psychologist who was researching Ugandan attitudes towards psychosis for her Ph.D., and who thought it might be useful for me to see how mental health services were organized in remote areas.

On our arrival in Mbarara, we had met up with Marjolein van Duyl, a young Dutch psychiatrist, who ran a clinic in the small medical school that had recently been established by the Ugandan government. Accompanied by a couple of local nurses, the three of us left the town

---

* I am indebted to Joanna Teuton for her helpful advice about the contents of this chapter.

in a pick-up truck and, after venturing along a dirt track for about three quarters of an hour, arrived at a small cluster of brick buildings, surrounded by a huge expanse of open grassland. At the sound of our engine, people began to filter out of doorways into the sunlight. Disembarking, we made our way along a small footpath into a field where the healers were gathering. There were about fifteen in total, men and women, young and old, some standing, some squatting on two old benches that had been dragged into the sharply defined shade of a solitary tree. Some of those present, Marjolein explained, were traditional birth attendants, some were spiritual healers, some specialized in diseases of the gut and others in diseases of the mind. 'Hello-how-are-you-I-am-well-thank-you', spoken almost as one word, seemed to be the customary Ugandan greeting even among those who did not speak English and, as each of the traditional healers found it necessary to greet each of the visitors, it was some time before we were all settled.

The discussions that took place over the following hour were facilitated by one of the nurses, who proved to be a gifted translator. It was not the first time the healers had met Marjolein, who had worked hard to build a good relationship between them and the medical school. By fostering a climate of mutual respect, Marjolein hoped to help the healers give front-line medical care, while she provided European-style psychiatric treatment to those who failed to benefit from the traditional methods.

We began by exploring the healers' ideas about psychiatric problems. The most severe disorder that they recognized, called *irraro* in Runyankole (the local language), made people aggressive and violent. People who suffered from this disorder typically threw stones, ran about naked and refused to eat food. Addiction to alcohol was also seen as a serious problem. Surprisingly, the healers regarded hallucinations and delusions as much less worrying. As the afternoon wore on, we shuffled around to stay in the shade and discussed treatment methods. Some of those who specialized in psychiatric problems said that they would use herbs, grown especially for the purpose. Others said that they would use spiritual methods. For example, when asked how he would treat a patient who was suffering from voices, one man said that he would summon his spirits and ask them to speak with the spirits who were tormenting the afflicted person.

Throughout the discussions, the healers responded politely to the questions that Joanna and I put to them. The healers also asked questions about the kinds of treatment that would be offered to emotionally distressed people in Britain. I found myself trying to explain my role to an audience that had never before encountered a psychologist and began by attempting to outline, in simple terms, how I might set about helping a patient who suffered from auditory halucinations.

The healers listened thoughtfully. They did not seem to find my ideas ridiculous, or necessarily incompatible with their own. In their efforts to compare the two approaches, they asked intelligent questions about the effectiveness of my techniques. Although the conversation was conducted via a translator, and despite the unusual circumstances, it seemed fairly typical of the kinds of discussions that take place whenever clinicians gather to discuss their cases.

Is Madness Universal?

In the middle of the nineteenth century, Samuel Butler, the rebellious son of an English rector, left his homeland to rear sheep in New Zealand. At the time, large areas of that country were still unmapped. Butler's experiences gave him a distant perspective on his own society, which he affectionately mocked in his utopian fiction *Erewhon* (Nowhere), which was published in 1872.[2] In the novel, he described a civilization in an undiscovered corner of the world, chanced upon by an explorer, where many of the values of Victorian society were inverted. Attitudes towards crime and health were prominent among the topsy-turvy features of Erewhonian culture. In Erewhon, ill health was considered a crime and was severely punished, whereas immoral behaviour was regarded as a cause for pity and professional treatment. Butler's satire raises an important question about the nature of mental health and illness: Are psychiatric disorders universal phenomena, or are they culturally determined?

This question needs some unpacking. Horacio Fabrega, Professor of Psychiatry and Anthropology at the University of Pittsburgh, has argued that all cultures, past and present, have recognized *human behavioural breakdowns* – anomalous behaviours that are sustained and judged negatively, and which are regarded as disruptive to organized social life.[3] However, this does not mean that madness, as defined within the Kraepelinian paradigm, is a universal phenomenon. Perhaps different societies single out different kinds of behaviours and experiences as evidence of madness? We must therefore divide our question about the universality of psychiatric disorders into two separate questions. First, do psychotic experiences and behaviours, as defined by neoKraepelinian criteria, appear everywhere we look? Second, do different cultures draw the boundaries between sanity and madness in the same or in different places?

My encounter with the traditional healers illustrates some of the difficulties involved in answering these questions. It seemed to me that *irraro* did not obviously correspond to any category of illness recognized by psychiatrists from the developed world, but it was possible that closer study of the disorder would have shown me to be mistaken. John Orley, a psychiatrist who spent some time with the Baganda (the largest tribe in Uganda), documented, in addition to this kind of madness (known as *eddalu* to the Bagandans), other locally recognized disorders, some of which, like *obusiru* (foolishness), are regarded as diseases of the head whereas others, for example *emmeme etyemuka* (fright), are regarded as diseases of the heart. Some, such as *ensimbu* (fits), seem to correspond very closely to Western medical concepts (in this case, epilepsy) whereas others, for example *emmeme egwa* (a general weakening of the body and failure to eat), do not.[4]

In practice, cross-cultural studies of madness have been pursued by two different groups of researchers, who have started out with different assumptions. Psychiatrists, for the most part, have tried to use Western medical concepts to explain the behaviour of people in developing countries. Orley, for example, argued that many cases of *eddalu* are in fact people suffering from schizophrenia. Social anthropologists, in contrast, have been interested in exploring concepts of normality and abnormality in different cultures.*

---

* There have been, of course, some notable researchers who have straddled both camps, for example Horacio Fabrega and Arthur Kleinman in the United States, and Roland Littlewood and Maurice Lipsedge in the UK.

Are Psychotic Symptoms Found in All Societies?

As we have already seen, Kraepelin was one of the first people to investigate whether psychotic symptoms could be found in non-Western cultures. Although he concluded that both dementia praecox and manic depression occurred in Java, he qualified this observation by suggesting that delusions and hallucinations were less common among the Javanese than among Europeans, and that states of mania and depression in the Far East seemed to be milder and more fleeting. Speculating about the likely causes of these differences, he argued that:

It is, of course, an open question whether the underlying processes there are basically the same as those which produce similar clinical pictures in our hospitals at home. Perhaps it will be possible to settle the matter by anatomical studies, but from the clinical point of view, based on a comparison between the phenomena of disease which I found there and those with which I was familiar at home, the overall similarity far outweighed the deviant features ... The relative absence of delusions among the Javanese might be related to the lower stage of intellectual development attained, and the rarity of auditory hallucinations might reflect the fact that speech counts far less than it does with us and that thoughts tend to be governed more by sensory images.[5]

Studies conducted by anthropologists and doctors working for colonial administrations during the first half of the twentieth century reported low rates of psychosis in non-Western countries, leading some observers to doubt whether schizophrenia could occur in societies that were close to a 'state of nature'. C. G. Seligman, for example, in a report published in 1929, commented of the people of Papua New Guinea: 'There is no evidence of the occurrence of mental derangement, other than brief outbursts of maniacal excitement, among natives who have not been associated with White Civilisation.'[6] Foremost among those who elaborated on this theme was John Carothers, a young physician who, in 1938, was appointed senior medical officer in charge of Mathari Mental Hospital in Nairobi, following the dismissal of James Cobb from the same position.[7] (Cobb, who unlike Carothers, had received a formal training in psychiatry, had scandalized Nairobi society by his drinking, his open homosexuality and his bizarre attachment to two pet lion cubs, with whom he was rumoured to have enjoyed sexual relations.)

Believing his appointment to be a temporary one, and mindful of his lack of experience in psychiatry, Carothers was at first reluctant to record any scientific observations about his patients. However, after working alongside a group of British army psychiatrists who passed through Kenya during the Second World War, and following a short period of training in London afterwards, he began to see parallels between European schizophrenia patients and ordinary African citizens. Both seemed self-absorbed, morally lazy, preferred to live in a world of fantasy and projected their own qualities and emotions on to the world around them. Because 'the step from the primitive attitude to schizophrenia is but a short and easy one', he believed that ordinary Africans would remain psychologically healthy in the simple and unstructured environment of the rural village but that, on coming into contact with European rule in the urban centres, ran the risk of becoming psychotic.

Such was Carothers' reputation that, in 1952, he was commissioned by the World Health Organization to write a report on the African mind, and, in 1954, by the British government to write a psychological analysis of the Mau Mau rebellion. The former, in which he attributed the African personality to poorly developed frontal lobes, was surprisingly well received by anthropologists. The latter attempted to pathologize the motives of a revolutionary movement and failed to mention the land disputes that had triggered the insurrection. Looking back from our vantage point at the beginning of the twenty-first century, it is easy to see that Carothers' ideas were taken seriously because they were consistent with the assumed inferiority of Africans, rather than because of the quality of his research. Not surprisingly, a rather different picture became apparent when the first systematic cross-cultural research on psychosis was conducted several decades later.

The new cross-cultural psychiatry

This new picture emerged from a series of investigations sponsored by the World Health Organization. In the International Pilot Study of Schizophrenia[8] and the subsequent International Follow-up Study of Schizophrenia,[9] patients in nine countries were examined and were assigned diagnoses according to local and Schneiderian criteria. It was these studies that confirmed that psychiatrists in the United States and the Soviet Union had very broad conceptions of schizophrenia in comparison with psychiatrists from the other participating countries. This aside, the main finding was that disorders recognizable to Western psychiatrists as 'schizophrenia' could be found throughout the world, an observation that was widely interpreted by the psychiatric community as evidence that schizophrenia is a tangible phenomenon that exists independently of the observer. However, as American psychiatrist and anthropologist Arthur Kleinman pointed out, the strategy employed by the WHO investigators was almost bound to filter out cross-cultural differences in psychopathology.[10] Indeed, the researchers' conclusion that schizophrenia is similar the world over was inevitable, as only patients meeting Western criteria for schizophrenia were included in the cross-cultural comparisons.

This criticism applies with even greater force to the more recent WHO study of the Determinants of Outcome of Severe Mental Disorders (DOSMD).[11] The researchers who undertook this ambitious project reached the remarkable (and much trumpeted) conclusion that the incidence rate of schizophrenia (the proportion of the population that succumbs to the disease in a given period) does not vary across the world. They therefore inferred that there must be a uniformly distributed liability to schizophrenia and that 'This liability must have a genetic basis.'

The logic of this argument is baffling. As British psychologist Richard Marshall once remarked before his untimely death, market capitalism is the dominant worldwide economic system but few people believe that there are uniformly distributed genes for capitalism. On the other hand, many diseases of known genetic origin do vary in incidence across the world. (Sickle-cell anaemia, to take but one example, is an inherited blood disorder that is common in African people, or people of African descent, but which rarely affects other ethnic groups.)

In fact, the DOSMD data did not demonstrate that incidence rates for schizophrenia are culturally invariant, as the researchers claimed. The team of over 100 investigators, led by Professors Norman Sartorius and Assen Jablensky, studied people experiencing their first psychotic breakdown at twelve sites (Aarhus in Denmark, Agra and

Chandigarh in India, Cali in Columbia, Dublin in Ireland, Honolulu and Rochester in the USA, Ibadan in Nigeria, Moscow in Russia, Nagasaki in Japan, Nottingham in the UK and Prague in the former Czechoslovakia). To be included in the study, an individual had to be experiencing at least one psychotic symptom, or showing at least two kinds of abnormal behaviour suggestive of psychosis. The researchers made great efforts to find people who were psychotic but who had sought help from non-medical agencies or traditional healers, in this way hoping to catch all new cases who failed to contact local medical services. Whether this strategy was successful is debatable. Occasional 'leakage' investigations, in which local informants were asked whether they knew of any psychotic people who had slipped through the net, failed to reveal many previously unidentified cases. However, the evidence we considered in the last chapter suggests that many people experience psychotic symptoms cheerfully and in silence. Certainly, it is difficult to be sure that all new cases have been detected without interviewing a random sample of the population.

In the end, incidence rates were only calculated for seven sites for which adequate data were available, with the Chandigarh site divided into urban and rural subsites. Of course, a further difficulty faced by researchers conducting this kind of study is the choice between the many different definitions of schizophrenia. Rates for both a broad and narrow (Schneiderian) definition of schizophrenia were therefore reported. Not surprisingly, there was considerably more variation in the rates for the broad definition than for the narrow definition (see Figure 6.1). Even for the narrow definition, however, the annual incidence rate reported for Nottingham (1.4 cases aged between 15 and 54 years per 10,000 population) was twice that for Aarhus (0.7 cases). It seems amazing that such a large difference was not considered important by the researchers, but this was because the statistical calculations they carried out on their data suggested that this difference could be due to chance factors (for example, random variations in the numbers of new cases occurring at each site). However, given the relatively small numbers of Schneiderian patients, it seems likely that the study was not large enough to detect reliably even quite big differences between the numbers at each site.[12]

In fact, statistically significant differences between the sites were observed for the broad definition and, as Kleinman has noted:

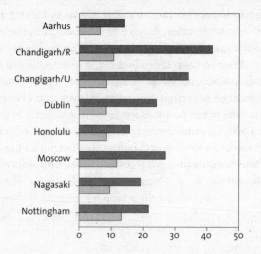

Figure 6.1 Incidence rates at seven different sites for two different definitions of schizophrenia detected in the DOSMD study (from A. Jablensky, N. Sartorius, G. Ernberg, M. Anker, A. Korten, J. E. Cooper, R. Day and A. Bertelsen (1992) 'Schizophrenia: manifestations, incidence and course in different cultures', *Psychological Medicine*, Supplement 20: 1–97). Dark columns show data for a broad definition of schizophrenia (S, P or O categories according to the CATEGO system of computerized diagnoses) and light columns show data for a narrow Schneiderian definition (CATEGO S+).

The 'broad' sample from the anthropological perspective is the valid one, since it includes all first-contact cases of psychosis meeting the inclusion and exclusion criteria. The 'restricted' sample is a 'constructed' sample, since it places a template on the heterogeneous population sample and stamps out a homogeneous group of clinical cases. The restricted sample demonstrates to be sure that a core schizophrenic syndrome can be discovered amongst first-contact cases in widely different cultures. This is an important finding, but it is not evidence of a uniform pattern of incidence.[13]

Other cross-cultural investigators, weighing data from a number of epidemiological studies, have usually concluded that schizophrenia-like psychoses are less common in non-Western societies than in the developed world, and continue to debate the possible causes of these apparent differences.[14] For example, New Zealand anthropologist John Allen has recently proposed that schizophrenia occurs less often in non-Western societies because life is *more* stressful in those societies than in the industrialized nations.[15] (On this view, life close to a state of nature is not so idyllic after all.) Like Paul Meehl, Allen accepts that schizophrenia is a stress-related disorder, but notes that episodes of psychotic illness are associated with reduced reproductive fitness. Therefore, he argues, precipitation of an increased number of schizophrenia episodes in the past will have resulted in a gradual weeding out of schizophrenia genes throughout the undeveloped world, leading to fewer episodes in the present. Ingenious though this argument is, it is, of course, an evolutionary just-so story, and difficult to test scientifically.

Incidence rates of psychosis within one country: the British Afro-Caribbeans

When attempting to make sense of the inconsistent results that have emerged from comparisons between countries it is easy to forget that many modern industrialized nations contain multiracial populations. In fact, some of the clearest evidence of cross-cultural differences in the incidence rates of psychosis has emerged from the comparison of different ethnic groups in Britain.

For many years it has been known that black Afro-Caribbeans are over-represented in British psychiatric hospitals, and are especially likely to be diagnosed as suffering from paranoid schizophrenia[16] or mania.[17] Not surprisingly, the reasons for this over-representation have been the subject of heated debate. One possible explanation might be that white psychiatrists, ignorant of Afro-Caribbean culture, often misunderstand the experiences of Afro-Caribbean people, and thereby misdiagnose many as schizophrenic.[18] To check for this possibility, researchers at the Institute of Psychiatry in London invited a Jamaican psychiatrist, Fred Hickling, to re-evaluate their diagnoses of Afro-Caribbean patients.* Although there was poor agreement

---

* We will see in a later chapter that the stresses associated with racial discrimination may play a role in the excess of psychotic breakdowns in British Afro-Caribbeans. It is therefore of some interest to note that Dr Hickling was stopped by the police for no apparent reason when driving in his hire car from his hotel to the Institute of Psychiatry. On being unable to prove his identity, he was arrested (Robin Murray, personal communication).

between Hickling's diagnoses of schizophrenia and those made by the white British psychiatrists, the overall rate at which Hickling and the British psychiatrists diagnosed schizophrenia in the patients did not differ much.[19] Therefore, it seems unlikely that the high rates of psychosis in British Afro-Caribbeans can entirely be accounted for by misdiagnoses made by culturally insensitive white clinicians.

Another possibility is that Afro-Caribbean people express distress in a culturally idiosyncratic way that often culminates in violence, leading to especially prompt intervention by psychiatric services. It is certainly true that Afro-Caribbean people are more likely to be compulsorily admitted to psychiatric hospitals in the UK than other ethnic groups.[20] However, as early as 1988, Glyn Harrison and his colleagues found a higher than expected rate of psychosis in a *community* sample of Afro-Caribbeans living in Nottingham, assessed using standardized criteria.[21] This finding has been replicated several times, notably by psychiatrists Dinesh Bhugra, Julian Leff and their colleagues in London.[22]

Studies conducted in the Caribbean have found lower incidence rates for psychosis in Trinidad[23] and Barbados[24] than in the British Afro-Caribbean community. Therefore, the Afro-Caribbean population as a whole does not appear to be especially vulnerable to psychosis, and a racially specific genetic sensitivity to madness can be ruled out. More intriguingly, several studies in Britain have found that the excess rates of psychosis are most evident in the children of Afro-Caribbeans who have moved to Britain, rather than in the generation that migrated.[25]

In a later chapter, we will see that this over-representation of psychosis in the British Afro-Caribbean community has provided important clues about environmental determinants of madness. For the present, however, we can note that this finding convincingly establishes that the incidence of psychosis is *not* identical in all ethnic groups in all regions of the world.

Cross-cultural differences in the outcome of psychosis

Ironically, although the DOSMD study obscured differences in incidence rates, it succeeded in its main purpose, which was to confirm a suspicion that cross-cultural differences exist in the *course* and *outcome* of psychosis. This suspicion arose in earlier research, in particular the five-year follow-up of patients recruited to the International Pilot Study of Schizophrenia.[26] In that study, it was reported that 27 per cent of patients in the developing nations experienced only one psychotic episode, followed by complete recovery, compared to only 7 per cent of patients from industrialized nations. Nor was this difference in outcome confined to symptoms; 65 per cent of patients in the developing countries compared to 56 per cent of patients in the industrialized countries were judged to have no or only mild social impairment at the end of the follow-up period. Arthur Kleinman described these observations as 'arguably the single most important finding of cultural differences in cross-cultural research on mental illness'.[27]

The DOSMD data broadly replicated these observations. In the two-year follow-up data from the study, 37 per cent of patients from the developing countries suffered one episode, followed by complete recovery, compared to only 16 per cent of patients from the developed world. Nearly 16 per cent of patients in the developing countries showed impaired social functioning throughout the follow-up period, whereas the corresponding figure for the developed countries was nearly 42 per cent. Despite the undoubted limitations of the WHO programme of cross-cultural research, the evidence that madness is more benign outside the industrialized world is quite compelling. On the basis of these findings, Ezra Susser and Joseph Wanderling of Columbia University in New York proposed the term *non-affective acute remitting psychosis* (NARP) to describe a clinical picture in which there is a rapid onset of symptoms followed by complete recovery. True to the spirit of the DSM, they argued that it should be considered a diagnostic entity distinct from schizophrenia. They calculated the incidence of this type of clinical presentation to be ten times greater in the developing world than in industrialized nations.[28]

Unfortunately, as critics of the WHO studies have pointed out, the researchers who designed the studies defined culture simply in terms of geography, and almost completely neglected to measure cultural factors that might be responsible for the observed differences.[29] The reasons people who experience psychosis in the developing world do so much better than those in the West must therefore remain a matter of speculation. It has been pointed out that developing societies have many positive characteristics in comparison with developed countries.[30] These include families who are more supportive and less critical; greater opportunities for employment; less competitiveness and impersonality in the workplace; and lower levels of stigma associated with psychiatric disorder. In later chapters we will encounter evidence that some of these factors really do help to determine the long-term prospects of psychiatric patients.

Cross-cultural differences in symptoms

So far, we have seen that there is evidence of cross-cultural differences in both the incidence and outcome of psychosis. However, all the studies we have so far considered have taken the Kraepelinian paradigm for granted. Further evidence of cross-cultural differences comes to light when we consider symptoms, rather than broad and scientifically questionable diagnostic concepts such as 'schizophrenia'. For example, the DOSMD researchers found that visual hallucinations were much more frequently reported in the developing than in the developed countries. This observation received little attention compared with the researchers' more contentious claims about incidence rates, but has been repeated by other investigators.[31] Studies of delusions also point to cross-cultural and historical differences. For example, although the most common type of delusion reported by modern patients is persecutory,[32] patients admitted to US hospitals during the Great Depression of the 1930s more commonly suffered from delusions of wealth and special powers.[33]

To these observations must be added the so-called *culture-bound syndromes* – disorders that are apparently restricted to particular societies.[34] Examples include *koro* (an illness suffered by Chinese people, usually males, who believe that their sexual organs are shrinking), *latah* (experienced by Indonesians, who develop an exaggerated startle response, which includes shouting rude words and mimicking the behaviour of those nearby) and *witiko psychosis* (a rare disorder in which Algonquian-speaking Indians of Canada believe themselves to be possessed by vampires). Western psychiatrists have sometimes attempted to account for these syndromes by arguing that the form of mental disorder remains constant across cultures but that the content varies, so that the culture-bound syndromes are locally shaped expressions of disorders that are universal (for example, witiko psychosis might be seen as an unusual variant of schizophrenia).[35] When doing so, they have typically ignored culture-specific factors that have shaped the observed behaviour (for example, there is evidence that *latah* evolved as a way of mimicking the unintelligible demands of European colonialists).[36] A further problem with this approach is that it assumes that Western psychiatry somehow 'knows best', and has discovered an accurate taxonomy of abnormal behaviours that can be applied without difficulty to non-Western cultures. The research we have reviewed in previous chapters suggests that this kind of psychiatric imperialism has no merit. Given the paucity of evidence supporting the Kraepelinian paradigm, it is not obvious why we should regard it as superior to that of the Baganda.

Are Psychotic Experiences Normal in Some Cultures?

Extract from my field diary:

> Dorze, Southern Ethiopia,
> Sunday 24 viii 69

Saturday morning old Filate came to see me in a state of great excitement: 'Three times I came to see you, and you weren't there!'
  'I was away in Konso.'
  'I know. I was angry. I was glad. Do you want to do something?'
  'What?'
  'Keep quiet! If you do it, God will be pleased, the Government will be pleased. So?'
  'Well, if it is a good thing and I can do it, I shall do it.'
  'I have talked to no one about it: will you kill it?'
  'Kill? Kill what?'
  'Its heart is made of gold, it has one horn on the nape of its neck. It is golden all over. It does not live far, two days' walk at most. If you kill it, you will become a great man!'
  And so on . . . It turns out Filate wants me to kill a dragon. He is to come back this afternoon with someone who has seen it, and they will tell me more . . .

Dan Sperber[37]

We must now turn to the second of our two questions. Because different cultures embrace starkly different taxonomies of mental disorder, there is clearly a possibility that the boundaries drawn between madness and normal functioning vary with geography. It just might be possible to be mad in one culture but at the same time sane in another.

Roland Littlewood, one of the few British psychiatrists with an interest in anthropology, has lamented that the most common question he is asked by his medical colleagues is, 'Is this a delusion?'[38] Certainly, as the above excerpt from anthropologist Dan Sperber's field diary demonstrates, the apparently irrational beliefs of other cultures present a challenge to those who seek a clear dividing line between normal and abnormal beliefs. What, for example, is the psychiatrist to make of the Fataleka of the Solomon Islands, who maintain that the Earth occupies the fifth of nine parallel strata, that reflections are in stratum three, flutes are in stratum four, crocodiles are in stratum seven, and stratum eight is empty? In a thoughtful discussion of these kinds of beliefs, Sperber has noted that they can sometimes be understood as proto-scientific theories.[39] For example, the West African notion that the mind is the meeting place of multiple souls is similar to Freud's theory of psychoanalysis. At other times the beliefs seem to be metaphors. The assertion by Bororo males that they are red macaws can be understood when it is known that red macaws are taken as pets by Bororo women, who play a dominant role in Bororo society. Sperber goes on to argue that much of the remaining puzzlement experienced by Westerners when encountering the beliefs of other cultures can be resolved by recognizing that often they are not literal statements of observed facts. When people are asked about these kinds of beliefs, they often justify them in terms of tradition or knowledge passed to them by others, much as a modern-day Christian might justify belief in the resurrection by referring to the Bible.

Unfortunately, this analysis does not help us very much. In later chapters, we will see that processes similar to those described by Sperber can be seen at work in the beliefs of many Western psychiatric patients. Some delusions, like West African beliefs about the mind, seem to be patients' rational attempts to explain their experiences. Others, like the Bororo males' identification with red macaws, may be metaphors. (As I write this passage, I am reminded of a young black man I once saw who had been raised by white adoptive parents and who claimed that he was an abandoned visitor from another planet who would one day be rescued by a flying saucer.) Others do not seem to be statements of fact at all, as witnessed by patients' failure to behave accordingly (for example, the patient who asserts that his food is poisoned but who can easily be encouraged to eat it).[40]

The standard psychiatric response to this conundrum is to rule the beliefs of other cultures non-delusional by definition. For example, the definition of delusions given in DSM-IV notes that 'The belief is not one ordinarily accepted by other members of the person's culture or subculture.'[41] Others, for example Roland Littlewood and Maurice Lipsedge, have argued that there is a spectrum of beliefs running from widely held religious convictions, through the beliefs of obscure sects, to individual psychotic delusions.[42] Both of these moves seem to make the answer to the question, 'Is this a delusion?' a matter of consensus. (If enough people locally share the belief it is not a delusion.) Although they have been proposed in order to allow psychiatrists to distinguish between 'true' delusions and unusual but culturally determined beliefs, they seem to let cultural relativism in by the back door.

The evidence on cultural variations in the acceptability of hallucinations is more clear-cut. Anthropologist Erika Bourguignon found that hallucinations played a role in the ritual practices of 62 per cent of the 488 societies for which she was able to obtain adequate data. For example, Mohawk Indian hunters are forbidden to eat their own game, and are visited by spirits if they do so.[43] American psychologist Ihsan Al-Issa has suggested that cross-cultural differences in hallucinatory experiences reflect culturally embedded beliefs about the boundaries between imagination and reality, so that experiences that would be regarded as imaginary in one culture are regarded as real in another.[44]

Failure to appreciate the cultural context may prevent clinicians from responding appropriately to the distress experienced by their patients. An example of this kind of mistake has been reported by Scott McDonald and Chester Oden, two clinical psychologists practising in Hawaii, who have described their misdirected efforts to help two men who suffered from hallucinations of dead relatives. They later discovered that this kind of experience, known as *aumakua*, is quite common among Hawaiians of Polynesian ancestry, and usually occurs when someone has violated a cultural taboo. Instructing their patients to make amends for their transgressions was sufficient to bring the hallucinations to an end.[45]

Some social scientists have suggested that experiences that would be regarded as psychotic in the West are afforded a normal status in the activities of traditional healers and shamans (holy people who experience altered states of consciousness).[46] For example, Robert Edgerton has discussed the work of Abedi, in Tanzania:[47]

Abedi's specialization in mental illness began during his apprenticeship when he first hallucinated ('hearing voices of people I could not see') and ran in terror to hide in the bush. He was discovered and returned to his father's care, but lay ('completely out of my senses') for two weeks before being cured. The cause was diagnosed as witchcraft and since the cure, Abedi has never been sick again. The experience initiated Abedi's interest in mental illness, and the subsequent mental disorders of his sister and his wife reinforced it. At different times, both women became violently psychotic, but Abedi cured them both. These two cures not only heightened Abedi's interest in psychiatric phenomena, but they led to his reputation as a skillful psychiatrist.

Similarly, of ten Ugandan traditional healers interviewed in depth by Joanna Teuton as part of her Ph.D. research, two had clearly been inspired to take up their vocations by psychotic episodes. For example, a woman from the Luganda tribe said that she had become a healer after a difficult period during which she had heard voices and entertained paranoid beliefs, experiences that she described with great lucidity.

Nor is this phenomenon restricted to the developing world. Historical figures from the West who might justifiably be regarded as shamans because their claims to religious leadership were associated with psychotic experiences include Francis of Assisi, Joan of Arc, John Bunyan and Ann Lee (the founder of the Shaker Movement in the United States), all of whom experienced hallucinations. Even today, some citizens from the developed world are able to pursue shamanistic careers on the basis of such experiences, as the following case-vignette from Holland demonstrates:

A 42-year-old divorcee, mother of two children, who has a private practice as a psychic healer, has heard voices for as long as she can remember. She hears the voices via her ears. The voices are located both inside and outside her head. One voice began in childhood and is still present, but she also hears other voices. The initial voice talks to her in the second person. She communicates with this voice, consulting it for the benefit of her clients. Her voices also talk amongst themselves. Although her voices are not actual voices she has heard in daily life, she is not afraid of them and does not feel restricted by them. Rather, she feels that they are protective: they give her advice, comfort and care. She considers her voices as protective ghosts. She also regularly experiences visual, tactile, and olfactory hallucinations.[48]

Anthropologists have often rejected the suggestion that many healers and shamans are psychotic, perhaps because this idea seems to devalue the contribution that they make to their own cultures.[49] They have argued that the healer's role requires a degree of organization that would be difficult to achieve by someone suffering from a full-blown psychotic illness, that most societies clearly distinguish between shamanistic states and behaviour believed to be evidence of madness, and that the experiences of shamans and Western schizophrenia patients are not so similar on close examination.

American anthropologist Jane Murphy of Harvard University studied local psychiatric concepts in a village of Yupik-speaking Eskimos on an island in the Bering Sea, and among Yorubas living in rural Nigeria.[50] The languages of both cultures included words for madness. Among the Eskimos, *nuthkavihak* refers to a sickness of the soul or spirit in which sufferers talk to themselves, and scream at people who do not exist. Among the Yoruba, *were* refers to a condition involving hearing voices, laughing at nothing in particular, picking up leaves for no purpose, throwing off clothes and defecating in public.

Another American anthropologist, Richard Noll, compared reports of altered states of consciousness, mainly collected from Native American shamans, with the description of schizophrenia in DSM-III.[51] He argued that, 'By far the most important distinction between shamanic states and schizophrenia is that the shaman voluntarily enters and leaves his altered states of consciousness while the schizophrenic is the helpless victim of his.' Moreover, according to Noll:

The phenomenology of schizophrenia contained in DSM-III ... indicates clearly that the shamanic state of consciousness ... cannot be mistaken for schizophrenic states if the current diagnostic criteria of the latter are assumed to be reliable and the experiential descriptions of the former are accurate.

But, of course, as we have seen in previous chapters, the current diagnostic criteria for schizophrenia are not reliable, and give a biased picture of psychosis. As the majority of people in Western societies who experience psychotic states never come into contact with psychiatric services, many must be capable of the degree of organization necessary to be a healer.

Perhaps the dispute about the relationship between psychosis and shamanism approaches our question about the boundaries of madness in the wrong way. Rather than ask whether psychotic experiences can be valued in some circumstances, we should step backwards and ask *why* certain types of behaviour and experience are singled out as evidence of insanity. As Horacio Fabrega points out, human behavioural breakdowns are nearly always recognized when individuals are unable to participate and function in social life.[52] The apparent consensus between different cultures about madness therefore concerns behaviours and experiences that are associated with an inability to cope with the demands of living. There seems to be an equal lack of consensus about how to describe similar behaviours and experiences when the individual is nonetheless able to lead a fruitful life and get along with others. According to the Kraepelinian paradigm embraced by psychiatrists in the developed world, such people are nonetheless psychotic or schizophrenic. Other cultures, in contrast, allow such people to find valued roles that prevent them from being dismissed as crazy.

Moving the boundaries of madness

Fortunately, we do not have to rely on cross-cultural studies for evidence that the boundaries of madness are culturally determined. Disputes about the positioning of these boundaries have been fought between Western psychiatrists since the earliest days of their profession.

Not many people today would take seriously a suggestion by Dr Samuel Cartwright, published in the *New Orleans Medical and Surgical Journal* of 1851, that *dreapetomania* (an uncontrollable urge to run away observed in American Negro slaves) should be regarded as a medical disorder.[53] More recently, the psychological problems of combat veterans have been variously described as evidence of low moral fibre, nostalgia, shell-shock, battle fatigue, brainwashing or post-traumatic stress disorder (the currently favoured diagnosis) in response to changing attitudes towards warfare.[54] Psychiatric theories about minority sexual preferences have shifted even more dramatically. Homosexuality was listed as a psychiatric disorder in DSM-II but was removed from the diagnostic manual following a referendum of members of the American Psychiatric Association in 1974.[55] Although it might be thought that the psychoses involve such a clear break from reality, and such obvious disability, that they would be immune from similar attempts to redraw the boundaries of psychiatric disorder, a recent experiment in Holland has shown that this is not the case.

Maastricht, a charming city of cobbled streets surrounded by thirteenth-century battlements, was catapulted into the limelight in 1992, when it hosted the signing of the European treaty that now bears its name. In addition to being a venue favoured by European bureaucrats, it is home to the University of Limburg where, until his recent retirement, Marius Romme was a professor of social psychiatry. A tall, white-haired and gentle man, Romme developed his unusual approach to helping people suffering from hallucinations after attempting to treat a 30-year-old female patient whose 'voices' gave her orders, forbade her from doing things, and dominated her life.[56] Severely distressed, she had been diagnosed as suffering from schizophrenia. Neuroleptic drugs had no impact on the voices, but marginally reduced her anxiety. A course of psychotherapy was similarly ineffective. Her attitude towards her hallucinations was unexpectedly transformed, however, by a chance encounter with a book written by an American psychologist, Julian Jaynes.[57]

The book (something of a cult classic in psychology) is called *The Origins of Consciousness in the Breakdown of the Bicameral Mind*, and has a strikingly original thesis. Jaynes proposes that self-reflective consciousness is a recently evolved faculty of the human mind that did not exist in Ancient Greece. According to Jaynes, because the Greeks lacked a concept of 'I', or the self-as-agent, the things they said to themselves when engaged in verbal thought were experienced as being said by gods (which is why they had so many gods).[58] Jaynes noted the similarity between the Ancient Greeks' experiences, and the experiences of modern-day schizophrenia patients, and it was this aspect of the book that had such a dramatic impact on Marius Romme's patient. Embracing the view that hearing voices was an entirely normal experience for the Ancient Greeks, she no longer saw her own experiences as pathological.

Romme and his patient appeared on a popular Dutch television programme and invited viewers who had experienced voices to write to them. Approximately one third of the 450 people who responded said they had little difficulty coping with their voices. As might be expected from the epidemiological evidence that we considered earlier, many had never received psychiatric treatment. When those who had avoided becoming patients were compared with those who had not, the two groups appeared to be remarkably similar. The main difference was that the non-patients saw themselves as stronger than their voices, whereas the patients saw themselves as weaker.[59]

Working with his partner Sondra Escher, a journalist, Romme has organized a national network for Dutch people who hear voices. This provides a forum in which they can meet to discuss their experiences and share ideas. The organization, known as Resonance, encourages people to accept their voices as part of normal human variation rather than as manifestations of disease, and encourages independence from psychiatric services whenever this seems possible.

This startling and quite deliberate attempt to move the boundaries of madness demonstrates that even the experiences normally attributed to schizophrenia *do not have to be* considered pathological. It may be true that hallucinations and delusions are found throughout the world, but whether or not these experiences are seen as evidence of illness appears to vary according to local customs and beliefs.

The NeoKraepelinian Paradigm as a Cultural System

Not surprisingly, anthropologically minded psychiatrists often objected to the picture of psychiatric disorders embodied in early editions of the DSM, not necessarily because they perceived its classification system to be invalid, but because it barely acknowledged the influence of cultural factors on mental health. In response to these kinds of criticisms, the US National Institute of Mental Health set up a task force to develop proposals for including cultural information in

DSM-IV.[60] As a consequence, the fourth edition of the manual contains notes on how culture can influence the expression of psychiatric disorders, and an appendix listing some culture-bound syndromes reported in developing countries. However, many of the recommendations made by the task force were not incorporated.[61] There is very little discussion of the way in which differing social norms can influence the experience and interpretation of symptoms, and the inclusion of culture-bound syndromes in an appendix appeared to give them a marginal status within the system as a whole. The task force's suggestion that two diagnoses widely used in the West, anorexia nervosa and chronic fatigue syndrome, should be described as culture-bound was not taken up.

However, even if the editors of DSM-IV had followed the advice of the task force to the letter, it is not obvious that they would have produced a manual that would be entirely satisfactory from an anthropological perspective. Indeed, the evidence that we have considered in this chapter suggests a radical reappraisal of the entire DSM enterprise. We can now see that *this enterprise is, itself, culture-bound*. It represents the efforts of members of one particular culture to make sense of human behavioural breakdowns.

In an insightful analysis of the relationship between medicine and culture, Arthur Kleinman has argued that medical concepts are always embedded within a cultural system, so that theories of disease (maladaptions or malfunctionings of biological or psychological processes) and illness (the individual's experience of disease) can never be separated from the cultural background.[62] On Kleinman's view, the health care systems of different cultures serve functions that are common to all. They enable individuals to communicate about their experiences; they sanction certain types of behaviour (for example, staying away from work when ill); they guide the choice of health care interventions; and they influence health care practices *per se* (for example the use of herbs, manufactured drugs or psychotherapy).

Kleinman points out that the explanatory models that are used to account for disease and illness often vary between different social groups occupying the same location at the same point in time. In African countries, for example, discrepancies often arise between the explanatory models of ordinary people, traditional healers and a professional elite trained in Western medicine. Kleinman believes that these discrepancies may be impediments to the provision of adequate health care in the poorest regions of the world. In his opinion, Western-trained doctors must therefore attempt to work with indigenous concepts of disease and illness in order to achieve mutually respectful and effective relationships with their patients.

Kleinman's research has focused on explanatory models of psychiatric disorder that are indigenous to China and the Far East. For example, as we shall see later, he has shown that Chinese concepts of mood disorder differ markedly from Western concepts, placing less emphasis on psychological symptoms such as low self-esteem and more emphasis on physical symptoms such as fatigue. Because of this focus, it is all too easy to assume that Kleinman's analysis applies only to non-Western cultures. However, the analysis is just as relevant to the European and North American context as it is to Africa or the Far East. The Kraepelinian paradigm, like the diagnostic system of the Baganda, is a product of a particular social and historical context (the period of German expansionism in the late nineteenth century) and has been moulded into its latest incarnation, DSM-IV, by North American psychiatrists imbued with the values of a powerful scientific and industrialized economy. (Leafing through DSM-IV, it is hard not to feel that the hand of Henry Ford has helped to shape it.)

Towards a Post-Kraepelinian Psychiatry

This chapter concludes the first part of this book, in which I have tried to show the limitations of the Kraepelinian approach to explaining and understanding psychiatric problems. I am sure that social constructionists or extreme cultural relativists, who regard 'reality' as nothing more than an invention of the dominant culture, will particularly welcome the conclusions I have reached in the last few pages. According to this kind of reasoning, a scientific account of madness could never be constructed because there are no facts, free of social interpretation, on which to build a theory.[63]

My own view is that this kind of nihilism is self-defeating. All scientific theories, even those in the physical sciences, are developed in a particular cultural context. Although the context may help to explain the persistence of a theory in the face of apparently falsifying evidence, the fact that a theory arises from a particular context is not sufficient to condemn it. Theories and paradigms must be accepted, modified or rejected on the basis of evidence. Indeed, if we swallow the postmodernist dogma that any theory is as valid as any other, and thereby reject the assumption that standards of scientific evidence lead to the tangible advance of knowledge, it is difficult to see why the arguments I have so far marshalled against the Kraepelinian approach should carry any weight. The main purpose of criticizing outdated theories is not to abandon theories altogether but to replace them with theories that are more useful and more scientific.

The persistence of Kraepelin's paradigm in the face of such overwhelming negative evidence reflects the difficulty of finding an alternative. It is one thing to criticize a theoretical system and quite another to offer something in its place. Despite various proposals for an alternative system (by making diagnoses more sensitive to cross-cultural distinctions, by classifying patients using dimensions rather than categories, by lumping together the psychoses under an *einheitspsychose* concept) none has been enthusiastically embraced by large numbers of clinicians or researchers, mainly because practical versions of these systems have yet to be devised. Although we cannot entirely exclude the possibility that a future Linnaeus of psychiatry will achieve what others have so far been unable to accomplish, I am sceptical whether any new system will succeed where Kraepelin's has failed.

In the remaining chapters of this book, I will therefore describe a more radical alternative. The fundamental principle guiding this approach can be simply stated as follows: *We should abandon psychiatric diagnoses altogether and instead try to explain and understand the actual experiences and behaviours of psychotic people.* By such experiences and behaviours I mean the kinds of things that psychiatrists describe as *symptoms*, but which might be better labelled *complaints*, such as hallucinations, delusions and disordered speech. I will argue that, once these complaints have been explained, there is no ghostly disease remaining that also requires an explanation. Complaints are all there is.

An advantage of this approach is that it does not require us to draw a clear dividing line between madness and sanity. Indeed, when constructing explanations of complaints it is not necessary to assume that they are always pathological. By 'complaint', I just mean any class of behaviour or experience that is singled out as sometimes troublesome and therefore worthy of our attention.

The approach I am advocating has been given various names, none of which is entirely satisfactory. It is most commonly labelled the *symptom-orientated approach*; although I will occasionally use this name in the following chapters, I feel uncomfortable with it because of the medical connotations of the word 'symptom'. The term *cognitive neuropsychiatry* has been suggested by British psychologist Haydn Ellis to describe the attempt to understand psychiatric symptoms using the theories and techniques of cognitive and neuropsychology[64] (we will see what these are in later chapters). Although there is now a journal of this name, and although brains clearly play an important role in unusual behaviours and experiences, I think that the prefixes *cognitive* and *neuro* presume too much. If the new approach needs a label (and perhaps it does not) then *post-Kraepelinian psychiatry* is perhaps as good as any.

Manifestos are probably best left to political parties, but Gerald Klerman's attempt write one for the neoKraepelinian movement[65] has tempted me into constructing one for my fellow post-Kraepelinians. The manifesto (which is given in Table 6.1, and which matches Klerman's almost point by point) tries to accommodate the lessons we have learnt in the past few chapters, and anticipates some ideas that I will introduce later on. It is designed to stimulate debate, and perhaps should not be taken too seriously.

An initial objection that I must overcome

The fundamental idea that I am advocating in this book – studying complaints and abandoning psychiatric diagnoses – is hardly new. It was anticipated in the ideas of Adolf Meyer but, to my knowledge, was first clearly articulated by the British psychologist Donald Bannister in the late 1960s.[66] When I first began to investigate hallucinations and delusions in the mid-1980s, many of my colleagues still seemed to feel that this approach was slightly batty. Recently, however, an increasing number of psychologists and psychiatrists in Europe and North America have begun studying complaints, and this kind of research has been in danger of becoming absorbed into the mainstream of psychiatry. One indication that an idea has arrived is the emergence

Table 6.1 A post-Kraepelinian manifesto.

1. The understanding and treatment of psychiatric problems must be approached from multiple perspectives, including those of the neurosciences, psychology, sociology and anthropology. None of these approaches alone provides a sufficient framework, or has precedence over the other. (Psychiatry is not just a branch of medicine, except in the trivial sense that laws in many countries allow only medical practitioners to call themselves psychiatrists.)

2. Psychiatric practice should use modern scientific methodologies and be based on scientific knowledge.

3. Psychiatric practice involves the treatment of people who are distressed by psychological complaints, or who are having difficulty coping with the demands of everyday life. In some circumstances, experiences such as hallucinations, unconventional beliefs, or thinking that appears bizarre to others, occur in people who are not distressed, and who are functioning well. Such people should not be encouraged to seek psychiatric treatment.

4. There is no clear boundary between mental health and mental illness. Psychological complaints exist on continua with normal behaviours and experiences. Where we draw the line between sanity and madness is a matter of opinion.

5. There are no discrete mental illnesses. Categorial diagnoses fail to capture adequately the nature of psychological complaints for either research or clinical purposes.

6. There is no inseparable gulf between the psychological and the biological. Adequate theories of psychological complaints must show how psychological and biological accounts are interrelated. (An exclusive focus on biological determinants of psychological complaints is bad science and leads to treatments that fail to meet the needs of psychiatric patients.)

7. Research into psychological complaints must start from a detailed description of those complaints. Such descriptions should be reliable and valid.

8. Efforts should be made to understand the psychological mechanisms underlying psychological complaints. Specification of those mechanisms is likely to lead to an understanding of the aetiological role of both social and biological factors.

9. Psychological complaints must be understood as endpoints of developmental pathways, which are determined by complex interactions between endogenous and environmental processes.

of a thoughtful critical response. As I was completing the first draft of this chapter, an article criticizing symptom-orientated research appeared in the *British Journal of Psychiatry*.

Ramin Mojtabai and Ronald Rieder, two psychiatrists working at the College of Physicians and Surgeons at Columbia University in New York, make three general points.[67] Their first concerns reliability – they argue that clinicians and researchers often show less agreement when deciding whether a patient has a particular symptom than when deciding whether a patient fits a particular diagnosis. Second, they argue that genetic studies show that the heritability of symptoms is less than the heritability of diagnoses (in other words, clearer genetic effects are found when patients are selected according to diagnoses rather than according to symptoms). Finally, they argue that studies of symptoms have revealed nothing about the aetiology of psychiatric disorders. The second and third of these arguments will be addressed in later chapters. However, it is important to deal with the question of reliability here because, if Mojtabai and Rieder are correct, this objection would be fatal to my argument. Obviously, an approach focusing on complaints will get nowhere if we cannot decide who is experiencing which complaint.

Mojtabai and Rieder present data from three American studies in which the reliability of symptoms yielded average kappa values of 0.62, 0.40 and 0.49. At face value, these results are certainly disappointing. Fortunately, they almost certainly underestimate what can be achieved, even with conventional psychiatric interview schedules. A recent study using the Positive and Negative Syndromes Schedule, a widely used interview-based method for rating the severity of psychotic disorders, showed that the reliability of symptom ratings improves when clinicians are given appropriate training. After five sessions of training, kappa exceeded 0.90 for seventeen out of thirty symptoms, and exceeded 0.70 for all but one.[68]

When instruments especially designed to measure specific complaints have been evaluated, high levels of inter-rater reliability have consistently been achieved. At the Mental Health Research Institute of Victoria, in Melbourne, Australia, a group led by Professor David Copolov has developed an interview schedule for assessing unusual perceptions, particularly hallucinations; a study showed that kappa values for each of the subscales (measuring different aspects of hallucinations, for example physical and emotional characteristics of hallucinated voices) varied between 0.81 and 0.98.[69] In Britain, a somewhat simpler interview-based scale for rating features of hallucinations and delusions has been developed by Gill Haddock, a clinical psychologist based at the University of Manchester. In field trials, this instrument has been shown to yield levels of inter-rater reliability for its various subscales that reach a minimum of 0.79.[70] Several instruments are available to measure the thought, language and communication disorders of psychotic patients, for example Nancy Andreasen's Thought, Language and Communication Scale[71] and Nancy Docherty's Communication Disturbance Index,[72] both of which have been shown to have acceptable levels of reliability. Mojtabai and Rieder's pessimism about the measurement of complaints seems to reflect a biased reading of the evidence.

No doubt many readers will be as sceptical about focusing on complaints as Mojtabai and Rieder, although perhaps for different reasons. In the following parts of this book I will therefore lay out the framework of post-Kraepelinian psychiatry in some detail, describing research on depression, paranoia, mania, hallucinations and disordered speech. I will then explore the implications of this research for aetiological theories of psychosis. In this way, I will attempt to demonstrate that the approach that I am advocating leads to a richer understanding of the nature and origins of psychiatric disorder than has been possible within the Kraepelinian paradigm.

Part Two

A Better Picture of the Soul

7

The Significance of Biology

We are not interested in the fact that the brain has the consistency of cold porridge.

Alan Turing[1]

In the first part of this book I have offered a damning portrait of Kraepelinian psychiatry. By examining the taxonomic assumptions that have underpinned modern theories of psychosis, I have argued that the conventional approach to understanding madness is deeply flawed. This is the reason why there has been so little progress in the treatment of psychiatric disorders since the time of Kraepelin. Most researchers and clinicians have been stuck at the end of the blind alley into which he led us over a century ago.

It is now time for me to make good my earlier promise that I would demonstrate a workable alternative to the Kraepelinian system. In the remaining parts of this book, I will therefore show how psychological theories can be used to explain many of the strange behaviours and experiences ('symptoms') encountered both inside and outside the psychiatric clinic. As I have already stated, my approach will be to examine each of these behaviours and experiences in turn. I will therefore make no attempt to explain schizophrenia, manic depression or any of the other myths of twentieth-century medicine. Instead, I will show how psychological research can cast light on phenomena such as hallucinatory voices, depressed mood, delusional beliefs, manic episodes and incoherent speech.

Before we start, however, we should do some groundwork. In earlier chapters I have argued that psychotic behaviours and experiences lie on continua with normal behaviours and experiences. One implication of this argument is that the processes that govern ordinary mental life may well play an important role in psychosis. Indeed, it seems very unlikely that we will be able to develop a useful account of madness unless we first have an adequate understanding of human nature. The purpose of the next few chapters is to provide the framework for such an understanding.

Unfortunately, there is not space within these pages to give the reader a comprehensive review of what is known about human psychology, a field that is in any case changing daily. However, what I can do is focus on a small number of topics that have important implications for the way in which we attempt to explain madness. In the process, I will demonstrate how some of the theories of schizophrenia and manic depression proposed by neoKraepelinians have often failed, not only because they have been based on an unworkable system of classification, but also because they have accepted, as self-evident, assumptions about the human mind that are in fact erroneous. The general theme that I want to address is that the brain, the mind and human emotions cannot be understood in isolation from their social context.

We will begin by considering what many regard to be the most fundamental question in psychology: the relationships between brain, behaviour and experience. This topic is important because any coherent account of psychosis must accommodate both the findings from neurobiological research and the results of psychological investigations. That this is not a trivial problem is attested to by the fact that most researchers who have studied psychiatric disorders have treated these two types of explanation as irreconcilable.

The Interminable Debate

From the very beginnings of their calling, many psychiatrists have assumed that biological explanations of psychosis should somehow take precedence over psychological accounts. For example, when Wilhelm Griesinger founded the *Archives for Psychiatry and Nervous Disease* in 1867, he penned an opening editorial, which stated that:

Psychiatry has undergone a transformation in its relation to the rest of medicine. This transformation rests principally on the realization that patients with so-called 'mental illnesses' are really individuals with illnesses of the nerves and brain.[2]

Nearly a century later, in their famous account of *Th*
Years of Psychiatry, published in 1963, psychiatrists Ri
and Ida MacAlpine argued that: 'The lesson of the history
is that progress is inevitable and irrevocable from psychol
ogy, from mind to brain, never the other way round.'[3] Similarly, in
the 1975 edition of an influential British textbook of psychiatry, the
following remarks can be found:

It would be absurd to maintain that psychology can be to psychiatry what
physiology is to medicine, not only because the claim would be exaggerated,
but also because it implies that psychiatry and medicine are mere cousin-
sciences ... The primary concern of the psychiatrist is the morbid mental
states; and however much is known about the psychology of the normal
individual, in the pathological field new laws will be found to operate.[4]

More recently, Samuel Guze, a prominent neoKraepelinian, has simply
stated that: 'There can be no such thing as a psychiatry that is too
biological.'[5] It is clear, therefore, that psychiatrists' recent preoccupation with biological determinants of psychosis, emphasized in proposition 6 of Gerald Klerman's manifesto (see Table 3.3, p. 59), was
the culmination of a historical trend within the profession.

A curious parallel exists between these assertions and the arguments
put forward by some prominent anti-psychiatrists. Both groups, it
seems, have assumed that the criterion for disease is some kind of
pathology in the brain, and that disputes about the boundaries of
madness can therefore be solved by reference to biological data. However, whereas the biological psychiatrists have assumed that neuropathology will inevitably be found in patients (if it has not been found
already), the anti-psychiatrists have assumed that it is non-existent.
Thomas Szasz, perhaps America's most controversial critic of
psychiatry, is best known for taking this position.

Born in Budapest in 1920, Szasz qualified as a psychiatrist and
psychoanalyst in the United States and has been Professor of Psychiatry
at the State University of New York, Syracuse, since 1956. He first
stated his now infamous position in a 1960 paper entitled 'The myth
of mental illness',* which was published in the *American Psychologist*,

---

* According to Kleinman's distinction between illness and disease (as discussed in
the last chapter), Szasz's argument is against the concept of mental *disease*.
However, I will stick with Szasz's terminology here.

ιe professional journal of the American Psychological Association.[6] This has been followed by a long series of articles and books that have addressed the same theme in different ways. In contrast to those of Ronald Laing, Szasz's ideas appear to have been little influenced by his clinical experience; he offers few insights into the nature of psychosis. Rather, his arguments have been directed against the *logic* and ethics of biological psychiatry. Because Szasz's opponents have often misunderstood these arguments, it is worth examining them in detail.

The argument outlined in 'The myth of mental illness' falls into two parts. Szasz's first and most important claim is that the concept of mental illness is incoherent. His starting point is the work of the nineteenth-century physiologist Rudolf Virchow, who defined illness in terms of the presence of a lesion in the body. According to this definition, if mental illness is truly illness, it should be associated with some kind of physical pathology, which is most likely to be located in the brain. So far, Szasz's position is entirely consistent with that of the neoKraepelinians. However, Szasz further notes that, in modern times, disorders of the brain are usually considered to be the province of neurology and therefore that the defining feature of a *mental* illness is the absence of physical pathology. For this reason, he claims, mental illness cannot be illness in any real sense of the word 'illness'. On Szasz's view, talk of mental illness is self-contradictory, in much the same way that describing someone as a 'married bachelor' or a 'meat-eating vegetarian' would be self-contradictory.

Szasz's second claim concerns the role that the concept of 'mental illness' plays in industrialized societies. Following his argument that this concept is incoherent, Szasz is moved to ask why it has been so readily accepted by mental health professionals and the general public. He argues that a diagnosis of mental illness allows a kind of moral sleight-of-hand, apparently justifying the control of individuals who are a nuisance to others but who are not law-breakers. Once diagnosed as 'mentally ill', such individuals can be coerced into undergoing 'treatment' so that they will conform more fully to the social norms. On this view, psychiatrists, psychologists and psychiatric nurses belong to a kind of police force that controls and limits the amount of deviance within society.

This second part of Szasz's argument has often been erroneously identified with the political left. In fact, Szasz's views build on a tradition of right-wing libertarianism that is familiar to North Americans but which often seems alien to Europeans. Szasz believes that the state should have a minimal role in regulating the conduct of individuals. He therefore argues that recreational drugs should be legalized,[7] and that the right to commit suicide should be respected.[8] At the same time, he opposes the use of the insanity defence in court cases, because 'Excusing a person of responsibility for an otherwise criminal act on the basis of inability to form conscious intent is an act of legal mercy masquerading as an act of medical science.'[9] Although he has objected to compulsory psychiatric treatment, he has stated that he has no objection to psychiatry between consenting adults.[10]

Not surprisingly, Szasz's ideas have earned him the opprobrium of many of his colleagues. Five years after the publication of 'The myth of mental illness', Frederick Glaser wrote in the *American Journal of Psychiatry*: 'The question will inevitably be raised whether sanctions of some form ought to be taken against Dr Szasz, not only because of the content of his views but because of the manner in which he presents them.'[11]

Some saw Szasz's arguments as part of a wider anti-establishment conspiracy. Commenting on the anti-psychiatry movement in general, British psychiatrist Sir Martin Roth (co-author of the 1975 textbook that sought to distance psychiatry from psychology) suggested that:

The anti-medical critique of psychiatry represents one approach within a wider movement which has assumed international proportions and adopts a critical or derogatory stance towards psychiatry's methods, aims and social role; it is anti-medical, anti-therapeutic, anti-institutional and anti-scientific, either by expressed aims or implicitly through the dogmatic, hortatory, diffuse and inconsistent character of its utterances.[12]

Of course, these objections are very emotional and tell us little about the merits of Szasz's position, which deserves a more dispassionate analysis.

Scientific evidence that madness is associated with neuropathology should be problematic for Szasz and other critics of the Kraepelinian paradigm but comforting to neoKraepelinians. Few of Szasz's early opponents rose to this obvious challenge, perhaps because biological research into madness was still in its infancy at the time that 'The myth of mental illness' was written. In the four decades since, however, there have been substantial advances in the technologies available to biological researchers and there can be no doubt that these have provided encouragement to those who have continued to see psychiatry as a branch of physical medicine. It will be helpful to take a look at some of these developments, not only to facilitate our evaluation of the merits of the contrasting positions taken by Szasz and the neoKraepelinians, but also so that we can form an opinion about the achievements of biological psychiatry.

Before commencing this task I should point out that the following review is not intended to be comprehensive. Studies of brain biology have become so complex that it would be difficult to encompass them within a single book, let alone a single chapter. In the present context we must therefore focus more on the implications of biological investigations of psychosis than on the details of individual studies. In particular, what we need to establish is whether studies that point to apparent abnormalities in the brains of psychotic patients leave any room for theories of madness that have a more psychological flavour.

Psychotic Brains

Although it has long been known that the brain is the organ responsible for thought and feeling, its anatomy and physiology only began to be properly appreciated in the nineteenth century, largely as a result of the efforts of the early biological psychiatrists. Their work revealed that the brain consists of billions of small nerve cells, known as *neurones*, which are connected together into circuits of almost unimaginable complexity. These are surrounded by an even larger number of *glial* cells, which have metabolic functions, and which help to determine the overall structure of the brain.

At the time of these major advances in neuroscience, it was widely believed that electrical impulses were responsible for the transmission of information within the brain, a belief that had been fostered by Galvani, Volta and others in the eighteenth century, who had shown that nerves could be stimulated by electricity. The invention of the electroencephalogram (EEG) by the German psychiatrist Hans Berger in the 1920s allowed the first recordings of electrical activity from electrodes placed on the human scalp, which appeared to confirm this hypothesis. Our current understanding that the transmission of information *within* the neurone is electrical, but that neurones communicate by means of chemicals, known as *neurotransmitters*, is therefore surprisingly recent. Although Otto Loewi and Henry Dale received the Nobel Prize for medicine in 1936 for their demonstration that the peripheral nervous system utilizes noradrenaline and acetylcholine,[13] the idea that neurotransmitters played an important role in the central nervous system only became widely accepted in the 1960s.[14]

At the moment, neuroscience is again a rapidly expanding field of inquiry, and many different methods of investigation are currently being employed. In what follows I will restrict myself to the three approaches that have been pursued most vigorously by modern biological psychiatrists: studies of the gross anatomical structure of the brain, investigations of activity in different brain regions, and finally examination of the brain's biochemical composition. I will also focus mainly on studies of schizophrenia patients, as other diagnostic groups within the psychotic spectrum have been much less intensively investigated.

The anatomy of madness

Perhaps the most obvious way of searching for a biological substrate of madness is to look at the brains of mad people. Kraepelin advocated post-mortem studies for this purpose, and encouraged his colleague Alois Alzheimer to pursue this line of research. Although he accepted Alzheimer's conclusion that the brains of dead psychotic patients looked more or less normal, this did not stop him from asserting that, in dementia praecox, 'Partial damage to, or destruction of, cells of the cerebral cortex must probably occur, which may be compensated for in some cases, but which mostly brings in its wake a singular, permanent impairment of the inner life.'[15]

Since Kraepelin's time, post-mortem studies have been pursued with sporadic enthusiasm but without consistent results. This is no doubt partly because, as we have seen, schizophrenia is an incoherent concept, so that patients who receive the diagnosis are likely to have acquired their symptoms as a consequence of a number of distinct aetiological processes, but also because of the methodological difficulties encountered in this kind of work. The brains studied, which are usually taken from the bodies of elderly patients, may not represent psychotic brains in general, and may have been damaged by whatever factors were responsible for the patients' deaths. Following death, decay progressively alters brain tissue and these changes become more marked with time. Add in the difficulty of finding comparable brains from ordinary people who died at the same age of similar causes, and which have been stored after death for a similar period under identical conditions, and it is easy to see why repeatable findings have been elusive.[16]

Interestingly enough, the observation that has been most often replicated is a negative one. At any stage in life after the end of the second trimester of foetal development, neuronal damage (for example, as a consequence of infection or injury) leads to a proliferation of glial cells, accompanied by a rise in associated enzymes and proteins – a process known as *gliosis*. Most studies that have looked for gliosis in the brains of patients have failed to find it,[17] suggesting that damage to the brain after birth is unlikely to play an important role in psychosis. This inference, which is not uncritically accepted by all neuropathologists who agree with the basic observation,[18] has in turn led to the suggestion that some kind of foetal brain damage prior to the end of the second trimester may be responsible (a proposal we will consider in detail in a later chapter).

A more promising approach is to study the brains of living patients. Early methods of imaging the living nervous system followed from Röntgen's discovery of X-rays in 1895.[19] These included angiography (in which an X-ray-opaque medium is injected into the cerebral arteries), which was developed in the 1930s by the Portuguese neurosurgeon (and one time foreign minister) Egas Moniz. Moniz's invention was an important medical breakthrough, because it allowed neurosurgeons to locate cerebral tumours with precision for the first time. The same cannot be said of his more famous invention, the prefrontal leucotomy operation given to thousands of unfortunate schizophrenia patients, for which he was awarded a Nobel Prize in 1949. (In one of the more ironical twists in the history of psychiatry, Moniz was shot dead by a disgruntled leucotomy patient in 1955.)

Godfrey Hounsfield, a British engineer whose work for Electrical and Musical Industries (EMI) Ltd heralded the modern era of brain imaging, was a more deserving recipient of the Prize. In 1970,

Hounsfield introduced computed tomography (CT) scanning, which allowed X-ray information taken from different angles to be integrated into a single image depicting a slice through the body. Although this was a revolutionary step forward, the achievements of CT scanning have recently been surpassed by even more advanced technologies, which make similar use of computers to construct complex images. Perhaps the most important of these is magnetic resonance imaging (MRI), which uses strong magnetic fields to provoke a discharge of radio waves from the body, and which is better than CT at imaging the soft tissues of the brain. MRI scans now generate breathtakingly beautiful three-dimensional pictures of the brain that can be rotated and inspected from different angles.

Studies employing these *structural imaging* technologies have reported a variety of abnormalities in the brains of psychotic patients, including enlargement of the sulci (crevices in the folded tissue of the cortex), focal lesions in different cortical areas, and atypical asymmetries of the cerebral hemispheres. Most researchers, however, have focused their attention on the fluid-filled ventricles in the centre of the brain, perhaps because these were the only anatomical structures that were adequately revealed by early CT scans (see Figures 7.1 and 7.2).

The earliest CT study of psychotic patients was carried out by

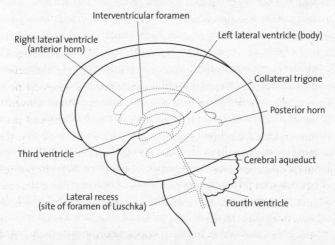

Figure 7.1 The cerebral ventricles (reproduced from K. W. Walsh (1978) *Neuropsychology: A Clinical Approach*. Edinburgh: Churchill Livingstone).

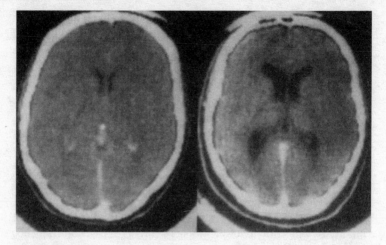

Figure 7.2 CT scans showing the cerebral ventricles in a healthy individual, left, and a patient with a diagnosis of schizophrenia, right (reproduced from N. C. Andreasen (2001) *Brave New Brain: Conquering Mental Illness in the Era of the Genome*. Oxford: Oxford University Press).

Eve Johnstone, Tim Crow and their colleagues at Northwick Park Hospital, near London, who used the first scanner to become available in Britain.[20] They reported that a small group of chronically ill schizophrenia patients had significantly larger lateral ventricles than a comparison group of ordinary people. Later studies conducted in several different countries appeared to replicate this finding, implying that schizophrenia patients suffer from some kind of loss of volume in the cerebral cortex.[21] As some of these findings were obtained from patients who had only recently become ill and who had not been treated with medication,[22] some researchers have inferred that brain disease is present at the very beginnings of psychosis. In the light of the inconsistent neuropathological evidence, it has also been argued that this loss of volume reflects a reduction in the size of neurones and the interconnections between them, rather than a loss of neurones *per se*.[23]

On closer inspection, however, the CT and structural MRI data are more ambiguous. In all studies, substantial variations in ventricular size have been observed in both patients and ordinary people. Moreover, some studies have failed to find evidence of significant ventricular enlargement, presumably because people who receive the diagnosis of schizophrenia form a heterogeneous group.[24] However, enlarged ventricles have been recorded in studies of bipolar patients and patients suffering from unipolar (simple) depression, although, again, findings have varied substantially from study to study.[25] When mood disorder patients and schizophrenia patients have been compared, little evidence of difference has been found.[26] It is therefore unlikely that ventricular enlargement (even if we can be sure that it is present in some patients) is uniquely associated with schizophrenia.

Some of the inconsistencies in the data probably reflect problems that are unique to this kind of research. For all the precision of CT and MRI, it can be difficult to calculate the exact volume of the cerebral ventricles. A further and perhaps more fundamental obstacle is the difficulty of finding appropriately matched non-psychotic people who are willing to be scanned. In 1986 two Canadian researchers, Geoffrey Smith and William Iacano, highlighted this problem by reanalysing the results from twenty-one studies then available, splitting them into those studies that had found differences between schizophrenia patients and controls and those that had not.[27] The average ventricular size of the *patients* in the two sets of studies was about the same, but the control participants in the studies that did report a difference had smaller ventricles than the control participants in the studies that did not. It seemed that those studies that reported abnormally large ventricles in schizophrenia patients did so because they recruited controls (often patients attending hospital for neurological tests whose brain scans were judged to be normal) who had ventricles that were unusually small! Not surprisingly, later studies, using larger samples and more carefully matched controls, have found more modest differences between patients and ordinary people.[28]

The importance of recruiting adequately matched controls is underscored by studies which have shown that ventricular volume is affected by factors such as sex, age, head size, educational achievement, social class, ethnicity, alcohol consumption, water retention and even pregnancy.[29] As some of these sources of variation can change with time, it should not be surprising that ventricular volume can vary between one occasion and another. A recent study found that some psychotic patients who at first appeared to have large ventricles showed a *reduction* of ventricular volume to within normal limits when scans were repeated at a later date.[30]

By offering an unapologetically sceptical account of the research on ventricular enlargement, I do not mean to imply that structural imaging studies are always uninformative. As investigations have become progressively more sophisticated, subtler differences between the brains of psychotic patients and ordinary people have been reported.[31] However, even if these findings – or any other observations of atypical brain structure – prove to be replicable, we should be cautious when making inferences about the aetiology of psychosis. Psychological changes are always accompanied by changes in the brain. Each new skill, or piece of information that we learn, is accompanied by the creation of new neural circuits that make new patterns of behaviour possible.[32] These changes reflect the endless interaction between ourselves and the physical and social environment in which we live. Put crudely, our brains are constantly being rewired in response to our experiences.

This process can result in anatomical changes that are large enough to be detected by a scanner. For example, several studies have shown that the volume of the hippocampus (an area of the brain that plays an important role in memory) is reduced in people who experience post-traumatic stress following warfare or sexual assault.[33] Other studies have shown that the corpus callosum and other anatomical structures are reduced in volume in children who have been victims of sexual or emotional abuse.[34] Experience can also cause brain structures to *increase* in size. As I was completing this chapter, a research group at the Institute of Neurology in London published the results of a study of London taxi drivers. They reported that the posterior hippocampus becomes enlarged as taxi drivers struggle to acquire a detailed knowledge of the geography of London.[35]

Plainly, these findings do not imply that post-traumatic stress can be adequately understood as a disorder of the brain. It is better thought of as a psychological reaction to adverse events that manifests itself, at the biological level, as changes in brain structure. Perhaps some of the structural abnormalities observed in the brains of psychotic patients are similarly products of unfortunate experiences. (It is not difficult to believe, for example, that the richness of the early social environment affects cortical volume and thereby the size of the cerebral ventricles, a hypothesis that would be consistent with the lack of gliosis observed in neuropathological studies, and the suggestion that the loss of volume observed in some patients reflects changes in the synaptic connections between neurones rather than in their number.) Only research that focuses specifically on aetiological factors (which we will consider later in the book) can establish whether this is the case, or whether the abnormally shaped brains of psychotic patients are evidence of some kind of early biological insult.

The glimmer of enlightenment

The second type of biological investigation that we will consider involves measuring brain activity in the hope of discovering which regions are involved in different psychological functions. Surprisingly, perhaps, studies of this kind considerably predate the development of the new neuroimaging technologies. For example, Anglo Mosso, a nineteenth-century Italian physiologist, was able to observe blood pulsations in a peasant who had suffered damage to an area of the skull lying over the frontal lobes.[36] Mosso asked his subject to perform mental calculations, observed an increase in the pulsations, and concluded that this was probably caused by increased blood flow to this region of the brain.

Hans Berger's invention of the electroencephalogram at the beginning of the last century enabled regional brain activity to be quantified for the first time. Recall that neurones create electrical potentials, which are involved in the transmission of information within the cell. The synchrony or asynchrony of this activity in many cells results in gross electrical potentials that can be detected on the scalp. It is possible to use these potentials to gain some general indication of changes in activity in the underlying regions of the cerebral cortex. Often the results of these investigations are fairly uninformative. (When I worked in a high security hospital after qualifying as a clinical psychologist in the mid-1980s, EEGs were routinely taken from patients. The reports made by the electroencephalographer usually made vague reference to 'possible' and 'non-specific' abnormalities and were almost always useless for clinical purposes.) However, under well-controlled experimental conditions, EEGs can reveal quite specific information about brain functioning. One approach is to measure the *evoked potentials* that are detected in different brain regions when a stimulus is presented many times over. By averaging across the many presentations, it is possible to remove random noise from the EEG record, and thereby obtain a recording of the specific neural response evoked by the stimulus.

Functional imaging has been revolutionized by more recent developments in scanning technology. Two methods now widely used by researchers are positron emission tomography (PET)[37] and functional magnetic resonance imaging (fMRI).[38] In the case of PET, the volunteer is injected with a radioactive substance (for example, glucose that has been 'radio-labelled'), which is drawn to those parts of the brain that use most energy. From there, the substance emits positrons, which almost immediately decay into two photons travelling in opposite directions. These are detected by a scanner surrounding the skull, which consists of a large number of crystals that scintillate when struck by the photons. By detecting which pairs of crystals scintillate together, the scanner is able to 'see' where the photons originated from, thereby identifying those brain regions to which the substance has been drawn. Although very precise, PET has several disadvantages. Because the radioactive isotopes employed by PET have very short half-lives, they have to be created on-site using expensive equipment. Also, of course, there are health hazards associated with introducing radioactive substances into the body, however short-lived.

The more recently developed fMRI approach, which capitalizes on the relationship between blood flow and brain activity first described by Mosso, is less hazardous than PET. As in structural MRI, a strong magnetic field is used to stimulate molecules in the body. However, fMRI makes use of the fact that oxygenated blood, which surges to different parts of the brain as they become active, responds with a stronger MRI signal than deoxygenated blood. It is therefore possible to use this blood-oxygen-level-dependent (BOLD) response to detect those brain regions that are most active at any point in time. In practice, the process of experimentation is rather similar to that for PET. Typically, a volunteer is asked to lie in a scanner and to perform a series of tasks in response to various cues and instructions. Outside the scanner, the researchers watch a video monitor and see an image of the volunteer's brain, which is coloured to indicate which regions are most active.

PET and fMRI are such dazzling technologies that it is easy to regard them as a kind of magic. A person thinks and regions of her brain begin to glow. In fact, the successful conduct of this kind of experiment requires considerable forethought. Tasks must be chosen to reflect the kinds of psychological functions that are of special interest. Moreover, the brain activity measured when the volunteer performs the task must be compared with the activity observed when the brain is doing something else. (The choice of the 'off-task' can dramatically affect the observations made when the volunteer performs the 'on-task'. The best kind of off-task is identical to the on-task except that the psychological function of interest is not involved.) In short, the success of functional imaging studies usually depends on having a reasonable understanding of the psychological processes that are being imaged. In the absence of such an understanding, functional neuro-imaging research is somewhat reminiscent of the nineteenth-century pseudoscience of phrenology, which tried to locate mental functions in different regions of the brain by mapping bumps on the scalp.

Psychiatrists and psychologists have attempted to use these technologies to test theories about the role of abnormal brain activity in psychosis. One line of research has been driven by the observation that the left and right sides of the normal brain have different functions. This phenomenon, known as *cerebral lateralization*, was known to neurologists in the nineteenth century, and was enthusiastically researched by neuropsychologists throughout the 1970s and 1980s. (Roger Sperry, the only psychologist to receive the Nobel Prize for medicine, was responsible for many of the most important studies of lateralization carried out during this period.) Looking downwards from above the brain, the two cerebral hemispheres stand out as the most prominent anatomical structures. In most people, the left hemisphere is said to be dominant because language functions are located there (damage to the right side of the brain usually results in much less language impairment than damage to the left) and because most people are right-handed (each hemisphere controls the hand on the opposite side, so right-handedness implies left dominance). In 1969, a Canadian psychiatrist, Pierre Flor-Henry, suggested that epileptic patients who had schizophrenia symptoms usually had left hemisphere or bilateral damage to their brains, whereas those that had mood disorder usually had damage to the right. This led him to argue that cerebral lateralization might be abnormal in psychotic patients.[39]

The idea that atypical lateralization is implicated in psychosis is still favoured by some researchers. However, there is now a plethora of theories about how this leads to symptoms. Some have argued that dominance may be less marked or even reversed in psychotic people, so that the functions of the hemispheres are less clearly differentiated than in ordinary people. One version of this hypothesis suggests that schizophrenia patients hear voices when the left hemisphere detects speech emanating from the normally silent right.[40] Another theory suggests that it is not the relative dominance of the hemispheres that is important, but the way in which they are connected and work together. Perhaps the boldest account of the relationship between lateralization and psychosis has been proposed by Tim Crow, who argues that schizophrenia is a price paid by humanity for the gift of language.[41] According to Crow, the genes that are responsible for determining language specialization by one hemisphere (usually the left) are also responsible for schizophrenia. (Crow takes the much disputed WHO claim that the incidence of schizophrenia is constant across the world, which we considered in Chapter 6, to support his view that it is 'a disease (perhaps the disease) of humanity',[42] and that the genetic mutation that leads to psychosis is as old as humanity itself.)

One observation that seems to be consistent with the abnormal lateralization hypothesis is a high rate of mixed-handedness in schizophrenia patients compared to ordinary people.[43] Also consistent with Crow's particular version of the theory is recent structural scanning study data indicating that the slight anatomical differences between the hemispheres seen in ordinary people are absent in some schizophrenia patients.[44] However, studies using EEG have yielded complex findings that do not lead to any simple interpretation, so that, in the words of Raquel Gur of the University of Pennsylvania, 'One may vacillate . . . between being overwhelmed by the amount of data that have converged on the issue of laterality in schizophrenia and feeling some exasperation at the paucity of solid answers for questions that seem quite rudimentary.'[45]

In an attempt to make sense of this evidence, including the results of his own research conducted over several decades, psychologist John Gruzelier of Imperial College London has suggested that different kinds of abnormal lateralization are related to different types of complaints.[46] He has argued that *active symptoms* of psychosis (by which he means over-activity, pressure of speech, mania and paranoia) reflect the excessive dominance of the left-hemisphere functions, and an under-activation of the right. He attributes symptoms of social and emotional withdrawal, on the other hand, to the excessive dominance of right-hemisphere functions and an under-activation of the left hemisphere. Interestingly, Gruzelier's analysis of the evidence led him to conclude that these abnormal patterns of activation are reduced when patients' symptoms improve following drug treatment.

Strangely, studies of brain lateralization in psychosis have rarely been conducted using the newer functional imaging techniques. These technologies have been associated with a quite different theory of abnormal brain function, known as the *hypofrontality hypothesis*. In a study published in 1974, Swedish researchers David Ingvar and Goran Franzen used an early version of PET to obtain crude measures of regional blood flow in the brains of a small group of chronically ill schizophrenia patients. Although the results from the patients were broadly normal, two important observations were noted. First, there seemed to be reduced blood flow to the anterior (front) portions of the brains of the schizophrenia patients in comparison with the healthy controls (hypofrontality). Second, the increase in blood flow to these regions detected when the controls were asked to perform certain mental tasks was not observed in the schizophrenia patients.[47]

The hypofrontality hypothesis has enjoyed mixed support since Ingvar and Franzen's initial observations. In a recent review, Peter Liddle was able to find thirty-five studies in which blood flow had been measured while schizophrenia patients were resting, and found that hypofrontality was reported in only a minority of these.[48] However, Ingvar and Franzen's report of attenuated activation when schizophrenia patients engage in some kind of mental task has, to some extent, been supported by later investigations.

In an influential study by Daniel Weinberger and his colleagues at the National Institute for Mental Health in Washington, schizophrenia patients and normal controls were administered a psychological test, known as the Wisconsin Card Sort. This test requires participants to sort cards marked with complex shapes according to a rule known by the tester. The tester gives feedback as the test proceeds, allowing the participant gradually to formulate a hypothesis about the unknown rule. Consequently, their performance gradually improves. However, every so often, the tester changes the rule without informing the participant. The ability to shift to the new rule in these circumstances is thought to involve neural circuits located in the frontal cortex, as patients with damage to this area lack this kind of cognitive flexibility. Consistent with the hypofrontality hypothesis, the schizophrenia patients in Weinberger's study performed poorly on the Wisconsin test and, in comparison with ordinary people, showed less increased activation of the frontal cortex as they attempted it.[49] Other researchers have since reported similar findings, but have also demonstrated that hypofrontality is only present when patients are acutely ill, and is absent (or at least much reduced) when patients have recovered.[50] It is not yet clear whether hypofrontality is restricted to schizophrenia patients, as adequate investigations have yet to be conducted with patients diagnosed as suffering from bipolar disorder.[51]

It would be foolish to underestimate the impact that functional neuroimaging is having on our understanding of the brain. As these technologies have become more routinely available, studies of abnormal neuroactivations in psychiatric patients have become more fashionable. Recent investigations have often focused on specific symptoms of psychosis rather than poorly defined diagnostic categories, and are therefore consistent with the approach that I am advocating in this book. (Although the main thrust of this book is psychological, in later chapters I will describe some of these experiments.) However, once again, caution is required when attempting to infer the causes of psychosis from the results of these experiments.

Most importantly – and this may seem an elementary point – the results of functional neuroimaging studies depend on how the participants attempt the prescribed psychological tasks. Abnormal activations in patients may simply reflect the fact that they are not cooperating, are poorly motivated, or are doing something else. In fact, as we will see in the next chapter, psychiatric patients often are poorly motivated when attempting psychological tests such as the Wisconsin Card Sort, and their performance can sometimes be dramatically improved by providing them with an incentive. Suspicion that this kind of problem can affect neuroimaging research is fuelled by the observation that hypofrontal patients sometimes show normal brain activations after a course of appropriate training on the relevant psychological tests.[52]

As in the case of structural abnormalities, abnormal brain activity may, in the end, turn out to be a consequence of adverse experience rather than a product of some kind of biological insult or malfunction. Evidence that supports this supposition is available from studies of people who have suffered from early trauma. It has been found, for example, that survivors of sexual and emotional abuse show abnormal left-hemisphere activity as measured by EEG, and reduced activation of the left hemisphere compared to the right as measured by fMRI.[53]

The chemistry of madness

We turn finally to the chemical processes that underlie the changing neural activity detected in functional imaging experiments. For readers who are not already familiar with the basic facts of neurotransmission, the following is a brief summary (and see Figure 7.3).

We have already seen that neurones influence other neurones by means of chemicals known as neurotransmitters. These are secreted across the special junctions where one neurone meets another, known as *synapses*. At the receiving end of each synapse there are structures, known as *receptors*, which are proteins to which the neurotransmitter binds. Complex biochemical processes are then involved in the 're-uptake' of the neurotransmitter from the synaptic gap. When a post-synaptic neurone is stimulated by a neurotransmitter in this way, an electrical potential is created within the cell. These potentials, summating from several firings of a pre-synaptic neurone or of a number of pre-synaptic neurones, determine whether the post-synaptic neurone fires in turn, releasing neurotransmitters where it synapses with other neurones further along the circuit. It is the combined action of large numbers of neurones, working together in this way, which allows the brain to process input from the environment, integrate information, and command co-ordinated behaviour.

Different brain circuits use different neurotransmitters. The most intensively researched are acetylcholine, gamma-aminobutyric acid (GABA), glycine, serotonin (5-hydroxytryptamine), noradrenaline and dopamine. However, a large number of peptides may also function as neurotransmitters (a recent textbook of biological psychiatry[54] lists twenty-nine candidate substances). Until only a few years ago, it was thought that each neurone used only one type of neurotransmitter. However, it now appears that some neurones use both a classical neuro-

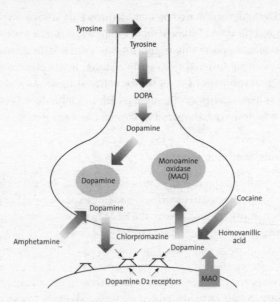

Figure 7.3 The structure and function of the dopamine synapse (reproduced from R. W. Heinrichs (2001) *In Search of Madness: Schizophrenia and Neuroscience*. Oxford: Oxford University Press). Dopamine is synthesized from tyrosine and stored in vesicles. When released into the synapse, it binds with receptors on the post-synaptic membrane. Monoamine oxidase breaks dopamine down to yield homovanillic acid. Dopamine is also taken back into the pre-synaptic cell. Drugs such as amphetamine and cocaine release and prevent the uptake of dopamine. Anti-psychotic drugs such as haloperidol and chlorpromazine occupy post-synaptic receptors and thereby block dopamine occupancy.

transmitter and a peptide. To complicate matters further, there are also a number of different kinds of receptors for each neurotransmitter. For example, in the case of dopamine, five main types are known, which, by convention, are labelled D1 to D2.

The biochemical approach to psychosis attempts to explain how dysfunctional neurotransmission can lead to symptoms. Theories of this kind have usually been stimulated by the accidental discovery of drugs that either mimic psychosis or ameliorate patients' symptoms. For example, in 1938 the Swiss chemist Albert Hoffman first synthesized the powerful hallucinogen, lysergic acid diethylamide (LSD). At the time he was exploring the therapeutic properties of compounds derived from naturally occurring ergot in the hope that these would prove useful for controlling muscle spasms during pregnancy. Animal tests indicated that LSD had no unusual behavioural effects, and there the matter might have rested had Hoffman not accidentally inhaled a dose of the drug (it is active in microgram quantities) some years later. He described his experiences afterwards as follows:

In the afternoon of 16th April, 1943 . . . I was seized by a peculiar sensation of vertigo and restlessness. Objects, as well as the shapes of my associates in the laboratory, appeared to undergo optical changes. I was unable to concentrate on my work. In a dreamlike state I left for home, where an irresistible urge to lie down overcame me. I drew the curtains and immediately fell into a peculiar state similar to drunkenness, characterized by exaggerated imagination. With my eyes closed, fantastic pictures of extraordinary plasticity and intensive colour seemed to surge towards me. After two hours this state gradually wore off.[55]

Not surprisingly, this discovery encouraged some researchers to argue that schizophrenia might be caused by some kind of endogenous (self-created) hallucinogenic substance.[56] In 1962, a dramatic breakthrough was reported which seemed to support this theory. Researchers saw a 'pink spot' (which was later found to be the chemical 3, 4-dimethoxyphenylethylamine) when the urine of schizophrenia patients was allowed to diffuse on chromatography (blotting) paper. The spot was absent when the procedure was repeated with urine from ordinary people.[57] Unfortunately, it later turned out that the spot was of dietary origin and could be found in the urine of anyone who ate institutional food.

Following the discovery that LSD interferes with the neurotransmitter serotonin, some neurochemists embarked on a search for abnormalities in the relevant neural pathways of schizophrenia patients.[58] However, this approach rapidly fell out of favour for two main reasons. First, as will be discussed in detail in a later chapter, the experiences induced by hallucinogenic drugs are quite dissimilar to those reported by psychotic patients.[59] Second, and more importantly, the serotonin hypothesis was displaced in the minds of most scientists by an alternative theory, which seemed to promise a simple and complete biological account of madness. This theory was, of course, the famous *dopamine hypothesis*, which was stimulated by Laborit's accidental discovery of the anti-psychotic properties of chlorpromazine.

Arvid Carlsson, a pharmacologist at the University of Lund in Sweden, first discovered the neurotransmitter function of dopamine in 1957. Soon afterwards, with his colleague Margit Lindqvist, Carlsson obtained evidence from animal studies that chlorpromazine and haloperidol (another neuroleptic) occupied dopamine receptors, blocking them from being stimulated by dopamine.[60] Subsequent experiments by the pharmacologist Paul Jannsen and others confirmed that the potency of the various neuroleptic drugs that had, by that time, become available, correlated with their capacity to do this.[61] The more readily they occupied the receptors, the lower the dose required to produce an anti-psychotic effect. This discovery led a number of researchers to conclude that schizophrenia must be caused by some kind of abnormality in the dopamine system.

A parallel observation that seemed to support this hypothesis concerned the effects of abusing the stimulant drug amphetamine. Early reports that this sometimes led to a psychotic reaction were confirmed in 1958 when a British psychiatrist, Philip Connell, published a monograph describing forty-two patients who had become ill in this way. Usually, the patients became paranoid and experienced visual hallucinations, but these symptoms typically remitted within a few days of discontinuing the drug.[62] Connell's observations were later supported by the results of a remarkable series of experiments conducted in the United States by Burt Angrist and Samuel Gershon, in which normal volunteers were persuaded to take large hourly doses of amphetamine. The effects of this procedure were sometimes dramatic. For example, a volunteer:

who had taken 465 mg of amphetamine over 22³/₄ hr abruptly experienced a florid paranoid psychosis. Before the experiment he had made a 'deal' with the attendant on the ward, to whom he owed several dollars. As he became psychotic, he 'heard' a gang coming on the ward to kill him (sent by the attendant). His paranoid feelings included the experimenter who he assumed had 'set up' the 'trap'. He was at times quite hostile. Explanations that his feelings were amphetamine-induced were rejected with sardonic mock agreement ... He had visual hallucinations of gangsters, of doors opening and closing in the shadows, and visual illusions, in which papers on the bulletin board 'turned into' 'a gangster in a white coat'.[63]

As it was known that amphetamine causes a functional excess of dopamine in the brain, the irresistible conclusion was that over-activity of the dopamine system causes psychosis whereas dampening down the system by blocking dopamine receptors makes psychotic patients better. This theory not only neatly explained the benefits of neuroleptics, but also some of their negative effects as well. Parkinson's disease, characterized by stiffness, tremor and other movement disorders, is caused by a depletion of the brain's supply of dopamine. Neuroleptics often cause Parkinsonian symptoms as side effects, which is precisely what should be expected if they act by dampening the dopamine system. Conversely, the drugs used to treat Parkinson's disease (for example, levo-dopa, which is metabolized into dopamine after crossing the blood–brain barrier) sometimes cause hallucinations and delusions in people who have previously had no experience of psychosis.

Unfortunately, time has not been particularly kind to the dopamine hypothesis. As we saw in Chapter 4, one problem is that the theory has rested on a false premise – the specificity of neuroleptics for schizophrenia. For this reason, Carlsson has recently acknowledged that the theory should be renamed 'the dopamine hypothesis of *psychosis*'.[64] Unfortunately, other deficiencies of the theory are much less easily overcome.

Whereas blockade of the dopamine receptors is usually achieved within an hour or so of taking a single dose, patients normally have to take their medication for several weeks before experiencing any benefit.[65] More embarrassing for the theory is the fact that some psychotic patients fail to obtain any benefit at all, even after many months of treatment.[66] In the 1980s it became possible to use PET scans to estimate the extent to which receptor blockade is achieved in individual patients. This was accomplished by detecting photon emissions from patients who had been injected with a neuroleptic that had been 'radio-labelled' (made radioactive). Studies using this technique established that receptor blockade is as complete in non-responding patients as in responding patients.[67] To make matters even more complicated, a number of atypical neuroleptic compounds have since been discovered and, although effective at reducing symptoms, these drugs do not seem to have the same affinity for dopamine receptors as the older, more established compounds.[68] Taken together, these findings add up to compelling evidence that dopamine receptor blockade is not a sufficient condition for bringing about a reduction in psychotic symptoms.

An even greater problem for the theory is researchers' failure to demonstrate direct evidence of dopamine abnormalities in the brains of patients, despite several decades of hard labour. According to the most obvious interpretation of the theory, schizophrenia should be associated with an excess of dopamine. Some investigators have attempted to test this prediction by measuring dopamine levels in the brain at post mortem, but the results have been inconsistent. Others have therefore attempted to measure homovanillic acid (HVA, a metabolite or breakdown product of dopamine) in the cerebrospinal fluid of living patients. These levels should be high if there is excessive dopamine in the brain. However, the majority of studies that have addressed this issue have reported no difference between schizophrenia patients and ordinary people.[69]

A second interpretation of the dopamine hypothesis, which follows logically from the failure of the first, suggests that psychosis is associated with an excess of dopamine receptors. Although early post-mortem studies seemed to support this version of the theory, it later transpired that increased receptor density could be the consequence of consuming neuroleptics for many years. (Animal studies have confirmed that the brain responds to prolonged neuroleptic treatment by sprouting more receptors.)[70] This objection led to an experiment which British psychiatrist Peter McKenna has (wrongly, in my view) described as, 'arguably the most important . . . in the history of psychiatry'[71] – the attempt to measure the density of dopamine receptors in living patients who have never received drug treatment.

This was first achieved in 1986 by a group of researchers at Johns Hopkins University in the USA, who used PET to assess ten drug-naive patients after they had been injected with a radio-labelled neuro-leptic in sufficient dose to ensure complete dopamine receptor occupancy.[72] Their announcement that DA_2 receptor density was elevated in the patients appeared to herald a major breakthrough in the search for the biological origins of mental illness, but within months this was followed by a report from another group who were unable to obtain the same result.[73] Several years later, the Johns Hopkins University group announced that they had found increased DA_2 receptor density in bipolar disorder patients who were suffering from psychotic symptoms.[74]

More recent research has far from clarified these findings. For example, in a longitudinal investigation, a group of researchers in Finland administered PET scans at intervals of between six and twenty-four months to four schizophrenia patients who had never taken neuroleptic drugs. Two patients who were highly psychotic at the outset showed a considerable reduction in their symptoms between scans. One showed a corresponding 24.7 per cent decrease in the density of his DA_2 receptors, whereas the other showed an *increase* in receptor density of 13.5 per cent. The remaining two patients experienced only very modest changes in their symptoms, but one showed a 56 per cent reduction in DA_2 receptor density, while the other showed a 24.6 per cent increase.[75]

As the dopamine hypothesis has unravelled, investigators have studied the role of other neurotransmitters in psychosis, although with equally inconclusive results.[76] It is therefore difficult to escape the conclusion that biochemical research into psychiatric disorders has failed to live up to its initial promise. Of course, we should not therefore infer that this type of research is doomed to failure. Anyone who has ever visited a pub knows that changes in the chemistry of the brain can bring about dramatic changes in behaviour and experience. However, even if biochemical peculiarities can be found in psychiatric patients, they may tell us very little about the origins of psychosis.[77] Consider the results of two recent studies. In the first, researchers at the Department of Psychiatry at Columbia University used functional imaging techniques to record the brain's biochemical reaction to a dose of amphetamine. They reported that the consequent increase in dopamine synthesis was excessive in schizophrenia patients who were currently ill. However, the responses of patients who were currently well were quite normal.[78] This finding suggests that, although dopamine abnormalities may be associated with the generation of symptoms, they may not be of primary aetiological significance. In the second, researchers at the Ralf H. Johnson Veterans Affairs Medical Centre in Charleston, USA, measured dopamine beta-hydroxylase (an enzyme that converts dopamine to noradrenaline) in the plasma of patients suffering from post-traumatic stress. Higher levels of the enzyme were found in a subgroup of the patients who were suffering from psychotic symptoms.[79] This finding suggests that, when dopamine abnormalities are present in psychotic patients, they may be part of the brain's response to emotional trauma.

The Limits of Biology

We embarked on this review of biological studies of madness in order to answer two questions. First, we wanted to establish whether the discovery of brain abnormalities in mad people precludes a psychological analysis of their problems. Second, we wanted to evaluate the competing claims about the disease status of psychosis made by the neoKraepelinians and Thomas Szasz (recall that both presume that this issue hangs on whether or not neuropathology can be demonstrated in patients). A sceptic might attempt to address both of these questions by asserting that the presence of biological abnormalities in psychosis remains unproven (the position taken by Szasz). But to make this claim is to doubt too much. Whereas many of the biological hypotheses that we have considered appear to be unsupported by data, it does appear that the brains of psychotic patients are (perhaps subtly) different from the brains of ordinary people. The most compelling evidence is that obtained from structural imaging. Whereas early studies clearly exaggerated the extent to which the cerebral ventricles of patients are enlarged in comparison with those of ordinary people, the less dramatic differences found in recent and more carefully conducted investigations cannot be dismissed so easily.

In order to address the first of our two questions, therefore, we need to think more carefully about the implication of these observations. Many biological psychiatrists have argued for a crude form of biological reductionism in which it is assumed that brain abnormalities reflect aetiological processes that are unconnected to the social environment. However, this assumption is plainly false, because, as we have also seen, brain abnormalities alone provide few clues about aetiology. Because our brains are affected by our experiences, peculiarities in the size of its anatomical components, in neuroactivations when we perform particular tasks, or in the biochemical transactions between neurones, can be as readily attributed to the impact of the environment as to causative biological factors such as early brain damage, viruses or endogenous neurotoxins. (This is not to say that brain damage, viruses or endogenous neurotoxins play no role in psychosis, but that other kinds of evidence – which I will discuss in later chapters – will be required to demonstrate that they do.) Curiously, this limitation of brain research was better understood by Emil Kraepelin than by many contemporary psychologists and psychiatrists. It was for this reason that Kraepelin regarded aetiology and pathological anatomy as providing, in principle at least, *independent* methods of classifying patients.

The problem here seems to be a persisting naivety about the relationship between the biological and the psychological, which has deep roots within our culture. Its origins predate Descartes, who, three and a half centuries ago, articulated the philosophical doctrine of *dualism*, which holds that the mind and brain are different kinds of substances, the former non-material and the latter physical. This idea is so entrenched in our language and our folk psychology that, even today, many people find it difficult to think in any other way. It is this prejudice that has led both biological researchers and anti-psychiatrists to assume that the processes underlying abnormal behaviour must be attributed *either* to biology *or* to psychology. The remedy for this confusion is, of course, a better understanding of relationships between the brain, mental events such as thoughts and feelings, and the social and physical environment. Clearly, it will not be possible to provide a completely satisfactory account of these relationships in a few paragraphs. (The problem of consciousness is particularly intractable, and continues to test the best minds in the business.) For present purposes, it is sufficient to note that most attempts to solve this problem assume that statements about brain biology and statements about mental processes represent different levels of descriptions of the same phenomena – in other words, that the mind and the brain are one.

One implication of this unity is that we are likely to make more progress in understanding the biology of psychosis if we first attempt to understand the psychology. Once we know how the environment influences patients' complaints, and the mental processes that underlie them, we will be in a much better position to make sense of the data obtained from biological investigations.

Szasz's error

Some of the implications of the foregoing account of the relationship between the mind and brain may not be apparent until we consider psychotic phenomena in detail later. However, an immediate implication is that we should not accept the terms on which psychiatrists and anti-psychiatrists have debated the disease status of psychosis.

The more carefully we examine the scientific evidence, the more difficult it is to decide which brain abnormalities are really 'pathological'. What are we to make of increases in ventricular volume that may be the consequence of adverse life experiences? Or of dopamine abnormalities that come and go, and which are only present when an individual experiences hallucinations or delusional fears? Or of either of these abnormalities when we know that people experiencing voices or strange beliefs often suffer no detriment to their quality of life?

These difficulties are resolved when we recognize that the distinction between the pathological and the non-pathological inevitably involves some kind of implicit reference to human values. As the British philosopher Peter Sedgwick pointed out two decades ago,[80] it is not enough that a physical characteristic is shown to be statistically unusual in order for it to be regarded as pathological; *it must also be perceived as undesirable, or at least to have consequences that are perceived as undesirable.** If this is not obvious in the case of physical disease it is because there is almost universal agreement that the consequences of particular kinds of biological abnormality are disagreeable. The pain-

---

* In an attempt to make this point humorously, I once wrote an article entitled 'A proposal to classify happiness as a psychiatric disorder' (*Journal of Medical Ethics*, 18: 94–8, 1992). In the article I was able to point to evidence that happiness often leads to irrational or reckless behaviour; that some people are genetically disposed to be happier than others; and that states of happiness are accompanied by abnormal activity in the right cerebral hemisphere of the brain. Of course, my proposal was not a serious one, and was meant to illustrate the problems involved in discriminating between disease and health. Unfortunately, the joke was lost on a number of British journalists who were alerted to the article by a press release from the publisher of the journal. The magazine *New Scientist* devoted a whole page to suggesting that I was making poor use of the salary at that time paid to me by the University of Liverpool. However, my favourite headline from this period was from the *Daily Star*, which said, TOP DOC TALKS THROUGH HIS HAT! From this I could at least take some comfort that I was a top doc.

ful death that can follow a rapid swelling of the appendix is bad by anyone's standards. (If, instead, the only consequence of appendicitis was a doubling of the patient's IQ, it might be regarded differently.) In the field of psychiatry, by contrast, the role of values in determining diagnostic judgements is made obvious by diverse opinions about the relevant behaviours and experiences, which might be attributed to illness, regarded as evidence of harmless eccentricity or creative energy, or described as spiritual phenomena.

The implications of this analysis of the nature of diagnoses have recently been worked out in more detail by Bill Fulford, a British psychiatrist who is also a professional philosopher.[81] Fulford has suggested that, far from threatening the scientific status of psychiatry, acknowledging the role that values play in psychiatric judgements would help to make psychiatric diagnoses *more* reliable and scientifically valid. He argues that the descriptive and evaluative components of each diagnosis should be explicitly separated out, so that, for example, a diagnosis of schizophrenia would require not only that the patient experiences certain symptoms, but also that the symptoms are experienced as distressing or unwanted. Such a step would make it clear that it is impossible to create a value-free theory of mental illness as hoped for by the neoKraepelinians, and would obviously go some way towards solving some of the cross-cultural disagreements about psychiatric disorders that we encountered in the last chapter.

It follows from this argument that Thomas Szasz is *correct* in asserting that psychiatric diagnoses inevitably involve a degree of value judgement, but mistaken in assuming that this is a feature of diagnosis that is unique to psychiatry. It is perhaps ironic that Szasz accuses mental health professionals of using the concepts of 'disease' and 'illness' to justify coercive practices, when the right of patients to refuse unwanted treatments is widely recognized by practitioners of physical medicine.[82]

The future of biological psychiatry

Some years ago, I was invited to speak at a Dutch symposium about controversies in psychiatric research. My talk was followed by a presentation by a highly respected Spanish neurologist who responded angrily to my attack on the Kraepelinian paradigm. 'Some people may say that schizophrenia is a myth, but *we know* that it is brain disease,' she exclaimed. She did not quite strike the table with her fists, but everything else about her demeanour suggested that she found my analysis offensive. She then proceeded to talk about her own structural neuroimaging studies, as if these settled the matter for all time.

Biological findings about madness have often been greeted by a dramatic suspension of the critical faculties of both researchers and bystanders. (In recent years, my enjoyment of the Sunday newspapers has often been impaired by articles claiming that biologists have at last found *the* cause of one psychiatric disorder or another.) New discoveries are announced triumphantly, but with the passage of time are often found to be either unreplicable or to be consequences of some aspect of psychiatric treatment (for example, drug therapy or a hospital diet). Of course, part of the problem is that investigators continue to labour within the framework of the Kraepelinian paradigm. As neoKraepelinian diagnoses group together individuals who have very little in common, it is no wonder that biological research has yielded inconsistent and confusing data. However, just as important is researchers' unreflective hunger for the rewards and plaudits that go with genuine scientific progress. It is as if they are mesmerized by the scent of the Nobel Prize that will be given to the person who finally finds the *real* cause of schizophrenia.

It would obviously be wrong to extrapolate from these criticisms to the conclusion that brain research is fundamentally misguided. The unravelling of the mysteries of the central nervous system remains one of the most challenging and exciting tasks for science in the twenty-first century. Almost certainly, this effort will eventually lead to dramatic improvements in the quality of human life and perhaps revolutionize the way that we think about ourselves as sentient beings. For this reason, it is especially disappointing that so many biological psychiatrists have approached this quest in a naive way. In order to fulfil the promissory notes now routinely handed out by neuroscientists in their scientific papers and public statements, future investigators will surely have to engage with other disciplines, and abandon the assumption that discoveries about the brain somehow obviate the need to understand individuals from a social or psychological perspective.

8

Mental Life and Human Nature

The human being is the best picture of the human soul.

Ludwig Wittgenstein[1]

In the last chapter I established that research into the neurobiology of madness leaves ample room for psychological analysis. In this chapter I will develop this argument further by examining the long tradition of psychological research into psychosis that has been conducted from within the Kraepelinian paradigm. I will not deny that this research has led to useful discoveries. However, I will try to show that the insights that have been gained have been limited, not only by a misleading approach to diagnosis, but also by a failure to recognize the social origins of human mental life.

Psychological Research from the Kraepelinian Perspective

It has been known for many years that psychotic patients perform badly on most psychological measures. This much was understood by Kraepelin, who pioneered the use of psychological tests in psychiatric settings. A vast number of tests have since been devised for administration to psychiatric patients, the majority of this work being carried out with patients diagnosed as suffering from schizophrenia. (For reasons that are unclear to me, much less research has been carried out with patients with a diagnosis of bipolar disorder.) However, a number of problems have to be resolved before the data from these kinds of investigations can be interpreted properly.

An obvious difficulty is that test performance can be affected by factors that have very little to do with patients' symptoms. As early as the 1930s, psychologist David Shakow at the Worcester State Hospital in Massachusetts showed that the performance of schizophrenia patients on a range of psychological measures varied according to their co-operation, motivation and interest, so that, under optimum conditions, their scores sometimes equalled those of ordinary people.[2] This effect of motivation on performance has recently become obvious in a number of experiments using the Wisconsin Card Sort Task (WCST), the measure of frontal lobe function briefly introduced in the last chapter. The WCST is one of a wide range of *neuropsychological tests* devised by psychologists to enable the detection of damage to particular regions of the brain.*

As we have already seen, the WCST has been used to test the hypothesis that the frontal lobes of schizophrenia patients are underactive, especially in response to environmental demands. Consistent with this hypothesis, numerous studies have shown that schizophrenia patients typically perform poorly on the test.[3] There have also been reports that patients diagnosed as suffering from manic depression find the task difficult, although these have been less consistent.[4] However, studies by Alan Bellack and his colleagues in Maryland, by Michael Foster Green and his colleagues in California, and more recently by Heidi Nisbet and her colleagues in New Zealand,[5] have shown that the scores of psychotic patients on the WCST can be improved by paying them for performing well, or by simply giving them feedback on their performance. Clearly, therefore, the poor performance of patients on this test must be explained, at least in part, by motivational problems.

The effects of medication on psychological test performance must also be considered. American psychologists Herbert Spohn and Milton Strauss have shown that these effects vary according to the type of medication prescribed and the type of tests administered.[6] For example, the anti-cholinergic drugs used to control some of the side effects of neuroleptic medication adversely affect memory. On the other hand, there is consistent evidence that performance on tests of attention usually improves following the administration of neuroleptic drugs to acutely ill patients. In order to control for these effects, investigators

---

* These tests are devised by finding out how different types of brain damage affect the ability to solve different kinds of problems. Not all psychological tests can be used to identify a specific locus of brain damage in this way.

sometimes try to administer tests to patients while they are free of drugs. However, this is often hard to achieve, as doctors usually give their patients medication at the earliest signs of illness.

A further problem is that psychotic patients have performed poorly on just about every test that anyone has ever administered to them. For this reason, it is sometimes impossible to decide whether poor performance reflects specific psychological processes that are affected in the patient, general intellectual deficits, or the more general effects of demoralization and institutionalization. There is no simple solution to this problem. One approach is to administer several tests, in order to show that performance is more abnormal in some than others. For example, if the difference between patients and controls is greater on a test of perception than on a test of memory, this can be considered evidence that perception is specifically affected. Many years ago, Loren and Jean Chapman of the University of Wisconsin pointed out that this strategy is only reliable when the tests are equally difficult for normal individuals.[7] To see why this is the case, imagine the consequences of administering a test (say a simple measure of general knowledge) that was so easy that almost everyone would do well on it. Such a test would fail to discriminate between patients and controls. The same would be true of a very difficult test (say a questionnaire measuring knowledge of the mathematical principles underlying quantum mechanics), which both patients and ordinary people would fail. In general, tests are most sensitive to differences between patients and control groups when they are designed so that normal individuals of average intelligence will make errors on 50 per cent of opportunities. Returning now to our hypothetical experiment in which patients and controls are administered a test of perception and a test of memory, imagine what would happen if the perception test was moderately difficult but the memory test was either very hard or very easy. Under these conditions, the patients would appear to be specifically handicapped on the measure of perception but not on the measure of memory. However, this result would be entirely an artefact of the relative difficulty of the tests.

This problem is most severe when tests are designed to measure gross deficits in cognitive ability.[8] A *deficit* is said to be present when there is a general failure in an individual's mental processes. We will see, for example, that there is evidence that psychotic patients often have difficulty attending to things that are happening, irrespective of what those things are. It is often assumed that deficits are the product of some kind of general malfunction of the central nervous system, although this is not always the case, because, as we have seen, poor performance on general measures of mental functioning may be caused by poor motivation.

It is very important to recognize that *not all psychological abnormalities are deficits*. A cognitive *bias* is said to be present when someone preferentially processes (attends to, remembers or thinks about) some kinds of information as opposed to others. For example, we will see that people who feel depressed generally remember positive life experiences less easily than negative experiences. Their failure to recall good events cannot be attributed to a deficit, or poor motivation, because they can recall bad events exceptionally well. Because there is no general malfunction of the nervous system, but rather a skew in the way that the mind is orientated towards the world, biases are sometimes assumed to be the products of adverse learning.

For reasons that are not obvious (at least to me), psychological studies of psychosis have, until recently, focused almost entirely on deficits, whereas research on non-psychotic conditions has usually measured biases. In later chapters, we will see that both types of abnormality contribute to psychotic symptoms.

Psychosis and attention

In fact, although many different mental processes have been assessed in psychotic patients, the most consistent observations of deficits have been made using measures of *attention*, which can be thought of as the ability to focus on and respond to some stimuli in the environment in preference to others. Kraepelin provided the following strikingly modern account of the process of attention, and of the abnormal distractibility experienced by psychotic patients:

The content of consciousness of the child is hopelessly dependent upon its chance environment; it only perceives the strongest stimuli, not taking into account the inner connection of things, for it is lacking those general conceptions which also distinguish the less obtrusive perceptions as essential links in the chain of experience. In the adult, on the other hand, the process of perception is increasingly controlled by the special inclinations which gradually develop from his personal life experience. We *exercise* ourselves chiefly in taking notice of certain impressions by a progressively increasing responsiveness of our imagination to these impressions, so that even slight suggestions suffice to meet with a vivid inner resonance. On the other hand, we *become accustomed* to disregard everyday stimuli and to deny them any influence whatsoever on the course of our psychic processes . . .

The slightest degree of increased distractibility can be observed as a temporary phenomenon in the state of distraction as it occurs in progressive fatigue. In spite of all efforts we are no longer able methodologically to follow a series of coherent sensory impressions, but realize again and again that we are diverted by other impressions or ideas and that we can only grapple with the task in a fragmentary way. This disorder is developed to a higher degree in chronic nervous exhaustion, in the period of convalescence following severe mental or physical diseases, to an even higher degree in acute exhaustion psychoses strictly speaking moreover in mania, often also in paralysis and dementia praecox. Here in many cases, an exclamation, a single word, even the exhibition of an object suffices for immediately diverting the direction of attention and suggesting quite complex conceptions.[9]

Interest in the attentional difficulties of psychotic patients was renewed sixty-two years after Kraepelin's account, following the publication of a study by Andrew McGhie and James Chapman, who were working at the Royal Dundee Mental Hospital in Scotland.[10] They interviewed twenty-six schizophrenia patients who had recently become ill, and found that the majority reported subjective cognitive difficulties such as problems of attention, increased distractibility, heightened sensory impressions, and awareness of processes and actions that would normally be automatic. For example: 'My concentration is very poor. I jump from one thing to another. If I am talking to someone they only need to cross their legs or scratch their heads and I am distracted and forget what I was saying.' And: 'I have to do everything step by step, nothing is automatic now. Everything has to be considered.' Chapman and McGhie later reported that schizophrenia patients performed poorly on a variety of psychological measures designed to assess attention. Although other researchers criticized their methods,[11] later studies broadly supported their conclusions.

The assessment of attentional processes is a complex and technical field, and I will therefore limit the present discussion to the three most widely used tests. In the first and simplest, the *Digit Span with Distraction Test* (DSDT), the participant listens to recorded strings of numbers, which he then repeats. Sometimes a second voice in the background reads out distraction numbers, which the participant is required to ignore. To ensure that the conditions are equally difficult for ordinary people, the number of digits presented is greater in the non-distraction than in the distraction condition. In the late 1970s, American psychologists Thomas Oltmanns and John Neale studied the DSDT performance of patients who were classified according to a loose hospital diagnosis of schizophrenia and according to the Research Diagnostic Criteria. When patients with the hospital diagnosis were compared with those with other diagnoses, no differences were found. However, when the patients who met the narrower RDC for schizophrenia were compared with those who did not, they were found to perform particularly badly in the distraction condition, indicating that schizophrenia patients are unable to screen out stimuli that are irrelevant to their current needs. Oltmanns and Neale studied the symptom profiles of their patients and found that distractibility was specifically associated with disordered speech.[12] Their observations have been replicated many times since, with various refinements. American psychologist Mark Serper and his colleagues have recently shown that performance on the DSDT usually improves when patients are given anti-psychotic drugs, and that this improvement precedes and correlates with later improvements in symptoms.[13]

A second measure that has been widely used in studies of schizophrenia patients is the *Continuous Performance Test* (CPT). The CPT measures sustained vigilance, a phenomenon that first became of interest to psychologists during the Second World War, when the Royal Air Force commissioned a series of experiments to discover the optimal length of time that a radar operator could function effectively when on anti-submarine patrol.[14] To a person tested on the CPT, the experience is a bit like watching a radar display. Letters are briefly presented on a computer screen, usually at the rate of one every second or so. The participant has to press a button immediately after seeing particular targets, which may be simple (e.g. the letter 'T') or complex (e.g. the letter 'X' but only when it follows the letter 'T'). When ordinary people are administered the test, their performance usually decreases over a relatively short period of time as their attention fades. Many studies, such as those conducted by Keith Nuechterlein and his colleagues at the University of California at Los Angeles Clinical Research Center for the Study of Schizophrenia, have shown that this performance decrement is greater in psychotic patients than in normal people.[15] By studying the effects of varying some of the characteristics of the CPT, for example the complexity of the target and how clearly it is presented on the screen, Nuechterlein and his colleagues have been able to study more precisely the attentional difficulties experienced by their patients. For example, they observed that patients with predominantly negative symptoms performed very poorly on 'high load' (difficult) versions of the test.[16]

A third test which we will consider here measures the very earliest processes involved in perception, and is best described in the words of Michael Foster Green, who also works at the UCLA Clinical Research Center:

Imagine that you are seated in front of a screen and an experimenter is presenting letters to you one at a time with a type of projector. Although the duration of each letter is very brief (perhaps 10 msec.), you can easily identify each letter with perfect accuracy. The experimenter pauses and tells you that he/she will continue to show you letters at the same duration, but there will be one difference: after you are shown each letter, the screen will go blank for a short time and some crossed lines will appear where the letter had been. Your job is only to report the letter and ignore the crossed lines. The task probably sounds quite easy because you had no difficulty identifying the letters before, and the duration of the letters will not change. However, when the stimuli are presented, you might find that you can see the crossed lines, but no letter at all. This is the backward masking effect.[17]

The *backward masking effect* occurs because visual information is briefly held in a sensory store (sometimes called the *iconic memory*) prior to being passed on to later brain centres for more detailed processing. If the 'mask' of crossed lines is presented very soon after the initial letter, it displaces the information about the letter from the sensory store before it can be passed on. As the later processing is required for us to be aware of the letter, we are unable to identify it.

By varying the interval between the presentation of the letters and the mask until the letters can be seen, it is possible to measure the amount of time the sensory store requires to pass on the letter for later processing. In 1981, Dennis Saccuzzo and David Braff, two researchers at the University of California at San Diego, showed that this interval was longer for schizophrenia patients than for normal controls, indicating that the speed with which the visual information was being passed on was slower for the patients.[18] It was later observed that unmedicated patients' performance on the test improved after they had been given anti-psychotic drugs.[19]

In this short space it has been difficult to do justice to the large volume of research on the performance of psychotic patients on attentional tests, and the attempts that have been made to account for these findings. Of the many models of attentional dysfunction that have been proposed I will mention just one, developed over a number of years by Keith Nuechterlein and his colleagues at UCLA.[20] On the basis of a detailed theory of the processes involved in normal attention, they have argued that the patterns of results observed in their patients can best be explained in terms of two separate types of abnormality.

First, they argue that poor performance on the backward masking task and on certain versions of the CPT (especially versions in which the stimuli are blurred and difficult to identify) is caused by deficits in the very earliest and most automatic stages of information processing. Interestingly, these deficits seem to be present in patients who are enjoying a remission of their symptoms, and Nuechterlein and his colleagues therefore argue that the deficits are enduring psychological characteristics that cause people to be vulnerable to breakdown under times of stress.

Second, they argue that poor performance on other versions of the CPT (especially versions in which complex targets are employed) and also on the DSDT is best explained by an inability to use active memory to guide the selection of information. When we try to focus on some types of stimuli to the exclusion of others, we have to hold a representation of the target stimuli in an active 'on-line' memory store (the same memory system that you use when performing mental calculations). The content of this store – sometimes known as *working memory* – therefore exerts control over our voluntary attention. Nuechterlein and his colleagues argue that the poor performance of patients on the complex versions of the CPT is caused by a failure of this kind of control, probably caused by some kind of deficit in the working memory system. As performance on the complex versions of the CPT is usually worst during periods of active illness, and usually improves during remission, Nuechterlein and his colleagues argue that this type of deficit is directly involved in the onset of symptoms.

Impressive though this work has been, it suffers from three important limitations. First, the reader will not be surprised when I question the specificity of the findings. Although much less effort has been made to study cognitive deficits in bipolar patients than in patients with a diagnosis of schizophrenia, when those efforts have been made, similarities between schizophrenia and bipolar patients have been more apparent than differences. For example, bipolar patients have been found to perform poorly on the DSDT,[21] the backward masking task,[22] and on other measures of working memory and attention.[23] Poor performance on the CPT has been found, not only in bipolar patients[24] but also in unipolar depressed patients who are experiencing psychotic symptoms.[25]

Second, gross cognitive deficits appear to be only tenuously linked to the behaviours and experiences that most people would regard as prototypical of psychosis. In a recent review of the relevant evidence, Michael Foster Green has pointed out that *poor scores on most deficit measures seem to be unrelated to positive symptoms* (see Figure 8.1)![26] Although most patients perform poorly, little difference is observed between those with hallucinations and delusions and those with other symptoms or – on many tests – even between patients who are currently ill and those who are in remission. In contrast, performance on neuro-psychological and cognitive deficit measures seems to be a much better predictor of patients' social and occupational functioning. Patients with severe deficits generally fare less well when living in the community, are poor at dealing with social problems, and experience very great difficulty when attempting to learn new skills.

Green's response to this *paradoxical lack of association between positive symptoms and deficits* is surprising. Evoking Bleuler's distinction between primary and secondary symptoms of schizophrenia, he has concluded that cognitive deficits are the core of schizophrenia, and that positive symptoms are peripheral features. To put this proposal another way, he has suggested that we redraw the boundaries of the disorder to put deficits in the centre, so that positive symptoms are no

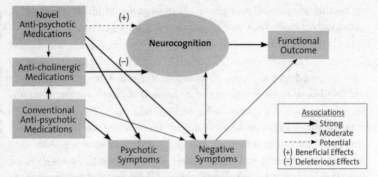

Figure 8.1 Relationship between cognitive deficits, drug treatment, symptoms and social functioning (functional outcome) according to Michael Foster Green and Keith Nuechterlein ('Should schizophrenia be treated as a neuro-cognitive disorder?', *Schizophrenia Bulletin*, 25: 309–19, 1989). The strength of causal relationships is indicated by the type of arrows shown.

longer attributed much importance. Of course, even if we were to accept this proposal, it would still be necessary to identify those processes that, in addition to cognitive deficits, are responsible for delusions and hallucinations. After all, it is usually these symptoms, however peripheral, that drive patients and their families to seek psychiatric help.

A final limitation of the research we have reviewed concerns the type of mental functions studied. Most psychologists have chosen to focus on gross mental functions, especially perception and attention, and have employed stimuli that have been essentially meaningless (for example, strings of numbers in the DSDT, sequentially presented letters in the CPT, and abstract patterns in the WSCT). Because they knew that performance on psychological tests is influenced by the content of the test materials, early test designers regarded meaning as a dangerous complication. This was not an entirely senseless attitude, as the poor performance of patients on attentional measures is presumably telling us something quite important. However, it should be obvious that *these tests do not measure the kinds of tasks that the human mind performs in ordinary life*. We are likely to get a more complete picture of the psychological mechanisms involved in psychosis if we focus not only on raw deficits but also on those processes that are known to be important in everyday functioning. In the remainder of this chapter, I will briefly review some of these processes, particularly those which will prove important when we come to look more closely at symptoms in later chapters.

The Social Brain

So far as the brain is concerned, any stimulus is not the same as any other. Its operations are content-specific, which is to say that the brain processes different kinds of information in different ways. This preference for certain kinds of stimuli in contrast to others is a requirement for intentionality (the 'aboutness' that connects the contents of our thoughts to the external world) and underlies the cognitive biases which, we will see in later chapters, play an important role in symptoms.

Recent studies have shown that the normal brain has specialized to deal with one particular class of stimuli above all others. These stimuli are the most complex and demanding objects in our everyday environment, namely other human beings. Unless you are a Nobel-prize-winning rocket scientist, the problems that demand most of your attention, in all likelihood, involve your relationships with others, a fact that is reflected in popular culture, from songs and novels to films and television soap operas. (The characters of *Neighbours*, *Friends* and *Coronation Street* are constantly falling out with each other, making up, finding new lovers or losing old ones. We almost never see them sweating over some intractable problem at work, or struggling to complete their tax returns.)

The idea that the human mind has evolved to preferentially process social information is sometimes called the *social brain hypothesis*. Considerable evidence in its favour can be found in both the biological and the psychological literature. Let us begin by considering anatomical comparisons of human beings and other species. Compared with other vertebrates, we have a disproportionately sized cerebral cortex. Across the vertebrate species, brain volume increases on average as a two-thirds power of body mass (in other words, in proportion to the surface area of the body), reflecting the increased processing capacity needed by big organisms with large numbers of sensory receptors and muscle fibres.[27] However, when this relationship is taken into account, it is evident that some species have brains that are larger than would be expected from their body size, a phenomenon known as *encephaliz-ation*. The most encephalized species is, of course, ourselves, with other primates following closely behind. The evolutionary pressures responsible for encephalization remain a matter of some controversy. Robin Dunbar, an evolutionary psychologist working at the University of Liverpool, has suggested that group size made an important contri-bution to this process. The members of each species relate to each other in groups of characteristic size, and Dunbar has shown that this size correlates reasonably well with encephalization. Larger groups, according to this hypothesis, demand larger brains, and so our own brains have evolved to cope with social systems that are more complex than those of any other species. If Dunbar's theory is correct, the majority of our brain's 'computing power' is dedicated to processing social information.[28]

Leslie Brothers, a psychiatrist working at the University of Cali-fornia in Los Angeles, has argued that neurophysiological investi-gations provide a second important strand of evidence about the social brain. In studies carried out mainly on monkeys, Brothers and her colleagues have recorded the responses of specific neurones following the presentation of different kinds of stimuli. In these experiments, some neurones have been found to be specifically responsive to social information. For example, neurones have been identified which fire only when the animal sees a hand, a face, eye movements or other bodies walking. These are mostly located in the temporal lobes, in areas such as the inferotemporal cortex and the amygdala. Brothers has suggested that these structures function as an 'editor', which highlights social information for preferential processing by other areas of the brain, thereby determining which stimuli are personally signifi-cant.[29] (Interestingly, other researchers have argued that the amygdala plays an important role in emotion, a proposal that is consistent with Brothers' theory, as emotional responses are most often elicited when we encounter social problems.)[30]

A third source of evidence about the social brain comes from psycho-logical studies of ordinary human beings. If the human brain has evolved to deal with social stimuli, we should find tasks that employ these stimuli easier to perform than tasks that do not. There is an abundance of evidence supporting this prediction (much of which was collected before the social brain hypothesis was first proposed) but there is only space enough in these pages to describe one example, taken from the field of child psychology. In the 1950s, the famous Swiss child psychologist Jean Piaget reported a series of studies that appeared to demonstrate that young children are unable to 'decentre' their imagination from their experience.[31] In some of these studies, children were shown a model of three mountains, and a doll was placed on one corner of the model. When children below the age of 9 were asked to choose a picture that showed how the mountains looked from the position of the doll they almost always failed, the younger children typically choosing a picture taken from their own perspective. At first sight, this seems to be powerful evidence in favour of Piaget's account of the cognitive limitations of young children. However, British child psychologist Martin Hughes later carried out a similar study in which much younger children seemed to perform better than Piaget's 7- and 8-year-olds. In this task, two toy policemen were placed on a table, divided by two intersecting walls. When asked to place a third doll in a position where it could not be seen by either policeman, children were able to do this with 90 per cent accuracy, implying that they could simultaneously think about the perspectives of both policemen. Margaret Donaldson, a psychologist at the University of Edinburgh, has accounted for this apparent discrepancy with Piaget's work by pointing to the socially realistic nature of Hughes's task.[32] Young children know what it is like to be naughty and to hide from adults. The motives and the intentions of the characters in Hughes's task were therefore comprehensible to them. For this reason, they were able to complete the task successfully, unlike the older children confronted with the more abstract task devised by Piaget.

A final source of evidence about the social brain concerns the impairments seen in some neuropsychological disorders. If the brain has evolved specific mechanisms for dealing with social information, it would not be surprising if some conditions turned out to be the consequence of the loss of or inability to develop specific kinds of social reasoning. Autism is a disorder that seems to reflect this kind of problem. The main features of the condition, which usually become evident within the first few years of life, are an inability to engage in imaginative play, impaired development of language and a failure to form even rudimentary relationships.[33] In many cases, these difficulties are so severe that the autistic person requires lifelong care. Although the causes of the disorder are poorly understood, a high proportion of autistic children have demonstrable brain damage, suggesting that some kind of disruption of specific neural circuits may be implicated.

Psychological research conducted over the last two decades has suggested that the inability to understand the mental states of other people may be a core feature of autism, and that the symptoms that lead to its diagnosis may be a consequence of this deficit.[34] The ability to guess what people think, and to anticipate what they might do (in other words, to use folk psychology effectively), is a vital ingredient of normal social life. In adulthood, it enables us to recognize our friends and enemies, and to predict what will happen when we try to interact with them. When talking to another person, it allows us to adjust our speech to match the perceived needs of the listener. Children who acquire this ability are often said to possess a *theory of mind** (for this reason, psychologists sometimes speak of people having ToM skills), a term which has been rightly described as 'a daft expression because it [misleadingly] suggests that a child theorizes about the nature of feelings, wishes, beliefs, intentions, and so on'.[35] It might be more correct to say that we can '*mentalize*'.

Mentalizing or ToM skills are usually assessed by means of tests in which the individual is required to infer that someone else holds a false belief about the world. A simple example used with children is the so-called 'Sally–Ann' test in which a story is enacted with two dolls, Sally and Ann, who are shown with two boxes, one of which contains an object. In the story, Sally leaves the room, and Ann switches the object from one box to the other. The child who is being tested is then asked to say in which box Sally looks for the object when she returns. In order to answer this question correctly it is, of course, necessary to understand that Sally's belief about the world when she returns is at variance with reality. Ordinary children begin to pass this kind of test during their fourth year of life (although they may show evidence of more rudimentary mentalizing skills – for example, the ability to direct the gaze of others, or to distinguish between pretend and reality – as

---

* The origin of this terminology is the paper that started this line of research, written by the distinguished American primatologist David Premack and his colleague Guy Woodruff, which was entitled 'Does the chimpanzee have a theory of mind?' (*Behavioral and Brain Sciences*, 4: 515–26, 1978).

young as 2 years of age).[36] In autistic children, the development of mentalizing skills is severely delayed, and perhaps permanently impaired, even though they may perform normally on other types of tests.[37]

It is possible to draw two important conclusions from these findings. First, the terrible consequences of the autistic person's inability to understand the minds of others demonstrates how important social cognition is in everyday life. Second, the fact that many autistic children score relatively normally on conventional IQ tests suggests that at least one type of social cognition may be relatively independent of the kind of gross cognitive abilities usually measured by psychologists investigating psychosis.

Uniquely Human

Many psychologists have proposed that the human mind's specific ability to deal with social information reflects the evolution of specific mental modules dedicated to this purpose. On this view, there may be, for example, brain modules dedicated to recognizing faces, detecting the emotional states of other people, guessing their intentions, and predicting what they will do. This view is taken by many researchers studying autism, mainly because of the striking evidence that ToM skills can be severely impaired in individuals of average or above average intelligence.[38]

In fact, evidence that the mind is organized in this way is far from clear cut. The American philosopher Jerry Fodor has suggested several criteria that might be used to identify modular information-processing systems. He has argued, for example, that they are unconscious, respond quickly and in an obligatory fashion (predetermined inputs lead to predetermined outputs), develop in a characteristic sequence in the child, are neurologically localized (that is, implemented by dedicated neural circuits), and deal with only specific types of information.[39] However, many of these characteristics are true of acquired skills that have been practised to the point of becoming automatic. For example, champion chess players often choose moves intuitively, without being aware of the mental processes that guide their decisions. As the ability to master chess no doubt depends on the individual's level of cognitive development, it is likely that children learning chess from an early age will develop their skills in a characteristic sequence. Moreover, functional neuroimaging studies have shown that specific areas of the brain 'light up' as grand masters progress through a game.[40] Despite these observations, it obviously would be a mistake to assume that the human brain has evolved a chess-playing module.

A more serious problem for extreme versions of modularism concerns the relationship between genes and brain circuits.[41] Presumably, the modular architecture of the brain is determined genetically. However, as I completed this chapter, the latest estimate of the number of genes in the human genome (calculated as the Human Genome Project came towards an end) was 30,000, whereas there may be up to 100,000,000,000,000 synapses in the human brain. For this reason, it is simply not plausible that neural circuits are precisely predetermined by the genetic code. Of course, this argument does not imply that there can be nothing module-like in the human brain – modules may develop without the precise genetic specification of specific circuits. However, it does suggest that the development of the neural circuits responsible for social cognition, whether or not they are ultimately organized into discrete modules, must depend on complex interactions between the developing individual and the environment. In later chapters of this book, we will see that this observation has some important implications for our understanding of the origins of psychosis.

Perhaps the human faculty that has the best claim to being modularized is language. As we have already seen, there is extensive evidence that specific regions of the brain are involved in generating and understanding speech. Moreover, the fact that language is a species-specific ability strongly suggests that the development of this ability is genetically controlled.[42] Even so, the environment also plays an obvious role. Children grow up to speak the language they hear from their caregivers rather than the language of their ancestors. Children who are not exposed to the speech of others as their brains develop grow up to be, tragically, severely linguistically and intellectually disabled in later life.[43]

The ability to speak has a profound effect on all other aspects of the human mind, and therefore must be considered when we attempt to understand the role of cognition in psychosis. When thinking about the function language plays in human life, it is only natural to regard it as a means by which information is passed from one individual to another. Psychologists who have speculated about the origins of language have usually assumed that the advantages thereby conferred provided the major selection pressure for language evolution.[44] For example, it has been argued that language evolved because it enabled our ancestors to cope with the complex relationships entailed by our membership of large social groups.[45] Another, not incompatible suggestion is that our rapid specialization for language was fuelled by some kind of evolutionary arms race.[46] The ape-like ancestor who can say to another something like, 'Hide behind that rock over there, jump out with your stick and attack the intruder as he passes by!' is clearly going to have better survival prospects than one who lacks this skill. However, even this simple example suggests that language also has an intellectual function. By framing problems in a verbal form we can organize our ideas, and plan what we are going to do.

When I was young, it was commonly said that talking to oneself was the first sign of madness, but a case can be made for asserting the opposite. I think all readers will be aware of the internal dialogue that runs through the mind from the moment of waking until sleep resumes. Talking to ourselves, we debate events, plan actions, issue chastisements to ourselves when things go wrong and exclaim inwardly with delight when things go well. While it is certainly not the case that the stream of consciousness is entirely verbal, for much of the time our thoughts are dominated by words.

The intellectual function of language was recognized in the early years of the twentieth century by the Russian physiologist and psychologist Ivan Pavlov. Pavlov argued that this use of words has conferred on human beings mental powers that separate us from other species. Because we can think in words, we are to some extent free from being controlled by the simple conditioning processes that dominate the behaviour of non-human animals.* Building on this idea, his student Lev Vygotsky studied the way in which communicative speech is

* Intriguingly, this observation led Pavlov to what may seem a most unPavlovian conclusion: 'On the one hand, numerous speech stimulations have removed us from reality, and we must always remember this in order not to distort our attitude towards reality. On the other hand, it is precisely speech which has made us human' (I. P. Pavlov (1941) Conditioned Reflexes and Psychiatry (trans. W. H. Gantt). New York: International Publishers).

transformed into verbal thought. Unfortunately, because he died of tuberculosis at the age of 37 in 1934, and because Stalin suppressed his work, Vygotsky's observations did not become known to Western child psychologists until the early 1960s.

In his now famous book *Thought and Language*,[47] Vygotsky summarized the relationship between language and thought at different stages of child development as follows:

1) In their . . . development, thought and speech have different roots. 2) In the speech development of the child, we can certainly establish a preintellectual stage, and in his thought development, a prelinguistic stage. 3) Up to a certain point in time, the two different lines grow independently of each other. 4) At a certain point these lines meet, whereupon thought becomes verbal and speech rational.

Vygotsky studied the different ways that children make use of language, in order to discover the psychological processes involved in this merging of the lines of thought and speech. He observed that the growing child first learns to produce and understand speech in the context of his relationship with caregivers. During this stage, the child and adult are constantly issuing instructions or asking questions of each other so that, for the child, the whole process of speaking becomes bound up with attempts by the two parties to control each other's actions. Later, towards the end of the second year of life, children discover that they can instruct themselves by speaking aloud about what they are doing. (This is often preceded by a period in which they ask questions of their parents and then immediately answer for themselves.)[48] At this stage, children spend a lot of time talking to themselves out loud (a phenomenon known as *private speech*) and language becomes a powerful mechanism for self-regulation. Finally, at about the age of 4 years, social and private speech become differentiated from each other. Children of this age learn the neat trick of talking silently to themselves, resulting in *inner speech* that is inaudible and undetectable to others.

During the 1920s, Jean Piaget disagreed with this account because he was reluctant to believe that the private speech of 2-year-olds had an intellectual function. Piaget believed that young children talk out loud when on their own because they are too egocentric to realize that no one is listening to them.[49] However, observational studies of children have consistently supported Vygotsky's contention that the young child who talks when on his own is communicating effectively with the person who really matters – himself.[50] Moreover, recent studies by American developmental psychologist Laura Berk have confirmed that children who can use private speech effectively when learning new skills acquire those skills most quickly.[51]

By adulthood, inner speech has lost many of the characteristics of social speech, and become a highly condensed form of silent verbal activity. When using inner speech, we rarely have to state the subject of our thoughts, because it is already known to us. Elements of speech that allow propositions to be linked meaningfully together so that they appear coherent to the listener (known to linguists as *cohesive ties*) become redundant. At the same time, inner words expand their symbolic function and develop multiple and complex associations. Although the measurement of this kind of thinking is fraught with difficulty,[52] studies in which immediate recollections of inner speech have been compared with the full expression of the same thoughts have suggested that one minute of inner speech can equal up to 4000 words of overt speech.[53]

As we spend much of our time talking about ourselves to ourselves, inner speech is an important vehicle of self-awareness.[54] It tends to be evoked in social situations that are personally challenging or emotionally arousing. In some circumstances during adult life, we may lazily forget the habit of silent speech acquired during childhood, and speak out loud. This may happen if we have a particularly demanding task to perform (I have been intermittently mumbling to myself while writing this book), when we are under stress, or when we think we are alone (anyone doubting this should stand by a roadway intersection and watch unaccompanied drivers talking to themselves as they wait for traffic lights to change). However, even when we speak silently to ourselves, there is a neuromuscular echo of the time in childhood when we could only speak aloud. Surprising though it may seem, when we think in words, our lips and speech muscles are active.

The idea that activity in the speech muscles accompanies verbal thought is almost as old as the idea of inner speech itself. The American behaviourist J. B. Watson tried to measure this activity in the 1920s, but his efforts failed because he had inadequate equipment (he experimented with comical devices that used wires and pulleys connected to suction caps fastened on the lips). The invention shortly afterwards of a device, known as an *electromyogram* (EMG), which directly measures electrical activity in the muscles, soon led to the unequivocal detection of *subvocalization*, as this silent activation of the speech muscles is now called. In a typical electromyographic study, electrodes are attached to the lips and larynx in order to measure electrical currents in the muscles beneath the skin. Sometimes electrodes are also attached to non-speech muscles (for example, the pectorals) in order to ensure that any increase in muscle activity is limited to those involved in speech. The participant in the experiment is then asked to perform various mental tasks. Countless EMG experiments conducted in the past fifty years or so have demonstrated that subvocalization* accompanies virtually any kind of mental process that requires us to think in words.[55] (Interestingly, both psychological and EMG studies have shown that deaf people who have acquired sign language use inner speech in the form of silent signs. As they think, microcurrents are detectable in their finger muscles.)[56]

Not surprisingly, in adults subvocalization is particularly evident when we think about ourselves, or when we are ruminating about matters that are emotionally important to us.[57] As we have seen, it is precisely these circumstances that most readily elicit inner speech.

The Brain and its Self

I want to conclude this brief tour of the human mind by considering a topic that, until recently, has been regarded as more the province of philosophers than psychologists. Indeed, to any hard-nosed biological scientists reading this book, 'the self' may still seem a vague and almost metaphysical concept. However, we will see that it can be subjected to scientific analysis.

In a commendably concise attempt to shed light on the nature of

---

* The phenomenon of subvocalization does not imply that speech muscles are necessary for verbal thought. The subvocalization is an echo of activity occurring in the language centres in the brain. For this reason, if you are unfortunate enough to lose your speech muscles in some kind of dreadful accident, your intelligence will not be affected.

the self, the American social psychologist Roy Baumeister has made the following observation:

Providing a satisfactory definition of the self has proven fiendishly difficult. It is what you mean when you say 'I'. Most people use 'I' and 'self' many times each day, and so most people have a secure understanding of what the self is – but articulating that understanding is not easy.[58]

It would be wrong, therefore, to regard the self as a thing, as supposed by Cartesian dualists. It is instead a set of ideas, pictures, or beliefs (or, to use a generic term, *mental representations*) about who we are. Some of these representations are explicit and available for contemplation, but others are implicit and take the form of vague assumptions or 'schemas'. Like most mental representations, the self has fluid boundaries and overlaps with other kinds of thoughts and feelings, which is why it defies precise definition. When we talk about or imagine ourselves, we can generate verbal descriptions of our attributes, talents and deficiencies; remember defining moments in our lives; consider how we match or fail to match our moral, social and material aspirations; contemplate the quality of our relationships; compare ourselves to other people; and imagine how those other people see us. Each of these activities evokes one or more aspects of the self but none encompasses the self in its entirety. To borrow a metaphor from the philosopher Dan Dennett, the self is the centre of narrative gravity, which, like the centre of gravity of a physical body, cannot be isolated and touched, but around which our memories, the stories we tell about ourselves, and the decisions we make, all revolve.[59]

The pivotal role of the self in human cognition is demonstrated by a deceptively simple phenomenon, known as the *self-reference effect*. Our ability to remember information depends on how we 'encode' information when we encounter it. For example, if we look at a list of words, we can pay attention to whether they are written in upper- or lower-case letters (feature encoding) or what the words actually mean (semantic encoding). In general, we will tend to recall more of the information if we pay attention to its meaning. However, it seems that people are most likely to recall information later if they encode it according to its relevance to the self.[60] For example, if we are asked to fill in a questionnaire about our own personality characteristics, and we are then given a surprise memory test of the items on the questionnaire, we will tend to remember the questions we answered 'yes' to. The brain, it seems, prioritizes the processing of information that is perceived to be important to the self.

Because we do not arrive in the world knowing who we are and how we are different from other people, it is pretty obvious that there must be a developmental story to tell about the self. Some child psychologists have traced its origins to the first few weeks of life, when the infant initially learns to distinguish between himself and his caregiver during 'proto-conversational' exchanges that precede the emergence of language.[61] Once we can speak, we acquire increasingly elaborate descriptions of the self, some of which we learn from what we are told about ourselves by significant others, and some of which we tell ourselves as we contemplate our triumphs and disasters. Alongside these descriptions, we accumulate memories of what has happened to us and the things that we have done. This stored reservoir of knowledge about the self is the bedrock from which all other aspects of the self are derived. It allows us to define our individual identity ('I am a slightly overweight family man with a good sense of humour'); our membership of groups of like-minded people ('I belong to the tribe of clinical psychologists'); claim our rights ('I want my medical colleagues to acknowledge the wisdom of my views about madness'); plan our future achievements ('I have the skills and motivation to write a book'); and acknowledge our limitations ('. . . but not to climb Mount Everest').

Inevitably, when constructing a self, the child internalizes historically and culturally determined values. It is therefore possible that the self as known to people of the past may have been quite different from the self as known to people living in the modern world. Roy Baumeister has argued that for medieval Europeans, the self was relatively transparent, and was equated with visible manifestations and actions. As life on earth was, at that time, believed to be a preamble to eternal bliss, there was no need to search for self-fulfilment.[62] In modern Western societies, in contrast, the self is often viewed as a hidden territory that can only be known with difficulty, but which must be explored (perhaps with the technical assistance of a psychotherapist) if its special talents are to be fostered and self-actualization achieved.

Although anthropological studies suggest that people across the globe today share a common preoccupation with the self,[63] even modern human beings may think about the self in diverse ways. American psychologists Hazel Markus and Shinobu Kitayama have noted important differences between the way in which the self is construed in *individualist* societies such as North America, in which people tend to define themselves and evaluate their self-worth in terms of their achievements, and *collectivist* societies such as Japan, in which individuals tend to define their identity in terms of harmonious relationships with other people.[64] In the former, people tend to describe themselves in terms of traits and the self is largely context-free whereas, in the latter, people tend to describe themselves by reference to particular social relationships or situations (for example, 'I care for my sister').

Given that the self plays such a pivotal role in human life, it would not be surprising if thinking about ourselves were to involve the activation of specific neuroanatomical structures. Of course, we should avoid the error made by Descartes, who decided that the pineal gland was the communication gateway that linked the brain to the soul. It would be foolish to assume that the self has a specific physical embodiment of this sort. Nonetheless, when we contemplate ourselves in any of the ways that I have described above, we are clearly doing something 'brainy'.

In recent experiments, Professor Tony David and his colleagues at the Institute of Psychiatry in London have tried to determine whether particular regions of the brain are involved in self-recognition. They used computer techniques to blend photographs of ordinary people with photographs of strangers, creating a series of pictures running from 'other' to 'self' in twenty-one steps. The participants were then shown the pictures while lying in an fMRI scanner, and were asked to say at which point they believed that the pictures were of themselves. All of the pictures activated the posterior fusiform gyrus, a region of the brain known to play a role in the recognition of faces. More interestingly, when the participants recognized a face as 'me' neuroactivations were detected in the dorsolateral prefrontal cortex, an area of the brain known to play a role in complex semantic judgements.[65]

The Social Nature of Psychosis

The reader may be forgiven for thinking that much of the material covered in this chapter has been something of a digression from our main business of explaining madness. As we have covered quite a lot of ground, the reader might also be feeling a little breathless. I would like to finish off by attempting to draw from this diverse material a few simple but important implications.

The findings we have considered in the last few pages paint a picture of the mind–brain that is dramatically different from that assumed by many psychologists investigating psychosis. Most of these researchers have been heavily influenced by the computer metaphor, which sees the brain as a machine that processes information in much the same way that a food processor processes food – without much regard to its meaning or significance for the individual. On the contrary, we have seen that the mind–brain is very unlike a typical computer. Indeed, the things that it does well (for example, recognizing faces, speculating about why other people act in the way that they do) are precisely those things that a typical computer does badly, whereas the things that most computers do well (for example, discovering the square-root of 5876.9) are things that the average human mind finds daunting. The mind–brain is a biologically evolved but flexible cognitive system, which adapts to its environment by learning from other mind–brains (notably its caregivers), and which prioritizes its current activities according to both short-term and long-term goals. To summarize these properties in a single statement that is as profound as it is blindingly obvious: *the mind–brain is a living system*.

This picture is entirely consistent with an important conclusion that we arrived at towards the end of Chapter 7. Remember that, in that chapter, we found strong evidence that the brain is (literally) shaped by experience. The anatomical structures that form subcomponents of the adult central nervous system change in size according to the demands placed on them by events. The structure and function of the adult brain are not simply products of some pre-ordained genetic program (although genes must have an influence) but are the results of a complex series of interactions between the individual and the social environment. It follows that psychiatric theories that consider the brain in isolation from the social world are unlikely to lead to a proper understanding of the origins of psychosis. The neoKraepelinian project of an exclusively biological psychiatry has been doomed to failure from the outset.

The failure of researchers working within the Kraepelinian framework to consider psychological mechanisms that are important in ordinary life has had at least two unfortunate consequences. First, a huge explanatory gap remains between observations of gross cognitive deficits in patients and an understanding of their symptoms. It is simply not obvious how attentional impairments, no matter how real, can lead to hallucinations, paranoid ideas or incoherent speech. Second, as we will see in a later chapter, the findings from studies of gross deficits have had few implications for treatment. Indeed, they have reinforced the neoKraepelinian prejudice that schizophrenia and bipolar disorder are nothing more than brain diseases, and so impeded the development of treatments that address patients' psychological and social needs.

By trying to give a more realistic account of the human mind than that assumed by the neoKraepelinians, I have attempted to provide the conceptual tools with which we will later fashion a more adequate account of madness. To elaborate too much on this point at this stage would be premature. However, even without considering specific complaints in detail, it is not very difficult to see the relevance of the topics we have discussed in the preceding pages.

It is perhaps most obvious that there must be a close relationship between language and psychosis. The three psychotic complaints that have been most intensively investigated – delusions, auditory hallucinations and communication disorder – manifest themselves as forms of speech. (Although we may question Tim Crow's speculative theory that psychosis is genetically associated with cerebral lateralization, there must surely be some truth in his assertion that language and madness are inextricably linked.)[66] It may be less apparent that madness is inherently social in a broader sense. Of course, social cognitive deficits affect patients' ability to negotiate the social world. (American psychologists David Penn, Patrick Corrigan and others have shown that the social competence of patients is better predicted by their performance on measures of social cognition than by their performance on tests of general deficits.)[67] However, there is also good reason to suppose that abnormal social cognition is directly implicated in the behaviours and experiences that are the most obvious manifestations of madness.

Invariably, psychotic complaints reflect concerns about the self, or relationships with other people. Psychotically depressed people, for example, often believe that they are inadequate, or guilty of imaginary misdeeds. Manic patients, in contrast, often feel that they are superior to others, and are capable of achievements that will amaze the world. The delusional beliefs usually attributed to schizophrenia are particularly redolent with social themes. Patients rarely profess bizarre ideas about animals or inanimate objects. Instead they believe that they are being persecuted by imaginary conspiracies, that they have been denied recognition for inventing the helicopter or the pop-up toaster, that they are loved by pop stars or by their doctors, or that their partners are conducting numerous affairs despite compelling evidence to the contrary. Although some patients experience pleasant hallucinations, many report that their voices comment adversely on their actions, or goad them to perform acts that will harm themselves or frighten others. Michael Musalek, a psychiatrist at the University of Vienna, has suggested that psychotic symptoms therefore reflect the core existential dilemmas experienced by ordinary people.[68] To put this observation another way, the unusual beliefs and experiences of psychiatric patients all seem to reflect preoccupations about the position of the self in the social universe.

9

Madness and Emotion

Reason is, and ought only to be the slave of the passions, and can never pretend to any other office than to serve and obey them.

David Hume[1]

Emotions play a pivotal role in human nature. On the one hand they colour the moments when we feel most human – falling in love, witnessing birth or death, achieving our ambitions or accepting humiliation and defeat. On the other hand, because we share them with other species, they ground us in the biological world. Yet, curiously, they are not usually considered to be important features of some of the extreme forms of mental suffering that are the focus of this book. In this chapter, I wish to redress this neglect and argue that psychotic symptoms are above all emotional phenomena. This argument will entail an examination of what we know about the psychology of emotions, which will prepare the way for our more detailed examination of individual psychotic complaints in later chapters.

Some readers may be surprised by this approach. When most psychologists and psychiatrists think about extreme emotions, they usually focus on the spectrum of neurotic disorders, perhaps because non-psychotic depressions and anxieties are among the most common symptoms reported by patients visiting general physicians.[2] When research has been carried out into the role of negative emotion in psychosis, much of it has adhered to the Kraepelinian paradigm, and has therefore focused on patients with a diagnosis of bipolar disorder rather than schizophrenia. This is unfortunate because emotion probably plays as important a role in the experiences of schizophrenia patients as it does in the lives of patients diagnosed as suffering from manic depression.

Some studies have shown that as many as 65 per cent of schizophrenia patients complain of being depressed.[3] Others have observed comparable levels of anxiety.[4] Canadian psychiatrists Ross Norman and Ashok Malla measured both depression and anxiety in a large group of schizophrenia patients and found that the two emotions were highly correlated. High levels of both emotions were associated with delusions and hallucinations but, surprisingly, not with negative symptoms such as apathy or social withdrawal.[5]

Other studies have shown that negative emotions are prominent in the early stages of psychotic breakdown, often preceding the emergence of positive symptoms. American psychiatrists Marvin Herz and Charles Melville interviewed the relatives of schizophrenia patients in order to discover *prodromal* symptoms that typically occur before a full-blown episode. Depression was reported in 76 per cent of cases, and anxiety in 86 per cent.[6] A similar study conducted in Britain by clinical psychologist Max Birchwood and his colleagues at All Saints Hospital in Birmingham found that depression was reported in 57 per cent of cases, and anxiety in 62 per cent.[7]

Further evidence that emotion plays an important role in schizophrenia symptoms has recently been gathered by American clinical psychologist Nancy Docherty of Kent State University in Ohio. Docherty has pointed out that many (although perhaps not all) schizophrenia patients find that their symptoms worsen when they are emotionally stressed. Positive symptoms (hallucinations and delusions) and also symptoms of cognitive disorganization (psychotic speech) are particularly affected in this way. Negative symptoms, on the other hand, appear to be relatively unaffected.[8]

Taken together, these observations have two important implications. First, the presence of negative mood in so many schizophrenia patients, especially those suffering from positive symptoms, is yet further evidence that the Kraepelinian distinction between schizophrenia and the mood disorders is misleading. Second, because negative emotions are usually present before a recurrence of hallucinations or delusions, it seems unlikely that they are mere consequences or by-products of psychosis.

So, What is an Emotion?

Surprisingly, although the problems treated by psychiatrists are often called 'emotional disorders', most textbooks of psychiatry have nothing to say about the nature of emotions. As British psychologists Mick Power and Tim Dalgleish have recently commented:

A worrying truth about the psychology of emotion literature is that the majority of theories of normal, everyday emotions make little or no reference to emotional disorder. Similarly, there are a host of theories of emotional disorder, which are only loosely anchored, if indeed they are anchored at all, to theories of emotional order.[9]

Two assumptions

It is in fact quite difficult to distinguish between emotions and other feelings such as pain or hunger, or other types of mental contents such as attitudes and beliefs. Textbooks of psychology routinely observe that emotions have affective (feeling), cognitive (thoughts and beliefs) and behavioural components, which should alert us to the possibility that the ordinary language word 'emotion' does not refer to a single process. Two other assumptions about emotion commonly held by psychologists are worth noting before proceeding further.

First, many psychologists have assumed that emotions involve some kind of evaluation or appraisal of events. We tend to be happy when we know that we are loved by someone special or when we believe that we have achieved something important, sad when we have lost someone or suffered a setback to our ambitions, and anxious when we anticipate that something unpleasant will happen in the future. During the 1980s, a protracted debate about the role of appraisals in emotion was conducted between two American psychologists, Robert Zajonc and Richard Lazarus. Zajonc argued that feelings are the primary component of emotion, and that emotional reactions can occur without a conscious appraisal of the environment. (An obvious example would be our sudden reaction when we catch a brief glimpse of a large object moving dangerously towards us.)[10] Lazarus, on the other hand, argued that cognitive processes are primary, and that emotions are always triggered by the belief that something positive or negative has happened or is about to happen. According to Lazarus, each emotion therefore has a specific meaning or 'core relational theme' – an offence against the individual in the case of anger, or the experience of irrevocable loss in the case of sadness.[11] To some extent this dispute was more semantic than substantial – not all cognitive processes are conscious and some kind of rapid appraisal of the environment is presumably involved even when we automatically throw ourselves out of the path of an approaching car.

Mick Power and Tim Dalgleish have noted that, when emotional responses are triggered automatically, this is often because the appraisal process has taken place at some point in the past. For example, a man whose memories of childhood are shrouded with fear may immediately feel frightened on hearing his elderly father's raised voice. In this case, the sound of the father's voice automatically elicits fear because it has previously been appraised as signalling danger. They also note that emotions often involve cycles of appraisal, rather than a single appraisal event. The experience of anger when insulted by a friend may lead to reflections about the relationship, modulating further encounters with the friend, and thereby leading to further appraisals.

A second, widely held assumption about emotions is that their behavioural manifestations have a long evolutionary history, and serve important functions in our lives. Not surprisingly, people who are suffering from anxiety or depression often find this a difficult proposition to accept. However, it is obvious that at least some emotional states help us to respond effectively in emergencies. When we see the car moving towards us, the rush of adrenalin prepares us to make the physical effort that will save our lives and, when we feel anxious, we can brace ourselves for the calamities to come.

It is less obvious that emotions have important cognitive benefits. We usually have to juggle many competing goals in life. Our emotions enable us to prioritize our mental resources rapidly in order to face the changing demands of our environment, so that we can focus on those goals that are most immediately pressing.[12] The decisions we make in these circumstances are often influenced, not by a labour-intensive analysis of the likely outcomes of different actions, but by a much quicker anticipation of the emotional consequences of each choice.

(People selecting between risky options choose the option that they think will lead them to feel better.)[13] Mr Spock, the character in the science fiction television series *Star Trek* who hails from the planet Vulcan and who, in the absence of emotion, can only reason logically, would be mentally paralysed when faced with many everyday dilemmas.[14]

Of course, extremely negative emotions do not *appear* particularly adaptive. However, the neural mechanisms responsible for emotional behaviour presumably evolved a long time in the past. Therefore, although the situations that typically elicit emotions – 'fighting, falling in love, escaping predators, confronting sexual infidelity, and so on'[15] – have occurred innumerable times in evolutionary history, the most appropriate way of responding to these challenges today may differ from the ways that were most adaptive in the past. British psychologist Paul Gilbert has argued, for example, that many of the behaviours associated with depression (particularly reduced aggression to more dominant individuals and increased anger towards more submissive persons), although apparently maladaptive in a modern context, allowed our ancestors to adapt following a loss of rank in a simple hierarchical society.[16]

The two faces of emotion

In practice, psychological research on emotions has focused on two quite separate phenomena. Many ethologists and social psychologists, following Charles Darwin, have focused on the expression of emotions, particularly on the face. These investigators have sometimes argued that emotional expressions are special forms of communication that are universal, and therefore probably inherited.[17] Other researchers, particularly clinical psychologists, have been more concerned with subjectively experienced emotions as revealed by first-person reports such as 'I feel depressed', 'I feel anxious', or 'I feel ashamed.' It is easy to assume that there is a special relationship between these two types of phenomena, that each facial expression is associated with a particular subjective feeling. Consistent with this assumption, there is obviously some degree of correspondence between feelings and expressions – when we feel depressed we are more likely to frown than to smile. However, we should not therefore leap to the further assumption that expressions and subjective experiences are different manifestations of a single underlying process, that there is a discrete number of *basic emotions* that are reflected on our faces and in our minds.

The idea of basic emotions seems so natural and self-evident that it has dominated research on normal emotions, and also on the abnormal emotions encountered in psychiatric practice. It has particularly influenced research on facial expressions. In an important series of studies, Paul Ekman and his colleagues at the University of California in San Francisco have collected evidence that common expressions of anger, fear, enjoyment, sadness, disgust and possibly surprise are recognized in diverse societies of the world.[18] However, not all psychologists have accepted this evidence uncritically. Canadian researcher James Russell has carefully scrutinized the work of Ekman and others, and has noted that most studies have employed forced-choice procedures in which informants are shown photographs of faces and are then asked to select from a list of possible emotions. Russell has argued that these procedures minimize disagreements and that there is less agreement when more open-ended procedures are used.[19] Even when forced-choice procedures have been employed, differences between cultures are greater than Ekman has supposed. (For example, Japanese and American informants generally agree that certain expressions are best described as happiness, sadness and surprise, but show less agreement when asked to describe expressions corresponding to North American notions of anger, disgust or fear.)

Subjective emotions

In the case of subjective experience, the idea of basic emotions is closely related to the idea that we discover our emotions by a process of introspection. According to this theory (and, no matter how natural and self-evident it may appear, it is a theory), when I say that I feel depressed something happens along the following lines. First, I notice some kind of internal state or sensation; second, I recognize that inner state or sensation as the feeling of 'depression'; and, third, I report it to anyone who is likely to be interested.

Some elements of this theory are uncontentious. For example, there is nothing wrong with the idea that we are influenced by events occurring inside our bodies. Writing in 1948, the influential American behaviourist B. F. Skinner observed that:

The response 'My tooth aches' is partly under the control of a state of affairs to which the speaker alone is able to react, since no one else can establish the required connection with the tooth in question. There is nothing mysterious or metaphysical about this; the simple fact is that each speaker possesses a small but important world of private stimuli.[20]

Some psychologists have suggested that this private world is the source of our emotional experiences. For example, in his celebrated two-volume *Principles of Psychology* published in 1890, the American psychologist and philosopher William James argued that:

Bodily changes follow directly the perception of the exciting fact, and our feeling of the same changes as they occur *is* the emotion. Common sense says ... we meet a bear are frightened and run ... The hypothesis here to be defended says that the order of the sequence is incorrect, that the one mental state is not immediately induced by the other [the perception of the bear], that the bodily manifestations must first be interposed between them, and that the more rational statement is we feel ... afraid because we tremble.[21]

Recent versions of this theory have implicated various types of internal stimuli in subjective emotions, including arousal of the autonomic nervous system,[22] feedback from motor responses involved in facial and bodily expressions,[23] and even changes in brain blood temperature resulting from the disruption of vascular flow by facial muscle movements.[24] Overall, there is quite convincing evidence that each of these processes does have some influence.[25] For example, if people are persuaded to adopt particular expressions, their feelings tend to be affected in predictable ways. However, as long ago as 1927, the American physiologist Walter Cannon pointed out that bodily sensations are too diffuse to account for the rich variety of emotional experiences reported by ordinary people. More importantly, even if it was to transpire, following further physiological studies, that the range of internal stimuli is sufficiently varied, the problem of how people can learn to notice and report these stimuli as emotional states represents an insuperable obstacle to James's theory.

In order to see the power of this criticism, we must consider how individuals come to possess a vocabulary of feelings and internal states. This question was considered by the Austrian-British philosopher Ludwig Wittgenstein, and was famously debated in his posthumously published book *Philosophical Investigations*, which first appeared in 1953.[26] However, Wittgenstein's analysis was anticipated in a less well-known paper published by B. F. Skinner in 1945.[27] Although written in the terse jargon beloved by American behaviourists of the period, Skinner's account is much simpler than Wittgenstein's, and so it is his version of the argument that I will outline here.

Having established that we each possess an internal world of stimuli to which we have exclusive access (no one else can feel our toothache), Skinner points out that the way we learn to label those stimuli is far from obvious. The problem is that speaking is a social process in which the appropriate use of words depends on rules and conventions that we learn from other people.* These conventions can only be discovered in the context of the right kind of relationship between the person who is learning to speak and what Skinner describes as the wider 'verbal community'. To take a simple example, learning object names like 'cow' or 'dog' presents no particular problem as both the learner and the verbal community have access to the stimuli that prompt these names (cows and dogs). I can correct you if you call a dog a cow, and my failure to respond appropriately to your request to 'pat the cow' may alert you to the fact that you have used the wrong name. However, these possibilities are absent in the case of internal stimuli. I cannot point to a particular profile of physiological states inside you, no matter how complex, and teach you to call it 'depression'. Nor am I in a position to disagree with you should you label a physiological state as 'depression' on the grounds that I would call the very same state 'anxiety'.

Nonetheless, we plainly do talk about internal states and Skinner discusses a number of indirect ways by which we can acquire the necessary vocabulary. Any publicly observable event that regularly accompanies a private stimulus may be exploited by the verbal community in much the same way that a sighted person might use visual

---

* This argument that *names* are learnt from others does not contradict the view, now widely held among linguists, that some aspects of language – particularly syntax – are wired into the architecture of the brain.

cues when teaching a blind person to name objects. For example, a child's protest, 'That hurts', may be responded to appropriately if it occurs following a fall resulting in a grazed knee. Similarly, the verbal community may encourage statements that are made together with particular types of non-verbal behaviour (groaning and clutching the jaw in the case of 'toothache', smiling and related gestures in the case of 'happiness'). Nor must we assume that some kind of overt reinforcement is required for these kinds of learning to occur – children have many opportunities to observe in others associations between particular types of emotional statements and the relevant public stimuli.

Sometimes we are able to learn terms that appear to describe internal states because those states occasionally occur in a public form. For example, the word 'murderous' may be used to describe an emotional state that typically accompanies murderous behaviour. Other emotion words, for example 'agitated' or 'ebullient', began their life referring to public events but have been extended to the psychological domain by a process of analogy. Recently, the British psychologist Graham Richards devoted an entire book to this phenomenon, and the following is just one of the many examples that he cites:

Fire-control terms have proved especially useful for the encoding of what we now term arousal states, and constitute an extension of the temperature-based PL [psychological language] (hot, cold, tepid, frigid, lukewarm, icy). They include the following:

to blaze up, to burn, to be burnt up/out/into one's memory, to burn one's fingers, to dampen down, to douse, dying embers (e.g. 'her smile rekindled the dying embers of passion'), fiery, flaming, to fan the flames, to flare up, to fuel, to ignite (e.g. 'his words ignited the passions of the crowd'), inflammatory, to kindle, to light (e.g. 'I just want to light a flame in your heart'), to rake over the ashes, red hot, to rekindle, scorched, searing (e.g. especially in the phrase heart-searing), singed, to smoulder/smouldering, to spark off, to stoke up.[28]

The word 'depression' began its life in just this way. Until the early years of the nineteenth century, doctors labelled negative emotional states as 'melancholia', 'neurasthenia' or 'moppishness' (the last term being reserved for the uneducated classes). 'Depression' was first used in physical medicine to describe a reduction in cadiovascular function and was afterwards adopted by early psychiatrists to indicate emotional states that were considered to be the opposite of excitation.[29] During the early years of the twentieth century the term intruded into the language of ordinary people, so that we now think of 'depression' as a natural label for how we feel during times of loss.

This account suggests the possibility that different cultures will describe subjective emotions differently. Collating the evidence that addresses this question, James Russell has demonstrated that societies vary dramatically in the range of words they allocate to emotional states.[30] For example, the English language contains over 2000 emotion words, whereas most languages contain fewer than 200. Emotional states that appear quite fundamental from the perspective of an English speaker are not always mirrored in the lives and languages of other cultures. In some African languages, the same word covers what in English would be described as anger and sadness whereas the Gidjingali aborigines of Australia do not discriminate between fear and shame. Prototypical emotions that have a central place in Western concepts of psychopathology appear to be entirely absent in some cultures. For example, there is no word equivalent to depression in many non-Western cultures and no word equivalent to anxiety among Eskimos or Yorubas.

Even when emotion concepts do appear to translate from one language to another the relevant words in the two cultures may not be precisely equivalent in meaning. A number of studies have been carried out in which the Japanese equivalents of the English words 'anxiety' and 'depression' have been identified by the process of back-translation (translating the English words into Japanese and then checking that independent translators translate them back to their original English expressions). However, further studies of the meanings of these words (for example by asking people for other words they associate with them) have revealed substantial differences in the way that they are used in the two cultures.

Cultures even appear to differ in where they draw the line between emotional and non-emotional internal states. For example, the Japanese word 'jodo' has been translated as the equivalent of the English word emotion, but includes states that translate as considerate, motivated, lucky and calculating. To take another example cited by Russell, the Chewong of Malaysia, who are apparently limited to only seven words that clearly translate as emotion states, group together both thoughts and feelings, locating them in the liver. Of course, one possible way of interpreting these findings would be to assume that Japanese and Chewong informants are simply wrong about their emotional states. However, in pursuing this argument, we would be making the chauvinistic assumption that the structure of the human mind is uniquely and accurately reflected in the vocabulary of English.

The dimensional structure of subjective emotion

Despite the different ways in which cultures describe internal states, it is possible that a considerable degree of cross-cultural consistency exists when emotions are considered within a dimensional framework. The idea here is that, underlying the diverse ways in which different cultures describe their emotions, there may be a relatively small number of emotional dimensions that are universal. Various statistical methods have been used in an attempt to discover such dimensions, the most common being multidimensional scaling in which informants are asked to rate the similarity of various emotion words. The informants' ratings are then analysed using a complex mathematical procedure, which tries to account for the ratings in terms of a minimum number of dimensions. (This approach is similar to the technique of factor analysis, which I briefly described in Chapter 4.)

This type of research has consistently shown that ratings of emotions can be plotted as a circular pattern or circumplex in a two-dimensional space. This structure has been found not only using words but also using photographs of facial expressions, and with people from such varying places in the world as North America, Greece, Spain, Vietnam, Hong Kong and Haiti. The two dimensions that define this space have in turn have been interpreted in different ways by different researchers. Russell has taken what might seem to be the commonsense view, and has suggested that the two dimensions are, first, pleasantness versus unpleasantness and, second, the degree to which the individual is physiologically aroused. On this view, pleasure is the opposite of *dysphoria* (negative emotion).[31] In contrast, American psychologists David Watson and Auke Tellegren have argued that the same structure is better described in terms of two independent dimensions of positive and negative affect, which are revealed by rotating Russell's model through 45 degrees[32] (see Figure 9.1).

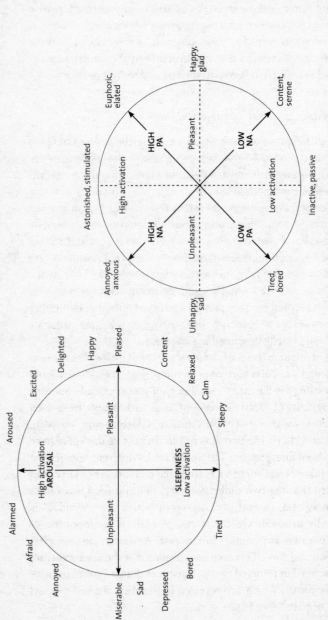

Figure 9.1 The two emotional circumplexes (adapted from B. Parkinson, P. Totterdell, R. B. Briner and S. Reynolds (1996) *Changing Moods: The Psychology of Mood and Mood Regulation*. Harlow: Longman). Russell's model, on the left, proposes two dimensions of affect – positive vs negative and arousal vs sleepiness. Rotating this model through 45°, we arrive at Watson and Tellegren's model of independent positive (PA) and negative affects (NA), which is on the right.

These systems are clearly inter-translatable (for example, a state of high positive affect according to Watson and Tellegren corresponds with a state of high arousal and high pleasure according to Russell). The debate about which system is preferable is therefore quite technical and, to some commentators, the differences between them are largely arbitrary. However, to my mind at least, Watson and Tellegren's system has several compelling advantages.

Least importantly, Watson and Tellegren have argued that the majority of emotion words in most languages describe the regions of the circumplex that they have characterized as high positive affect and high negative affect. Therefore, they argue, these two types of subjective emotion are the most salient, and the most psychologically real, to most people in the world.

More importantly, Watson and Tellegren's model of positive and negative affect clearly maps on to two fundamental psychological processes that are common to all animal species, and which govern much of our behaviour. *Reinforcement* (or reward in ordinary language) refers to the process by which behaviours tend to be repeated if they lead to stimuli that have positive consequences for the individual. Stimuli of this sort are known as *reinforcers*. The most basic reinforcers satisfy biological drives such as hunger and the need for sex. Not surprisingly, organisms (whether human or non-human) tend to approach reinforcing stimuli, and the accompanying emotion experienced by human beings is positive affect. Punishment, in contrast, refers to the process by which organisms (whether human or non-human) tend to desist from actions that lead to negative consequences, such as painful stimuli. The emotion we experience when encountering such stimuli is negative affect. The neurophysiological systems responsible for these two processes are beyond the scope of this book; suffice it to say that there has been an impressive accumulation of evidence indicating that distinctive brain mechanisms are responsible for these processes and hence, presumably, for the two types of emotion.[33]

An important implication of Watson and Tellegren's model is that, contrary to folk wisdom, positive and negative emotions can occur independently of each other. This claim has sometimes been regarded as controversial, partly because, in most circumstances, positive and negative affect are negatively correlated.[34] (Stimuli that evoke positive affect tend not to evoke negative affect and vice versa, so that they often *appear* to lie at opposite ends of a single dimension of emotion.) However, even in ordinary life the two types of emotion sometimes occur together – for example during periods of transition between one phase of life and another, such as when starting at college or when moving to a new job.[35] In a later chapter we will see that this model helps to make sense of the experiences of manic patients, who often experience positive and negative affect simultaneously.

It should be emphasized that nothing in this dimensional account of emotion detracts from the fact that we are able to use a sophisticated emotional vocabulary. Presumably, our choice of emotion words when experiencing positive or negative affect is influenced by additional information that is available at the time. This information may include some of the physiological cues we considered earlier (for example, the butterfly sensation in our stomach that we associate with fear), our knowledge of our recent history (we are unlikely to feel ashamed unless we know that we have transgressed a moral code or caused insult to others), together with various environmental stimuli (for example, the behaviour of other people who are present).

The emotional circumplex and abnormal mood

As I noted at the beginning of this chapter, most psychiatrists and clinical psychologists have uncritically accepted the theory of basic emotions as reflected in the English language. For example, the neuroses have traditionally been divided into depression and anxiety disorders in much the same way that ordinary English distinguishes between being depressed and being anxious. In the past few years, this classification of the neuroses has been challenged by a number of researchers in Britain and the United States who have used arguments similar to those I employed in Chapter 4 when criticizing the neo-Kraepelinian account of the psychoses.[36] For example, patients rarely experience depression or anxiety alone, and clinical studies using questionnaire[37] and interview measures[38] have consistently found that these symptoms are highly correlated. Moreover, when patients have been studied over long periods of time, mood symptoms often shift so that what seems to be mainly depression at the outset may later appear to be an anxiety disorder or vice versa.[39] Not surprisingly, as we have seen, parallel observations have been made by researchers interested in the moods experienced by schizophrenia patients. Although some researchers have focused on depression and others on anxiety, high levels of *both* emotions are usually reported during psychotic episodes and also during the prodromal phase that precedes them.

David Watson and his colleague Lee Anna Clark have argued that these problems of classifying abnormal mood can be explained by locating them on the emotional circumplex.[40] All negative emotions, they have argued, involve strong negative affect or dysphoria. Feelings of anxiety typically also involve physical tension (the body's natural preparation for fight or flight in the face of an emergency). Depression, on the other hand, usually involves not only the presence of negative affect, but also the absence of positive affect. Psychiatric patients who have been administered questionnaires designed to measure these different components of emotion have been found to score as the theory predicts.[41]

Do Some Psychotic Patients Lack Emotions?

Although the experiences of patients diagnosed as suffering from bipolar disorder provide the most obvious point of contact between madness and theories of normal emotion, I will focus in the remaining parts of this chapter on symptoms more usually attributed to schizophrenia. The apparent absence of emotions sometimes observed in patients with this diagnosis presents an obvious but hopefully not insuperable difficulty for my claim that emotion plays a central role in psychosis.

Schizophrenia patients' apparent lack of emotional expression is sometimes described as *flat affect* or *affective blunting*. However, patients sometimes complain of a lack of subjective pleasure, known as *anhedonia*. These symptoms are usually included in the broader class of negative symptoms that emerges from factor-analytic studies such as those we considered in the first part of this book. The appearance of these symptoms in the same factor suggests that they occur together in real life, so that someone who complains of anhedonia is also likely to show flat affect, and vice versa.

However, they are separable phenomena nonetheless. The Scale for Assessment of Negative Symptoms (SANS), a widely used symptom-rating scale devised by American psychiatrist Nancy Andreasen,[42] describes the following features of flat affect: unchanging facial expression ('the patient's face appears wooden, mechanical, frozen'); decreased spontaneous movements; paucity of expressive gestures ('the patient does not use his body as an aid in expressing his ideas'); poor eye-contact; affective non-responsivity ('failure to smile or laugh when prompted') and lack of vocal inflections ('speech has a monotonic quality, and important words are not emphasized through changes in pitch or volume'). All of these descriptors concern the expression of emotion.

In contrast, the same scale describes *anhedonia-asociality* as comprising a lack of recreational interests and activities; a loss of sexual interest and activity; an inability to feel intimacy and closeness; and impoverished relationships with friends and peers. This description emphasizes the failure to obtain subjective pleasure from relationships, a phenomenon that is sometimes called *social anhedonia* to differentiate it from the inability to experience physical pleasure, known as *physical anhedonia*. Psychologists Loren and Jean Chapman of the University of Wisconsin have devised questionnaires for measuring these types of anhedonia separately in both patients and ordinary people and have shown that they are usually highly correlated.[43]

It is also important to note that flat affect and anhedonia do not exhaust the negative symptoms commonly attributed to schizophrenia patients. For example, other negative symptoms listed in the SANS manual include *alogia* (impoverished thinking); *apathy*; and *attentional deficits*. With the exception of the last of these, which we considered in the previous chapter, these symptoms have been the subject of almost no psychological research, and so I will say almost nothing more about them in the present context.

The status of negative symptoms

Before proceeding to consider flat affect and anhedonia in detail, it is worth briefly considering the status of the negative symptoms in general.

Different psychiatrists have emphasized the negative features of psychosis to varying degrees. For example, Kraepelin's account of dementia praecox clearly emphasizes the intellectual and emotional deficits he observed in his patients, whereas Schneider placed much more emphasis on what we now regard as positive symptoms. Modern theories of negative symptoms, which, in the absence of a substantial volume of psychological research, have sometimes tended to be rather speculative, have turned on two controversies. First, some psychologists and psychiatrists have debated whether negative symptoms are products of some kind of underlying intrinsic (in medical terms, morbid) process and, second, others have debated whether they can be distinguished from depression. These debates are not entirely unconnected as, clearly, if negative symptoms are just an unusual variant of depression they are less mysterious than they might otherwise appear.

The problem of whether negative symptoms are caused by some kind of process intrinsic to the individual is raised by the suspicion that they may be environmentally determined or iatrogenic (doctor-caused) conditions. Until recently, patients commonly spent many years languishing in large hospitals where they received very little stimulation. Not surprisingly, many patients treated in this way fell into a state of learned helplessness, in which they lacked the skills to interact with others or the motivation to look after themselves. In the 1970s, British social psychiatrist John Wing, working with the sociologist George Brown, observed that providing institutionalized patients with appropriate support and stimulation could bring about a reduction in what we now call negative symptoms, although they cautioned that overstimulating patients might cause an exacerbation of their delusions and hallucinations.[44] More recently, some authors have made comparisons between the fate of institutionalized patients and other marginalized or victimized individuals such as the long-term unemployed or the victims of concentration camps.[45] Psychiatrist and anthropologist Richard Warner, based at the University of Colorado, has examined historical records to show that recovery rates in psychotic patients are lower in periods of poor economic opportunity such as the Great Depression of the 1930s, so this comparison may not be entirely far-fetched.[46] However, not all studies have found an association between institutionalization and negative symptoms. Eve Johnstone, Tim Crow and others failed to find differences in negative symptoms between patients living in the community and those who had experienced long-term hospitalization.[47]

Whereas evidence on the relationship between negative symptoms and an adverse environment is inconsistent, the evidence that negative symptoms can be exacerbated by the medications administered to patients is clear-cut. Although biological psychiatrists have been slow to recognize the negative psychological impact of their treatment methods, a *neuroleptic-induced deficit syndrome* (NIDS), characterized by emotional blunting and reduced motivation, has been well documented. It is often difficult to distinguish between this syndrome and negative symptoms that are not drug-induced.[48] As neuroleptics are also known to make some patients depressed, side effects of medication may also contribute to the difficulty in distinguishing between negative symptoms and depression. In a study conducted by psychologist Martin Harrow and his colleagues at the University of Illinois, schizophrenia patients were studied for a period of five years. Patients who were taking neuroleptics, in comparison with those who were not, were more likely to experience both depression and anhedonia during the follow-up period, even when initial levels of symptomatology were taken into account.[49]

Other researchers have concluded that negative symptoms, while overlapping with depression, cannot simply be explained by negative mood. In the study by Ross Norman and Ashok Malla described earlier, depression was more closely associated with positive than negative symptoms.[50] In another study, carried out by psychiatrist Steven Hirsch and others in London, in which a group of schizophrenia patients who were currently depressed was compared with a group that was not currently depressed, no difference was found in the SANS scores of the two groups.[51] If these findings seem inconsistent with those reported by Martin Harrow and his colleagues it is perhaps because they have not been interpreted in the context of a well-thought-out theory of emotion. As we will see later, when researchers have focused specifically on patients' emotional responses, a clearer picture of the mechanisms responsible for some negative symptoms has begun to emerge.

The discovery that some of the cognitive deficits found in schizophrenia patients are specifically associated with negative symptoms might seem to be consistent with the notion that they are intrinsic characteristics of the individual. In the last chapter we saw, for example, that negative symptom patients perform particularly poorly on high-load versions of the Continuous Performance Test. However, as we have also seen, test performance may not be a reliable indicator of an intrinsic morbid process. Indeed, there is nothing implausible about the idea that cognitive deficits arise from an impoverished environment. (Remember David Shakow's observation that the performance of schizophrenia patients on psychological tests could match that of ordinary people if they received an appropriate level of support and encouragement.) Better evidence that negative symptoms are more than just an adverse reaction to an unsupportive environment is the finding that they are sometimes present during the earliest stages of psychosis, especially in those patients whose premorbid functioning (as reflected by occupational or school reports) is poor.[52] This observation suggests, first, that there is a continuum between poor social functioning and negative symptoms and, second, that whatever mechanisms are responsible for negative symptoms may be present before the onset (and treatment) of full-blown psychosis.

In an attempt to resolve the debate about the intrinsic nature of negative symptoms, psychiatrist William Carpenter and his colleagues at the University of Maryland have proposed that only a proportion of patients suffer from what they describe as a core *deficit syndrome*.[53] They have argued that the symptoms that define the deficit syndrome are enduring features of the patient that are not caused by extrinsic factors such as depression or demoralization. The six symptoms which they believe often meet these requirements are: restricted emotion as evidenced by facial expression, gestures and vocal inflection; diminished subjective emotional range; poverty of speech; curbing of interests; a diminished sense of purpose; and diminished social drive. However, the crucial feature of their definition is the exclusion of possible causes such as anxiety, depression or drug side effects, which they argue can be achieved with a high degree of reliability if information about the long-term course of an illness can be obtained from a suitable informant, for example a close relative of the patient.[54] Although this approach is surely an important advance on previous attempts to make sense of negative symptoms, it suffers from disadvantages that we have already encountered in other categorial classification schemes. First, the division of patients into those with or without the deficit syndrome does not allow for the possibility that patients suffer from deficit symptoms by degrees (that is, that deficit symptoms, like other symptoms we have considered, may lie on a continuum with normal functioning). Second, the approach does not help us understand the role of psychological processes in negative symptoms. It is possible that these problems can be avoided by focusing on particular symptoms without trying to prejudge, for the moment, their causes.

Flat affect

The danger of equating outward expression with the subjective experience of emotion was vividly illustrated by a remarkable paper written by Jean Bouricius, a retired social worker and mother of a 32-year-old schizophrenia patient.[55] Suspicious that objective ratings of psychopathology failed to capture adequately her son's experiences, she asked five professionals (two doctors, two social workers and a psychologist) who knew him well to assess his symptoms using the SANS. All five returned moderately high ratings, especially for affective blunting. However, Ms Bouricius was able to show that her son's diary notes for the same period were rich with emotional material. For example, he described a visit to his doctor in the following manner:

Went to see my doctor but couldn't talk. Kept saying, 'I don't know,' to his questions. Started crying. Felt pity and love for Rhoda [a friend] because she has fear, because she has to take medication, because she is a mental patient like me, because I want to marry her, but I think I never can. I started saying that I had lost my memory. Then I got up and left.

And a few days later:

Rhoda asked me if I were spoiled and I angrily said no, but I feel hurt, as if I was born for a purpose I hide from, covering myself with warm blankets. Go to hell, World! I cannot die in peace and safety. I cannot face the slightest breath of real life or death or ugliness. But I hurt for being such a coward. I was always a coward — socially, physically, mentally, sexually, emotionally. If I go insane, am I brave? I will, because then, and only then, I am brave, not a coward. I hate all people. They compete and want stimulation. I hate them all, all. None loves, none cares, none understands or ever will understand. I am dead, dead — very, very limited, afraid and hurt. Go to hell, World!

The relationship between flat affect and patients' subjective experience of emotion has been more formally investigated in a number of studies which have broadly supported Ms Bouricius' observations. Howard Berenbaum and Tom Oltmanns showed emotionally blunted schizophrenia patients, non-blunted schizophrenia patients, depressed patients and ordinary people film clips that had been selected for their ability to elicit emotional reactions. The participants were asked to report the extent to which they felt happy or disgusted by the content of each clip. As expected, the blunted patients were rated as less expressive than the normal controls when watching both positive and negative clips. They were also less expressive than the non-blunted schizophrenia patients, but only when watching the positive clips. However, when the participants' subjective ratings of their emotions were examined, the blunted patients did not differ from those of any of the control groups.[56]

Ann Kring, Sandra Kerr, David Smith and John Neale of the State University of New York at Stoney Brook carried out a very similar experiment, but studied patients who were drug-free in order to exclude the confounding effects of neuroleptic medication. Using a questionnaire designed to measure positive and negative affect as defined by Watson and Tellegren's circumplex model, they also found that their schizophrenia patients experienced just as much positive and negative emotion as ordinary people, despite being less emotionally expressive.[57] More recently, a group of researchers at the University of Maastricht in Holland have taken the study of patients' subjective emotions out of the laboratory and into everyday life by using a technique known as *experience sampling*, in which a small electronic device is used to prompt patients to fill in simple diaries at random points in the day; in this study, schizophrenia patients as a whole were found to experience more intense and variable negative emotion than healthy controls, and emotionally blunted patients did not differ from patients who were not showing evidence of flat affect.[58]

The overall picture that emerges from these studies is of normal subjective emotion in schizophrenia patients. Flat affect, therefore, appears to reflect a difficulty of expressing rather than feeling emotions. Consistent with this hypothesis, Cecile Sison, Murray Alpert and others at the New York University Medical Center have observed that patients with flat affect show more hesitations in their speech, and less activity in their facial muscles (as measured by electromyography), than schizophrenic patients without flat affect, or depressed patients.[59]

It remains unclear why some psychotic patients experience this difficulty. In a study reported by Meredith Mayer, Murray Alpert and their colleagues it was found that flat affect was associated with severe side effects of neuroleptic medication, length of hospitalization, and poor performance on neuropsychological tests designed to assess the functioning of the right half of the cerebral cortex.[60] As the right cerebral hemisphere is believed to be involved in the regulation of emotional expression, this last finding might seem unsurprising. Unfortunately, later researchers, using more sophisticated right hemisphere tests, have not been able to replicate these results.[61]

Intriguingly, whether or not flat affect is associated with poor functioning of particular brain regions, it may most accurately be described as a problem of social communication. Heiner Ellgring, a psychologist at the University of Würzburg in Germany, studied the facial expressions of schizophrenia patients as they watched emotion-provoking films and, like the American researchers, found that they were under-expressive. However, she found that the patients showed reduced activity specifically in those muscles of the upper face that are normally active when we are talking to other people (for example, when we raise our eyebrows in response to a juicy piece of gossip). In another study, she calculated the rate at which facial expressions occurred while speaking and when not engaged in conversation. Ordinary people are most expressive when talking to others. However, in the case of the schizophrenia patients studied by Ellgring, no differences were observed in the rates at which expressions were generated while speaking and not speaking. Ellgring argues that these findings show that, in schizophrenia patients, facial expressions have become dissociated from their communicative function. Clearly, this could be caused by some kind of damage to the social brain. Equally, it is possible that the long periods of social isolation often experienced by schizophrenia patients might cause them to lose the skill of expressing their emotions to other people.[62]

Anhedonia

Like affective blunting, the inability to experience pleasure has long been regarded as an important feature of schizophrenia. In the mid-1950s, the Hungarian-born psychoanalyst Sandor Rado, who had joined the great European exodus of intellectuals to America in the years preceding the Second World War, argued that anhedonia was not merely a symptom of the disorder, but a core deficit that led to loss of motivation, a vulnerability to irrational fears, an incoherent sense of self, and an inability to form adequate relationships.[63] This idea was developed further in Paul Meehl's speculative 1962 paper on the relationship between schizophrenia and personality.[64] Meehl suggested that anhedonia might be a primary cause of the disorder, present before the onset of illness, and responsible for patients' social isolation and aberrant interpersonal behaviour. One problem with this idea is that anhedonia is not restricted to schizophrenia patients. Martin Harrow and his colleagues in Chicago interviewed psychiatric patients about their experiences of joy and pleasure, and found that, although anhedonia was most often reported by schizophrenia patients, it was also frequently reported by patients with other diagnoses.[65] Similarly, Joanna Katsanis and colleagues at the University of Minnesota studied patients who were experiencing their first episode of psychosis, and found that high levels of anhedonia were reported, not only by those diagnosed as suffering from schizophrenia, but also by patients diagnosed as suffering from schizoaffective disorder, depression or bipolar disorder.[66]

This last observation may seem particularly surprising, as bipolar patients are said to experience both extreme positive and negative emotions. For this reason, American psychologists Jack Blanchard, Alan Bellack and Kim Mueser examined levels of anhedonia in schizophrenia and bipolar patients more carefully. They found that high levels of anhedonia were reported by depressed bipolar patients but not by those who had recently suffered from an episode of mania. Therefore, whereas anhedonia may be a stable or trait-like characteristic of some schizophrenia patients, it appears to vary with time in patients with a bipolar diagnosis.[67] Consistent with this hypothesis, Katsanis and her colleagues found that anhedonia correlated with premorbid social functioning in schizophrenia patients (those who functioned poorly prior to illness showed high levels of anhedonia when ill) but not in patients with other diagnoses.[68]

These findings tell us very little about the emotional life of anhedonic patients. Again, the circumplex model of emotion provides a useful framework. In a recent study, Blanchard, Mueser and Bellack measured physical and social anhedonia, as well as positive and negative affect, in schizophrenia patients and normal controls. As expected, the schizophrenia patients reported higher levels of anhedonia and lower levels of positive emotion in comparison to the controls. However, they also reported high levels of negative emotion and social anxiety. These differences remained when the participants were retested three months later. When the anhedonia scores of the schizophrenia patients were examined, it was found that they were negatively correlated with positive emotion. Social anhedonia scores, but not physical anhedonia scores, were positively correlated with negative emotion. It therefore appears that anhedonic patients suffer not only from a deficiency of positive emotion, but also from a surfeit of negative emotion.[69]

Disorders of affect-logic

Negative symptoms are among the least researched facets of psychosis. As we will see in later chapters, much more effort has been directed towards understanding the psychological mechanisms involved in more flamboyant symptoms, such as delusions, hallucinations and unusual forms of speech. Perhaps because they have been ignored, negative symptoms have appeared all the more mysterious, or have simply been dismissed as reflecting the impoverished output of a wounded brain. However, we have seen that, when some of these symptoms are examined in the context of what is known about normal emotions, the picture of a type of madness in which the individual is aloof or indifferent to the social world is revealed as largely myth. The negative symptoms become more understandable, if as yet not completely explained.

The misleading view that negative symptoms reflect a lack of emotion has underpinned the assumption that schizophrenia is an intellectual disorder whereas manic depression is a disorder of affect.

Objecting to this assumption, the Swiss psychiatrist Luc Ciompi has suggested[70] that all psychotic illnesses are disorders of *affect-logic*, a term which he uses to highlight the inseparable relationship between cognition and emotion.* In the next part of this book, in which we consider the most commonly reported symptoms of psychosis, we will see that this principle holds for delusions, mania, hallucinations and disordered speech.

---

* According to Ciompi ('Is schizophrenia an affective disease?', in W. F. Flack and J. D. Laird (eds.), *Emotions in Psychopathology*. New York: Oxford University Press, 1998):

The term affect-logic is not an entirely satisfactory translation of an appropriated German neologism meaning, simultaneously, 'the logic of affectivity' and 'the affectivity of logic'. It points to the central conceptual basis of the model, which postulates that in all normal and most pathological mental functions, emotions and cognitions – or affective and cognitive functions, feeling and thinking, affectivity and logic – are inseperably connected and interact in regular but not yet sufficiently well understood ways.

Ciompi's theory is a complex blend of Piagetian developmental psychology, biological studies of emotion and non-linear dynamics. There is clearly considerable overlap between his approach and the approach taken in this book. The main difference is that Ciompi has paid less attention to the psychological processes involved in specific symptoms.

Part Three

Some Madnesses Explained

Depression and the Pathology of Self

O God, I could be bounded in a nutshell and count myself a king of
infinite space, were it not that I have bad dreams.

Shakespeare, *Hamlet*

I can vividly remember beginning the first draft of this chapter on a cold February morning in 1999. My wife Aisling sat nearby on a sofa, cuddling our children, Keeva and Fintan, who had been born a few weeks earlier. Although they were breast-fed in the daytime, at night we gave them bottles so that we could share the burden imposed by their arrival. The night before, we had fed them at two o'clock and again at half past four. On the second of these occasions, I had stared at Keeva while in the semi-psychotic state that lies at the boundary between wakefulness and dreaming, and it had occurred to me that she might *really* be an angel. It would not have surprised me if, at that moment, fluffy wings had unfurled from behind her back.

In many ways, the period immediately following the birth of the twins was extremely stressful. Aisling and I survived on vanishingly small amounts of sleep. Naturally, my academic productivity was affected (later, I calculated that the year 2000 saw my lowest number of publications since the mid-1980s). Yet, I was probably as contented as I have ever been.

My life had not always been so happy. The years that followed my twenty-ninth birthday were especially difficult. Looking ahead a year or two earlier, the omens had seemed good. In short order, I had married my first wife, obtained my doctorate in experimental psychology, qualified as a clinical psychologist, and secured my first job in the National Health Service. And yet, in the few years that followed, my father died in a road accident, my brother committed suicide, and

I walked out of my marriage in favour of an old girlfriend who immediately disowned me. When I struggled to make sense of these events, they seemed to be inexplicably connected, as if fruits of some kind of curse.

Leaving my small house in Chester, I found myself homeless. For almost twelve months I lived from a suitcase and drifted between friends. At my worst during the year of 1986, I probably met the DSM-IV criteria for major depression. However, I cannot remember a point at which I thought of myself as 'ill' or a specific moment when I seemed to have become 'better'. Instead, my feelings seemed appropriate to the dismal sequence of events that had befallen me. I saw myself drinking from a well of emotion that I shared with others suffering similar difficulties, a common reservoir of misery which is part of my species' collective experience. Many of us, when confronted by these kinds of events, pick ourselves up and struggle onwards. In my own case, I was helped by a good psychotherapist, to whom I was referred by a colleague who could see that I was not coping.

Although it is not usually included among the symptoms of psychosis, there are several good reasons for beginning our detailed examination of psychotic phenomena with depression. First, as American psychologists David Rosenhan and Martin Seligman have observed, depression is 'the common cold of mental illness'.[1] The very familiarity of negative mood will make it more understandable to most readers than some of the other symptoms that we will encounter later. Second, depression is very commonly experienced by schizophrenia patients, both during acute episodes and also during the prodromal phase that precedes the appearance of positive symptoms. Third, it is also an important facet of manic depression as described by Klaus Leonhard, who observed that mania rarely occurs in its absence. Moreover, unipolar depression can, in its own right, become psychotic, which is to say that it can be accompanied by other psychotic symptoms such as delusions and hallucinations. And finally, many of the concepts that we will explore when attempting to explain depression will serve us well in later chapters, when we attempt to get to grips with other types of symptoms.

Before we can begin, we must first address a complication. I have thus far talked about 'depression' as if what I mean by this term is self-evident. Indeed, most of us accept the idea of depression as if it can be easily differentiated from other types of unpleasant feelings. However, as we saw in the last chapter, the landscape of emotion is not so easily charted. To take my own experiences fifteen years ago, I suffered not only deep feelings of dysphoria, but I also had a very low opinion of myself and felt very pessimistic about the future. I had difficulty sleeping, and would ruminate in the dark hours about how other people saw my change of circumstances. During the daytime I felt tired and lacking in energy. So preoccupied was I with my own difficulties that my capacity to empathize with my patients was severely blunted. (With the benefit of hindsight I can now see that I should have given up clinical work for the duration.)

People diagnosed as depressed often have experiences such as these, but suffer them to varying degrees. At its worst, the pessimism associated with depression can be so severe that the person does not believe that there is any point to getting up, and may languish in bed for days on end. Other symptoms are also commonly reported. The first depressed patient I was asked to treat when I was a trainee clinical psychologist was a recently divorced and lonely middle-aged woman whom I will call Clare.* Consistent with my own experience, she felt severely demoralized and made gloomy predictions about what would happen to her in the years ahead. However, in contrast to many patients who complain of anhedonia, her interest in food and sex were heightened, making the lack of a partner even more difficult to bear. In common with many other patients, she felt very tense. However, less commonly, she found that she could relieve her tension by taking a knife and making shallow cuts across her breasts and arms.

In psychotic depression, the content of the accompanying symptoms is usually congruent with the patient's mood, so that hallucinations make derogatory remarks, and the patient feels guilty of improbable crimes, or becomes convinced that he is doomed to some kind of horrific fate. George, an extremely successful engineer, could survive with equanimity the stresses of his demanding job, but became severely

---

* When clinicians write about their work there is a tension between being truthful and preserving the anonymity of their patients. In all the brief case studies reported in this book, I have gone to some length to disguise patients' backgrounds and circumstances in order to render them unrecognizable. However, without exception, I have tried to be accurate when describing their complaints. Inevitably, the result is an uneasy blend of fiction and reality.

dysphoric after travelling abroad (a fact that did not deter him from taking his family on regular foreign holidays). During these episodes, which sometimes lasted for several months, he would develop the delusion that his employers were about to sack him and reclaim his salary from the preceding years (in fact, they were amazingly tolerant of his long absences). He also believed that he had somehow mislaid the very substantial savings that he had accumulated, and that his family were about to be evicted from their home and would eventually starve. Efforts to reassure him, for example by showing him his bank statements and building society accounts, were all to no avail. For weeks, he would avoid brushing his teeth, in order to 'conserve energy', and would spend his time sitting around his house in his pyjamas, remaining as motionless as possible.

Investigators studying cross-cultural differences in depression have noted that cognitive symptoms – especially guilt and low self-esteem – are less evident in developing countries than in the West. In contrast, patients in developing countries tend to complain more of somatic symptoms, such as fatigue, loss of weight, or headaches and dizziness. Not surprisingly, beliefs about the nature and causes of these symptoms also vary between cultures. In a vivid example of this kind of difference, Arthur Kleinman has described the case of Mrs Lin, a 28-year-old primary school teacher he met at Hunan Medical College in south central China in 1980:[2]

Mrs Lin, who has suffered from chronic head-aches for the past six years, is telling me about her other symptoms: dizziness, tiredness, easy fatigue, weakness, and a ringing sound in her ears. She has been under the treatment of doctors in the internal medicine clinic . . . for more than half a year with increasing symptoms. They have referred her to the psychiatric clinic, though against her objections, with the diagnosis of neurasthenia. Gently, sensing a deep disquiet behind the tight lips and mask-like squint, I ask Mrs Lin if she feels depressed. 'Yes, I am unhappy,' she replies. 'My life has been difficult,' she adds quickly as a justification. At this point Mrs Lin looks away. Her thin lips tremble. The brave mask dissolves into tears. For several minutes she continues sobbing; the deep inhalations reverberate as a low wail.

Further inquiry revealed that Mrs Lin's parents had been killed during the Cultural Revolution. A teenager at the time, she and her four siblings had been dispersed to different rural areas. She had difficulty adapting to her new environment, which was much harsher than the city in which she had been raised. During the following years, she felt cold and hungry and had only one friend. She later learned that one of her sisters had committed suicide and that her brother had been paralysed in a tractor accident. Unable to pass the entrance exam to her chosen university, she agreed to an arranged marriage. Her husband and mother-in-law later subjected her to physical and psychological abuse following the stillbirth of a nearly full-term foetus. Kleinman remarks:

For a North American psychiatrist, Mrs Lin meets the official diagnostic criteria for a major depressive disorder. The Chinese psychiatrists who interviewed her with me did not agree with this diagnosis. They did not deny that she was depressed, but they regarded the depression as a manifestation of neurasthenia, and Mrs Lin shared this viewpoint. Neurasthenia – a syndrome of exhaustion, weakness, and diffuse bodily complaints believed to be caused by inadequate physical energy in the central nervous system – is an official diagnosis in China; but it is not a diagnosis in the American Psychiatric Association's latest nosology.

Kleinman's view is that Western depression and Chinese neurasthenia are the same condition, which is expressed in different ways in response to local cultural influences. Chinese neurasthenia is therefore somatized depression. However, as Richard Shweder of the University of Chicago has pointed out, we might just as well describe North American depression as emotionalized neurasthenia.[3] The solution to this cross-cultural conundrum is to recognize that Western depression and Chinese neurasthenia are different but overlapping clusters of symptoms. There is no need to think of an underlying disease entity that is the 'middle man', or to give primacy to one diagnosis or the other.[4]

Given this degree of variation – both within and between cultures – between people who are all said to suffer from the same condition, it is not surprising that some psychologists and psychiatrists have suggested that the concept of depression has outlived its usefulness.[5] As I agree with this conclusion, writing this chapter has presented me with a series of dilemmas. First, although I would like to focus specifically on dysphoric mood, I am hampered by the fact that nearly all the relevant research has been conducted on individuals from developed countries who are described as depressed rather than dysphoric. To some extent I will be able to get around this problem by making the dangerous assumption that negative mood is the common symptom experienced by these individuals. Unfortunately, there is not much that I can do about the cultural biases inherent in the research (although I will speculate a little about cross-cultural differences wherever this seems appropriate).

Second, most of the published research on depression has been carried out either with ordinary people (typically university students) who are temporarily distressed, or with patients who are diagnosed as suffering from non-psychotic depression. Fortunately, there are good reasons to believe that the findings obtained can be generalized to psychotic patients. When experiments have been carried out both on ordinary people and on psychiatric patients, comparable results have usually been obtained. In the case of patients who are diagnosed as suffering from unipolar depression, the main difference between those who are psychotic and those who are not (other than the presence of hallucinations and delusions) seems to be the severity of their negative mood, those patients who are most dysphoric being most likely to experience delusions and hallucinations.[6] When bipolar depression has been compared with unipolar depression, the results again reassure us that we are not dealing with fundamentally different phenomena.[7]

There is one final caveat I must offer before proceeding with my account of the psychology of depression. As the term 'depression' applies to a loosely connected group of symptoms, of which dysphoria is the most obvious, it is unlikely the experiences of every depressed patient can be explained in the same way. We should therefore expect to find that depressive symptoms are influenced by a network of interacting psychological mechanisms, which play more or less decisive roles in different individuals. It follows that there may be several different pathways to depression. In this chapter, I will attempt to identify two such pathways (there may well be others), taking the reader step by step through the evidence that is relevant to each.

From Appraisal to Distress

Anyone who has failed to avoid the ordinary tragedies of life will recognize that many events can provoke a dysphoric mood – the death of a loved one, the collapse of a relationship, humiliation in the eyes of one's peers, or the failure to achieve a cherished ambition. However, it is equally obvious that individuals react to these experiences in different ways. Some shrug them off after a few days of emotional discomfort while others plummet into an extended period of despair. These differences reflect the role of appraisals in modulating emotional reactions. A relatively positive interpretation of the death of a loved one ('He had a good innings; he was loved by his family until the end; at least he is no longer suffering') is likely to lead to better emotional adjustment to the loss than a negative appraisal ('He never had a chance to fulfil his potential; I did not love him as much as I should have; he died a painful and lonely death'). Of course, appraisals are partly determined by the facts of the situation – a loved one might really have died a lonely and painful death – but, in most situations, there is usually some degree of freedom in the kind of interpretation that can be offered.

There have been many attempts to define the kinds of appraisals that lead to dysphoria, but most have assumed that they involve some kind of pessimistic interpretation of events. Psychiatrist Aaron Beck of the University of Pennsylvania (who is best known for his pioneering efforts to develop effective psychological treatments for psychiatric patients) has observed that the thinking of depressed people is dominated by a negative view of the self, the world and the future. Beck refers to this cluster of attitudes as 'the negative cognitive triad'. According to Beck, automatic or unbidden thoughts that reflect these themes are the immediate precursors of dysphoric mood.[8] These thoughts are presumably part of the stream of inner speech, which, we saw in Chapter 7, tends to be evoked whenever we are emotionally aroused.

Although Beck's theory has enormously influenced clinical practice, most research on the appraisals of depressed patients has focused on a slightly different but not incompatible theory developed by American psychologists Martin Seligman, Lyn Abramson, Lauren Alloy and various collaborators. In a landmark paper, Abramson and Seligman, together with British psychologist John Teasdale, noted that we usually experience negative emotions when we are exposed to unpleasant events that are beyond our control.[9] However, they argued that full-blown depression only develops when we hold certain beliefs about the causes of those events.*

The theory developed by Seligman and his colleagues built on an observation, made some years earlier by the social psychologist Fritz Heider, that human beings act for much of the time like intuitive scientists.[10] As we navigate our way through the challenges of everyday life, we usually attempt to find explanations for noteworthy events, particularly those that involve other people. An unpleasant disagreement with a friend might be attributed to some characteristic of the friend ('She's bad tempered and argumentative'), the situation ('We've both been under stress lately'), oneself ('It's because I offended her when we met last week'), or some combination of these causes. In the jargon of social psychology, these kinds of causal statements (made to other people or to ourselves while thinking) are known as *attributions* (because they involve us attributing events to particular causes). So readily do we generate attributions that they might be thought of as one of the defining characteristics of our species – Seligman and his colleagues have estimated that most people make at least one causal statement (a sentence including or implying the word 'because') in every few hundred words of ordinary speech.[11]

To understand how attributions are involved in the experience of negative mood, imagine that you have failed an exam. (Young readers will not find this too difficult. Readers who are as old as myself may have to think back a few years.) You might explain your performance in a number of ways. For example, you might say to yourself: 'It's

---

* This theory is a revision of an earlier account of depression, known as 'the theory of learned helplessness', proposed by Seligman in his book *Helplessness: On Depression, Development and Death* (San Francisco, CA: Freeman, 1975). To confuse matters further, the revised model has undergone some further revisions, most notably by Lyn Abramson and her colleagues (see L. Y. Abramson, G. I. Metalsky and L. B. Alloy (1989) 'Hopelessness depression: a theory-based subtype of depression', *Psychological Review*, 96: 358–72). Details of the differences between the various versions of the theory are not important in the present context.

because I didn't work hard enough', 'I had bad luck', or 'The examination was unfair.' According to Abramson, Seligman and Teasdale, your failure will only lead to lasting distress if you attribute it to a cause that is *internal*, *global* and *stable*.

An internal cause is something to do with you, whereas its opposite, an external cause, is something to do with other people or circumstances. A global cause is something that will affect all areas of your life, as opposed to a specific cause, which will have an effect only on specific kinds of events. A stable cause is something you cannot change and which will be present in the future, whereas an unstable cause is something that is only likely to have an impact at this particular point in time. According to Abramson, Seligman and Teasdale's recipe for depression, if you fail an exam the best way of ensuring enduring misery is to say or think to yourself, 'It's because I'm stupid.' This attribution is internal (it locates the fault within yourself), global (it will adversely affect not only your performance in this exam but also your performance in others and, ultimately, your ability to earn a good living) and stable (there is not much you can do about being stupid; if you are stupid today the chances are that you will be stupid in the future). If you make any other kind of attribution you may still be miserable, but your misery will be short-lived.

The attributional theory of depression is a type of *stress-vulnerability model*. According to Seligman, we each have an individual *attributional style* that remains relatively fixed throughout our adult lives. Individuals with a pessimistic style (those who usually explain negative events in terms of causes that are internal, global and stable) may go for many years without experiencing depression. It is only when they encounter a severe negative event, and explain it pessimistically, that they become markedly dysphoric.

Unfortunately, the measurement of attributional style has not been devoid of problems. With Christopher Petersen at the University of Michigan, Seligman developed a questionnaire for this purpose, known as the Attributional Style Questionnaire (ASQ, see Table 10.1). People completing the ASQ are asked to imagine a range of positive and negative events and are asked to write down their most likely cause. It is assumed that the kinds of attributions people make about these hypothetical scenarios are indicative of the kinds of attributions they make in everyday life. After writing down each cause, they are

Table 10.1 An item from the Attributional Style Questionnaire (C. Peterson, A. Semmel, C. von Bayer, L. Abramson, G. I. Metalsky and M. E. P. Seligman (1982) 'The Attributional Style Questionnaire', *Cognitive Therapy and Research*, 3: 287–300).

You meet a friend who acts hostilely toward you.

1. Write down one possible cause of this event

_____

2. Is the cause of your friend acting hostilely toward you due to something about you or something about other people or circumstances?

   Totally due to other people   Totally due to me
   or circumstances
                        1 2 3 4 5 6 7
                        (circle one number)

3. In the future, when interacting with friends, will this cause again be present?

   Will never again be present   Will always be present
                        1 2 3 4 5 6 7
                        (circle one number)

4. Is the cause something that just influences interacting with friends or does it also influence other areas of your life?

   Influences just this   Influences all situations
   particular area   in my life
                        1 2 3 4 5 6 7
                        (circle one number)

asked to rate it on seven-point scales of internality–externality, globalness–specificity and stability–instability. These characteristics of attributions are therefore viewed as dimensions rather than categories.

Although widely used in research, the ASQ suffers from a number of shortcomings,[12] some of which we will consider when we think about delusions in a later chapter. For this reason a number of alternative approaches have been proposed. One strategy involves using judges to score attributions recorded from samples of everyday speech (a tech-nique that Seligman calls the Content Analysis of Verbal Explanations, or CAVEing). Seligman and his colleagues have imaginatively employed this strategy to analyse patients' mood changes during psychotherapy (less pessimistic attributions precede positive changes in mood),[13] voter-preferences in elections (Americans, it seems, prefer to elect presidential candidates who make optimistic election speeches)[14] and even political decision-making (optimistic shifts in Lyndon John-son's press statements preceded bold decisions in the Vietnam War).[15]

Does attributional style predict future dysphoria in the way suggested by Seligman? It has turned out to be surprisingly difficult to answer this question. To begin with, there can be no doubt that depressed patients make excessively internal, global and stable attributions for negative events as predicted by the Abramson, Seligman and Teasdale theory. As early as 1986, psychologist Paul Sweeny and his colleagues at Indiana University were able to summarize the results of no less than 106 studies, most of which provided evidence that was consistent with the theory.[16] Subsequent research has mostly replicated these findings.[17] Although most of these studies have involved non-psychotic people, with Helen Lyon and Mike Startup at the University College of Wales in Bangor I have looked at the attributions of patients diagnosed as suffering from bipolar disorder.[18] The scores of our participants, shown in Figure 10.1, illustrate some general points about attributional style.

The panel on the left of the figure shows internality scores. High scores indicate that attributions are relatively internal (self-blaming) and low scores indicate that they are relatively external (blame is attributed to others or to circumstances). Average scores are given separately for hypothetical positive events (for example, being awarded a pay rise) and negative events (for example, going on a date that turns out badly). Note, first, that the scores of ordinary individuals (people without psychiatric problems) who took part in the study are not exactly fair-minded. Although the reader might expect that we tend to blame ourselves equally for positive and negative events, in fact we usually take more credit for things that turn out well than for things that turn out badly (if I fail an exam it's probably because I've been handicapped by various problems beyond my control; if I pass it's because I am a genius). This attributional distortion, which social psychologists call the *self-serving bias*, and which has been documented

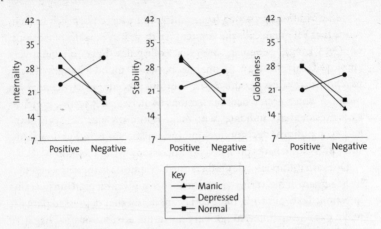

Figure 10.1 Internality, stability and globalness data for bipolar-manic, bipolar-depressed and normal participants (from Lyon et al., 1999).

in numerous experiments,[19] was accurately described by William Shakespeare in *King Lear* nearly four centuries ago:

This is the excellent foppery of the world, that, when we are sick in fortune, – often the surfeit of our own behaviour, – we make guilty of our disasters the sun, the moon, and the stars; as if we were villains by necessity, fools by heavenly compulsion.

The stability and globalness data, shown in the right two panels, provide further evidence of a lack of fair-mindedness in ordinary people. Positive events are attributed to causes that are more stable and global than negative events. In order to maintain our mental health, it seems, we have to make unrealistically optimistic appraisals about the likelihood that good things will happen in the future and about our power to bring such events about.[* 20]

* The flip side to this observation is the claim that dysphoria often reflects a realistic appraisal of events. This idea, first proposed by Lauren Alloy and Lyn Abramson (see, for example, L. B. Alloy and L. Y. Abramson (1988) 'Depressive realism: four theoretical perspectives', in L. B. Alloy (ed.), *Cognitive Processes in Depression*. New York: Guilford), has become known as the *depressive realism hypothesis*. It suggests that depressed people are more in touch with reality than ordinary people but that, unfortunately, reality is a very unpleasant place to be in touch with.

There is plenty of evidence that seems to be consistent with this hypothesis. For

Although I will discuss mania in detail in the next chapter, it is interesting to note that those suffering from this condition showed a robust self-serving bias, just like the normal controls. They were also, like the controls, optimistic in attributing positive but not negative events to stable and global factors. In contrast, the depressed patients blamed themselves more for negative than for positive events. As in previous studies of unipolar patients, the bipolar-depressed patients also believed that factors responsible for negative events were likely to be more enduring, and to affect more areas of their lives, than the factors responsible for positive events. Similar findings have been obtained from patients with other psychiatric diagnoses involving high levels of dysphoria, particularly anxiety disorders.[21] As might be expected in the light of the circumplex model of emotion, the pessimistic style is therefore associated with negative mood, rather than any specific diagnosis.

So far, so good for Abramson, Seligman and Teasdale's theory. However, it has proved more difficult to find evidence that a pessimistic attributional style *precedes* the development of dysphoria. Most researchers who have attempted to show that this is the case have begun by identifying people who have a high probability of experiencing some kind of disappointment or failure (for example students who are about to take an exam) or a stressful life event (for example, women who are about to give birth). Although some studies have found that a pessimistic attributional style predicts a bad emotional response to adverse events,[22] others have produced either negative or equivocal results.[23]

Clearer evidence has emerged from a different kind of prospective study, which has recently been reported by Lauren Alloy, Lyn Abramson and their colleagues at Temple and Wisconsin Universities in the USA.[24] In this study, known as the Temple–Wisconsin Cognitive Vulnerability to Depression (CVD) Project, the researchers attempted

---

example, depressed people seem to make more realistic appraisals of other people's opinions about them, and their attributions have sometimes appeared more even-handed. However, these findings can often be interpreted in ways that are inconsistent with the hypothesis (see R. Ackermann and R. J. DeRubeis (1991) 'Is depressive realism real?', *Clinical Psychology Review*, 11: 565–84). My own view, for what it is worth, is that the hypothesis holds for moderately but not severely dysphoric patients.

to identify students who were apparently psychologically well but vulnerable to abnormal mood. Over 5000 students were assessed using a measure of attributional style, together with a measure of abnormal attitudes towards the self which we will consider in detail later in the chapter. From this sample, 173 students were identified who showed strong evidence of a pessimistic cognitive style, but who were not currently dysphoric. These students, together with a matched group who were not thought to be vulnerable to mood disorder, were followed up every six weeks for two years and then every four months for a further three years. The main finding from the first two years of the project was that the vulnerable students were much more likely to experience severe dysphoric episodes than the control students (17 per cent versus 1 per cent for major depression as defined by DSM criteria and 39 per cent versus 6 per cent for minor depressive symptoms).

Although these findings may seem inconsistent with the results obtained from the earlier prospective studies, this impression is probably inaccurate. The students in the high-risk group of the Temple–Wisconsin Project represented under 4 per cent of the total sample – a very highly selected, and probably very highly vulnerable group. It is not surprising that much weaker effects were detected in the earlier studies carried out with unselected participants. In this context it is important to note that the selection policy adopted in the Temple–Wisconsin Project was not only one of its strengths, but also a weakness. Although the project appears to confirm that a pessimistic attributional style can precede depression, the high-risk students who were identified were probably not representative of dysphoric people in general. If negative mood is indeed the common cold of psychiatry, it is a fair bet that the majority of those who become dysphoric do not fall into this high-risk group.*

Overall, therefore, there is some evidence that attributional style can predict future negative mood, as illustrated in Figure 10.2. How-

---

* In fact, the data from the Temple–Wisconsin Project support this conclusion. Approximately 17 per cent of the 173 high-risk participants were subsequently diagnosed as depressed, yielding 30 'cases' of illness. However, if we assume that about 1 per cent of the remaining 4827 participants became ill (the figure obtained for the low-risk group), we find that this yields 48 cases of illness. Therefore, more cases of illness probably occurred among the low-risk than the high-risk participants.

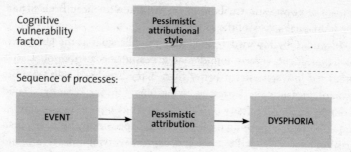

Figure 10.2 Relationships between negative events, attributional style and dysphoria.

ever, we are not therefore entitled to conclude that attributional style is the sole, or even most important, psychological characteristic implicated in mood disorders. Nor should we rush to accept a simple stress-vulnerability model of dysphoria of the kind proposed by Seligman. Those who have debated the causal status of attributions have often assumed that attributional style is either a trait (an enduring personality characteristic) or a state (a transient phenomenon, perhaps a symptom of negative mood). As we will see shortly, the truth may be more complex than this.

The Self Worth Living with

A pessimistic appraisal of events probably has an impact on mood for several reasons. Aaron Beck, it will be recalled, suggested that people who feel depressed harbour negative thoughts about themselves, the world and the future. Lyn Abramson has focused on the last element in this negative cognitive triad, arguing that excessively stable and global attributions for negative events lead to a sense of hopelessness – a pervasive conviction that life cannot get better which in turn saps the individual's motivation to cope with adversity.[25] It is certainly true that many depressed people experience a profound sense of hopelessness about the future, and the greater this sense of hopelessness the greater the likelihood that they will attempt suicide.[26] (Hopelessness has also been found to be a strong predictor of suicidal tendencies in schizophrenia patients.)[27] However, at least as important must be the impact of pessimistic attributions on the first element in Beck's triad: the individual's view of the self.

In studies by Howard Tennen and his colleagues at the University of Connecticut, it was found that a pessimistic attributional style predicted low self-esteem better than it predicted scores on a more general measure of depressive symptoms.[28] More recently, David Romney of the University of Calgary used a complex statistical technique known as path analysis to explore specific relations between attributional style, self-esteem and depressive symptoms. He found that the attributional dimensions of internality, stability and globalness did not affect depressive symptoms directly, but that each had an impact on self-esteem, which in turn had a strong impact on depression.[29] On this evidence, then, pessimistic appraisals of events lead to problems of self-esteem, which in turn lead to negative mood.

How appraisals influence the self

In Chapter 8 we saw that the self is a dynamic, multifaceted phenomenon that is unlikely to be adequately captured by a single dimension varying between the extremes of grandiosity and self-loathing. Indeed, as British psychiatrist Philip Robson has lamented, self-esteem is 'an idea rather than an entity and the term signifies different things to different people'.[30] One problem is that it is not immediately obvious how we go about making global assessments of our self-worth. For example, it seems likely that positive self-esteem (the sum of all the good things an individual thinks about himself) and negative self-esteem (the sum of all the bad things that the individual thinks about himself) are not necessarily opposites – it is as easy to imagine that someone holds both extreme positive and negative opinions about herself as it is to imagine that someone holds exclusively positive or negative opinions, and, indeed, these types of beliefs can be measured separately.[31] Although most ordinary people seem to hold beliefs about the self that are so predominantly positive that any objective assessment would deem them unrealistic, people who score low on self-esteem questionnaires rarely harbour exclusively negative opinions but, rather, tend to believe a mixture of positive and negative things about themselves.[32]

The specific beliefs about the self that we are immediately aware of have been described as the *actual self*. The depressed patient's tendency to include more negative attributes in this description than ordinary people can be easily demonstrated by means of questionnaires, but it has also been shown using the *self-reference effect* (the general tendency to recall information that is directly relevant to the self), which I described in Chapter 8. When given a list of trait words that are either negative (for example, 'stupid', 'unloved', 'weak') or positive ('successful', 'dynamic', 'confident'), and asked to say whether they are self-descriptive, unipolar depressed patients not only endorse more negative words as true of themselves in comparison with ordinary people, but later recall more of the negative words if given a surprise memory test.[33] Helen Lyon, Mike Startup and I recently found exactly the same result with bipolar patients who were currently depressed.[34]

Of course, beliefs about the self are not always present in our minds. For much of the time, we direct our thoughts towards other things. Moreover, it appears that some people's beliefs about themselves are more subject to change than others. When social psychologist Michael Kernis of the University of Georgia asked ordinary people to record their current feelings about themselves at random intervals over an extended period (usually about a week) he found that self-esteem remained relatively stable in some people whereas, in others, it fluctuated dramatically.[35] Surprisingly, stability of self-esteem seems to be relatively independent of average level of self-esteem (that is, some people with unstable self-esteem have high self-esteem on most days whereas others have low self-esteem on most days). Kernis found that individuals with unstable self-esteem are more vulnerable to feelings of depression than individuals with stable self-esteem. He also found that individuals with unstable but typically high self-esteem are especially likely to react angrily to negative information about themselves.

Beliefs about the self change over time because they have to be provoked into consciousness ('activated' or 'primed' in the language of cognitive psychology) before they can affect us. This is why appraisals have such a powerful effect on mood – because they determine whether or not the events we experience activate positive or negative representations from our reservoir of stored knowledge and beliefs about ourselves. Not surprisingly, stability of self-esteem seems to be, at least in part, determined by the extent to which people make extreme appraisals for everyday events; individuals who make more extreme appraisals tend to have very unstable self-esteem.[36] However, our beliefs about ourselves are also dependent on the information about ourselves that we have acquired and stored away earlier in our lives. The more negative information about ourselves we have stored in our long-term memory, the more vulnerable we will be to experiencing negative thoughts and ideas about ourselves. Conversely, if we have learned only positive things about ourselves, it is unlikely that even the most challenging of experiences will persuade us to think about ourselves in a very self-critical way.

If this account is correct, individuals who are depressed should have an abnormal tendency to recall negative information about themselves. This kind of memory bias has long been recognized by clinicians, for example Aaron Beck,[37] who have observed that unipolar depressed patients organize their memories in a 'depressogenic fashion'. In an early empirical study, G. W. Lloyd and W. A. Lishman at the Institute of Psychiatry in London asked depressed people and non-depressed people to think of either a pleasant or an unpleasant memory when they heard a series of cue words, and to signal to the researchers when suitable memories came to mind. They found that depressed patients tended to recall negative events more rapidly than positive events, but that this was not the case for non-depressed controls.[38] This finding has been replicated many times. For example, John Teasdale and Sarah Fogarty at Oxford University experimentally induced negative moods in normal volunteers by asking them to read depressing statements and found that they were slower to recall positive events as a consequence.[39]

Standards and discrepancies

Even if the account of the self I have so far given seems half plausible, a moment's reflection will reveal that it must be incomplete. Although we have assumed that the discovery of undesirable aspects of the self will provoke feelings of distress, we have not explained how individuals know that particular attributes are undesirable. After all, it is quite possible to imagine a person who knows that he is vicious and heartless, but who believes that these characteristics are valuable, or at least acceptable (the Nazis deliberately cultivated this kind of self-image, and hence were able to commit atrocities against civilians while remaining emotionally unscathed).[40] We therefore need to consider not only the actual self, but also the internal standards against which the self is evaluated.*

American social psychologist E. Tory Higgins of New York University has pointed out that most of us can describe how we think we would like to be (the *ideal self*) and how we think we ought to be (the *ought self*).[41] According to Higgins, these self-standards help us to define our goals in life and are sources of two different types of motivation – the striving for desired outcomes in the case of the ideal self and the avoidance of undesired outcomes in the case of the ought self.† To further complicate matters, Higgins also points out that we can consider the self from different *perspectives*. For example, I can imagine how my mother thinks I actually am (the 'mother-actual self'), how she would like me to be (the 'mother-ideal self') and how she thinks I ought to be (the 'mother-ought self'). (Of course, I cannot read my mother's mind to find out what she really thinks about me, but have to guess on the basis of the quality of our relationship.) In principle, there are as many perspectives on the self as there are people whose opinions we can imagine.

You can get a snapshot portrait of your actual self by simply writing down the first ten words that come to mind when thinking about 'myself as I actually am'. Similarly, a snapshot of the ideal self can be recorded on paper by writing down ten words that come to mind when you think of 'myself as I would like to be'. Next try 'myself as I ought to be', 'how my mother/father thinks I am', 'how my mother/father would like me to be' and so on. When carrying out this exercise, you will probably notice that many of the descriptions are very similar. However, you might also notice that some are different. For example, you might list the word 'industrious' when describing your ideal self and its antonym, 'lazy', when thinking about your actual self. Higgins refers to these kinds of differences as *self-discrepancies*, and has argued that it is our awareness of them that provokes negative mood.

* Readers familiar with Freud's theory will recognize this particular aspect of the self as the 'superego'. One important general implication of the material covered in this section, which I hope to examine further at a later date, is that moral values play a direct and important role in human psychology.
† In Higgins's terminology, the actual self, ideal self and ought self are described as different *domains* of the self. The ideal self and the ought self are also called *self-guides* because of their motivational properties.

A substantial body of research supports this idea. Tim Strauman of the University of Wisconsin has shown that ordinary people when depressed, as well as psychiatric patients with a diagnosis of unipolar depression, report a large number of actual–ideal discrepancies.[42] Socially anxious people, on the other hand, typically report substantial discrepancies between the actual self and the ought self. Not surprisingly, given the substantial overlap between depression and anxiety symptoms, most researchers have reported a strong correlation between the two types of discrepancy, leading some to question whether they are qualitatively distinct.[43]

Strauman and Higgins have also shown that strong negative feelings can be provoked by making people think about self-discrepancies they have revealed at an earlier time.[44] Not only does this lead to negative mood, but it also produces quite profound behavioural and physiological effects. For example, when people contemplate actual–ideal discrepancies, their speech becomes momentarily more sluggish, there is a change in the electrical conductivity of the skin (known as an 'electrodermal response' and caused by sweating, indicating that the autonomic nervous system is firing up in anticipation of stress) and, most dramatically of all, the efficiency of the immune system (responsible for protecting the individual from infection) is temporarily reduced.

Until recently, no attempt had been made to explore psychotic disorders from the perspective of Higgins's theory. However, in a recent study Peter Kinderman, Kerry Manson and I measured self-discrepancies in patients who had received a diagnosis of bipolar disorder, and who were divided into three groups – patients who were currently depressed, those who were currently manic and those whose symptoms were in remission. (Patients in this last group had experienced both depressive and manic episodes in the past but were currently well.) Also participating was a group of ordinary people for comparison purposes. As expected, we found that the bipolar-depressed patients, like previously studied unipolar patients, reported considerable discrepancies between their actual selves and their ideal and ought selves. Currently manic patients, on the other hand, reported even fewer discrepancies between their actual selves and their self-standards than either the healthy controls or the patients in remission.[45]

The quality of ideals

Obviously, the more exacting our self-standards, the more likely it is that we will experience self-discrepancies. Aaron Beck has argued that many of the problems experienced by depressed patients can be attributed to their abnormally perfectionistic standards, which place them at constant risk of experiencing failure. On Beck's view, such standards may lurk as barely articulated 'schemas', of which we are hardly aware until we are reminded that we have failed to meet them.[46] Sticking to the terminology we have adopted so far in this chapter, we can say that failure experiences have the potential to activate these schemas, so that they become available in consciousness as representations of the ideal self and the ought self.

To test this idea, many researchers have used the Dysfunctional Attitudes Scale (DAS), a questionnaire that asks people to consider the extent to which they agree with statements such as 'I should be able to please everybody' and 'My value as a person depends greatly on what other people think of me.'[47] Patients suffering from depression consistently score highly on this and similar measures. Although many patients who recover from episodes of depression score normally on the DAS,[48] there is also evidence that dysfunctional self-standards predict later episodes of mood disorder. In a study carried out by J. Mark Williams and his colleagues, it was observed that recovered patients who still scored highly on the scale were especially likely to relapse.[49] More recently, in the Temple–Wisconsin Cognitive Vulnerability to Depression Project, the DAS was used together with the Attributional Style Questionnaire to select individuals who were later proven to be at very high risk of depression.[50]

Beck has suggested that self-standards can be divided into two main types, reflecting different fundamental needs. *Sociotropy* refers to a strong need for care and approval from others, whereas *autonomy* refers to a need for independence and goal-attainment.[51] This idea that some people judge their self-worth in terms of the quality of their relationships, whereas others associate self-worth with freedom of choice and the achievement of goals, represents common ground between cognitive theorists such as Beck and some psychologists working from a neoFreudian perspective.[52] According to Beck, sensitivity to

different life stressors should reflect these different personality characteristics. Individuals high in sociotropy should feel especially miserable
when rejected by others, whereas individuals high in autonomy should
feel doubt, self-criticism and despondency when failing to live up to
their goals and expectations. In general, researchers have found that
individuals who are high in sociotropy are especially likely to become
dysphoric when faced with interpersonally threatening events. However, the evidence for a specific vulnerability to failure experiences in
individuals scoring high on autonomy has been more equivocal.[53]

The Attribution Self-Representation Cycle

The psychological structure of the self – the way in which different
kinds of self-representation interact with each other – is the subject of
enduring controversy, so the attempt I have made here to integrate the
various findings may be disputed by some of my colleagues. It is, of
course, possible that not only the content but also the structure of the
self varies across cultures. Perhaps cultural differences help to explain
why low self-esteem is less apparent in depressed patients from
developing countries than in patients from the West. These doubts
notwithstanding, we can take home two simple conclusions from
the evidence reviewed thus far. First, most people who are prone
to depression (including people diagnosed as suffering from bipolar
disorder) evaluate negative events with excessive pessimism. Second,
in perhaps the majority of cases, it is the belief that the self is wanting
that finally triggers negative mood. This belief, in turn, arises partly
because the individual at risk of depression holds unrealistic standards.
Building these observations on top of our previous findings (and including the pathway from life events to dysphoria via hopelessness proposed by Lyn Abramson) we arrive at the model of depression
illustrated in Figure 10.3.

This model leaves one important question unanswered. Although
we have assumed that the pathway from life experiences to dysphoria
is mediated by attributions, we have not explained where attributions
come from. Strangely, most researchers working on attributional
models of psychopathology have neglected this problem. Because attributional style has been assumed to be a stable trait, the mechanisms

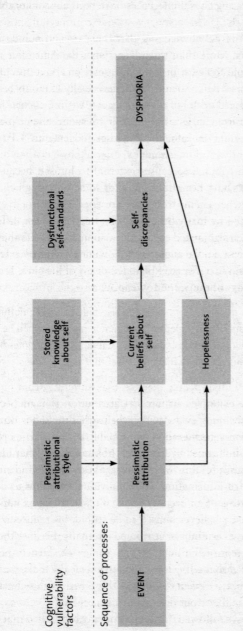

Figure 10.3 An elaborated model of dysphoria, showing the contributions of a pessimistic attributional style and dysfunctional self-standards. The pathway to dysphoria mediated by hopelessness, proposed by Abramson, is also sketched in.

involved in generating causal inferences have been almost completely ignored.

We can begin by acknowledging that most events include attributional signposts. More than thirty years ago, the American social psychologist Harold Kelley argued that information about the *consistency* (has it happened before?) and *distinctiveness* (does it only happen in particular circumstances?) of events, together with *consensus* information (does the event affect only me or everyone else?), may be particularly important in influencing causal judgements.[54] For example, an apparently random assault experienced by a civilian during warfare may be attributed to causes external to himself because he knows that attacks have been happening for some time (high consistency), occur only when enemy troops are present (high distinctiveness) and are experienced by many other civilians (high consensus). However, even such well signposted events allow some freedom in the kind of attribution generated. Consider the following attempt by a Jewish concentration camp survivor to explain the death of his older brother during the final days of the Second World War:

My brother died in my arms from dysentery. He faded away to nothing. A man who was a giant died a skeleton. I held him in my arms when he died. There was just nothing I could do. When I think about it, I sometimes blame myself. He did so much to keep me alive. I feel that had he saved some of that energy for himself he would have had a better chance to survive.[55]

In this moving example, an internal attribution is made despite apparently overwhelming evidence that the cause should be allocated elsewhere (his German tormentors), presumably because the speaker's judgement is also influenced by his beliefs about himself (that he was not strong enough). In this way, beliefs about the self form an additional source of information when individuals attempt to determine the causal locus of an event. To take a more trivial example, if an individual already believes himself to be stupid, his failure to pass an exam will almost certainly be attributed internally, because there is an available self-representation that 'fits' the event. Hence, people who score low on global self-esteem measures typically make internal attributions for negative events[56] whereas those with high self-esteem tend to make internal attributions for their successes.[57]

Readers who have followed this argument may be puzzled that I am now claiming that beliefs about the self influence attributions, whereas, only a few paragraphs ago, I was arguing that attributions affect beliefs about the self. Before resolving this gallinovular* problem, however, I want to consider two predictions that follow from my account of the way in which attributions are generated. The first concerns the time it takes to think of the likely cause of an event. If we assume that this process involves some kind of mental search that terminates when an appropriate explanation is found, and if we assume that the first step in this process involves searching current beliefs about the self, it follows that ordinary people who believe good things about themselves will more quickly generate attributions for positive events than for negative events (because they will more quickly find something good about themselves than something bad). On the other hand, people with psychiatric disorders who harbour negative beliefs about themselves should not show this bias, which may even be reversed if their negative beliefs about themselves outweigh their positive beliefs. This was the rationale for an experiment I carried out with Peter Kinderman and Kim Bowen-Jones in which we asked ordinary people, depressed patients and paranoid patients to read aloud descriptions of hypothetical events before saying what they thought their likely causes would be.[58] This method enabled us to measure precisely the interval between the time the participants finished reading each scenario and the time they began to generate an attribution (see Figure 10.4). As expected, the ordinary people more quickly generated internal attributions for positive events than for negative events. The depressed patients, on the other hand, just as quickly generated internal attributions for negative events as for positive events, which is consistent with the idea that they harbour a mixture of positive and negative beliefs about themselves. (I will discuss paranoia in detail in a later chapter; suffice it to say for the moment that the data obtained from this experiment are consistent with the hypothesis that patients who are paranoid, like depressed patients, hold more negative beliefs about themselves than ordinary people.)

The second prediction involves the effects of making people believe bad things about themselves. This can be temporarily achieved in a variety of ways, but one fairly reliable method involves creating a

* Gallinovular = chicken or egg. I am grateful to my good friend David Dickins for this contribution to the English language.

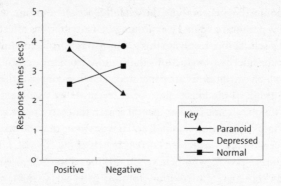

Figure 10.4 Response times needed to make internal attributions for positive and negative events by paranoid, depressed and normal participants (from Bentall, Kinderman and Bowen-Jones, 1999).

contrived failure experience.* If beliefs about the self influence attributions, people should make more pessimistic attributions about negative events as a consequence. In fact, this effect has been demonstrated by Stanford University psychologist Joseph Forgas in a series of experiments with ordinary people,[59] and more recently by Sue Kaney and myself in a study that also included depressed and paranoid patients.[60] In our version of the experiment, we asked our participants to make attributions for hypothetical negative events before and after they completed an anagram task, which included a mixture of some questions that could be solved (for example, IEPNCL, which can be solved as PENCIL) and some that could not be solved (for example, LSIDTL).

The impact of this experience is shown in Figure 10.5. At the outset, the depressed patients made more internal attributions for hypothetical negative events than the ordinary people who acted as controls. The paranoid patients, on the other hand, made more external attributions, a phenomenon that we will discuss in detail later. However, both psychiatric groups made more internal attributions following the contrived failure experience than beforehand, presumably because this experience activated negative self-schemas, which in turn influenced

---

* It would be understandable if readers had some ethical qualms about this kind of experiment. However, it should be borne in mind that the failure experiences contrived in these experiments are always very mild, and that participants are always fully debriefed afterwards.

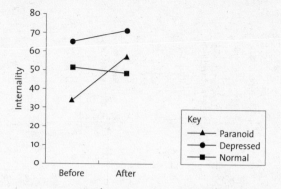

Figure 10.5 Normal, depressed and paranoid individuals' internality scores for hypothetical negative events before and after completing the insoluble anagrams task (from Bentall and Kaney, in submission).

their subsequent attributions. In this study, no change was seen in the attributional responses of the healthy controls, undoubtedly because they were less readily influenced by the failure experience than the two psychiatric groups. However, Forgas was able to produce a pessimistic shift in the attributions of ordinary people, presumably because they used a more potent contrived failure experience.

I will have more to say about the psychological mechanisms involved in generating causal explanations when I discuss the role of attributions in paranoid beliefs. For the moment, I want to point out an important implication of what we have discovered. *It seems that attributions not only influence self-representations, but that changes in self-representations affect future attributions.* The two processes are cyclically coupled in an *attribution–self-representation cycle*, so changes in either inevitably lead to changes in the other.

As a consequence, an individual's psychological response to a negative experience is likely to produce, not only an immediate change in mood, but also longer-term changes that may affect the way in which she appraises negative experiences in the future. *Indeed, this cycle, shown in Figure 10.6, appears to have all the hallmarks of a dynamic and non-linear system, in which the various components (beliefs about the self, attributions) are likely to fluctuate, perhaps dramatically and unpredictably, over time.*

If this account of the processes involved in generating attributions is

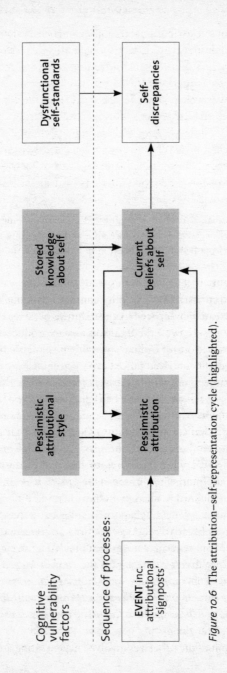

Figure 10.6 The attribution–self-representation cycle (highlighted).

correct, fluctuations in attributional responses and beliefs about the self should be observable in real life. In fact, we have already seen that this is so. Remember that, in studies in which attributions were extracted from recorded speech, it was discovered that Lyndon Johnson's decisions during the Vietnam War were predicted by his current attributional style,[61] and that changes in attributions during psychotherapy predicted changes in mood.[62] The implication of these findings is that (in the case of American presidents and psychotherapy patients, at least) attributional biases change detectably over time. Similarly, we have also seen that, even in ordinary people, self-representations (at least as reflected by global self-esteem measures) sometimes fluctuate quite dramatically.[63]

The theory of the attribution–self-representation cycle helps us to understand better two observations noted earlier in this chapter. First, recall that most people take greater credit for success than failure. The self-serving bias seems to be one of a number of self-enhancing strategies that most of us employ in our everyday lives.[64] (Another concerns the kinds of attributes we value most highly. People usually value those attributes on which they know themselves to excel. On the other hand, attributes that we do not possess are usually dismissed as relatively unimportant – overweight businessmen are rarely distressed by their inability to run marathons.) Ordinary people, it seems, actively strive to hold good opinions about themselves.

These strategies – which all involve self-serving appraisals – act as homeostatic mechanisms that maintain positive beliefs about the self in all but the most challenging conditions. Not surprisingly, research has shown that we tend to resort to these strategies when we feel that we are under threat,[65] when pressures to maintain self-esteem are particularly intense,[66] and when we are in the presence of other people who are relatively unknown to us and about whose opinions we are uncertain.[67] Without self-serving appraisals, negative events would always lead to more negative beliefs about the self, and these negative beliefs would lead to more negative appraisals in the future – ultimately culminating in a horrible spiral of increasing dysphoria.

Of course, this is exactly what seems to happen in people who are vulnerable to depression. Their pessimistic appraisals of negative events lead to negative beliefs about the self, which increase the probability that they will make further pessimistic appraisals in the future. They have no psychological defences. Hence, when suffering the slings and arrows of outrageous fortune, their self-esteem goes into free-fall.

This effect helps us to understand an unresolved problem about the role of attributions in depression. Remember that the evidence that a pessimistic attributional style always precedes depression is rather weak. On the one hand, the results from the Temple–Wisconsin Cognitive Vulnerability to Depression Project demonstrated fairly clearly that a pessimistic attributional style confers vulnerability to future dysphoria. On the other hand, many longitudinal studies have revealed at best equivocal evidence that a pessimistic style precedes the onset of low mood in the majority of people who become depressed. The account I have just given of the attribution–self-representation cycle neatly accommodates these apparently contradictory findings. As negative experiences will tend to increase the magnitude of a vulnerable individual's pessimism, highly pessimistic attributions need not be present at the onset of the descent into depression – it is sufficient that the individual's self-serving bias is not quite strong enough to counter the damage to self-esteem inflicted by a distressing life event.

It's Not What You Feel, it's the Way that You Feel it

At this point I would like to introduce a final set of concepts that will help us understand the link between appraisals and negative mood, and which will be useful when we come to examine other symptoms later on. So far, I have focused almost exclusively on psychological processes that seem to play a role in the *onset* of dysphoria. However, processes that *maintain* a dysphoric state may be just as important as processes that create a negative mood in the first place. Most of us become depressed occasionally; factors that determine the rapidity with which we bounce back may separate those of us who react to adversity with extreme distress from those of us who do not.

This insight leads to two simple ideas that we will encounter so often in later chapters that, together, they may well constitute a fundamental principle of psychopathology. First, people who are experiencing psychological distress are rarely passive victims of their emotional turmoil; rather, *they usually make active attempts to cope with it*. Second, whereas some of these attempts may successfully ameliorate distress, *other coping strategies may have the unfortunate effect of increasing the likelihood that the distress will persist.* Stating these ideas formally as *the reaction–maintenance principle*:

People do not react passively to distressing behaviours and experiences; the way in which they react plays a role in determining the duration and nature of these behaviours and experiences.

It is probable that there are many different ways in which we can respond to the experience of negative mood. However, two particularly important coping strategies have been identified by psychologist Susan Nolen-Hoeksema of the University of Michigan.[68] Some people, it seems, respond by *ruminating*; that is, by engaging in thoughts and behaviours that focus the individual's mind on their distress. People with this style of coping spend much of their time thinking about how badly they feel and pondering such questions as, 'Why am I in such a mess?' and 'Will I ever feel better?' Others, however, *distract* themselves by focusing their attention away from their unhappiness and its causes and on to pleasant or neutral stimuli that are engaging enough to prevent their thoughts returning to the source of their distress. For example, they may throw themselves into their work, or seek out pleasant social activities. Like all good research psychologists, Nolen-Hoeksema has developed her own assessment tool, the Response Styles Questionnaire (RSQ), which measures the tendency to use these strategies. (Early versions of the questionnaire also measured two other strategies – the tendency to engage in active problem solving and the tendency to rush into dangerous activities such as reckless driving or the taking of illicit drugs. These subscales were abandoned, the former because it correlated highly with distraction strategies and the latter because – surprisingly – it correlated highly with rumination. However, other researchers, unconnected to Nolen-Hoeksema, have since shown that depressed patients, whether diagnosed as unipolar or bipolar, perform poorly on measures of problem-solving ability.)[69]

That ruminative coping leads to prolonged periods of depression was demonstrated by Nolen-Hoeksema first in simple experiments in which depressed mood was induced in ordinary people by asking them to read depressing stories while listening to sad music. The participants were then instructed either to ruminate or to engage in distracting activities. Those who ruminated experienced longer and deeper periods of dysphoria. In these experiments, it was also shown that dysphoric participants who ruminated, compared to those who distracted, recalled more negative memories about their lives,[70] would interpret ambiguous situations more negatively, were more pessimistic about the future, and were less able to propose effective solutions to interpersonal problems.[71] In other words, rumination seemed to exacerbate processes which, we have already seen, are thought to be important determinants of dysphoric mood.

A unique opportunity to test the impact of the ruminating and distracting strategies was presented by the Loma Prieta earthquake, which hit the San Francisco Bay area on 17 October 1989, with a force measuring 7.1 on the Richter scale. Sixty-two people were killed in the disaster, nearly 4000 were injured, and 12,000 people were left homeless. Horrific pictures were played on news programmes over the next few days, most notably of the upper deck of a two-deck highway in Oakland, which had collapsed on to the lower deck, killing the occupants of cars travelling below. By chance, Nolen-Hoeksema had administered the RSQ to a class of Stanford University students just two weeks earlier.[72] She had also interviewed the students to determine whether they were experiencing symptoms of depression. Administering follow-up measures at ten days and at seven weeks after the earthquake, she found that those students who had been most exposed to danger, and who reported ruminating about the earthquake, were more likely to feel depressed afterwards. More importantly, she found that those students who were already depressed or suffering from stress symptoms, and who also reported a ruminative coping style on the RSQ, were especially likely to report depressive symptoms.

These findings have been confirmed in a more recent prospective study conducted under less dramatic circumstances by Nancy Just and Lauren Alloy, who found that reports of a ruminative response style in non-depressed college students predicted their later experience of dysphoric episodes over an eighteen-month follow-up period.[73] Nor have these kinds of observations been confined to samples of college students: Nolen-Hoeksema showed that a ruminative coping style predicted longer and more severe periods of depressed mood in gay men whose partners had died of AIDS,[74] and in the family members of recently deceased cancer victims.[75]

Overall, the weight of evidence about the impact of coping styles collected by Nolen-Hoeksema and her colleagues is impressive. However, two important questions remain to be answered. First, given the objections to the idea of basic emotions that I raised in the last chapter, it might be expected that rumination will affect a wide range of negative emotional states. This seems to be the case: Nolen-Hoeksema has recently shown that rumination can prolong episodes of anger[76] and also episodes of anxiety.[77] Second, although the negative impact of rumination has been well demonstrated, the effects of distraction remain relatively unexplored. We will return to this question in a later chapter.

Rhythms and Blues: from Fatigue to Depression

One obvious problem with the account I have so far given of the pathway from negative events to negative mood is that not everyone who is said to be depressed experiences negative beliefs about the self; indeed, we have seen that such beliefs may be relatively uncommon in some regions of the world. It is therefore time for me to make good my earlier promise to describe a second pathway that leads from negative experiences to the cluster of loosely related symptoms that we call 'depression'. In the process, I will attempt to explain how somatic symptoms such as loss of appetite might fit into the general framework I have constructed. We will begin by briefly plunging into an area of research that, on first sight, appears to be completely unconnected to everything that we have discussed so far.

At the same time as psychologically orientated investigators have attempted to understand the psychological processes involved in extreme forms of negative emotion, biologically orientated investigators with an interest in depression have pursued their own research agendas, most of which are too complex to describe in any detail here. A few of these avenues have directly paralleled the research we have already considered. For example, Richard Davidson at the University of Wisconsin has attempted to measure the way in which different emotional states reflect interactions between cortical areas of the brain and deeper brain structures in the limbic system.[78] Davidson's studies raise a range of issues that lie beyond the scope of this book. However, it is interesting to note that, in an experiment carried out in collaboration with Lyn Abramson, he found that ordinary people with an optimistic attributional style showed increased neural activation in the left frontal cortex.[79] Depressed people with a pessimistic style, on the other hand, showed greater activation in the right frontal cortex. Interestingly, these relationships seemed to be specific to attributional style; no such asymmetrical associations were found between dysfunctional attitudes towards the self and neural activity. If nothing else, these observations remind us that an adequate approach to psychopathology will eventually have to integrate psychological and biological findings within a single framework.

Other biological investigations have focused specifically on processes that may be responsible for some of the somatic symptoms reported by depressed patients. A particularly interesting although relatively neglected line of investigation concerns the effects of disrupting the biological rhythms that regulate our patterns of sleeping and waking. These *circadian rhythms* are reflected in subtle bodily changes (for example, changes in biochemistry and core body temperature) that occur throughout the day. Left to their own devices, they tend to become progressively longer, so that most people confined to a land without clocks or daylight would eventually settle down to a cycle of about twenty-five hours. (Readers who have experienced unemployment or other kinds of prolonged periods of inactivity may have noticed this effect, finding that they go to bed slightly later every day and that they get up progressively later in the morning.) However, our rhythms are usually kept in synchrony with the Earth's rotation by activities that expose us to regular stimuli, such as alarm clocks, journeys to work and meals. These stimuli are known as *Zeitgebers* (a German term that means clock-setting stimuli).

By way of an analogy, the reader might like to think of a person who is forced to keep time with a slow running watch, but who, at certain times of the day, is able to obtain information about the correct time. On each of these occasions, she moves her watch forward, thereby ensuring that it is always accurate within certain limits. When first encountered, this system of circadian rhythms and *Zeitgebers* seems strangely maladaptive – it is not immediately obvious why we have not simply evolved internal timekeeping devices that are more in tune with the rhythms of our planet. However, the system seems less maladaptive when we consider that, at most latitudes, human beings need to change their routines according to the seasons. It turns out that the circadian system has just the right degree of flexibility required to enable this to happen.

Now let us consider what happens if we are unable to access *Zeit-gebers*, or if our exposure to them becomes somehow irregular, so that our circadian rhythms become markedly desynchronized with the cycle of light and darkness. Many readers who have travelled abroad will have experienced this as the unpleasant but happily temporary phenomenon of jet lag. The symptoms of jet lag include fatigue and listlessness, disturbed sleep, loss of interest in food, and all too notice-able cognitive effects such as difficulty remembering, concentrating and finding words. These symptoms are, of course, caused by our circadian rhythms being out of synchrony with the place that we have travelled to, and resolve as they shift to the new cycle of activity that we impose on them. (Typically, jet lag is especially bad when we travel from west to east. This is because our naturally slow-running internal clock has greater difficulty adapting to the earlier waking which this kind of journey necessitates, compared to the later waking to which we have to adapt when travelling in the opposite direction.)

David Healy, a psychiatrist at the University of Wales College of Medicine, has noted that stressful life events often lead to a disruption of routine. He has argued that, if this disruption is severe enough, the consequence can be a form of chronic *circadian dysrhythmia*, in which our biological rhythms are persistently out of synchrony with the demands of daily living. It is as if the patient develops permanent jet lag.[80] This proposal goes a considerable way towards explaining those symptoms of depression – for example, sleep disturbance, fatigue, loss of interest in simple pleasures, and subjective cognitive difficulties – that are difficult to explain in terms of the psychological processes that we have considered earlier. Interestingly, as Healy himself notes, these are precisely the symptoms that are most prominent in non-Western descriptions of depression.[81]

Healy's suggestion is that circadian dysrythmia is the primary cause of depression, and that the psychological changes that we have con-sidered earlier are consequences of it. He argues that people who experi-ence persistent fatigue and the kinds of subtle cognitive deficits that follow from disrupted sleep will often fail to cope adequately with the demands of their work and social relationships, and will begin to blame themselves for these shortcomings. According to Healy, once the indi-vidual has made internal attributions for these negative experiences, all the other cognitive abnormalities that we have considered will follow.

Although this theory has not received the attention that it deserves, observations that many depressed patients suffer from sleep problems and have irregular rhythms of social activity[82] are clearly consistent with it.[83] Nonetheless, we should be suspicious of Healy's assertion that circadian dysrhythmia is always the *primary* cause of depression. This proposal seems to assume that depression is a single, coherent entity, and that it must be the product of a single causal pathway. In fact, as we have seen, depression is a term used to describe a range of symptoms, only some of which are easily accounted for by Healy's hypothesis.

In all likelihood, many dysphoric episodes start with the pessimistic interpretation of negative events and, if somatic symptoms are present, it is because patients respond to their dysphoric mood by withdrawing from social life and abstaining from the kinds of regular activities that would normally keep their circadian rhythms synchronized. In other cases, a loss of routine may indeed be primary, and loss of self-esteem may follow from the perception of persistent failure. (The example I gave earlier of George, the dysphoric engineer, fits this kind of pathway well; recall that his episodes of depression typically followed trips abroad, which presumably challenged his circadian system.) Even in such cases, however, we probably need to assume that some kind of cognitive vulnerability, for example a pessimistic attributional style or dysfunctional attitude towards the self, is present beforehand. Why else would people interpret their fatigue and lethargy as evidence of their own inadequacy, rather than as a natural consequence of stressful life events?

In short, it seems reasonable to assume that more than one pathway leads to the disturbances of cognition and emotion that we lump together under the label of 'depression'. The sequence of cognitive changes that follows a pessimistic appraisal of an adverse life event constitutes one such pathway, the consequences of a severe disruption to routine another. There may be others that I am not aware of. Putting together what we have learned in this chapter into a single flow diagram, we arrive at the model shown in Figure 10.7.

In the following chapters we will see that many of the processes described in this diagram also contribute to other symptoms.

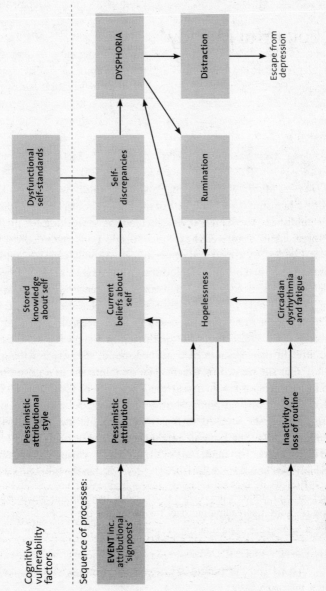

Cognitive
vulnerability
factors

Sequence of processes:

Figure 10.7 The final model of depression.

A Colourful Malady*

As an experience, madness is terrific . . .   Virginia Woolf[1]

An Unquiet Mind,[2] written by the American clinical psychologist Kay Redfield Jamison, is probably one of the bravest books about madness ever published. The daughter of a meteorologist working for the US air force, Jamison suffered the frequent dislocations that are often the lot of families of armed forces personnel. Although moody during childhood, she first became manic during her senior year at high school, when she experienced a period of intense excitement and disorientation that was followed by weeks of depression and exhaustion. At the time, it did not occur to her that she might be suffering from a psychiatric disorder. Even years later, after qualifying as a clinical psychologist, and after further episodes of disturbed mood, she was unwilling to believe that she needed treatment. Her appointment to a position in the Department of Psychiatry at the University of California in Los Angeles was a turning point. Shortly afterwards, following a period during which she worked furiously and without sleep, she began spending wildly. She bought watches, unnecessary furniture, books and (for some reason) numerous snakebite kits. Eventually she became 'ravingly psychotic', an experience she described in the following way:

One evening I stood in the middle of my living room and looked out at a blood-red sunset spreading out over the horizon of the Pacific. Suddenly, I felt a strange sense of light at the back of my eyes and almost immediately

* I am grateful to my Ph.D. student Justin Thomas for suggesting some of the ideas in this chapter.

saw a huge black centrifuge* inside my head. I saw a tall figure in a floor-length evening gown approach the centrifuge with a vase-sized glass tube of blood in her hand. As the figure turned around I saw to my horror that it was me and that there was blood all over my dress, cape and long white gloves. I watched as the figure carefully put the tube of blood into one of the holes in the centrifuge, closed the lid, and pushed a button on the front of the machine. The centrifuge began to whirl.

Then, horrifyingly, the image that previously had been inside my head now was completely outside of it. I was paralysed with fright. The spinning of the centrifuge and the clanking of the glass tube against the metal became louder and louder, and then the machine splintered into a thousand pieces. Blood was everywhere. It spattered against the windowpanes, and the walls and paintings, and soaked down into the carpets. I looked out towards the ocean and saw that the blood on the window had merged with the sunset; I couldn't tell where one ended and the other began. I screamed at the top of my lungs. I couldn't get away from the sight of the blood and the echoes of the machine's clanking as it whirled faster and faster.

The main theme of *An Unquiet Mind* is Jamison's struggle to come to terms with her diagnosis. As the story unravels, she tells of her reluctance to accept the fallibility of her own mind, and of the anxiety she felt when forced by circumstances to reveal her condition to other people. The decision to write about her experiences is portrayed as the culmination of a gradual and frightening processes of 'coming out', facilitated at various points by sympathetic colleagues, friends and lovers. Early in her career, she made use of her experiences by presenting her own story at conferences as if she had heard it from a patient. Only later, after finding a type of medication that seemed to suit her, was she able to admit publicly that her life had been punctuated by periods of madness so severe that they had necessitated hospital treatment.

Jamison's research has mostly focused on the link between abnormal moods and creativity. (We considered some of her findings in Chapter 5.) She is such a good example of the triumph of ambition over adversity (and therefore an excellent role-model for psychotic patients) that it

---

* A piece of laboratory equipment that separates out different components of a sample of blood (or other bodily fluid) by spinning it at high speed.

will probably seem uncharitable to pass judgement on her account. And yet, throughout *An Unquiet Mind*, Jamison accepts the Kraepelinian paradigm uncritically. She hints at difficulties in her own life (her father was prone to moods that became so extreme that they eventually made him unemployable; her parents divorced, as she did later; a lover died tragically) but, for reasons that are easily inferred, she says very little about how these events contributed to her psychosis. The 'illness' in *An Unquiet Mind* is an invading army that imposes its will upon her. She endures its occupation with dignity. It does not appear to be the product of her psychology, a response to circumstances, or the outcome of a process of development.

This attitude is very common among psychologists and psychiatrists, who regard mania as such an extreme phenomenon that it is assumed to be impenetrable to psychological analysis. And yet, given that mania is typically experienced by people who also have a history of depression, it is reasonable to ask whether processes similar to those we have considered in the last chapter could be implicated in manic episodes. To begin to answer this question we must look more closely at what happens in a manic episode.

A Paradoxical Condition

Surprisingly, in her account of her illness, Kay Jamison nowhere describes in detail what it is like to experience mania. The closest she comes is her account of a terrifying hallucinatory episode, which I have reproduced above. Perhaps mania is too frightening to recall. Or more likely there is something about the manic state that makes it almost impossible to portray in words. Although I have spent many hours listening to recovered manic patients attempting to describe their experiences, their accounts have often seemed curiously incomplete. It is as if the break from normal functioning during an episode is so severe that the mind, on returning to sanity, cannot comprehend it.

This amnesia may be explained by a phenomenon known as *state-dependent memory*. We are most likely to remember something if we are in a similar state to that in which we learnt it. Howard Weingartner and his colleagues at the US National Institute of Mental Health demonstrated this effect in bipolar patients by asking them to learn simple word lists when manic and when in remission, finding that they were better able to recall the lists when in the same mood state.[3] In a case study that illustrates this effect more vividly than any experiment, J. Mark Williams and H. R. Markar have described a patient who hid several thousand pounds when manic. Recovering, he could not remember where he had put the money. Some months later, when manic again, he tried to hide something else and, choosing the same place, found it.[4]

The difficulty experienced by patients when attempting to recall mania is matched by the poor descriptions offered in the classic literature of psychiatry. Even modern researchers have harboured gross illusions about the manic state. For example, the term 'bipolar disorder' gives the quite misleading impression that mania lies at the opposite pole to depression on a spectrum of emotion. Interestingly, some ancient physicians were more acute observers than their modern counterparts. The second-century physician Aretaeus, who lived in Cappadocia in Asia Minor, was probably the first person to suggest that mania is an extreme end-state of depression,[5] a hypothesis that is consistent with much of the evidence that we will consider shortly.

The symptoms of mania

One of Kay Jamison's most remarkable achievements is her encyclopaedic textbook *Manic-Depressive Illness*, which she co-authored with American psychiatrist Frederick Goodwin.[6] Within its pages, Goodwin and Jamison gather together data on the emotions reported by patients suffering from mania or its milder variant *hypomania* (defined in DSM-IV as a period of 'abnormally and persistently elevated, irritable or expansive mood' accompanied by at least three additional symptoms such as inflated self-esteem, non-delusional grandiosity, decreased need for sleep, flight of ideas, distractibility or 'excessive involvement in pleasurable activities that have a high potential for painful consequences'). Collating the data from fourteen studies involving over 700 patients, they found that euphoria was reported by 71 per cent of the patients examined, a finding that at first seems consistent with the bipolar concept. However, 72 per cent of patients were described as depressed, and 80 per cent of patients were described as irritable. Simple arithmetic reveals that some patients must be both dysphoric and euphoric. The DSM system recognizes this phenomenon by describing three types of bipolar episodes: depression, mania, and mixed episodes in which both manic and depressive symptoms are evident. However, the concept of a mixed episode remains controversial.[7] Some researchers have suggested that the apparent co-occurrence of depression and euphoria in fact reflects ultra-rapid transitions between one mood state and the other, so that patients are euphoric one moment and depressed the next. Others have suggested that different moods predominate as manic episodes unfold. Frederick Goodwin, for example, has argued that most manic patients progress through three distinct phases, with euphoria dominant only in the first, whereas depression, panic and irritability dominate in the third and most severe stage (see Figure 11.1).[8]

The paradox of co-existing euphoria and depression in manic patients becomes less paradoxical when viewed from the perspective of the circumplex model of emotions, described in Chapter 9 (pp. 215–19). Recall that, according to this model, negative mood and positive mood are independent dimensions of emotion. Therefore, although we would expect these emotions to be negatively correlated for much of the time (because events which make us feel bad tend not to make us feel good and vice versa) there is nothing to stop both types of mood states occurring together under exceptional circumstances.

This explanation is consistent with the results of a factor-analytic investigation of manic and mixed episodes recently reported by Frederick Cassidy and his colleagues at Duke University in North Carolina.[9] Prior to their analysis, they collected detailed information about the symptoms of more than 200 patients. They discovered that these symptoms fell into five separate groups. Two of the factors were dysphoric mood and 'increased hedonic function' (euphoric mood, increased humour and an increased interest in sex), which were therefore shown to be independent of each other. The remaining three factors were psychomotor pressure (racing thoughts, rapid speech and increased activity), psychosis (mainly grandiose and paranoid delusions) and irritability.

One reason why the emotional component of mania may have been so badly misunderstood is that it is usually not an immediate source of concern to other people. More often it is non-mood symptoms that draw attention to the patient and precipitate an admission to hospital.

	Stage I	Stage II	Stage III
Mood	Lability of affect; euphoria predominates; irritability if demands not satisfied	Increased dysphoria and depression, open hostility and anger	Clearly dysphoric; panic-stricken; hopeless
Cognition	Expansivity, grandiosity, overconfidence; thoughts coherent but occasionally tangential; sexual and religious preoccupation; racing thoughts	Flight of ideas; disorganization of cognitive state; delusions	Incoherent, definite loosening of associations; bizarre and idiosyncratic delusions; hallucinations in 1/3 of patients; disorientation to time and place; occasional ideas of reference
Behavior	Increased psychomotor activity; increased initiation and rate of speech; increased spending, smoking, telephone use	Continued increased psychomotor acceleration; increased pressured speech; occasional assaultive behavior	Frenzied and frequently bizarre psychomotor activity

Adapted from Carlson and Goodwin, 1973

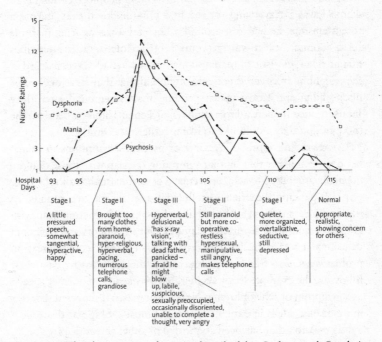

Figure 11.1 The three stages of mania described by Carlson and Goodwin (1973), reproduced from F. K. Goodwin and K. Jamison (1990), *Manic-Depressive Illness*, Oxford, Oxford University Press.

The reckless activity that is common in manic episodes can provoke alarm in friends and relatives, causing them to seek the advice of doctors and psychiatrists. One of my patients drove his car at frightening speeds down country lanes, convinced that he was invincible. The car rolled on a corner and was damaged beyond repair but my patient walked away from the accident unscathed, his conviction in his own indestructibility reinforced by the experience. Not surprisingly, his more realistic parents ensured he had an early appointment at a local psychiatric clinic.

Fortunately, life-threatening deeds of this sort are fairly unusual. It is also rare for patients to act on their heightened sexual feelings (experienced by 57 per cent of patients according to Goodwin and Jamison). When they do, they more often expose themselves (29 per cent) than make sexual advances towards other people. (A young man whom I was interviewing for the first time disclosed that, during a recent episode, he had run around a hospital ward wearing just one sock, adding, 'And it wasn't on my foot!') More mundane activities that are characteristic of mania or hypomania include excessive use of the telephone (recovered patients often find that they have enormous phone bills) and extravagant spending that is regretted later (Kay Jamison once bought a large number of Penguin books, because she thought that they would like to live together in a family).

Goodwin and Jamison's review of psychotic symptoms in manic patients reminds us that bipolar symptoms overlap with those that are normally attributed to schizophrenia. They estimate that about 15 per cent of patients experience hallucinations, which are usually in the auditory modality. Abnormal beliefs are more common, with grandiose delusions reported by 47 per cent of patients and paranoid delusions reported by 28 per cent. Language and communication problems are also frequently observed. Although most psychiatrists, following the example set by Bleuler, have regarded incoherent speech as a symptom of schizophrenia, Nancy Andreasen discovered that it is more often evident in patients with a diagnosis of bipolar disorder,[10] an observation that has been confirmed by other researchers.

From this evidence, it is obvious that mania, like depression, is not a symptom, but a complex group of symptoms (some of which are discussed in other chapters of this book). Unfortunately, the very limited psychological research that has so far been carried out with bipolar patients (including my own) has tended to treat mania as a lump, so it is not always clear which characteristics of manic episodes are associated with the processes that have been investigated.

An insight from psychoanalysis?

The earliest systematic contributions to the psychology of mania were made by psychoanalysts. Of those who studied the problem, the most important was Karl Abraham. Born in Bremen in 1877, Abraham became Bleuler's assistant at the Burghölzli Hospital in Zurich, where he fell under the influence of the Freudians, despite developing a strong dislike for Jung. Until his premature death from cancer in 1925, he was one of Freud's most loyal disciples. He was described by Freud's biographer Ernest Jones as, 'Certainly the most normal of the group. His distinguishing attributes were steadfastness, common sense, shrewdness, and a perfect self-control.' However, Jones qualified this observation by adding, 'One would scarcely use the term "charm" in describing him; in fact, Freud sometimes told me he found him "too Prussian".'[11]

In a paper published in 1911, Abraham argued that:

Viewed externally, the manic phase of the cyclical disturbances is the complete opposite of the depressive one. A manic appears very cheerful on the surface; and unless a deeper investigation is carried out by psychoanalytic methods it might appear that the two phases are the opposite of each other even as regards their content. Psychoanalysis shows, however, that both phases are dominated by the same complexes, and that it is only the patient's attitudes to these complexes that is different. In the depressive state he allows himself to be weighed down by his complex, and sees no other way out of his misery but death; in the manic state he treats the complex with indifference.[12]

Abraham's proposal was that the underlying psychological processes in mania are similar to those in depression, but that, in the manic state, these processes are experienced as intolerable and are therefore denied. This idea was later elaborated by Sandor Rado, the Hungarian-born psychoanalyst whose ideas about anhedonia we considered earlier. Rado argued that manic-depressive patients are highly narcissistic, and that the manic defence is therefore motivated by an abnormal need for approval by others.[13]

The *manic-defence hypothesis* has been neglected by psychological researchers, mainly because of persisting doubts about the scientific status of psychoanalysis. Because the early psychoanalysts were unable to frame their theories in ways that could be tested experimentally, and even refused to recognize the value of the experimental method, many modern psychologists have assumed that their ideas were not worth investigating.[14] In doing so, they have forgotten that the early psychoanalysts made perceptive observations about the behaviour of their patients, and have failed to recognize that many of their theories seem less bizarre when translated into ordinary language. This is certainly true of the idea of defence, which simply implies that we attempt to regulate our own emotions by avoiding thoughts that are exceptionally distressing. Evidence in support of this idea is not difficult too find, and we have already encountered some of it in the previous chapter.

In fact, there has been at least one attempt to restate the manic-defence hypothesis in the language of modern psychology. John Neale, working at the State University of New York in the late 1980s, suggested that people who are vulnerable to manic episodes suffer from unrealistic standards for success and unstable self-esteem. According to Neale's account, when negative events intensify the vulnerable person's underlying feelings of low self-regard, he responds with a cascade of grandiose ideas, which inhibit distressing thoughts about the self. These grandiose ideas in turn rapidly spiral out of control, causing mood elevation and eventually mania.[15]

Is There a Manic Defence?

Because so few data were available to him, Neale's reformulation of the manic-defence hypothesis was necessarily vague. In fact, the hypothesis can be expressed in various forms. A weak version implies that mania is triggered by incipient negative mood, or perhaps the threat of negative mood, and reflects patients' efforts to avoid negative emotion. A stronger version would also imply that the manic state consists of an underlying depression that is somehow masked by these efforts. (An ultra-strong version, consistent with the claims of psychoanalysis, would go still further, and suggest that these symptoms enable patients to avoid *awareness* of their underlying depression altogether. However, because of the considerable difficulties in establishing what patients are really aware of – as opposed to just ignoring – I will leave this issue to cleverer minds than mine.)

The remitted bipolar patient

If episodes of mania are triggered by incipient negative mood, it follows that remitted bipolar patients should have many of the psychological characteristics of depressed patients, and that the more they have these characteristics, the more likely it is that they will become manic. At least one piece of evidence seems, at first sight, inconsistent with these assumptions. When patients are asked to recall their experiences of the prodromal phase of the disorder, they usually report symptoms of excitement (for example, reduced sleep, increased activity, excessive talkativeness, euphoria and racing thoughts) rather than symptoms of depression.[16] However, this evidence is far from conclusive. As we have seen, patients often have difficulty recalling their symptoms, and, in any case, we probably need to look further backwards in time than the prodrome, which marks the beginning of the manic state.

Although it has often been assumed that remitted patients suffer from no symptoms of any importance, and function just as well as ordinary people, recent studies suggest that this impression has arisen simply because they usually live their lives beyond the sight of psychiatrists and clinical psychologists. 'Subclinical' depression, it seems, is the norm.[17] Remitted bipolar patients also appear to have many of the psychological characteristics of depressed patients, even if they are sometimes reluctant to reveal them. One of the earliest investigations to demonstrate this was conducted by Ken Winters and John Neale, who argued that, because patients would respond defensively, it would be misleading to study the psychology of the remitted state using conventional questionnaires.[18] They therefore devised a non-obvious or implicit test of attributional style, known as the Pragmatic Inference Task (PIT), which is disguised as a memory test. People taking the test are asked to listen to a series of brief stories such as the following:

You decide to open your own dry-cleaning shop in a small but growing town near the border. Your shop will be the only one of its kind for miles around. In the first year of business, the town's population doubles and your business prospers. Your advertising campaign is a big success and reactions from your customers indicate that the cleaning is of good quality. Your gross sales exceed expectations. You wonder whether it would be to your advantage to open a chain of shops, so you go to the bank and apply for a loan. As you had hoped, the bank approves the loan.

After each story, the participant is asked to answer a number of multiple-choice questions, some of which have clear right and wrong answers. (For example: What kind of shop did you open? A: Hardware or B: Dry-cleaning. The answer, obviously, is B.) However, one question after each story asks listeners to recall which of two causes (one internal and one external) was responsible for the good or bad outcome portrayed (What is the reason for the success of your business? A: You are a clever businessman or B: You have no competition). The stories are carefully constructed so that neither answer is more obviously correct than the other. Therefore, Winters and Neale argued, the answers chosen will reflect the way that participants feel about themselves. Winters and Neale found that, like unipolar depressed patients but unlike ordinary people, remitted bipolar patients made internal (self-blaming) attributions for negative events much more than for positive events.

Winters and Neale also measured a characteristic known as *social desirability*.[19] This slightly confusing term refers to the need to present a positive image of the self to others. Questionnaires that measure social desirability invite people to admit to undesirable but common dispositions and behaviours (for example, gossiping about others, playing sick to gain advantage). It is assumed that people who deny these characteristics are so defensive that they are unable to admit to even trivial shortcomings. Winters and Neale found that their remitted bipolar patients scored much higher on this measure than ordinary people.

This study, published in 1985, was largely ignored by other investigators. In the past few years, however, researchers have used other measures to confirm Winters and Neale's general observation of depressive processes in remitted patients. For example, Jan Scott and her colleagues in Newcastle recently administered the Dysfunctional Attitudes Scale (the measure of perfectionist self-standards that I briefly described in the last chapter) and found that remitted patients, like people suffering from depression, scored much more highly than ordinary people.[20]

My earliest research with bipolar patients attempted to detect underlying depressive processes in people who were vulnerable to bipolar symptoms, and made use of an obscure psychological phenomenon known as the *Stroop effect*. In 1935, a British psychologist, J. R. Stroop, reported an experiment in which ordinary people were asked to look at a series of colour words printed in incongruent ink colours (for example, the word 'red' might be printed in blue, the word 'green' might be printed in red, and so on). The people taking part in the experiment were asked to name the ink colour of each word but to ignore the word itself. Stroop observed that people find this task very difficult – the participants in his experiment were much slower at this kind of colour-naming than when colour-naming words in congruent ink colours (for example, 'green' printed in green) or meaningless strings of letters (for example, 'XXXXX') written in different ink colours.[21] The precise mechanisms responsible for this effect are still debated. However, it is safe to assume that people find it hard to suppress the habit of reading the word itself, creating an internal competition between reading and colour-naming. To anyone attempting the task, this urge to do two things at once creates the weird subjective sensation that the mind is filling with glue.

The Stroop effect is useful to clinical psychologists, because it occurs for any words that draw the individual's attention. This is especially the case for words that have some kind of emotional significance and which reflect a source of worry. Depressed patients but not ordinary people are much slower to colour-name depression-related words (for example, 'failure', 'sadness') than emotionally neutral words ('diamond', 'collector').[22] Similarly, anorexic patients are slow to colour-name food words[23] and anxious patients are slow to colour-name anxiety-related words.[24]

Michelle Thompson and I used the Stroop technique to test university students whom we selected according to their scores on a hypomania questionnaire. We gave the students a Stroop task with depression-related words (for example, 'dread', 'rejected'), euphoria-related words ('wonderful', 'glorious') and emotionally neutral words ('pod', 'tendency'). As predicted, the hypomanic students showed slowed colour-naming for the depression-related but not for the euphoria-related words, suggesting that the former words were emotionally troubling to them.[25] Although this finding might seem to be slightly counter-intuitive – after all, the hypomanic students did not show any evidence of depression – it has since been replicated by Chris French at the University of London, who started out by questioning some aspects of our methodology, but who ended up obtaining almost identical findings when using his own methods.[26]

In two more recent studies, conducted in Manchester with my students Julie Highfield and Tom Woodnut, we decided to investigate self-esteem in well-adjusted students with hypomanic personality traits, and also in a group of remitted bipolar patients.[27] Aware of the evidence that self-esteem is often highly unstable in people who are vulnerable to depression, we decided to measure it daily in both groups and matched controls, using the diary method devised by Michael Kernis.[28] Participants completed a very simple self-esteem questionnaire and also answered a series of questions twice a day for a week about what had been happening to them. We compared each of the target groups – the hypomanic students and the remitted patients – to control groups matched with them for age, sex and educational achievement and found that the self-esteem scores of both the hypomanic students and the remitted patients fluctuated more markedly than the scores of these comparison groups. Interestingly, although neither the hypomanic students nor the remitted patients scored very highly on a measure of depression, their scores exceeded those of their respective controls, and when we allowed for this difference statistically, the differences in stability of self-esteem were no longer evident. The unstable self-esteem of these groups therefore seemed to reflect 'bubbling' subclinical depression.

The manic-defence hypothesis suggests not only that individuals vulnerable to mania should experience incipient depressive symptoms, but also that the severity of their depressive psychological processes will predict the likelihood that they will become manic in the future. As yet, only one study has properly addressed this prediction. Lauren Alloy and her colleagues tried to extend the high-risk research strategy they have developed for the study of depression to bipolar symptomatology. They used a questionnaire followed by a psychiatric interview to screen 3000 students for a history of mood symptoms. This led them to identify 49 apparently bipolar students, most of whom were well when first assessed, and a group of 97 students with an apparent history of unipolar depression, most of whom were also well. After being tested on a range of psychological measures, including attributional style, these groups, together with a small control group, were reassessed one month later. Unfortunately, because of the small numbers in the study, the researchers did not report separate attributional style data for currently depressed and currently manic participants. However, in both the bipolar and unipolar group, there was evidence that a pessimistic attributional style predicted an increase in depressive symptoms at the follow-up assessment. More interestingly, in the bipolar group, a pessimistic style also predicted an increase in manic symptoms.[29]

Whether self-esteem measures foretell the onset of mania is less certain. Psychologist Sheri Johnson and her colleagues at the University of Miami have reported a small study in which they found that low self-esteem in remitted patients predicted later depression but not mania.[30] However, Jan Scott and Marie Pope in Newcastle, in a similar study, recently measured positive and negative self-esteem separately, finding that the negative component predicted both future depression and future mania.[31]

The psychology of mania

Very little psychological research has been conducted with actively manic patients, almost certainly because of the difficulty in getting them to sit still for long enough to complete a set of tests. However, Helen Lyon, Mike Startup and I decided to repeat my earlier Stroop experiment with bipolar patients who were attending psychiatric clinics in North Wales.[32] Consistent with my earlier findings, we found slowed colour-naming for depression-related but not euphoria-related words in both bipolar-depressed and bipolar-manic patients (see Figure 11.2).

Perhaps we should not have been surprised by this finding. After all, as we saw earlier, euphoria is usually evident only in the earliest stages of manic episodes, and dysphoria predominates in the later stages. Stronger evidence for the manic-defence hypothesis would require the demonstration that manic patients show depressive-like responding on some measures (preferably non-obvious or implicit

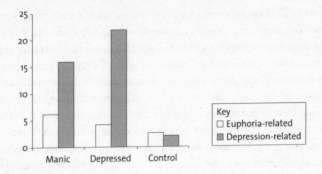

Figure 11.2 Stroop data reported for bipolar-manic, bipolar-depressed and normal participants by Lyon et al. (1999). The columns show interference indices (the extent to which the participants were slowed when attempting to colour-name emotionally salient words, calculated by subtracting the amount of time required to colour-name 50 emotionally neutral words from the time required to colour-name 50 salient words). This measure is shown for both depression-related (for example, *dread, rejected, suicide, depressing*) and euphoria-related words (for example, *wonderful, glorious, joy, jubilant*). Note that the two clinical groups show substantial interference for depression-related but not euphoria-related words.

measures, which might be relatively unaffected by defensive processes) while, at the same time, responding in a way that seems to be incompatible with depression on other measures (preferably obvious or explicit measures, which would be expected to be affected by defensive processes). In fact, this kind of evidence emerged from the same study. In the last chapter, I described the performance of bipolar patients on the Attributional Style Questionnaire (see Figure 10.1, p. 244), noting that patients suffering a manic episode appeared to make fairly normal attributions, in contrast to depressed patients, who made pessimistic (internal, global and stable) attributions for negative events. Figure 11.3 shows the performance of the same patients on Winters and Neale's Pragmatic Inference Task. Note that the performance of the normal and depressed participants on the PIT was concordant with their performance on the ASQ. The healthy controls showed a self-serving bias on both measures whereas the depressed patients showed a pessimistic bias, again on both measures. In contrast, the performance of the manic patients seemed to vary dramatically between the two tests. Whereas their performance on the ASQ showed a normal self-serving bias, their attributions on the PIT were highly pessimistic. In fact, on the implicit measure, little difference can be seen between their scores and the scores of the depressed patients.

Further evidence relevant to the manic-defence hypothesis can be obtained by looking at measures of self-representation. In the last chapter, I discussed a study of the self-discrepancies of bipolar patients conducted by Kerry Manson, Peter Kinderman and myself, in which we observed an abnormal *lack* of self–ideal discrepancies in manic patients. This finding is consistent with their apparent grandiosity and suggests that, on the surface at least, they harbour no doubts whatsoever about their attributes and talents, a finding that has been reported by other researchers using less complex measures of self-esteem.[33]

Evidence of a less positive view of the self in mania emerged from an additional measure included in the study that I carried out with Helen Lyon and Mike Startup. We exploited the *self-reference effect*, the tendency to recall information that is specifically relevant to the self. As I mentioned in the last chapter, many studies have shown that depressed people, when given a list of negative and positive words, say that more of the negative words describe their own personalities and, more importantly, recall more of the negative words if given a surprise memory test afterwards.[34] We therefore administered this kind of test

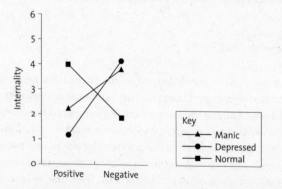

Figure 11.3 Internality data for manic, depressed and normal participants assessed using the Pragmatic Inference Task. These scores should be contrasted with the ASQ data from the same patients, shown in Figure 10.1, p. 244.

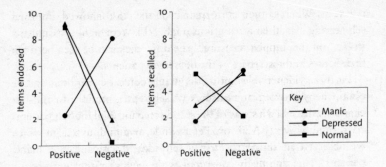

Figure 11.4 Left panel shows the number of positive and negative personality traits endorsed as 'true' by manic, depressed and normal participants. On the right is shown how many of the items were recalled by the participants when they were given a surprise recall test. From Lyon, Startup and Bentall (1999).

to our participants. Consistently with previous research, our bipolar-depressed participants endorsed and recalled more negative words than our well controls. However, our manic patients endorsed more positive words than negative words but recalled more negative words than positive words (see Figure 11.4).

Clearly, more psychological research must be carried out with manic patients. However, the evidence available to date supports *at least* the weak version of the manic-defence hypothesis, which assumes that mania arises from patients' attempts to avoid negative mood.

Becoming Manic

The account of the psychology of mania that I have given so far has focused on the remitted state, and on mania itself. However, a workable theory of mania requires a further vital ingredient: *a mechanism that enables patients to pass from the former state to the latter.*

We will begin considering this problem by examining two accounts of the processes that lead to mania which, at first sight, seem to be at odds with the manic-defence hypothesis. The first, which might be called the *excitability hypothesis* (a term which, so far as I know, is not used by any of its proponents), suggests that people who are vulnerable to mania are in some way hyper-excitable. The most carefully worked out version of this idea has been put forward by Richard Depue, of Cornell University in Ithaca, New York,[35] who based his model on a neurophysiological theory of personality proposed by British psychologist Jeffrey Gray.[36] On the basis of animal studies, Gray argued that two emotional systems could be identified in the brain, the behavioural inhibition system (BIS), which responds to stimuli associated with punishment or frustration, and the behavioural activation system (BAS), which responds to stimuli associated with reward. (Activation of the BIS is associated with negative mood whereas activation of the BAS is associated with positive mood, so the theory maps on to Watson and Tellegren's two-dimensional model of emotion, which we discussed in Chapter 9.) According to Depue, manic symptoms are a manifestation of a dysregulation of the behavioural activation system, which is why patients are highly sociable, desire excitement, and show high levels of motor activity, as if they are interminably over-reacting to a reward.

Sheri Johnson has reported two findings that fit this theory rather well. First, she demonstrated that hypomanic people score highly on a questionnaire designed to measure the subjective experience of BAS activation (items included, 'When good things happen to me, it affects me strongly'; 'When I want something I usually go all-out to get it'; 'I will often do things for no other reason than that they might be fun').[37] She also reported that patients with a diagnosis of bipolar disorder experience an increased risk of manic symptoms following the achievement of an important life goal.[38] This second finding can be interpreted in more ways than one, as Johnson also observed that positive events in general did not lead to an increase in manic symptoms (as might be expected from Depue's model), and as goal attainment often carries with it the threat of later failure (examples of goal attainments given in Johnson's paper include gaining admission to graduate school and obtaining a new job). A more important limitation of Depue's excitability hypothesis is that it does not seem to explain the close association between depression and mania.

The second apparent alternative to the manic-defence hypothesis implicates sleep disturbances. Many people feel energetic after a night without sleep, only to feel tired after the following night. David Healy has argued that, because of a disorder of the circadian clock, bipolar patients experience a magnification of this effect, so that they rapidly spiral into mania following a period of sleep deprivation. According to this account, the euphoria experienced by manic patients, and their grandiose ideas, are reactions to the high energy levels that they suddenly experience.[39] In an intriguing extension of this *sleep deprivation hypothesis*, Charles Raison and his colleagues at the University of California have recently suggested that old superstitions linking the full moon to insanity may be explained in this way.[40] Before the development of modern lighting, the moon was the main source of nocturnal illumination. People living before the development of electricity would therefore have been especially likely to experience sleep difficulties when the moon was full.

It is commonly observed that a period of sleep loss precedes an episode of mania.[41] For example, Thomas Wehr and his colleagues at the US National Institute of Mental Health have described a number of cases of people being provoked into a manic episode by a single sleepless night:

For the past 2 years, Mr. B, a 28-year-old bipolar patient, drove 800 miles to spend the Christmas holidays with his family. Impatient to return home and unable to find a motel room, he drove through the night without stopping. By the time of his arrival, Mr. B, who had been euthymic [that is, in a normal mood], became hypomanic. The first year the mania escalated and required hospitalisation; the following year it was possible to attenuate the severity of his mania through early treatment with adjunctive neuroleptic medications.[42]

Nocturnal physiological measurements have confirmed that loss of sleep is a characteristic of mania.[43] Several studies,[44] including one reported by Thomas Wehr's research group,[45] have also noted correlations between sleep duration and manic symptoms the following day. Taking this idea further, Susan Malkoff-Schwartz, Ellen Frank and their colleagues at the University of Pittsburgh School of Medicine have investigated whether manic episodes are typically preceded by what they term *social rhythm disruption (SRD) events*.[46] In their most extreme form, these events (for example, starting night work, the arrival of a new baby) completely disrupt sleep whereas, in their milder forms (for example, travelling between time zones, staying up to revise for an examination), the sleep–wake cycle is only partially disrupted.

When bipolar and unipolar patients were compared, it was found that about two thirds of patients who became manic had experienced an SRD event in the eight weeks preceding their mania, whereas no such effect was found for episodes of depression, either in the bipolar patients or in the unipolar patients.

It is important to remember that SRD events may be stressful for reasons other than their effect on sleep. For this reason, the best way to establish whether sleep deprivation *per se* leads to mania is to ask patients with a history of the disorder to volunteer to go without sleep. In general, the results of experiments of this sort suggest that only a minority of patients may be as sensitive to sleep deprivation as Thomas Wehr's case studies suggest. In perhaps the best study of this kind, reported by Christina Colombo, Francesco Benedetti and their colleagues at the University of Milan, over 200 bipolar-depressed patients underwent three nights of total sleep deprivation, interspersed with nights of normal sleep (it was hoped that this would benefit their depression). About 5 per cent of the patients became manic and a similar number became hypomanic. Only four of the patients became ill enough to require drug treatment.[47] Overall, then, the available evidence suggests that disruption to sleep *can* precipitate mania, but that this effect is not inevitable.

The excitability hypothesis and the sleep deprivation hypothesis should not be regarded as mutually exclusive. As we have seen, both are to some extent supported by research. However, unlike the manic-defence hypothesis, both seem to assume that the events leading up to mania are largely beyond patients' own control. We can incorporate both mechanisms within the framework of the manic-defence hypothesis if we assume that patients, faced with the threat of negative mood, sometimes choose to pursue activities that either cause them intense excitement or lead to sleep loss.

To see how this might happen we must return to the reaction-maintenance principle and some of the methods that people use to cope with negative mood, which we considered in the last chapter (see p. 262). Recall that, according to studies carried out by Susan Nolen-Hoeksema, people tend to react to being depressed in one of four ways. Some people ruminate about their feelings, others launch into attempts to solve the problems that they believe have led to their depression, some try to distract themselves and a few indulge in dangerous activities. Nolen-Hoeksema's research established that rumination leads to periods of depression that are deeper and more enduring.[48]

In a recent study, my Ph.D. student Justin Thomas administered Nolen-Hoeksema's questionnaire to a large group of students, who also completed questionnaire measures of depression and hypomanic traits.[49] Consistent with Nolen-Hoeksema's findings, we observed a strong correlation between rumination and depression. However, although we also found a weak association between rumination and hypomania, hypomania was more strongly predicted by the distraction and dangerous activities coping styles.

I think that anyone who has spent any time talking to bipolar patients will recognize these coping strategies (which include working around the clock, intense socializing, indulging in alcohol and drugs, and generally seeking novel experiences) from the patients' own accounts. Unfortunately, at the time of writing, only one study has systematically asked bipolar patients about their coping styles. Dominic Lam and Grace Wong at the Institute of Psychiatry in London divided patients into those who seemed to cope well with their symptoms, and who seemed to be able to control them, and those who did not. Many of the strategies reported by the poor copers ('continue to move about and take on more tasks', 'go out and spend money', and 'find more to do to fill out the extra minutes of the day') obviously involved some kind of distraction.[50]

Towards a Psychology of Mania

Less psychological research has been conducted into mania than into any other major psychiatric complaint. In this chapter, I have tried to weave together an account of the pathway from incipient negative mood to manic episodes that makes best sense of the limited evidence. This pathway, from distraction and risk-taking, to excitement, sleep loss and eventually mania, is shown in Figure 11.5, which is a modification of the final model of depression that we arrived at in the last chapter.

It is important to note that this tentative model seems to explain better some aspects of mania than others. Earlier, I explained that

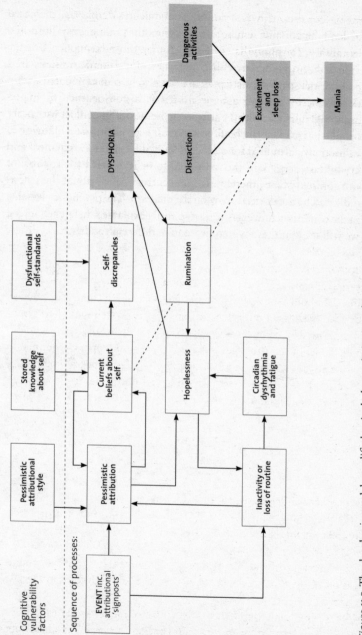

Figure 11.5 The dysphoria model, modified to include mania (unique features shaded).

mania consists of five separable components: dysphoria, increased hedonic functioning (euphoria), psychomotor pressure, psychosis and irritability. Dysphoria is accounted for by those components of the model that are shared with our earlier model of depression. It is possible that psychomotor pressure can also be accommodated within this framework if we assume that it is a consequence of hyper-excitability. Irritability may arise from the inevitable conflict with other people that manic behaviour provokes. It is possible that euphoria can be partially accounted for also, especially if feelings of excitement and boundless energy lead the individual to believe that he is capable of extraordinary feats, thereby affecting current beliefs about the self, as indicated by the dotted arrow on the diagram. The psychotic elements of the condition, however, are not so easily explained. In later chapters, we will see that these symptoms require different models.

Abnormal Attitudes

I am absolutely certain that in this regard I command experiences which – when generally acknowledged as valid – will act fruitfully to the highest possible degree among the rest of mankind ... You like other people may be inclined at first to see nothing but a pathological offspring of my imagination in this; but I have an almost overwhelming amount of proof of its correctness.

Daniel Schreber[1]

It remains for the future to decide whether there is more delusion in my theory than I should like to admit, or whether there is more truth in Schreber's delusion than other people are yet prepared to believe.

Sigmund Freud[2]

In the first chapter of this book I described how Emil Kraepelin's early career was influenced by an unsatisfactory encounter with Professor Paul Flechsig, a respected psychiatrist who worked at the University of Leipzig. Flechsig belonged to a generation of doctors who devoted more of their time to anatomical studies than to developing their clinical acumen. After they fell out, Kraepelin sought a new mentor, and thereby came under the influence of Wilhelm Wundt. The rest, as they say, is history.

Flechsig's contribution to the evolution of his discipline was not entirely negative. More at home with a microscope than with fellow human beings, he carried out important research on the localization of brain functions, helping to define the projection and association areas in the cerebral cortex.[3] However, he is rarely remembered for these efforts, or for his argument with Kraepelin. Instead he is most often remembered for his role in one of the most curious cases in the history of his calling.

Judge Daniel Paul Schreber experienced his first nervous breakdown in 1884, after failing to gain election to the Reichstag. He was 42 at the time. Very little is known about this episode, but he was treated by Flechsig and, after six months, recovered enough to resume a normal life. Eight years later he suffered a second breakdown, which was more enduring. He had just been appointed President of the Supreme Court of Saxony. One night he found himself wondering what it would be like to be a woman experiencing sexual intercourse. Several days later, he developed the first of an expanding set of delusional ideas. His subsequent psychosis lasted nine years, during which time he wrote his *Memoirs of my Nervous Illness*,[4] a book that was to make him one of the most frequently discussed patients in medical history.[5] The ideas that Schreber described in his autobiography defy easy summary, but began with hypochondriacal delusions, for example that his brain was softening, that he was decomposing and suffering from plague. These beliefs rapidly progressed to the conviction that Flechsig was transforming him into a woman in order to sexually abuse him. Later they evolved into a complex theological system, in which 'rays' from God, attracted by the highly excited nerves in Schreber's mind, would, he believed bring about a series of 'miracles' that would eventually feminize his body and induce a state of 'voluptuousness'. This process, he believed, would culminate in a state of heavenly bliss whereupon he would be reconciled with the Almighty. Examples of these imaginary events included the 'miracles of heat and cold' during which Schreber believed that blood was being forced to different parts of his body, and 'the head-compressing machine' into which Schreber believed his head was being forced by 'little devils'.

Memoirs of my Nervous Illness attracted the attention of the father of psychoanalysis, who wrote a speculative analysis of Schreber's delusions, thus cementing the judge's reputation with future generations of researchers. Undeterred by the fact that he had never met Schreber, his dissection of the case is vintage Freud.[6] Reading it today, it is impossible not to be impressed by the skill with which he marshalled various strands of evidence, until they pointed towards a conclusion that, in the cold light of day, seems quite implausible. In brief, Freud maintained that Schreber harboured homosexual feelings for his father, a well-known physician, which he had displaced on to his psychiatrist, Flechsig. According to Freud, in a further series of defensive manoeuvres, Schreber's love for his psychiatrist was then transformed into Flechsig's imagined hatred of Schreber, which eventually generalized into God's bizarre manipulations of Schreber's body. In this way, the judge was said to have avoided awareness of impulses that otherwise would be disturbing to his conscious mind.

Later writers who were inspired by psychoanalysis agreed with Freud that paranoid delusions have a defensive function, but took a less exotic view of the underlying emotions that were being defended against. Bleuler, for example, regarded all delusions as attempts to attribute unacceptable ideas to external agencies but disputed that these were necessarily homoerotic.[7] Over half a century later, Kenneth Colby, an American psychoanalyst who became a pioneer in the apparently unrelated field of artificial intelligence, created a computer simulation of paranoid thinking, which assumed that paranoid individuals are highly sensitive to threats to their self-esteem, but protect themselves from feelings of inadequacy by blaming disappointments on other people.[8]

Although Schreber's beliefs would not be completely out of place on a modern psychiatric ward, the delusions of today's patients are usually less complex, and therefore more easily summarized. Sometimes they straddle the fine line between tragedy and comedy as in the case of a young man called Ian, who suffered a breakdown shortly after leaving school and obtaining his first job. His most troubling symptom was a series of extraordinary beliefs about his abilities and achievements, on which he acted to the consternation of his long-suffering parents. Maintaining that he was a millionaire, he regularly telephoned a local bank to inquire about his savings, and struck up quite a good relationship with a sympathetic bank clerk. (At considerable cost to her employer, she would spend long periods on the telephone, reassuring him that his imaginary millions had not been stolen.) At other times he would ring military bases and inform them that he was a general who was about to carry out an inspection. One day, plausibly dressed in a well-cut suit, he left his ward and strayed on to another, where he announced that he was a new consultant psychiatrist. Searching for a job to match his perceived status, he awarded himself a knighthood and applied for the position of chief executive of a hospital in Wales. His requests for further information about suitable positions often culminated in the delivery of bulky envelopes addressed to 'Sir Ian . . .'.

Ian's delusions resisted his family's best efforts to challenge them. Neither logical argument, nor their increasingly exasperated efforts to point out the gap between his boasts and reality, seemed to bring about any change in his behaviour. This kind of incorrigibility has been considered a hallmark of delusions since clinicians first began to study them. It receives its most severe challenge when patients with incompatible delusions meet each other.

One such encounter was described by the French philosopher Voltaire who, in 1763, observed the meeting between two inhabitants of a madhouse, one believing that he was 'incorporated with Jesus Christ', the other believing that he was 'the eternal father'. The second of the patients was sufficiently shocked by the experience to recover his sanity temporarily. However, a less positive outcome was achieved in the only modern experiment of this sort, published in 1964 by Milton Rokeach. A social psychologist based at the University of Michigan, Rokeach was interested in the causes of dogmatism, and decided that the nearby state psychiatric hospital at Ypsilanti provided a wonderful opportunity to study rigidly held beliefs. Discovering that three of the patients at the hospital believed that they were Christ, he arranged for them to live together on a ward. Confronted by others who also claimed to be Jesus, two clung to their delusional identities. The third accepted the claims of his companions, but began to entertain a series of new beliefs that were just as bizarre, at one point claiming that he was a psychiatrist who was married to God. All three expressed sympathy towards the other two, apparently convinced that they were mad.[9]

Apparently not Beyond Belief

Although delusions vary, they tend to encompass a small number of themes. The most common type is persecutory or paranoid,* in which the individual feels himself the victim of some kind of malevolent plot.

* The terms 'paranoia' and 'paranoid' have a confusing history. They were first used by the Ancient Greeks to mean crazy or mad but were reintroduced to

In a study of patients who had recently been admitted to hospital in Denmark, it was found that 42 per cent of those with delusions had beliefs of this sort.[10] The imaginary persecutors are sometimes people known to the patient, but more often are institutions such as government bodies or criminal gangs, or ethnic, religious or ideological groups such as Catholics, communists or Jews. A patient I once saw had become psychotic after travelling to Australia, and had been deported back to Britain and hospitalized. He believed that he was the object of a conspiracy conducted by the British Home Office and the Australian secret service. It was, of course, part of the conspiracy that his psychiatrists should diagnose him as suffering from schizophrenia. As I attempted to interview him one day, he leaned forward and, whispering, asked me to admit that I knew about the plot, assuring me that no one would be able to overhear our conversation.

British psychologists Peter Trower and Paul Chadwick have argued that it is important to distinguish between those individuals who believe that their persecution is unwarranted (said to be suffering from 'poor me' paranoia) and those individuals who believe that persecution or anticipated persecution is richly deserved on account of some terrible sin they have committed (said to be suffering from 'bad me' paranoia).[11] Whether this distinction will prove to be useful remains to be seen; in Kraepelin's own classification, delusions of sin were listed separately from persecutory delusions, and it may be better to think of 'bad me' paranoia as belonging to a general category of depressive delusions in which the individual is tormented by extremely

---

describe a type of delusional disorder in the first half of the nineteenth century. As we have already seen, this usage was embraced by Kraepelin. During the post-Second World War era, when, under Adolf Meyer's influence, psychiatric diagnoses became unfashionable among US psychiatrists, the term 'paranoid' was often used to describe persecutory beliefs that were not necessarily delusional; hence the ordinary-language definition given in the *Shorter Oxford English Dictionary* (1993): 'A tendency to suspect or distrust others or to believe oneself unfairly used'. DSM-III used the term *paranoia* to refer to a pure delusional psychosis (Kraepelin's concept) but the term *delusional disorder* was used in its place in DSM-III-R and DSM-IV. However, *paranoid personality disorder* remains in DSM-IV as an axis-2 disorder, and is defined in a way that closely matches the ordinary-language definition given in the *SOED*. For the purposes of the present discussion, I will use the term 'paranoid delusion' to describe any delusional system in which themes of persecution are prominent.

negative self-evaluations. Certainly, delusions of guilt or badness are common in patients diagnosed as suffering from psychotic depression, who often believe that others share the negative opinions they hold about themselves.[12]

Grandiose delusions, such as those expressed by Ian and the three Christs, embrace four main themes: beliefs that the individual has special powers, is wealthy, has some kind of special mission, or has some type of special identity.[13] Often they occur with persecutory delusions. Another of my patients, who lived in very poor circumstances, asserted that he was the illegitimate heir to a fortune (special identity), had invented the helicopter and the pop-up toaster (special powers), and that the huge royalties from these achievements (wealth) had been stolen by the staff at the hospital he was reluctantly attending (persecution). My attempts to offer him help were confounded by his demands that I call in the police so that these crimes could be investigated.

Delusions of reference, in which innocuous events are held to have some special significance for the patient, are commonly observed but have been much less studied by psychologists and psychiatrists.[14] (Peter Chadwick, a psychologist who has suffered from a psychotic illness, has written a moving account of a delusional episode, which began when a radio programme he was listening to seemed to be directed at him.)[15]

Somatic or hypochondriacal delusions, in which the patient entertains bizarre beliefs about his body, are probably under-recorded, either because they are eclipsed by other symptoms, or because they are assumed to be complaints about side effects of medication. In a survey of 550 psychotic patients, psychiatrists Ian McGilchrist and John Cutting recorded this kind of belief in 55 per cent of those questioned, which would make them even more common than persecutory delusions. McGilchrist and Cutting have argued that somatic delusions can be subdivided into two main categories: elaborated beliefs about the body that have apparently been inferred from sensations, and beliefs that seem to involve the misinterpretation of sensory experiences.[16] Schreber's belief that he was changing sex presumably belongs to the first class, of 'cognitive' somatic delusions, whereas patients' assertions that they are burning, being sexually interfered with, or are blocked and filling with fluid would belong to the second, 'perceptual' category.

Much less common delusional themes include delusional parasitosis (in which the patient believes that he is infested by insects crawling under his skin),[17] dismorphobia (the belief that the individual is disfigured or ugly despite being completely normal in appearance), erotomania (in which the patient believes that she is secretly loved by someone who is in fact indifferent, usually a person who is famous or holds a position of authority)[18] and delusional jealousy (in which a loved one is irrationally believed to be unfaithful).[19] Some authors have cited this last type of delusion as evidence that a belief does not have to be false in order to qualify as delusional: partners often get so fed up with the restrictions placed upon them by their irrationally jealous spouses that they eventually run off with somebody else.[20]

A few rare but more colourful delusional systems have received more attention from researchers, some of whom have been rewarded by having obscure disorders named after them. An example is the Cotard syndrome, first described by the French psychiatrist Jules Cotard in 1882, following an encounter with a 43-year-old female patient who believed that she had 'no brains, chests or entrails and was just skin and bone', that 'neither God nor the Devil existed' and that she was 'eternal and would live forever' and therefore did not need to eat.[21] After Cotard's death, it was widely believed that he had identified a peculiar form of depression in which nihilistic delusions are the prominent symptom. However, a recent survey of 100 cases of Cotard syndrome reported in the literature found that there was considerable variation in the symptoms recorded, and that many of the patients met the criteria for conventional diagnoses such as depression, bipolar disorder and schizophrenia.[22]

Another unusual disorder is the Capgras syndrome, named after another French doctor, Joseph Capgras, who first described the delusion that a loved one had been replaced by an impostor, robot or *doppelgänger*.[23] This last type of belief belongs to a small family of delusional ideas in which misidentifications are the central theme. Other members of the family include the Frégoli delusion (named after a famous Italian impersonator of the 1920s), in which the individual believes that persecutors have disguised themselves as familiar people,[24] and the delusion of inanimate doubles,[25] in which emotionally significant personal items are believed to have been maliciously replaced by poor copies.

The reader will recall that Karl Jaspers held all truly delusional beliefs to be ununderstandable, by which he meant that they are meaningless and unconnected to the individual's personality or experience. I have already criticized this account for being far too subjective – the understandability of delusions seems to depend, to some extent, on the effort made to understand them. Indeed, when such efforts are made, it is apparent that the most common delusional themes observed in clinical practice, including most of those that I have just described, reflect patients' concerns about their position in the social universe. This much was recognized by Kurt Schneider, who argued that in all cases of delusion, 'Abnormal significance tends mostly towards self-reference and is almost always of a special kind: it is momentous, urgent, somehow filled with personal significance . . .'[26] This intuition has been supported by research conducted by Philippa Garety and her colleagues at the Institute of Psychiatry in London. They used a simple five-way classification to record the delusional beliefs of 55 patients. Consistent with the research in Denmark I mentioned earlier (p. 297), the most common type of delusion observed was persecutory (35 per cent) followed by abnormal negative beliefs about the self (32 per cent), and abnormal positive beliefs about the self (26 per cent). Less common were negative delusions about the world (only three patients) and positive delusions about the world (only one patient).[27]

Interestingly, this finding seems to have some cross-cultural validity. In a comparison of the delusions of psychiatric inpatients from Europe, the Caribbean, India, Africa, the Middle East and the Far East, persecutory delusions were the most common in all but one region, the exception being the Far East, where sexual delusions were more often reported.[28] Nevertheless, cultural, religious and socio-economic factors obviously influence the precise nature of the threat perceived by paranoid patients. For example, middle- and upper-class Egyptian patients typically report persecutory delusions that have scientific or secular themes, whereas the delusions of poorer patients often involve religious institutions.[29] Paranoid delusions in Korean patients tend to reflect fears of rape, whereas fears of vampires and poisoning are more common in Chinese patients.[30] There is also evidence that the content of delusions has changed over time. In the United States during the 1930s (a period of material deprivation and personal powerlessness), delusions of wealth and special powers were common, whereas delusions about threats of violence have been more common in recent decades.[31]

Defining delusions

Most modern definitions of delusions emphasize characteristics other than ununderstandability, but none distinguishes between delusional and ordinary beliefs in a manner that is entirely satisfactory. In DSM-IV a delusion is defined as:

A false personal belief based on incorrect inference about external reality and firmly sustained in spite of what almost everyone else believes and in spite of what usually constitutes incontrovertible and obvious proof or evidence to the contrary.[32]

As some sceptics have pointed out, this definition begs questions about what we mean by 'incorrect inference', 'external reality' and 'incontrovertible and obvious proof'.[33] Perhaps conscious of this limitation, the authors of DSM-IV go on to add, '[It] is not ordinarily accepted by other members of the person's culture or subculture', thereby opening up the possibility that a belief regarded as delusional in one culture might be considered perfectly rational in another.

Of course, much of the difficulty in defining delusions can be resolved if we accept that they exist on a continuum with ordinary beliefs and attitudes. In Chapter 5, we have already considered evidence that seems to support this idea. I think most readers will be able to think of acquaintances whose thoughts seem drawn to the same concerns that preoccupy psychiatric patients (the academic who suspects that rivals are stealing her ideas, the New Age enthusiast who sees special significance in coincidences, the unhappy young man who believes that a beautiful but indifferent woman will eventually admit to loving him).

Detailed studies have shown that delusional beliefs, like ordinary beliefs and attitudes, vary across a number of dimensions, such as their bizarreness, the conviction with which they are held, the extent to which the patient is preoccupied by them, and the extent to which they cause distress.[34] It is true, as psychologist Martin Harrow and his colleagues in Chicago have documented in carefully conducted long-term investigations, that delusions sometimes persist apparently unchanged for many years.[35] However, as Milton Rokeach recognized when conducting his 'three Christs' experiment at Ypsilanti Hospital, the same might be said of any beliefs that are important to an individual's identity, such as, for example, political and religious convictions. In fact, over short periods of time, the conviction with which delusions are held may fluctuate, so that beliefs that are held to be absolutely true on one day may be described as only possibly true on the next.[36]

Unfortunately, clinicians and researchers schooled in the biomedical approach to psychiatry have often assumed that delusions and ordinary beliefs are completely different. As recently as 1991, for example, the Cambridge psychiatrist German Berrios asserted that delusions are not beliefs at all, but 'empty speech acts, whose informational content refers to neither world nor self'.[37] Consequently, throughout most of the twentieth century, delusions were generally ignored by experimental psychologists.

My own work on this topic began a few years after I had qualified as a clinical psychologist, by which time I had published several studies of auditory hallucinations, and was keen to see whether my general approach could be brought to bear on other symptoms. Delusions seemed an obvious candidate, and I was amazed to discover the extent to which researchers had neglected them. Fortunately, I had just moved from a National Health Service post to a junior lectureship at the University of Liverpool, which ran a small fund for junior staff who wished to embark on new lines of research. My application was written in a couple of hours, without much optimism, was brief and could be summarized in two sentences: 'No one has done much research on delusions. Give me some money and I'll do some.' To my amazement, they did.

The funds provided to me by the University allowed me to employ a research assistant for six months. Sue Kaney, a recent graduate, was recruited and proved to have a knack for persuading suitable patients to co-operate. The initial studies that we completed together led to further experiments, which have kept me busy ever since. As psychologists in other universities had also spotted the dearth of research on delusions, by the late 1990s there had emerged a small cottage industry of investigators struggling to explain why psychotic patients hold unusual beliefs.

The Psychotic as Scientist

> Faced with the choice between changing one's mind and proving that there is no need to do so, almost everyone gets busy on the proof.
>
> John Kenneth Galbraith[38]

Most people probably regard delusional and scientific thinking as completely incompatible phenomena. After all, it is easy for scientific researchers to assume that there is something unique or special about the systematic way in which we approach our task. According to this orthodox view, the scientific approach involves the careful and dispassionate collection and evaluation of evidence, commonsense reasoning is open to all sorts of self-interested biases, fuzzy thinking and naked prejudices, and delusional reasoning exemplifies these biases in excess. Of course, it is not that simple. The inhabitants of this planet cannot easily be divided into different species on the basis of their scientific skills, any more than they can be easily divided into the mad and sane.

On the one hand, studies of what scientists actually do (as opposed to what undergraduate textbooks say that they do) have shown that research is far from an emotionless activity. In pursuit of the recognition of their peers, famous scientists have deviated from prescribed methods so frequently that some historians have suggested that the history of science should be X-rated.[39] At the same time, sociologists have observed that the language employed by modern scientists, when talking freely about their work, often reveals intense rivalries between different research groups, and portrays the scientific process as an epic struggle in which heroes and villains battle for high ground.[40] At moments when the scientific ego is especially threatened, the dividing line between the practice of science and paranoid thinking becomes almost undetectable. On opening the letter from a journal that tells us that the editor has on this occasion declined to accept our manuscript for publication, we scan the accompanying anonymous referees' reports to see if we can work out who to blame. ('It must be John Doe! He's always been envious of my work!')

On the other hand, ordinary people sometimes approach problems in their lives in ways that are no less systematic than the strategies of trained researchers, as highlighted in the following quotation from the clinical psychologist George Kelly:

One of my tasks in the 1930s was to direct graduate studies leading to the Masters Degree. A typical afternoon might find me talking to a graduate student at one o'clock, doing all those familiar things that thesis directors have to do – encouraging the student to pin-point the issues, to observe, to become intimate with the problem, to form hypotheses either inductively or deductively, to make some preliminary test runs, to control his experiments so he will know what led to what, to generalize cautiously and to revise his thinking in the light of experience.

At two o'clock I might have an interview with a client. During this interview, I would not be taking the role of the scientist but rather helping the distressed person to sort out some solutions to his life's problems. So what would I do? Why, I would try to get him to pin-point the issues, to observe, to become intimate with the problem, to form hypotheses, to make test runs, to relate outcomes to anticipations, to control his ventures so that he knows what led to what, to generalize cautiously and to revise his dogma in the light of experience.[41]

When exploring these parallels, a good starting point would be a simple framework for understanding how beliefs and attitudes are formed. Figure 12.1 shows a simple 'heuristic' model I devised in order to guide my own research when I obtained my small priming grant.[42] (I literally drew it up on the back of an envelope one day.) According to this model, beliefs about the world are not plucked out of the blue but are based on events (data). The events have to be perceived and attended to (those which we fail to notice cannot influence our thinking). Once we have noticed them, we can make inferences about their importance and meaning and this leads to beliefs about the world. Finally we may seek further information to either support or refute our beliefs, and so the cycle is repeated.

(The philosopher of science Sir Karl Popper argued that data that refute a hypothesis are nearly always more informative than data that appear to support it.[43] This is because negative evidence can be decisive whereas positive evidence may support several alternative hypotheses. Popper therefore suggested that scientists should vigorously seek evidence that disconfirms their pet theories in the hope that there will be no such evidence. Ordinary people, however, usually seek

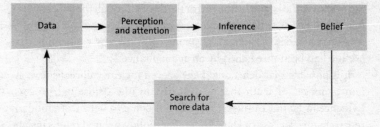

Figure 12.1 A simple heuristic model of the processes involved in acquiring and maintaining a belief (from R. P. Bentall (ed.) (1990) *Reconstructing Schizophrenia*. London: Routledge, pp. 23–60).

evidence that favours their ideas, a phenomenon known to psychologists as the *confirmation bias*.[44] Interestingly, some studies have shown this bias in professional scientists, although whether it has an adverse affect on their work remains a matter of debate.)[45]

It is probably worth noting that the model shown in Figure 12.1, although superficially different from the model of depression I developed in Chapter 10, is really quite similar to it (after all, an attribution could be described as a type of inference). Of course, it is *not* a model of delusions *per se*. It is a very crude account of the way in which beliefs and attitudes are acquired by scientists, ordinary people and psychiatric patients. However, by considering each part of this account in turn, we can begin to explore how different factors may lead an individual to develop beliefs that appear strange or unusual to other people.

The Nugget of Truth in Paranoia

When accused by Henry Kissinger of being paranoid about the Arabs, Golda Meir, the Israeli prime minister, retorted that 'Even paranoids have enemies.'[46] Of course, if patients' accounts of their lives were completely realistic, it would be wrong to regard them as delusional at all. In fact, it seems that clinicians sometimes do mistake patients' well-founded but unusual fears for delusions. A group of psychiatrists working on Long Island, USA, reported their attempts to help a distressed woman who had been brought into their clinic by friends. The woman said that 'something horrible' would happen to her if she did not leave the Island by the end of the day. Although the psychiatrists diagnosed her as suffering from a psychotic illness, she was later able to record a series of unpleasant phone calls, thereby confirming that her life had been threatened by an acquaintance.[47]

It is possible that delusional beliefs, even if clearly unrealistic, contain a nugget of truth that is distorted by the delusional process. Evidence in favour of this hypothesis has come to light from modern research into the case of Daniel Schreber. Following up Freud's insight that Schreber's delusions had something to do with his father, American psychoanalyst William Niederland investigated the judge's family.[48] Schreber's father, it transpired, was a well-known physician and educationalist who had unusual views about childrearing, which he proselytized in books that were widely read in his day. Believing that children should learn to hold rigid postures when sitting, walking or even sleeping, he invented a series of braces to force them to adopt the desired positions. For example, one brace was designed to make children sit upright while eating. Bolted to the table in front of the child, it consisted of an iron bar that extended up to the child's face, which it gripped by means of a leather strap under the chin.

Although subsequent research by the historian Zvi Lothane[49] has suggested a more positive view of the Schreber family than that painted by Niederland, it seems likely that the younger Schreber spent much of his childhood restrained by his father's devices. Moreover, the contents of the bizarre ideas he developed later in his life seem to reflect these experiences. For example, a delusion about a 'chest compression miracle' seemed to relate to his father's practice of securing the child to his bed by means of a specially designed strap. Similarly, the miracle of the 'head compressing machine' seems much more understandable when we known that Schreber's father invented a *kopfhalter* (head-holder, consisting of a strap, with one end clamped to the child's hair and the other to his underwear, so his hair was pulled if he did not hold his head straight) and a chin band (a helmet-like device designed to ensure proper growth of the jaw and teeth, see Figure 12.2).

Of course, it is difficult to gauge the extent to which real experiences colour most delusions, because it is hard to verify deluded patients' accounts of their lives. In an attempt to circumvent this problem, University of Illinois sociologists John Mirowsky and Catherine Ross studied persecutory beliefs (which they assessed by a brief interview)

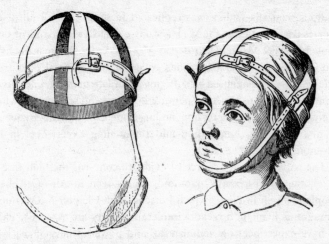

Figure 12.2 Schreber's chin band (reprinted from M. Schatzman (1973), *Soul Murder: Persecution in the Family*. London: Penguin Books).

in a survey of 500 randomly selected residents of El Paso, Texas, and Juarez in Mexico. As sociologists, Mirowsky and Ross were interested in objective circumstances that would encourage feelings of external control and mistrust, which, they believed, would lead to paranoid thinking. Such circumstances might include experiences of victimization and powerlessness which, previous research had shown, are very common in people of low socio-economic status who lack educational opportunities. Mirowsky and Ross were able to show that, in their sample, persecutory beliefs, beliefs about external control, and mistrust were connected to socio-economic status and educational attainment in roughly the manner they had expected.[50]

Although the sceptical reader might be forgiven for wondering whether Mirowsky and Ross's findings can be generalized to psychiatric patients, two further lines of evidence support this possibility. The first concerns the role of stressful experiences in psychosis. British sociologist Tirril Harris studied patients living in the community and found a high rate of events that she described as 'intrusive' in the weeks preceding psychotic and especially paranoid relapses.[51] These kinds of events, by Harris's definition, involve someone – not a close relative – imposing demands on the patient. Examples include threats from landlords, police inquiries, burglaries and unwanted sexual propositions. Harris's finding was replicated in some but not all of the centres participating in the WHO study of the Determinants of Outcome of Severe Mental Disorders.[52] More recently, Thomas Fuchs of the University of Heidelberg has collected biographical data from elderly patients diagnosed as suffering from *late paraphrenia* (a term sometimes used to describe paranoid-like psychotic illnesses which begin late in life) and depression, finding evidence of a higher frequency of discriminating, humiliating and threatening experiences in the paranoid group.[53]

The second relevant source of evidence concerns the high rate of psychotic, and especially paranoid, illness seen in Afro-Caribbean people living in Britain,[54] which I discussed in Chapter 6. Of course, immigrants living in a racially intolerant society are especially likely to have experiences of victimization and powerlessness of the kind described by Mirowsky and Ross. The evidence that this kind of stress is really responsible for the high rates of psychosis observed in British Afro-Caribbeans will be discussed in detail in a later chapter. For the moment, we can merely note that the elevated risk of psychosis experienced by this particular group can certainly be interpreted as consistent with the 'nugget of truth' hypothesis.

My own clinical experience is that delusional ideas rarely lack a nugget of truth. No matter how bizarre the ideas expressed by patients, it is usually possible to identify events in their lives that have contributed to their content. Of course, this observation does not imply that delusions are rational. (Very few people really are victims of government plots.) The nugget of truth is usually distorted in some way, and the challenge to psychologists is to discover how this happens.

Seeing is Believing

The next part of our back-of-an-envelope model concerns perceptual and attentional processes. The idea that delusions might be the product of rational attempts to make sense of anomalous perceptions was considered by Kraepelin, but later elaborated in detail by Harvard psychologist Brendan Maher. Maher's theory consists of two separable hypotheses. The first, which we will consider here, is that delusions are always a reaction to some kind of unusual perception. The second, which we will consider later, is that delusions are *never* the product of abnormal reasoning. Clearly the second hypothesis does not follow inevitably from the first, although Maher sometimes seems to suggest that it does.[55]

Maher has pointed to case study evidence that appears to support the first part of his theory.[56] For example, he has interpreted Schreber's delusions as attempts to explain unusual bodily sensations. (It seems likely that many somatic delusions develop in this way.) In clinical practice, it is not unusual to encounter patients whose delusions seem to be interpretations of other types of peculiar experiences. An unpleasant auditory hallucination, for instance, may be attributed to a malevolent spirit or to the Devil.

Most of the research on Maher's theory has focused on the effects of perceptual deficits. Following clinical observations of an apparent association between the slow onset of deafness in later life and paranoia, for example, it was suggested that elderly patients' failure to recognize that they have hearing difficulties might cause them to be mistrustful and suspicious of others (if you notice that your friends have begun to speak in whispers in your presence you might incorrectly infer that they are talking about you).[57] In an attempt to test this hypothesis, psychologist Philip Zimbardo and his colleagues at Stanford University in California used hypnosis to induce a temporary state of deafness in hypnotically susceptible students, allowing some to remain aware that they had been hypnotized. Those who were unaware of the source of their deafness, but not those who knew that they had been hypnotized, showed an increase in paranoid ideas, as indicated by their responses on various questionnaires, and their attitudes towards others who were present during the experiment.[58] Unfortunately, these findings are difficult to interpret because it is not clear how well hypnotic deafness simulates real hearing loss. Moreover, recent, more carefully conducted studies have failed to show the correlation between deafness and paranoid symptoms reported by earlier researchers.[59]

Clearer evidence in favour of the anomalous perception model exists for the Capgras delusion. The case of Madame M, described by Joseph Capgras and J. Reboul-Lachaux (and recently translated into English), is worth considering in some detail because it illustrates the complexity of the condition.[60] Mme M's illness began with the conviction that she was a member of the French aristocracy and had been dispossessed of her inheritance, having been replaced by an impostor. This grandiose delusion was transformed into a series of delusional misidentifications after the death of her twin sons and the deterioration of her marriage. Looking into the grave as a small coffin descended into the earth, she believed that she was witnessing the burial of a young boy who was not her own. Later, she came to believe that an impostor had been substituted for her husband and, furthermore, that the impostor had been replaced by further impostors on no less than eighty occasions. During the First World War, Mme M believed that tunnels beneath Paris contained thousands of people who had been abducted and replaced by substitutes, and that the aircraft that flew overhead were attempting to drive people below so that they would suffer a similar fate. It is not difficult to see why Capgras offered a psychoanalytical account of Mme M's illness. Many later psychologists and psychiatrists have similarly assumed that the delusion results from some kind of ambivalence towards the person who is believed to have been replaced.[61]

Haydn Ellis, a neuropsychologist at the University of Wales in Cardiff, has recently pointed to several reasons for doubting the psychodynamic account of the Capgras delusion.[62] The theory implies that the delusion should exclusively concern individuals who have a close relationship with the patient, whereas this is not invariably the case. Also, Capgras patients usually express no fears about the genuineness of voices heard over the telephone, suggesting that some difficulty in processing *visual* information is a crucial element of the disorder. Most importantly of all, about one third of Capgras patients are known to have suffered from some kind of brain damage that predates the appearance of their delusion.

With Andy Young, a psychologist at the University of York, Ellis has argued that the Capgras syndrome is caused by damage to brain systems responsible for recognizing faces.[63] When we encounter someone who is familiar to us, we normally experience a brief emotional response. This reaction, which is experienced as the feeling of familiarity, has considerable survival value, as it tells us whether we are meeting a friend or a foe. Not surprisingly, in most people it occurs automatically and very efficiently. (We may recognize a person as familiar after meeting him or her just once, many years ago.) In comparison, the skill of recalling specific information about a person, for example their name and occupation, is much less reliable. For this reason, most of us have had the embarrassing experience of meeting people who seem familiar to us without our being able to remember precisely who they are.

These two types of recognition seem to involve different pathways in the brain.[64] A pathway through the visual cortex to the limbic system is involved in the specific identification of individuals. A second pathway, which passes through the inferior parietal lobe, appears to be responsible for the feeling of familiarity. Capgras patients show subtle deficits when they are tested for their ability to recognize faces, indicating that they do not always gain a sense of familiarity on encountering people they know well, so that the second pathway is disrupted. The delusion seems to be an attempt to explain this experience.

Ellis and Young predicted that Capgras patients would show no emotional response when meeting people well known to them. Normally, when we greet someone familiar, our emotional reaction (however slight) results in a slight increase in sweat, leading to a transient change in the electrical conductivity of our skin (the electrodermal response) which can easily be detected from electrodes placed on the back of the hand. Ellis, Young and their colleagues tested five Capgras patients and found this response to be absent, just as they had predicted.[65]

It is not clear whether an anomalous face recognition experience on its own is enough to create a Capgras delusion. Some brain-damaged patients who suffer from impairment in their ability to recognize faces retain insight into their difficulties, know that they have a perceptual problem, and do not develop bizarre explanations of their experiences. On the other hand, as Andy Young points out, patients like Mme M very often entertain grandiose or paranoid ideas, indicating that some kind psychological disturbance may also be required for a full-blown Capgras delusion to develop.[66]

The evidence we have considered so far concerns the impact of perceptual *deficits* on delusional thinking. An interesting but nearly overlooked possibility is that delusions might arise as a consequence of perceptual skills that are *over-developed*. This possibility was tested in a strange experiment reported in 1978 by Canadian psychologist Lucrezia LaRusso. LaRusso persuaded a group of normal volunteers to allow her to film their facial expressions as she gave them brief electric shocks. She also filmed them as they pretended to receive the shocks. Showing the films to paranoid patients and to a second group of normal volunteers, she found that the paranoid patients were better able to tell the differences between the genuine emotional responses and the pretend responses.[67]

Similar findings have recently been reported by Penelope Davis and Melissa Gibson of Griffith University in Australia, who studied schizophrenia patients' ability to recognize genuine and posed facial expressions. While most of their patients were poor at recognizing posed expressions, their paranoid patients were better at recognizing genuine expressions of surprise and negative emotion than ordinary people.[68] These observations raise the intriguing possibility that over-sensitivity to other people's disingenuous communications might provoke paranoid thinking.

It is difficult to determine the extent to which the anomalous perception theory applies to delusions in general. One complication is that what counts as an *anomalous* experience may vary from person to person. Three American psychologists, William Johnson, James Ross and Marie Mastria of the University of Mississippi Medical Center, reported an extraordinary case study that illustrates this problem. Their patient complained that he was being sexually molested at night by 'warm forms'. A detailed history revealed that, from the age of 12, he had had numerous sexual partners and had never learned to masturbate. The warm forms appeared during a long period of sexual abstinence, occasioned by his contracting of a venereal disease. During this period, he experienced spontaneous episodes of sexual arousal at night-time, which seemed anomalous to him, but which would have seemed quite normal to anyone with a less colourful history. Because, previously, sexual arousal had always occurred in the presence of a partner, the patient had concluded that an invisible sexual partner (a warm form) was responsible for these experiences. The treatment, which was brief and successful, is left to the imagination of the reader.[69]

There have been few systematic attempts to address the extent to which delusions are products of anomalous experiences. In one study, Loren and Jean Chapman of the University of Wisconsin carefully interviewed students who scored very high on their questionnaire measures of schizotypy. They found that some expressed delusional ideas but reported no anomalous experiences, and that others reported anomalous experiences in the absence of delusional ideas. In only a few cases did there appear to be an obvious causal connection between anomalous experiences and unusual beliefs and, even in these, the steps leading from the anomalous experience to the delusion were often judged not to be 'reasonable'.[70] In a more recent three-year prospective study of eighty children who heard voices, Sondra Escher, Marius Romme and their colleagues found that only 9 per cent developed delusions during the follow-up period.[71]

On this evidence, at least, Maher's theory probably holds for only a minority of patients.

The role of attention

Despite the limited evidence for Maher's theory, it is possible that perceptual and especially attentional processes play a role in *maintaining* delusional ideas, once they have been formed. Our brains constantly scan the environment for information that is relevant to us and ignore information that is not. In the late 1960s, two American psychologists, Leonard Ullmann and Leonard Krasner, suggested that this process would lead deluded patients to notice selectively evidence that supported their beliefs.[72]

Sue Kaney and I used the emotional Stroop technique to investigate this hypothesis. (Recall that, in this type of test, described in detail in the last chapter (pp. 281–2), participants are required to look at words written in different ink colours and name the colours while ignoring the words. The difficulty they have in doing this indicates the extent to which they are selectively attending to the words.) We used four types of stimuli: paranoia-related words (for example, 'deceit', 'follow'), depression-related words (for example, 'defeat', 'failure'), neutral words (for example, 'bud', 'recipe') and meaningless strings of letters. The words and letter-strings were in five different ink colours and were printed on cards, five words to a line, in random order. As we had expected, paranoid patients took much longer to colour-name the paranoia-related words than the neutral words, indicating that the meaning of the words was grabbing their attention and interfering with their ability to name the ink colours. This effect was not found for a group of ordinary people or for a control group of depressed patients.[73] Perhaps this finding should be regarded as unremarkable. As we have already seen, people will show a Stroop effect for words relating to any topic that causes them concern.[74] Deluded patients are no exception to this rule.

In an interesting variant of this experiment, Kate Leafhead, Andy Young and Krystyna Szulecka studied a woman who was suffering from the Cotard delusion (she believed that she was dead). Their patient also suffered from a Capgras delusion that her brother and mother were impostors. She was tested on three occasions using words relating to death (for example, 'coffin', 'dead'), depression-related words, words relating to duplicates (for example, 'copy', 'double'), paranoia-related words, anxiety-related words and emotionally neutral words (see Figure 12.3). When very ill, on the first occasion that she was tested, the woman was slow to colour-name both the death-related and the duplicate-related words. On a second occasion, when she was beginning to improve, only the duplicate-related words caused her difficulty. By the third test, when she was nearly recovered, colour-naming was not impaired for any of the words.[75]

If people attend excessively to information relating to their delusions they should also recall this kind of information particularly easily. In several studies, Sue Kaney and I found that this was indeed the case. For example, after listening to a series of stories describing threatening and non-threatening social interactions, paranoid patients specifically recalled the threatening elements from the stories, but tended not to remember emotionally neutral elements.[76]

Interestingly, deluded patients do not seem to spend excessive time looking at stimuli relating to their delusions. Recently, Mary Phillips and Tony David at the Institute of Psychiatry in London studied the eye movements of patients as they looked at various pictures, some of which showed people making threatening gestures. Using sophisticated equipment to track the direction of gaze, they measured the amount of time spent visually scanning different parts of the pictures. Patients with paranoid delusions, compared with patients with other symptoms, spent *less* time looking at the threatening parts. Quick to identify stimuli in their environment that could be threatening, it seems they move rapidly to checking whether threats can be found elsewhere.[77]

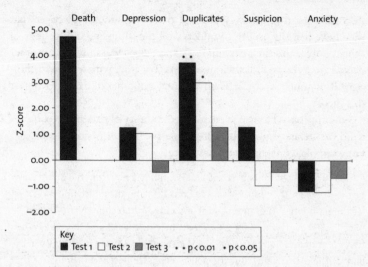

Figure 12.3 Extent to which a patient suffering both a Cotard delusion and a Capgras delusion had difficulty colour-naming death-related words, depression-related words, duplicate-related words, paranoia-related words and anxiety-related words when tested while ill (Test 1) and during recovery (Tests 2 and 3). Scores indicate the extent to which colour-naming for these words is slowed in comparison with colour-naming neutral words. From Leafhead, Young and Szulecka (1996).

What Happens in the Inference Box?

The third component of the back-of-an-envelope model concerns the process of drawing inferences from observations. Two lines of research have focused on this process in deluded patients. One was initiated by British psychologist Chris Frith,[78] and the other (which we will come to shortly) was started by myself.

Inferences about other minds

Frith has argued that a deficit in theory of mind (ToM; the ability to infer mental states in others, see Chapter 8), which is less severe than that found in autistic patients, and which is only present during episodes of psychotic illness, could lead to paranoid symptoms.

According to this theory, paranoid patients suddenly discover that they have lost the ability to understand the thoughts and feelings of other people, and then explain this experience by assuming that other people are trying to hide their intentions. Together with fellow psychologist Rhiannon Corcoran, Frith has used a number of strategies to test this theory.

One approach has involved testing the ability of patients to comprehend the beliefs and actions of people portrayed in simple stories.[79] For example, consider the following tale:

Burglar Bill has just robbed a bank and is running away from the police when he meets his brother Bob. Bill says to Bob, 'Don't let the police find me. Don't let them find me!' Then he runs off and hides in the churchyard. The police have looked everywhere for Bill except the churchyard and the park. When they come across Bob they were going to ask him: 'Where is Bill? Is he in the park or the churchyard?' But the police recognize Bob and they realize that he will try to save his brother. They expect him to lie and wherever he tells them, they will go and look in the other place. But Bob, who is very clever, and does want to save his brother, knows that the police don't trust him.*

The person being tested is asked 'Where is Bill really hiding?' to ensure that he can remember the story. If he answers correctly, he is then asked: 'Where will Bob tell the police to look for Bill – in the churchyard or in the park? Why?' Answering this second question requires the ability to make complex inferences about Bob's beliefs and intentions.

Frith and Corcoran found that two groups of schizophrenia patients experience problems with questions of this sort: paranoid patients and patients with mainly negative symptoms. In the latter group, ToM

---

* This kind of complex theory-of-mind conundrum is called a second-order test because, in order to answer it correctly, you have to be able to work out what Bob thinks the policemen are thinking. Similarly, third-order ToM problems require you to work out what X thinks Y thinks X (or Z) is thinking. I used to believe that multi-order ToM skills are rarely used in real life, but recently changed my mind because of the following incident. I was standing in a supermarket close to a (presumably married) couple, when a very beautiful young woman walked past. The man glanced towards her, and then looked sheepishly towards his wife. Responding to his expression, she said, 'You look as if you think that I'll be irritated because I know you think she's beautiful' – a statement that clearly required higher-order ToM skills.

performance correlated strongly with IQ, suggesting that their poor performance was probably caused by general cognitive deficits. In the paranoid patients, however, poor performance on the ToM questions seemed to be unrelated to IQ. Interestingly, as Frith had predicted, recovered paranoid patients performed normally in these studies, indicating that ToM deficits are present only in episodes of illness.

Further experiments conducted by Frith and Corcoran involved other ingenious methods of assessing ToM skills. For example, in one study they investigated the ability of patients to recognize simple hints (as when a husband in a hurry to leave for work glances at the ironing board and laments to his wife that none of his shirts is ironed). In this study, patients with persecutory delusions were poor at inferring intentions from hints, but schizophrenia patients whose symptoms were in remission performed the task as well as the ordinary people.[80]

Frith and Corcoran's ideas sparked off a series of studies by other researchers. Unfortunately, although these generally found that ToM skills are impaired in currently ill psychotic patients, the evidence that this kind of deficit is specifically associated with paranoid symptoms proved to be unclear. In studies carried out in France, Yves Sarfati and his colleagues have found strong associations only between ToM dysfunction and thought disorder,[81] while Robyn Langdon and Max Coltheart, working in Australia, have found evidence of ToM problems in groups of patients with negative symptoms but not in people with persecutory delusions.[82] Using a series of ToM tests, Val Drury and others in Birmingham found evidence of deficits in currently ill schizophrenia patients suffering from multiple positive and negative symptoms, but when they compared patients with persecutory delusions and those without they found no difference.[83] Some studies have even found that some paranoid patients perform better on ToM tasks than other groups of schizophrenia patients.[84] Overall, then, the evidence pretty decisively shows that ToM deficits are not specific to paranoia. Indeed, as one of my own postgraduate students, Natalie Kerr, found that both bipolar-depressed patients and bipolar-manic patients performed poorly on ToM tasks,[85] it seems likely that this kind of disability is present in acutely ill psychotic patients whatever their diagnosis.

Despite this negative evidence, I don't think we should give up on Chris Frith's theory. Indeed, there is obviously something *theory-of-*

mind-ish about persecutory delusions, which inevitably involve mistaken assumptions about the intentions of other people. It is as if the paranoid person can make inferences about the beliefs and attitudes of other people but, for some reason, reaches the wrong conclusions about what those beliefs and attitudes are. I will return to this idea later.

Inferences about causes

When I obtained my priming grant to study delusions in the late 1980s, an immediate difficulty was my embarrassing lack of hypotheses worth testing. After a few weeks thinking through this problem, I hit on the strategy of measuring the same processes that had been studied in depression, particularly attributions. After all, I speculated vaguely, Abramson and Seligman's attributional model of depression seemed to imply that dysphoric mood springs from some kind of delusional interpretation of events. Moreover, it seemed obvious just from listening to paranoid patients that many of their beliefs were, in fact, unusual causal statements. This intuition was reinforced by an almost trivial incident that occurred at about this time. One of my patients, Gerald, arrived half an hour late for an appointment and, as another patient was expected, I had to tell him that I would be unable to see him. Embarrassed, Gerald explained that a malicious neighbour had used supernatural powers to enter his mind and mess with his memory of the appointment. This explanation appeared to have all the characteristics of an external attribution, as the cause of Gerald's lateness was attributed to an external agent over which he had no control.

Readers will recall that the attributional model of depression was first tested by giving patients the Attributional Style Questionnaire (ASQ), which asks the person completing it to think of likely explanations for hypothetical positive and negative events (see Table 10.1, p. 242). In one of our first studies of paranoid thinking, Sue Kaney and I used this questionnaire to compare paranoid patients, depressed patients and ordinary people.[86] We found that paranoid patients, like depressed patients, tended to make excessively global and stable explanations for negative events. (In other words, when things went wrong they tended to assume that the cause would affect all aspects of

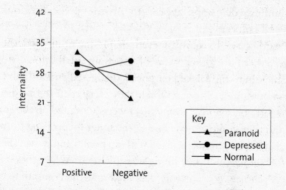

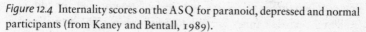

Figure 12.4 Internality scores on the ASQ for paranoid, depressed and normal participants (from Kaney and Bentall, 1989).

their lives and that they were powerless to change it.) However, we were more intrigued by their scores on the internality dimension of the questionnaire. Recall that this part of the scale measures whether the perceived causes of events are internal (to do with the self) or external (to do with other people or circumstances). Our findings are shown in Figure 12.4. Replicating the results of previous investigators, we found that depressed patients had lower internality scores for hypothetical positive events than for negative events – if something went wrong they tended to blame themselves whereas, if something good happened, they tended to assume that the cause was something to do with other people or circumstances. Again, as observed by other researchers, the ordinary people who served as controls tended to be more willing to attribute positive than negative events to themselves. This self-serving bias was markedly exaggerated in our paranoid patients, who appeared to be experts at blaming themselves for positive events and at avoiding blame for negative events.

This observation has been repeated by other investigators in Britain,[87] Canada,[88] Australia[89] and even South Korea.[90] However, an abnormal attributional style is not found in all deluded patients. In a study carried out in North Wales, Helen Sharp, Chris Fear and David Healy tested patients who expressed a variety of unusual beliefs. They observed an abnormal self-serving bias in patients with persecutory or grandiose delusions, but not in those who reported other kinds of delusional ideas.[91] This makes intuitive sense, because only paranoid and grandiose delusions appear to involve preoccupations about success and failure.

The studies we have considered so far have all used the ASQ. However, there are other ways of assessing attributions. In a later study, Sue Kaney and I asked paranoid, depressed and ordinary people to play a computer game in which they were required to discover a rule. On forty occasions, two pictures were presented on the computer screen and they could choose one or the other by pressing button 1 or button 2. The participants started with 20 points and, when they made a 'correct' choice, another point was awarded. When they made an 'incorrect' choice, a point was deducted and the computer made an angry chimpanzee noise. Of course, we had programmed the computer so that the participants' choices had no effect on whether they won or lost points. No matter what they did, one game (known to us as the 'win game') awarded more points than it deducted, leaving the player with 33 points at the end, whereas the other (known to us as the 'lose game') deducted more points than it awarded, leaving the player with 6. After each game the participants were asked to indicate on a 0–100 scale the extent to which they believed they had controlled the outcomes (see Figure 12.5). The depressed patients were sadder but wiser and claimed little control over either of the games (their judgements were therefore accurate). The normal control participants were thoroughly irrational, claiming control when they were winning but not when they were losing. As we had expected, the paranoid patients showed this self-serving bias to a significantly greater degree. (One of the paranoid patients, who played the win game first, was annoyed to discover that he was losing the second game and complained that we had 'rigged' it. As he was perfectly correct about this, he could be said to be suffering from paranoid realism.)[92]

So far in this discussion, we have assumed that attributions can be catalogued on a one-dimensional scale running from internal (self-blaming) to external (blaming other people or circumstances). However, many people find the distinction between 'internal' and 'external' difficult to comprehend[93] so it is not surprising that patients' judgements about internality are sometimes inconsistent.[94] Part of the problem seems to be that the ASQ and similar measures fail to distinguish between two types of external attributions that are different: explanations that implicate circumstances (which can be called *external-*

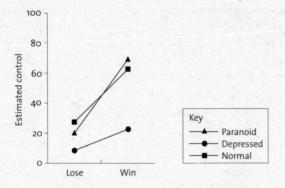

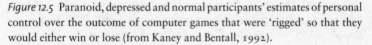

Figure 12.5 Paranoid, depressed and normal participants' estimates of personal control over the outcome of computer games that were 'rigged' so that they would either win or lose (from Kaney and Bentall, 1992).

situational attributions) and those which implicate other people (*external-personal attributions*). The importance of this distinction becomes obvious when we think about common events that provoke attributions. For example, most people explain being late for a meeting in situational terms ('The traffic was dreadful').* From what we learnt in Chapter 10, we might expect a depressed person to point to an internal cause ('I'm lousy at keeping track of time'). A paranoid person, however, might blame the police for maliciously setting all the local traffic lights to red. The implication of this simple thought-experiment is that external-situational attributions may be psychologically benign because they allow us to avoid blaming ourselves while, at the same time, blaming no one else. This is presumably why they are the essence of a good excuse. External-personal attributions, on the other hand, appear to be psychologically toxic: they allow us to avoid blaming ourselves only at the expense of blaming someone else.

Peter Kinderman and I conducted a series of studies to explore this distinction.[95] When we compared paranoid, depressed and ordinary people, we obtained the pattern of results shown in Figure 12.6. Although this figure may seem fairly complex, there are only three important features to focus on. First, as shown in the left panel of the

* Having discussed attributional processes with people in many countries, I can confirm that the traffic excuse is cross-culturally invariant.

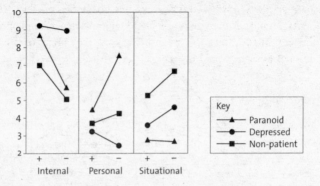

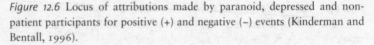

Figure 12.6 Locus of attributions made by paranoid, depressed and non-patient participants for positive (+) and negative (–) events (Kinderman and Bentall, 1996).

figure, the depressed patients we tested uniquely tended to blame themselves for negative events. Second, as shown in the centre panel, and as we had expected, the paranoid patients uniquely tended to blame other people for negative events. The right panel of the figure shows external-situational attributions. Although these might seem unimportant, a glance will reveal that the paranoid patients made fewer explanations of this sort, either for positive or for negative events, than the other groups. It was as if they just did not know how to make a good excuse. Their excessive use of external-personal (other-blaming) explanations can be partly understood in the light of this deficit. Unable to attribute negative events to situations, and with an excessive tendency to avoid attributing such events to themselves, the only choice left is to blame someone else.

The Epistemological Impulsiveness of the Deluded Patient

We can now move to the final box in the back-of-an-envelope model of belief acquisition that I introduced earlier in the chapter. This part of the model concerns the search for further information that might illuminate our beliefs, causing us to hold on to them more tightly, or to modify them on the basis of new evidence. Researchers have suggested two ways in which this process may be handicapped in deluded patients. First, they may be unable to adjust their beliefs appropriately in the light of additional information. Second, they may avoid seeking additional information altogether.

Evaluating hypotheses

When we try to figure out what is going on around us, the evidence rarely points exclusively in one direction. For example, imagine that you are struggling to make sense of a tense relationship with your employer. Perhaps she has taken a dislike to you. On the other hand, perhaps her occasional scowls reflect the constant pressure of her job. When you saw her earlier today she seemed irritable, but when you bumped into her last week she was cheerful and encouraging. Under these kinds of circumstances it can be very difficult to balance different strands of information to decide which explanation is most likely to be correct.

The ability of deluded patients to weigh up inconsistent evidence was first studied by clinical psychologists Philippa Garety and David Hemsley, at the University of London's Institute of Psychiatry. They argued that an inability to think clearly about the probable truth of incompatible hypotheses might lead people to hold on to bizarre beliefs and reject beliefs that are more reasonable.*[96] In order to test this theory, they conducted a series of experiments in which patients were asked to estimate the probability of a different hypothesis in the light of evidence that changed as the experiments progressed.

The task they chose for this purpose may seem very abstract and removed from the demands of everyday life. The people taking part in their experiments were shown two jars, each containing beads of the same two colours. In one jar, one colour far outnumbered the other (by a ratio of 85:15) whereas, in the other, the proportions were reversed. The jars were then hidden away, and the participants were shown a predetermined sequence of beads (some of one colour and

---

* This kind of reasoning is sometimes called 'Bayesian', after the mathematician who proposed a theorem that describes the optimum way in which to change one's conviction in a hypothesis in the light of new evidence. However, we will not consider the details of Bayes' model here, or the mathematical treatment of the research findings from deluded patients.

some of the other). Their task was to guess which jar the beads had been drawn from. (In some experiments, they made a guess after seeing each bead, in others they were required to guess whenever they had seen enough beads to feel confident about their decision.)

In their first study, Garety and her colleagues demonstrated that deluded patients made guesses on the basis of less evidence and with greater confidence, in comparison with a mixed group of psychiatric patients without delusions.[97] A more surprising result was obtained in a second study, in which the sequence of beads was designed so that it favoured one jar early in the sequence (when one colour appeared much more often than the other), but the other jar later (when most beads were of the colour which had initially been least frequent). In this experiment, Garety found that her deluded patients *more rapidly* changed their minds about the jar of origin than her non-deluded control participants.[98] This finding is paradoxical because it implies that deluded patients can sometimes be *excessively* flexible in their beliefs.

Garety's findings provoked other investigators to carry out experiments that have generally supported her initial observations. Yvonne Linney, Emmanuelle Peters and Peter Ayton at the Institute of Psychiatry in London found that ordinary people who scored highly on a questionnaire measure of delusional thinking also showed a tendency to jump to conclusions on a range of reasoning tasks.[99] Psychologists Caroline John and Guy Dodgson in Newcastle tested deluded patients and ordinary people using a variant of the well-known twenty-questions game, in which participants pose a series of questions (for example, 'Is it vegetable?') to elicit yes/no answers, until they have enough evidence to guess the identity of a hidden object. When taking part in this game deluded patients asked fewer questions than ordinary people before making their first guess.[100]

Some studies have also shown that this tendency in deluded patients is more pronounced when they are asked to reason about meaningful stimuli. Robert Dudley and his colleagues asked participants to guess whether a series of statements had been made by a person with mostly negative or mostly positive opinions about someone similar to themselves.[101] In a comparable study conducted by Heather Young and myself, we asked participants to guess whether a list of descriptions concerned someone who had mainly positive traits or someone who had mainly negative traits.[102] In both of these experiments, all of those who took part made more hasty and extreme judgements in these emotionally salient conditions than on Garety and Hemsley's original beads task.

Unfortunately, the cause of the deluded patient's *epistemological impulsivity* is unknown. One possibility, which might explain why they change their minds quickly when the weight of evidence on the beads task changes, is that they respond only to recent information. This explanation would be consistent with a neglected theory of schizophrenia proposed by American psychologist Kurt Salzinger, who argued that many of the cognitive deficits experienced by patients are a consequence of their tendency to respond to the most immediate stimuli in their environment.[103] Robert Dudley and his colleagues[104] and Heather Young and I[105] carried out experiments to test whether this kind of deficit could account for Garety's results, by seeing how patients managed when the balance of the evidence was less clear-cut. For example, Heather Young and I repeated the beads-in-a-jar experiment using colour ratios of 90:10, 75:25 and 60:40. We found that deluded patients, like ordinary people, become more cautious in their judgements as the ratio of the colours approached 50:50. This increasing caution in uncertain situations is completely rational and would not be expected if the patients based their judgements only on the last beads that they had seen.

A second possibility is that deluded people do not understand how to go about testing hypotheses. Earlier in this chapter, I discussed Sir Karl Popper's famous proposal that the most logical way of evaluating a theory is to look for evidence against it.[106] According to Popper, a single piece of disconfirmatory evidence can be enough to bring a theory to its knees, whereas confirmatory evidence may be equally consistent with rival theories. Although the observation that ordinary people typically seek confirmatory data when testing their hypotheses (the so-called confirmation bias) has sometimes been cited as evidence that we can be highly irrational, it has recently become clear that this bias may reflect 'sensible reasoning' strategies which, although illogical in the formal sense, are highly effective in real life.

Typically, the strategy we adopt when testing a hypothesis depends on the nature of the hypothesis. When some kind of choice is believed to have resulted in a good outcome (for example, when we believe that a cake is particularly nice because we used honey instead of sugar), it is sensible to test the hypothesis by looking for confirmatory evidence (for example, by baking another cake with honey but changing some of the other ingredients). This is because the result of the test is likely to be a further positive outcome (another nice cake). However, if the outcome is negative (for example, if we think that a cake tastes awful because we used margarine instead of butter) it is sensible to devise a disconfirmatory test (for example, by baking a cake with butter) as this will reduce the possibility of another disappointing result. Studies show that both children and ordinary adults vary their hypothesis-testing strategies according to the expected outcome in just this way.[107] When Heather Young and I asked paranoid patients, depressed patients and ordinary people to choose methods of testing a range of hypotheses about positive and negative outcomes, we found no differences. Like ordinary people, our deluded patients consistently chose confirmatory tests of positive outcomes and disconfirmatory tests of negative outcomes.[108]

Emotional and motivational factors provide a third possible explanation for the deluded patient's tendency to jump to conclusions. The idea that people vary in their ability to cope with ambiguous information was familiar to Milton Rokeach, who saw it as a cause of political dogmatism. More recently, this idea has been explored by American social psychologists Arie Kruglanski and Donna Webster, who have proposed the term *need for closure* to describe the general desire for 'an answer on a given topic, any answer compared to confusion and ambiguity'.[109] In experiments with ordinary people Kruglanski and Webster have shown that this need can be provoked by circumstances (most obviously, when we have to work against the clock) but also that some people tend to be less tolerant of ambiguity than others. In order to measure this tendency, they developed a simple questionnaire, which assesses a subjective need for order and structure, emotional discomfort in the face of uncertainty, decisiveness, the inability to cope with unpredictability, and closed-mindedness.

Do deluded patients have a high need for closure? One observation that we have already considered suggests that they might. In Chapter 5, I briefly described a study carried out by British psychiatrist Glen Roberts, in which deluded patients were compared with trainee Angli-can priests. Both the priests and the patients scored very high on a measure of their need for meaning in their lives. In the same study, the patients were asked whether they would welcome evidence that their delusions – which often caused them considerable distress – were false. Surprisingly, the majority said that they would not. Roberts interpreted this finding as evidence that, for the patients, their delusional worlds were 'preferred realities', embraced perhaps because they were more predictable than the real world.[110]

Direct evidence of a high need for closure in deluded patients has recently been obtained in a study conducted by my Ph.D. student Rebecca Swarbrick, who used Kruglanski and Webster's questionnaire to test patients suffering from paranoid delusions, patients who had recovered from paranoid delusions and ordinary people.[111] The currently deluded patients and those who had recovered scored very highly on the questionnaire compared to the ordinary people, suggesting that they experience emotional discomfort when confronted by uncertainty. This finding from the remitted patients is particularly interesting because it suggests that a high need for closure may be a trait that predisposes people to developing delusions, and which remains even after their delusions have remitted. However, whether a high need for closure can explain the findings obtained from Philippa Garety's beads-in-a-jar task seems doubtful. In a recent study, Emmanuelle Peters found that ordinary people who scored highly on a delusions questionnaire also scored highly on Kruglanski and Webster's need-for-closure questionnaire. However, in the same study no relationship was found between scores on the need-for-closure questionnaire and scores on Garety's beads-in-a-jar test.[112]

Back to the reaction-maintenance principle

It is possible that the ability of deluded patients to evaluate their hypotheses may be limited, not only by their inability to weigh evidence appropriately, but also by their avoidance of disconfirmatory information.

A few years ago, my colleague Tony Morrison noticed an interesting parallel between the behaviour of paranoid patients and the behaviour of patients suffering from phobias or anxiety disorders.[113] Patients suffering from these conditions often fail to notice that the object of their fear cannot harm them, because they avoid situations in which this would be obvious. Instead, they perform *safety behaviours*, which keep them in situations in which their fears never have to be confronted. For example, a man who is very seriously frightened of dogs may stay at home all of the time, thereby preventing himself from discovering that most dogs are friendly.

The concept of safety behaviours exemplifies, yet again, the reaction-maintenance principle (see p. 262). It is easy to see why persecutory beliefs in particular may lead to these kinds of behaviours, and why these behaviours in turn may help to keep the beliefs alive. It is fairly commonplace to find that patients who fear that secret organizations are conspiring to hurt them stay away from places where they believe that they may be vulnerable to attack, or that those who mistrust people living nearby avoid talking to their neighbours. An extreme example of this kind of behaviour studied by Tony Morrison concerned a woman who believed that she was being followed by the IRA, and who attempted to lose her trackers by wearing disguises, varying her routes to local shops, and by hiding behind cars at intervals while out walking. In a survey of a small group of paranoid patients recently carried out by Daniel Freeman at the Institute of Psychiatry in London it was found that the majority reported safety behaviours.[114]

Whether or not this concept can be extended to other types of delusions remains to be seen. There is evidence, for example, that dismorphobic patients (who believe that they are disfigured or ugly, despite being completely normal in appearance) avoid social situations in which they may be able to judge how other people look at them,[115] but it is difficult to see how, say, grandiose or somatic delusions could be maintained in this way.

An Embarrassment of Riches

By now, the reader will have appreciated that research on delusions has moved forward dramatically over the last decade. Whereas ten years ago there was hardly any evidence to discuss, we now have the opposite problem of trying to make sense of a wide range of research findings which can be interpreted in a variety of ways. The comparison between deluded patients and scientists that I have taken as my theme in this chapter seems to make some kind of sense (at least as a framework for organizing this information) but obviously leaves a lot of questions unanswered. For example, we can ask which of the many processes we have considered is most important in the causation of delusional beliefs. Of course it is possible that all play an important role but to different degrees in different people. (It is easy to imagine that somatic delusions arise primarily as an attempt to explain unusual bodily sensations, whereas what may be termed the *social delusions* – of persecution, grandiosity and jealousy – seem to involve the mental mechanisms responsible for generating causal explanations and understanding others' mental states.)

This idea raises the interesting possibility that it may one day be possible to construct a typology of delusions based on different psychological processes, rather than merely on content. However, it is equally possible that, in the case of some delusional systems, we will be able to construct a unifying theory that shows how these different processes interact. In the next chapter, I will try and construct such a theory to explain delusions of persecution.

On the Paranoid World View

When I was coming up, it was a dangerous world, and you knew exactly who they were. It was us vs. them, and it was clear who them was. Today, we are not so sure who they are, but we know they're there.
                                                    George W. Bush[1]

Only the paranoid survive.   Andrew Grove[2]

In this chapter I will attempt to bring together some of the ideas covered in the last three chapters and, at the same time, make good my promise to outline a detailed theory of paranoid (persecutory) delusions. The theory[3] that I will describe has evolved over more than a decade, during which time earlier versions[4] have been proposed and modified as they have confronted new data.* Of course, it is likely that further modifications will be required as new research findings become available.

I will begin with two assumptions. First, given that paranoid ideas involve worries about relationships with other people, they surely must have something to do with social cognition. Second, most people who have thought seriously about delusions in general have assumed that they arise from attempts to explain unusual or troubling experiences. This assumption seems to lie behind nearly every study that we considered in the last chapter.[5]

Together, these assumptions suggest that attributions must play a central role in paranoid ideas. And, indeed, we have already seen

---

* I sometimes think it would be helpful if researchers numbered different versions of their theories, in the same way that computer programmers number different releases of their software. The theoretical model of paranoia outlined in this chapter is, by my count, version 4.1.

evidence that this is the case. In the last chapter, we saw that paranoid patients show an exaggeration of the self-serving bias (the normal tendency to attribute positive events to the self and negative events to external causes) and that, when they make external attributions for negative events, their explanations usually implicate the intentions of others (they make *external-personal attributions*) rather than circumstantial factors (*external-situational attributions*). It is not difficult to see how complex conspiracy theories might arise from repeatedly explaining unpleasant experiences in this way.

The Paranoid Self

As the self-serving bias is a homeostatic mechanism that most of us use to regulate our self-esteem, the obvious inference from these findings is that paranoid patients are struggling excessively to protect themselves from negative beliefs about themselves. This idea is consistent with the account of paranoia proposed by psychoanalyst and computer scientist Kenneth Colby, which I discussed at the beginning of the last chapter, and *seems* to lead to the prediction that paranoid patients should score normally on self-esteem measures.[6]

In fact, the available evidence on self-esteem in paranoia is inconsistent and overall not favourable to this prediction. Daniel Freeman at the Institute of Psychiatry in London administered a questionnaire to a group of schizophrenia patients taking part in a treatment study and reported that many of the patients who had paranoid delusions had quite low self-esteem, although they also identified a small group in which self-esteem appeared to be normal.[7] B. Bowins and G. Shugar, two psychiatrists in Canada, also used a questionnaire to measure self-esteem in psychotic patients, reporting that deluded patients in general (although not necessarily patients suffering from persecutory delusions) had low self-esteem.[8] Most recently, Christine Barrow-clough and Nick Tarrier in my own university used a detailed interview to assess separately positive and negative self-esteem in a large group of schizophrenia patients, finding that paranoia was associated with high levels of negative self-esteem. This association remained even when the effects of depression and other symptoms were taken into account.[9]

Against these studies, several others have reported that self-esteem is relatively normal or even high in paranoid patients. For example, Carmie Candido and David Romney in Canada assessed global self-esteem in paranoid, depressed-paranoid and depressed patients. They reported high self-esteem in the paranoid group, low self-esteem in the depressed group, and intermediate scores in the depressed-paranoid group.[10] In one of my own studies, paranoid patients scored normally on a simple self-esteem questionnaire.[11] Perhaps the most interesting study to provide evidence of high self-esteem in paranoid patients was conducted by Thomas Oxman, Stanley Rosenberg and Paula Schnurr at the University of Washington in Seattle, who, instead of administering a questionnaire, simply asked paranoid patients and several other groups of patients to speak about anything they wished for five minutes. They then used a computer to analyse the frequency with which different concepts were expressed in the speech samples. The concepts expressed by the paranoid patients were judged to indicate 'an artificially positive, grandiose self-image, and a defensive abstractness'.[12]

When data are as inconsistent as this it is a fair bet that researchers have been asking the wrong question, or at least asking the right question in the wrong sort of way. In this case, a stumbling block seems to be the concept of self-esteem, which, as we saw in Chapter 10, fails to capture adequately the psychological processes involved in self-representation and can be measured in many different ways. Clearly, we need to turn to methods of assessing the self that more accurately reflect its dynamic nature.

Borrowing the ideas of American social psychologists E. Tory Higgins and Tim Strauman, Peter Kinderman and I asked paranoid patients, depressed patients and ordinary people to describe themselves as they actually were (the *actual self*), how they would like to be (the *ideal self*, a self-standard) and how they believed their parents saw them (the *parent-actual self*). (We began by asking our participants to describe how they thought their friends saw them. However, this strategy foundered because many of the paranoid patients reported that they had no friends!) We then examined the discrepancies between these different descriptions.[13] (Higgins and Strauman, it will be recalled from Chapter 10, showed that discrepancies between the actual self and ideals are associated with depressed mood.)

As other researchers had reported previously, we found that these descriptions were fairly concordant in our normal control group, who believed that they were more or less the sort of people they would like to be, and that their parents shared their positive self-perceptions. Like depressed patients in previous studies (see Chapter 10), our depressed group showed marked discrepancies between how they saw themselves and how they said they would like to be. In contrast, our paranoid patients showed very little discrepancy between their self-actual and self-ideal concepts but very marked discrepancies between their self-actual concepts and their beliefs about how their parents saw them. In general, they seemed to believe that their parents had extremely hostile attitudes towards them.

The observation that paranoia is associated with the belief that other people harbour negative attitudes towards the self might be regarded as a statement of the obvious. However, it is an observation that is consistent with the attributional data we considered in the last chapter. If paranoid patients consistently blame their misfortunes on the intentional actions of other people, it is not surprising that they believe that other people hate them.

Implicit beliefs about the self

So far we have considered immediate, conscious judgements about the self. However, many of our judgements about ourselves, for example when we make remarks that reflect our feelings without carefully thinking about what we are saying, are more implicit. These implicit judgements echo relatively enduring stored knowledge and beliefs about the self, rather than what we consider to be our virtues and deficits at the present moment in time. They may well be different from the kinds of opinions expressed when we actively reflect about the self, but (because they are ephemeral) can be difficult to capture.

Peter Kinderman devised an approach to this problem that exploited the Stroop effect, which I first described in Chapter 11 (pp. 281–2). He reasoned that people who are uncomfortable about themselves should be slow to colour-name self-descriptive words. He therefore showed paranoid patients, depressed patients and ordinary people a questionnaire consisting of high self-esteem words (for example, 'capable', 'wise') and low self-esteem words (for example, 'childish', 'lazy'). They were asked to indicate with a tick which of the words described themselves. As expected, ordinary people endorsed most of the positive words and very few of the negative words. The depressed patients, on the other hand, ticked about equal numbers of positive and negative words. The paranoid patients ticked mostly positive words but also slightly more of the negative words than the normal controls. In the second stage of the study, the participants completed a Stroop task in which they were asked to colour-name the same words. Peter Kinderman found that the normal people had little difficulty with this task and colour-named both the high self-esteem and the low self-esteem words about as fast as they colour-named a list of emotionally neutral words. However, the depressed patients showed slowed colour-naming for the high self-esteem words and especially for the low self-esteem words. This effect was even more pronounced for the paranoid patients, indicating that the words had special emotional significance for them (see Figure 13.1).[14] These findings were recently repeated in two studies carried out by Hon Lee in South Korea, one comparing students who scored high and low on a paranoia questionnaire, and one comparing clinically paranoid, clinically depressed and normal participants. In the first study, the paranoid students showed slow colour-naming only for low self-esteem words. In the second, paranoid patients showed slowed colour-naming for both positive and negative trait words.[15]

A second method of assessing implicit beliefs about the self involves studying *implicit attributions*. The ASQ asks people to make deliberate and thoughtful judgements about the causes of events, and it is therefore unsurprising that paranoid patients' responses on it are defensive. If patients could be led to make more implicit or thoughtless judgements, perhaps their responses would be more concordant with any underlying negative beliefs about the self. As we saw in Chapter 11 (pp. 279–80), a suitable measure – the Pragmatic Inference Task (PIT) – has been developed by researchers investigating bipolar patients.

Helen Lyon, Sue Kaney and I administered the PIT and a conventional attributional style questionnaire to paranoid patients, depressed patients and ordinary people. As we expected, the ordinary people showed a self-serving bias on both measures. In contrast, both the deluded and the depressed patients made more internal attributions

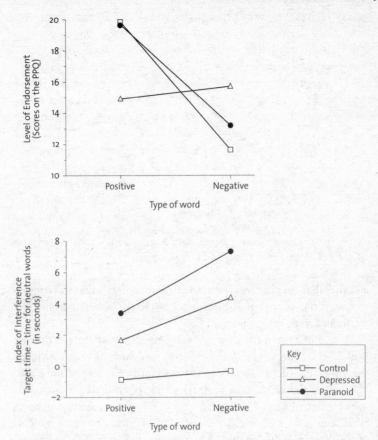

Figure 13.1 The upper panel shows the number of positive and negative trait words endorsed as true by paranoid, depressed and normal control participants on a questionnaire (PPQ). The lower panel shows the interference index (extra time taken in comparison with emotionally neutral words) for the same words in a Stroop colour-naming task administered to the same participants (from Kinderman, 1994).

for negative than for positive events on the PIT (see Figure 13.2). In the case of the depressed patients, this pattern corresponded with their scores on the conventional questionnaire, and is consistent with the research we considered earlier in this book. However, on the explicit measure the paranoid patients made more external attributions for

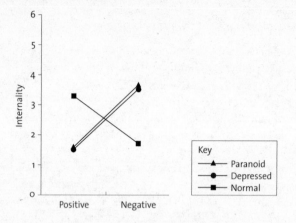

Figure 13.2 Internality scores for paranoid, depressed and normal participants on the PIT (from Lyon, Kaney and Bentall, 1994).

negative than for positive events, an attributional style that was consistent with our previous findings but completely different from their pattern of responding on the PIT.[16]

A final indirect method of assessing beliefs about the self that we will consider here concerns the enduring standards by which we judge ourselves. In order to measure these standards, Sue Kaney and I used the Dysfunctional Attitudes Scale (DAS), a widely used questionnaire, which I described in Chapter 10 (p. 253). Because paranoid patients often complain of being depressed, and because depressed patients typically score highly on the DAS, we wanted to ensure that any highly perfectionistic attitudes we detected could not be a mere consequence of negative mood. We therefore struggled hard to identify two groups of deluded patients, one with concurrent depression and a smaller group who were not depressed at the time of testing. As it turned out, both groups scored similarly to a group of depressed patients who were not suffering from delusions, and showed very high scores on the questionnaire.[17] Similar findings were obtained in a study by Chris Fear, Helen Sharp and David Healy, which was published at about the same time.[18] As perfectionistic self-standards presumably make individuals vulnerable to negative self-evaluations, these findings are consistent with the hypothesis that paranoid patients are strongly motivated to avoid threats to the self.

The dynamic nature of the paranoid defence

It is clear that paranoid patients do not consistently maintain a high level of self-esteem. Indeed, the findings obtained from the indirect measures that we have just considered seem more consistent with the opposite conclusion – that paranoid patients have *low* self-esteem. However, even this would be an over-simplification. The picture that emerges suggests a much more complex and dynamic relationship between attributions, different kinds of self-representations, mood and paranoid delusions, as if the paranoid patient is constantly fighting to maintain a positive view of the self, sometimes winning and but more often losing.

This picture is, of course, consistent with the idea of the *attribution–self-representation cycle*, which we arrived at a few chapters back (see Figure 10.6, p. 260). Remember that, according to this idea, attributions and self-representations are coupled in a cyclical relationship. Current beliefs about the self influence attributions, but attributions have the power to bring about changes in beliefs about the self (a psychological chicken-or-egg phenomenon).

To see how paranoid beliefs fit into this general model, let us look at the results of two experiments that Peter Kinderman and I carried out. The relatively minor differences between the experiments need not detain us here; suffice it to say that, in both, ordinary people described themselves, their ideals and their beliefs about other people's attitudes towards them *before and after* making a series of attributions for negative events. As we had expected from our existing understanding of depression (see Chapter 10) those who initially showed substantial discrepancies between their beliefs about themselves and their ideals tended to make internal attributions for the negative events, whereas those who had relatively few discrepancies tended to make external attributions. However, the most interesting finding emerged when we measured the *changes* in beliefs about the self that had occurred by the end of the experiments (see Figure 13.3). Again, as we had expected on the basis of previous research, those who made internal attributions tended to show even more substantial discrepancies between their beliefs about themselves and their ideals. However, the effects of external attributions depended on the precise nature of the attributions. *External-situational attributions* (the essence of

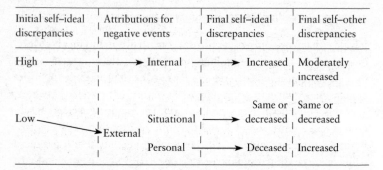

Initial self–ideal discrepancies	Attributions for negative events	Final self–ideal discrepancies	Final self–other discrepancies
High ⟶	Internal ⟶	Increased	Moderately increased
Low ⟶ External	Situational ⟶	Same or decreased	Same or decreased
	Personal ⟶	Deceased	Increased

Figure 13.3 Diagram indicating the influence of self-discrepancies on attributions, and the subsequent impact of attributions on later self-discrepancies, as found in two experiments by Kinderman and Bentall (2000).

good excuse-making, as in 'I'm sorry I'm late but the traffic was dreadful') led to few changes in discrepancies between beliefs about the self and ideals ('I'm still the sort of person I'd like to be') and very few discrepancies between beliefs about the self and beliefs about the opinions of other people ('and other people still think I'm wonderful'). However, *external-personal attributions* ('I'm sorry I'm late but the police deliberately set all the traffic lights to red to stop me from getting here on time'), although also resulting in few discrepancies between beliefs about the self and ideals ('I'm the sort of person I'd like to be'), led to increased discrepancies between beliefs about the self and the perceived beliefs of others ('but other people hate me'). Of course, as we have seen, it is precisely these kinds of attributions that are made in excess by paranoid patients.[19]

Paranoid patients can therefore be accommodated within the model of the attribution–self-representation cycle if we assume that, like depressed patients, their stored knowledge about the self is very negative but, unlike depressed patients, they have somehow learnt to avoid making internal attributions for negative events, and instead tend to make external-personal attributions. Because of the cyclic relationship between attributions and self-representations, these efforts to attribute negative experiences to external causes may not be sufficient to ensure that their current beliefs about themselves are always positive.

This theory neatly ties together the evidence on attributions and the paranoid self, but leads us to conclude that it may be impossible to make simple predictions about the way that paranoid patients will answer self-esteem questionnaires. Indeed, it is easy to see why some patients appear to have what Peter Trower and Paul Chadwick describe as 'poor me' paranoid delusions (they express relatively positive opinions about themselves and believe themselves to be the innocent victims of imaginary conspiracies) while others appear to have 'bad me' delusions (they seem to have low self-esteem and apparently believe that others have good reasons for wanting to harm them).[20] Depending on the precise nature of their stored self-knowledge, the circumstances in which they find themselves, and the extent to which they are able to attribute their most troubling experiences to external-personal causes, either of these types of delusional systems is a likely outcome of many iterations of the attribution–self-representation cycle.

Of course, sceptics might argue that a theory of this sort should not be trusted because it cannot be properly tested. (This is precisely the reason that many modern psychologists have rejected the theories of the early psychoanalysts.) Against this argument it can be said that some phenomena *just are* unpredictable (the weather is a familiar example), and establishing when this is the case is an important kind of scientific achievement. (This is one of the main goals of the mathematical science of non-linear systems theory, more popularly known as chaos theory.)[21] More importantly, as we saw in Chapter 10, it is possible to make other kinds of predictions that can be subjected to experimental investigation.

For example, the theory suggests that under some circumstances the attributions of paranoid patients will not always be excessively self-serving. If something happens to activate their underlying negative beliefs about themselves, their subsequent attributions should be temporarily more pessimistic. We have already seen evidence that this actually happens. Figure 10.5 (p. 259) shows the data from an experiment in which depressed patients, paranoid patients and ordinary people were asked to make attributions for hypothetical negative events before and after completing an anagram task that included impossible questions. Before the task, the paranoid patients made excessively external attributions for negative events, an observation that is consistent with the results of previous studies. However, *afterwards*, their attributions had shifted to become much more internal (almost like those of depressed patients), presumably because their failure on the anagrams task had brought some of their negative beliefs about themselves to the surface. It is difficult to see why these changes would happen if the attribution–self-representation cycle was not a real phenomenon.

Why External-Personal Attributions?

There is one remaining puzzle about the role of attributions in paranoia. Given that paranoid patients appear to avoid making internal attributions for negative events, why don't they just do what most of us do, and make external-situational attributions? After all, as we have seen, external-situational attributions are benign. They keep us from thinking bad things about ourselves, and from attributing malevolent intentions to other people.

There are two main explanations for the paranoid patient's failure to generate situational explanations. First, hyper-vigilance to threat-related information might lead the paranoid person to notice person-relevant information more than ordinary people. Second, paranoid patients may suffer from some kind of cognitive disability that prevents them from noticing situational information. As there is quite good evidence for both of these mechanisms, they are clearly not mutually exclusive.

Attention and attributions

In the last chapter, we saw that paranoid patients excessively attend to[22] and recall[23] threat-related information. More intriguingly, they seem to be more proficient than ordinary people at identifying negative emotional expressions on the faces of others.[24] The availability of this kind of information at the forefront of their minds is likely to make them attribute negative social interactions to something about the other people involved, rather than to themselves or to circumstances. For example, we can imagine a paranoid patient having a minor argument with an acquaintance and, detecting a subtle expression of suppressed anger, concluding that the acquaintance maliciously set out to provoke a disagreement.

If this idea is correct, it should be possible to influence ordinary people to make paranoid attributions for negative experiences by making them focus their attention on the actions of others. This effect has been demonstrated by social psychologists Ehud Bodner and Mario Mikulincer in a series of experiments conducted at Bar-Ilan University in Israel. In these experiments, ordinary people were asked to explain their performance after they had failed to solve a series of problems that were in fact unsolvable. When their attention was focused on themselves (for example, they could see a video camera pointing towards them, and their own faces on a nearby television screen), they made depressive attributions. However, when their attention was focused on the experimenter (because the video camera was pointing at the experimenter and the television screen was showing the experimenter's face) the participants in the experiments were especially likely to make paranoid attributions. Interestingly, these effects only occurred when the participants believed that they had uniquely failed to solve the problems. If they knew that everyone had failed to solve them, they made neither depressive nor paranoid attributions.[25]

The difficulty of understanding situations

The second possible explanation for the paranoid patient's tendency to make external-personal attributions is an inability to make situational attributions. To see why these kinds of attributions might present special difficulties, we need to look again at what happens when we try to explain things.

In Chapter 10, I argued that this process probably involves some kind of mental search that is terminated when a suitable explanatory construct is found. We rack our brains until we arrive at a satisfactory explanation and then stop. I also suggested that this search almost always begins with current beliefs about the self. In the case of ordinary people, if we can immediately think of aspects of the self that match the event we are trying to explain, we will attribute the event to an internal cause. On the other hand, if we are unable to find a character-istic of ourselves that matches the event, we will find ourselves search-ing for some other kind of cause, most likely something external to ourselves. (Paranoid patients going through the same process presum-ably reject most candidate internal attributions for negative events, and move smartly onwards in order to search for external causes.)

Studies carried out by social psychologist Daniel Gilbert at the University of Texas suggest that this further search for external causes does not happen in a single step. Gilbert required ordinary people to make attributions about the behaviour of other people in relaxed circumstances and also when their minds were being kept busy with a competing task. Without the competing task, the participants in these experiments tended to make external attributions that were situational whereas, when their minds were otherwise occupied, they tended to make attributions that implicated fixed traits in the other people. Gilbert concluded that, when accounting for the behaviour of other people, we first of all make external-personal attributions and then later discount these in favour of more situational explanations in the light of whatever information is available about the circumstances. This second step requires mental effort, so it tends not to occur when our minds are occupied with other tasks.[26]

There might be many reasons why paranoid patients lack the mental resources necessary to generate external-situational attributions. It is possible that, during a psychotic episode, some of the attentional and memory deficits we considered in Chapter 7 limit the extent to which they can think about situational factors. It is also possible that the tendency to jump to conclusions and a strong motivation to avoid ambiguity (characteristics of deluded patients that we discussed in the last chapter) result in a rush to attributional judgement, so that the second step described in Dan Gilbert's model is skipped. Another intriguing possibility is that the failure to understand other people's mental states contributes to this deficit.

When I earlier considered Chris Frith's suggestion that paranoid patients suffer from an impaired theory of mind (ToM),[27] we saw that, overall, the available evidence suggests that psychotic patients *in general* seem to suffer from difficulties of this sort (although only when they are ill). That is, these difficulties do not appear to be specifically connected to paranoia. Nonetheless, I would now like to suggest that ToM deficits, even though they may not be specific in this way, might indirectly influence paranoid thinking by limiting the ability of patients to make situational attributions.

To see why an inability to think about the mental states of others might have this effect, imagine that you are walking down a road and a friend passing in the opposite direction ignores you. What do you think? Most people considering this type of event generate some kind of excuse for the friend, such as 'She's having a bad day' or 'She's worried about something.' Many of these kinds of explanations have a situational flavour – they explain the friend's behaviour in terms of circumstances that are affecting her. Moreover, these kinds of explanations also require you to take your friend's point of view, in other words, to use your ToM skills. If you are unable to do this, and especially if you are anxious to avoid blaming yourself, you may well attribute your friend's behaviour to some kind of simple disposition or trait ('He's a bastard' or 'He's selfish and unreliable').*

In an attempt to test this prediction, Peter Kinderman, Robin Dunbar and I administered a ToM measure and also a measure of attributional style to a large group of students.[28] As we had predicted, students who performed relatively poorly on our ToM task made more paranoid-style external-personal attributions than students who performed well, a finding that has since been replicated.[29] Obviously, this study was limited by our use of students, rather than of people who were actually suffering from psychiatric symptoms. The necessary studies of the relationship between ToM skills and attributions in patients are currently being conducted by some of my postgraduate students.

More Understanding of the Ununderstandable

In this chapter I have argued that the paranoid world view arises from the tendency to make extreme self-protective attributions, together with the failure (for whatever reason) to take into account situational causes of events. Of course, this account does not mean that biological processes are not involved – attributions, self-representations and associated cognitive processes are presumably generated by circuits in the brain. Clues about the specific neural circuits that may be involved

---

* It is important to note that a dispositional attribution does not require ToM, as it does not involve taking someone's point of view. Even a simple attribution of malevolent intent, for example 'He hates me', may require less use of ToM than the more complex situational accounts we often give when friends behave in an unexpected manner.

have emerged from studies of patterns of regional cerebral blood flow in deluded patients,[30] and in patients with positive symptoms in general,[31] which have implicated the left lateral prefrontal cortex among other areas. More recently, Nigel Blackwood and Rob Howard at the Institute of Psychiatry in London have begun a programme of research (in which I am a collaborator) focusing specifically on paranoia, in which fMRI is being used to study relevant cognitive processes in both patients and ordinary people. Initial findings indicate that, in ordinary people, attention to threatening statements relevant to the self activates a neural network involving the left lateral inferior frontal cortex, the ventral striatum and the anterior cingulate.[32] It remains to be seen whether these areas are more highly activated in paranoid patients.

The reader will have noticed that many of the psychological processes implicated in the model I have described in this chapter are the same as those involved in abnormal mood. Indeed, the model is represented schematically in Figure 13.4 as a variation of the models of depression and mania previously presented in Figures 10.7 and 11.5. These parallels suggest a close relationship between depression, mania and paranoia, which bridges the Kraepelinian divide between dementia praecox and the affective psychoses.

In fact, I am not the first to suggest a close relationship between paranoid symptoms and depression. Previous researchers have noted that psychotic patients with paranoid symptoms are more likely to have a history of depression than those without.[33] Some studies have also shown that paranoid personality characteristics are frequently observed in the close relatives of patients diagnosed as suffering from an affective disorder,[34] but less commonly observed than might be expected in the relatives of patients diagnosed as suffering from schizophrenia.[35] Some years ago, American psychologists Edward Zigler and Marion Glick pointed out that preoccupation with the self is a central feature of depression, paranoia and mania, but not of other symptoms of psychosis.[36] Their own research also led them to conclude that social and occupational functioning is usually good before the onset of a paranoid or depressive illness, but typically poor in people who later develop other psychotic symptoms.

Zigler and Glick proposed that both paranoid schizophrenia and delusional disorder are therefore forms of camouflaged depression.

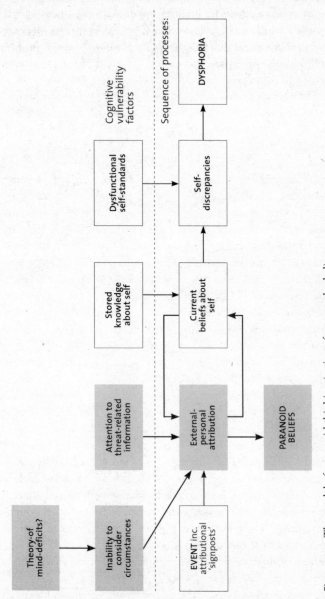

Figure 13.4 The model of paranoid thinking (unique features shaded).

This theory takes Kraepelin's distinction between schizophrenia and the affective psychoses for granted, but draws the line between the two types of disorder in a novel way. It will be evident from earlier chapters that I do not think that this is the right solution to the problem of classifying the psychoses.

14

The Illusion of Reality

Trintano: *Your Excellency, haven't we seen each other somewhere before?*

Rufus T. Firefly (Groucho Marx): *I don't think so. I'm not sure I'm seeing you now. It must be something I ate.*

Duck Soup (1933)

Hallucinations may seem unpromising candidates for psychological analysis. The hallucinatory experiences described by patients often seem so frightening and senseless that it is easy assume that they are exclusively the product of some kind of brain malfunction.

When I first attempted the psychological treatment of patients who heard voices, I was not convinced that I had anything useful to offer. I was just one year out of the Liverpool training course and going through my divorce, and my mind was more focused on personal problems than on clinical innovation. The Mersey Regional Forensic Psychiatry Service, where I was working, was responsible for the care of psychiatric patients who had committed criminal offences or who were considered to be dangerous to others. Most patients resident in the service's inpatient facility had been diagnosed as suffering from schizophrenia. However, before my arrival, the psychologists in the service had focused their efforts mainly on non-psychotic patients attending the outpatient clinic (mostly sex offenders), and had left work with the inpatients to nurses and psychiatrists. It was only because I had expressed a tentative interest in psychosis that one of the consultant psychiatrists encouraged me to see a few patients who were proving difficult to treat with medication.

Many years later, I can remember very little about the first patient I saw, a young woman who told anyone who cared to listen about her desire to kill old people. As she was at times quite paranoid, and had a history of violence, it seemed prudent to take this strange and frightening fantasy seriously. Unfortunately, although she freely admitted to an indiscriminate hatred of anyone above the age of 65, she was in other ways uncooperative. Unable to make any sense of her strange obsessions, or the voices she occasionally disclosed, I eventually admitted defeat and left decisions about her management to my wiser and more experienced colleagues.

It was the second patient who helped me to overcome my now growing therapeutic pessimism. Speaking to Brian[1] for the first time as we sat together in a small side room, it suddenly occurred to me that, during my lengthy training, no one had thought it necessary to instruct me in the best way of talking to mad people. I was not sure where to start. I need not have worried. Brian was charming and helpful. No doubt assisted by the many previous occasions on which he had told his story, he described how his problems had developed after he had failed at college, the years of periodic hospital treatment that had followed, and the violent confrontation with his father that had led to his recent admission. With hardly a pause for breath, he then proceeded to talk about his voices. He told me that they appeared to originate from inside his head, but seemed as real to him as my voice. They revealed to him evidence of a Jewish plot to confine Gentiles to concentration camps and, at the same time, tormented him with the simple refrain, 'Give cancer to the crippled bastard!'

Brian believed that the voices were being projected into his head by a team of parapsychologists, and asked me to use whatever influence I might have to end this bizarre and, to his mind, unethical experiment. Yet, even on the occasion of our first meeting, it was obvious that his voices were not merely the random product of a damaged nervous system. The 'crippled bastard' referred to by the voices was easily identifiable – Brian was sitting in a wheelchair, having crushed his legs in a bungled suicide attempt. (He had jumped from the top floor of a multi-storey car park.) I later learned that the girlfriend who had recently abandoned him was Jewish. I also learned that Brian's mother had died from cancer. No doubt 'Give cancer to the crippled bastard!' encapsulated a constellation of ideas linked by a common thread of guilt.

Emboldened by this insight, I tried to help Brian gain some understanding of his experiences. Over the following few months, we met regularly for periods of half an hour or so (any longer and he became exhausted). Sometimes I would sit in silence as Brian listened to his voices and described what they were saying, so that we could consider how their content might relate to events that had befallen him. At other times we considered the idea that his voices might be fragments of his mind that had somehow become separated from his conscious self. As the weeks passed, the voices became less frequent, and Brian's belief that he was the victim of a parapsychological experiment diminished. In retrospect, I realize that my efforts were not particularly well thought-out and, of course, it is possible (as a particularly cynical nurse enjoyed pointing out to me) that much of the improvement Brian experienced was due to simultaneous adjustments to his medication. However, Brian – a very gentle person who was happiest when idly strumming his guitar – seemed to gain something positive from our time together. Perhaps it was just the chance to have somebody listen to his point of view.

Impossible Perceptions

According to the historian German Berrios, 'Experiences redolent of hallucinations and illusions are part of the common baggage of humanity.'[2] Certainly, it is not difficult to find evidence of quasi-hallucinatory experiences in the historical record. As we saw earlier, American psychologist Julian Jaynes has attempted to account for the linguistic peculiarities of the *Iliad* by supposing that, in Ancient Greece, hallucinating was the normal mode of thinking.[3] Although this bold hypothesis has been disputed,[4] it is certainly true that hallucinatory experiences have been recorded since biblical times.[5] Socrates, to take one well-documented example, had a 'daemon' that spoke to him, offering moral and political advice. Unfortunately, researchers have been slow to consider the relationship between hallucinations and normal perceptual processes. As psychologists Theodore Sarbin and Joseph Juhasz have noted, 'Since the 1920s textbooks of general psychology have differentiated hallucinations from errors of perception by the simple expedient of locating them in separate chapters.'[6]

Before the efforts of the classificationists of the nineteenth century, hallucinations were considered to be independent diseases rather than symptoms of more general conditions. A French psychiatrist, Jean-Etienne Esquirol, first offered a definition of hallucinations in a paper published in 1832, observing that the hallucinating person, 'ascribes a body and actuality to images that the memory recalls without the intervention of the senses'.[7] In this way, he distinguished between hallucinations (roughly perceptions of objects not present at the time) and illusions (the misperception of objects which are present).

Modern definitions of hallucination are similar to Esquirol's. For example, DSM-IV states that a hallucination is 'A sensory perception that has the compelling sense of reality of a true perception but that occurs without external stimulation of the relevant sensory organ.'[8] In an earlier book, Peter Slade and I attempted to be more precise by suggesting that a hallucination is 'any percept-like experience which (a) occurs in the absence of an appropriate stimulus, (b) has the full force or impact of the corresponding actual (real) perception, and (c) is not amenable to the direct or voluntary control of the experiencer'.[9] Our emphasis on the absence of an *appropriate* stimulus acknowledges that the world external to the individual does impact on hallucinations, as we will see later. However, even this definition is not without its difficulties. What are we to make, for example, of rare individuals who say that they can make themselves hallucinate?

Karl Jaspers suggested that an important distinction could be made between 'true' hallucinations, which appear to be external to the individual (for example, a voice coming from somewhere beyond the boundaries of the body), and 'pseudohallucinations', such as those experienced by Brian, which are experienced as originating from inside the head.[10] However, the usefulness of this distinction has been disputed, and most modern psychologists and psychiatrists lump both types of experience together. In my own clinical work, I have often found that patients describe their hallucinations as external to themselves but, after being encouraged to think about them carefully, decide that they are occurring inside them. Oddly, this reattribution does not seem to alter the perception that these experiences are caused by some kind of external agency.

A phenomenon that appears to be a further step away from full-blown hallucinations is known as *thought insertion*. Patients who have this experience say that they have thoughts inside their heads that have been put there by someone else. For example:

I look out the window and I think that the garden looks nice and the grass looks cool, but the thoughts of Eamonn Andrews [a television presenter who was popular in Britain in the 1960s and 1970s] come into my mind ... He treats my mind like a screen and flashes thoughts onto it like you flash a picture.[11]

Intrusive or obsessional thoughts seem to lie still further down the scale of alienness. These kinds of thoughts, which are often the main complaint of non-psychotic patients given the diagnosis of obsessive-compulsive disorder, arrive unbidden in the head, and may vary from trivial memories (for example, an irritating advertising jingle that seems impossible to expel from the mind), to fears about violating social norms (for example, the worry that one might shout something out during a solemn ceremony, such as a marriage), to the self-critical automatic thoughts of the depressed patient. Surveys have established that just about everyone has these kinds of experiences, but that obsessional patients are unique in their fear of the consequences that might ensue (they may fear acting on thoughts that are socially unacceptable, for example,), and the efforts they make to suppress them.[12]

The most common type of hallucination encountered in the modern psychiatric clinic is auditory and consists of voices, like Brian's. As we have seen, these types of experiences, for example of voices telling the patient what to do or discussing the patient's behaviour, were thought by Schneider to be first-rank symptoms of schizophrenia.[13] Although some studies have shown that about three quarters of schizophrenia patients experience voices,[14] this no doubt reflects modern psychiatrists' adherence to Schneiderian diagnostic principles. Even so, hallucinations are often reported by patients receiving other diagnoses, particularly bipolar disorder and, more recently, dissociative disorder,* leading some researchers to lament that they have no diagnostic specificity whatsoever.[15]

* Dissociative disorder is a controversial diagnosis in which different facets of the individual's mind are supposed to become dissociated from each other, leading, in extreme cases, to multiple personalities. Unfortunately, the concept of dissociative disorder is often confused with the concept of schizophrenia, which has never included multiple personalities.

Cases of multiple personality were reported in the nineteenth century, for example by the French neurologist Pierre Janet and the American pioneer of

Often, the voices described by patients have a negative quality. They may insult the patient, or tell the patient to do something unacceptable (for example, to commit suicide). However, it would be wrong to assume that this is invariably the case. When three American psychiatrists, Laura Miller, Eileen O'Connor and Tony DiPasquale, interviewed a group of chronically hallucinating patients they found that many thought their voices were pleasant and they did not want them to disappear as a consequence of treatment. Some regarded their voices as important personages in their impoverished social networks, perhaps filling a gap created by the isolation they experienced as a consequence of their illness.[16]

Hallucinations may also be experienced in other modalities, such as visual hallucinations of people who are not really present. I have met a number of patients who have claimed to see the Devil. (As we saw in Chapter 6, these kinds of hallucinations are more often reported by patients in the developing world than by patients in the West.)[17] Others may have tactile hallucinations in which they believe that invisible people are touching them, or olfactory hallucinations in which they experience unusual smells that are not detectable by others.

Sometimes it is difficult to decide whether an experience really is a hallucination. For example, the term 'olfactory reference syndrome' has been used to describe a relatively circumscribed complaint in which the patient believes that he smells.[18] In practice, it can be difficult to decide whether this belief reflects a delusional explanation of social isolation ('People are avoiding me, and it's probably because I smell') or an olfactory hallucination. It may also be difficult to distinguish between a hallucination and ordinary mental imagery. I once saw a patient in a high-security hospital who complained of visual hallucinations in which he would 'see' himself having sex with naked women. When I suggested that it was not unusual for bored and sexually

---

abnormal psychology Morton Prince, but the diagnosis was used very rarely until recently. In a break from this historical trend, over the last decade large numbers of multiple personality cases have been reported by a small number of American psychiatrists and psychologists. It seems likely that many of these new cases are highly suggestible patients who have been encouraged to regard themselves as 'multiples' by their therapists. For a fascinating and sceptical account of the disorder, see Ian Hacking's book *Rewriting the Soul: Multiple Personality and the Sciences of Memory* (1995) Princeton: Princeton University Press.

deprived young men to have these kinds of experiences, he insisted that his visions could not be mere fantasies, because the women were unknown to him and, 'You can't imagine someone you've never met in real life.'

The idea that hallucinations exist on a continuum with normal mental imagery was suggested by American psychiatrist John Strauss in an influential paper published in 1969.[19] Strauss studied schizophrenia patients' accounts of their positive symptoms and concluded that they could be classified along four dimensions: the strength of the individual's conviction in the objective reality of the experience; the extent to which the experience seems to be independent of stimuli or cultural determinants; the individual's preoccupation with the experience; and its implausibility. 'Full-blown' hallucinations fall at the end of all of these dimensions. However, there is no doubt that some experiences fall midway along these dimensions (for example, you may think but not be certain that you have glimpsed someone you are hoping to avoid).

Back to the illness debate

In Chapter 5 we considered the possibility that there is a dimension of personality reflecting the extent to which people are likely to suffer from a psychotic illness.* On examining this evidence, we established that it is not necessary to assume that everyone who experiences a hallucination is suffering from an illness. Indeed, it was apparent that as many as ten times more people experience voices than receive treatment for psychosis. In Holland, Marius Romme and Sondra Escher have taken this discovery to its logical conclusion by forming a national society for people who hear voices.[20]

Nevertheless, it is clear that hallucinations can be provoked by disturbances of the nervous system. They are common consequences of many medical conditions, including progressive sensory loss

---

* It is easy to confuse the idea of a dimension of experience with the idea of a dimension of personality, but they are not the same. The first suggests that different kinds of experience (for example, vivid daydreams and hearing voices) may be related to each other, whereas the second indicates that people differ in their propensity to have those experiences. Of course, both types of dimension imply that there is no clear dividing line between normality and abnormality.

(blindness or deafness), fever, focal brain lesions, delirium and, most obviously, intoxication.[21] Although a variety of drugs (including alcohol if consumed in sufficient quantities) can cause hallucinations, the most potent known hallucinogen is lysergic acid diethylamide (LSD), first synthesized in 1938 by the Swiss chemist Albert Hoffman. As we saw in Chapter 7, the discovery of LSD provoked the hypothesis that schizophrenia might be caused by an endogenous neurotoxin. One problem for this theory is that drug-induced hallucinations are usually quite different from those reported by patients in the absence of intoxication. For example, the hallucinations induced by LSD and other drugs usually consist of intense visual experiences involving bright colours, and explosive, concentric, rotational or pulsating movements like those originally described by Hoffman.[22]

Careful medical investigations have revealed that only a very small proportion of psychiatric patients who experience hallucinations suffer from a recognizable medical condition. In a study by Eve Johnstone, Fiona MacMillan and Tim Crow at Northwick Park Hospital, near London, 15 out of 268 patients with an initial diagnosis of schizophrenia were found to be suffering from an identifiable medical disorder and, of these, 10 were experiencing hallucinations.[23] In a similar study in the United States, it was found that hallucinations associated with medical illness generally appear suddenly, and are usually visual.[24]

Learning to live with voices

When Marius Romme compared voice-hearers who had been diagnosed as suffering from a mental illness with others who had not, he found remarkably few differences in the experiences of the two groups. Both patients and non-patients experienced a combination of positive and negative voices, but the proportion of positive voices was greater in the non-patients. The non-patients in contrast with the patients often felt they had some control over their voices.[25] In Britain, a similar comparison conducted by Ivan Leudar and Phil Thomas found comparable results.[26] The majority in both groups reported that their voices played a role in regulating everyday activities, for example by issuing instructions. For many of those interviewed, their voices appeared to be aligned with significant members of the person's family, although this was less so for the patients. Overall, these similarities suggest that it is not hallucinations *per se* that determine whether people seek help from psychiatric services, but how well they are able to cope with these experiences.

Marius Romme and Sondra Escher have suggested that the process of adapting to hallucinations occurs in three distinct stages. They found that the majority of those they interviewed first heard voices during a period of emotional turmoil or following a traumatic experience of some kind. When the voices appeared, they typically provoked feelings of confusion, panic and powerlessness. However, this was usually followed by a phase, lasting months or even years, during which the person hearing voices struggled to find ways of coping. Some people learned to ignore their voices, others learned to listen to those that offered positive advice, and still others formulated some kind of 'contract' with the voices (for example, agreeing to listen to them for only a limited amount of time each day), which would limit their emotional impact. Eventually, some voice-hearers began to regard their voices as a positive facet of themselves.

Romme and Escher's observations have been echoed by recent studies carried out by clinical psychologists in Britain. Studies conducted by Paul Chadwick and Max Birchwood in Birmingham have shown that patients who believe that their voices are omniscient (all-seeing) and omnipotent (all-powerful) have greatest difficulty in coping with them, and that patients who appraise their voices as malevolent tend to resist them, whereas those who appraise their voices as benevolent tend to engage with them, by talking with them or taking seriously what they have to say.[27] Extending this work further, Birchwood has recently studied the origins of these kinds of appraisals, finding that patients who believe themselves to be less powerful and lower in social rank than most other people are especially likely to regard themselves as subordinate to their voices.[28] Patients' relationships with their voices, it seems, mirror their relationships with other people.

A slightly different approach to understanding patients' appraisals of their hallucinations has been taken by my colleague in Manchester, Tony Morrison, who has suggested that patients' interpretations of their voices might be influenced by their more general beliefs about the mind.[29] These kinds of *metacognitive beliefs* (literally, beliefs about beliefs) are known to play a role in obsessional thinking. For example, people who complain about intrusive thoughts often have excessive expectations of their mental efficiency, catastrophic fears about losing control of their thoughts, and superstitious beliefs about the consequences of this happening (for example, 'If I did not control a worrying thought, and then what I worried about really happened, it would be my fault'). In a recent study, he has compared patients who hear voices with patients suffering from persecutory delusions, patients suffering from panic attacks, and ordinary people, finding that the hallucinating group had more dysfunctional metacognitive beliefs than any of the other groups.[30]

Hear One Moment and Not the Next

Most people who hear voices do not hear them continuously or, if they do, the loudness and content of the voices vary. Research that has explored factors influencing these changes has provided important clues about the psychological mechanisms involved in experiencing hallucinations. Three factors appear to be particularly important.

Believing is seeing

The findings of Romme and Escher in Holland, and Chadwick, Birchwood and Morrison in Britain, suggest that patients' beliefs about their voices may influence how they are experienced, a conclusion that seems to be supported by the cross-cultural and historical studies that we examined at earlier in the book. American psychologist Ihsan Al-Issa has suggested that the positive attitude taken towards hallucinations in some developing countries reflects philosophical perspectives that differ markedly from the dominant philosophy of the Western world.[31] In Western societies, where scientific materialism prevails, the need to distinguish between what is 'real' and what is 'imaginary' seems self-evident whereas, in less materialistic cultures, this distinction is less important.

Al-Issa's survey of the cross-cultural evidence revealed that visual hallucinations are more commonly reported by psychiatric patients in non-Western countries than by patients in the developed world, a finding that was supported by evidence from the WHO study of the Determinants of Outcome of Severe Mental Disorders.[32] Similar differences have been observed in historical comparisons. Herman Lenz studied psychiatric records in Vienna that dated back over 100 years, finding that visual hallucinations were more often recorded at the end of the nineteenth century than in modern times.[33] There is also evidence that the typical content of hallucinations has changed with the passing of centuries. Hallucinatory experiences recorded during the Middle Ages were almost always religious in content, whereas those reported by modern psychiatric patients often have persecutory or technological themes[34] (one of my patients was convinced that the local police force was talking to him via a radio receiver that they had surgically implanted inside his head).

The suspicion that these kinds of cross-cultural and historical differences reflect differences in people's beliefs and expectations is fuelled by the results of studies in which hallucinations have been induced by suggestion. One of the first studies of this sort was carried out, not with psychiatric patients, but with students at a secretarial college. In the early 1960s, American social psychologists Theodore Barber and David Calverley attempted to demonstrate that most if not all hypnotic phenomena were caused by compliance with the hypnotist's unusual instructions, rather than by the induction of a special trance state. In one of a series of experiments, they simply asked their group of secretarial students to close their eyes and listen to the record 'White Christmas', but did not actually play it. When questioned afterwards, about 5 per cent of the students said that they had heard the record.[35]

When psychologists Sanford Mintz and Murray Alpert repeated this procedure with psychiatric patients in New York,[36] they found that the 'White Christmas' effect was more pronounced in patients who were experiencing hallucinations than in non-hallucinating patients or ordinary people, a finding that one of my postgraduate students, Heather Young, was later able to replicate.[37]

The role of external stimulation

The second factor that is known to influence hallucinations is external stimulation. Classical definitions of hallucination, for example Esquirol's, imply that hallucinations occur in the absence of any stimulus. Of course this cannot be strictly true; there is always some kind of stimulus around. Patients' accounts of their experiences often reveal the influence of this kind of background stimulation. For example, they may complain that their voices are worst when they are on their own at night, when they are in a crowd, or when they are close to electrical machinery such as fans and washing machines.

In one of the few experiments to assess systematically the impact of stimulation on hallucinations, Andrew Margo, David Hemsley and Peter Slade asked a small group of highly co-operative patients to sit in a sound-proofed room and listen to various kinds of sounds. The experiment included a sensory-restriction condition, in which the participants wore headphones through which no sound was played, and other conditions in which participants heard interesting speech, boring speech, speech in a foreign language, pop music, meaningless blips and 'white noise' (the kind of unpatterned hiss that can be heard from a mistuned radio). The main finding was that the patients' voices became worse (louder and longer in duration) during the sensory-restriction and white-noise conditions, but became less troublesome when the patients were listening to interesting speech. Margo and his colleagues also found that asking the patients to read aloud also seemed to suppress their hallucinations.[38] Figure 14.1 shows the results of an experiment that almost perfectly repeated these findings, which was recently carried out by Tony Gallagher and colleagues at Trinity College, Dublin.[39]

Stress and the impact of emotion

The third important factor that seems to affect hallucinations is emotional arousal. Clinical reports have documented cases of previously unaffected people who have experienced hallucinations following particularly stressful events, such as extended military operations,[40] being trapped in a coal-mine,[41] or after being taken hostage by terrorists. In the last case, a study by Ronald Siegel found that eight out of thirty-one terrorism victims experienced hallucinations varying from simple geometric shapes to complex memory images.[42]

However, perhaps the best evidence of a link between emotional stress and hallucinations has emerged from investigations of people who have recently suffered bereavement. In one study carried out in Britain it was found that over 13 per cent of recently widowed men and women had heard their dead spouse's voice.[43] In another, carried

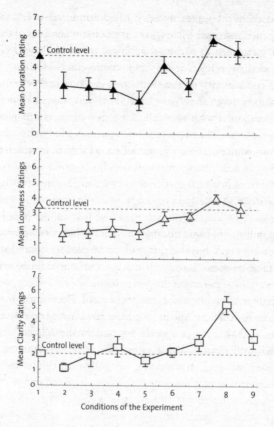

Key to conditions 1: control (sitting quietly); 2: reading aloud; 3: listening to interesting speech; 4: listening to boring speech; 5: listening to pop music; 6: listening to regular electronic blips; 7: listening to irregular electronic blips; 8: sensory restriction (wearing headphones and dark goggles); 9: white noise.

Figure 14.1 The effects of external stimulation on the duration, loudness and clarity of auditory hallucinations (from Gallagher, Dinin and Baker, 1994).

out in Sweden, 71 per cent of bereaved elderly people reported a hallucination, or hallucinatory-like experience, of their deceased partner.[44] The feeling that the deceased was present was particularly common. However, many of those surveyed reported seeing and talking to their dead spouse.[45] These kinds of experiences were usually comforting, and were most commonly reported by people who described their marriages as very happy. It is possible that many apparent encounters with ghosts are in fact hallucinations of this sort.[46]

As we have seen in earlier chapters, emotional arousal is usually accompanied by physiological phenomena, such as changes in the electrical conductivity of the skin (the electrodermal response). The relationship between these changes and hallucinations has hardly been investigated. However, one study has reported excessive fluctuations in skin conductance in hallucinating patients,[47] and, in another, these fluctuations were observed to coincide with the appearance of voices.[48]

Murmurings Within

We are now close to being able to construct a theory of hallucinations. Before we proceed, however, it will be helpful to remind ourselves about a facet of normal mental life that seems particularly relevant to the experiences of patients who hear voices.

In Chapter 8, I discussed the important phenomenon of inner speech, noting that we speak not only to other people but also to ourselves, and that silent speech directed to the self has important intellectual and emotional functions. We covertly comment to ourselves about what we have done, formulate our plans for the day ahead, keep transient memories (for example of telephone numbers) alive by rehearsing them, and wrestle with problems that we find emotionally challenging. However, despite the apparent silence of inner speech, it is accompanied by small activations of the speech muscles – a phenomenon known as *subvocalization*. These activations, which can be recorded using a machine called an *electromyograph*, occur because, in early childhood, we first learn to talk to ourselves out loud, and only later learn to suppress overt speech when no one else is listening. Subvocalization, therefore, is a neuromuscular echo of a time when we did not know how to speak silently.

By now the reader will have realized why I took the trouble to discuss inner speech at length. As Ivan Leudar and Phil Thomas noted from their interviews with people who heard voices, the most common form of auditory hallucination – a voice or voices issuing instructions – mirrors the most common form of inner speech, which is a stream of instructions issued to the self.[49] Other forms of auditory hallucination reflect less common forms of inner speech. For example, most people occasionally lapse into an inner debate or dialogue, in which different arguments or points of view are played off against each other. This form of inner speech is similar to the kind of auditory hallucination in which voices discuss the perceiver's actions among themselves. The inescapable conclusion is that auditory hallucinations *are* inner speech.

Hard evidence supporting this idea has been available since the late 1940s, when the first electromyographic studies of hallucinating patients were conducted at Norwich State Hospital in Connecticut by American psychiatrist Louis Gould.[50] In his first experiment, using equipment that must be judged crude by modern standards, Gould conducted EMG assessments of 100 patients, finding raised muscular activity in the lips and chins of those who experienced voices. In a later study, he was able to show that the onset of this activity coincided with patients' reports of hallucinations. This finding has since been repeated many times. Two Japanese psychiatrists, Tsuyoshi Inouye and Akira Shimizu, reported in 1970 that they had been able to time precisely the onset of increased activity in the speech muscles, and showed that this happened just a few seconds before their patients reported hearing voices. They also found that the duration and amplitude of the EMG activity they recorded corresponded with the duration and apparent loudness of their patients' voices.[51]

In two extraordinary case studies, researchers investigating the inner speech hypothesis even found that it was possible to *record and listen to* their patients' voices. The first was conducted by Louis Gould, who used a sensitive microphone and amplifier to detect rapid subvocal speech in one of his patients.[52] In a later study, British psychologists Paul Green and Martin Preston were able to record the whispers of a male patient who said that he was hearing the voice of a woman. When they amplified and played back their recordings to their patient this had the surprising (and as yet unexplained) effect of making his speech less and less silent, until both sides of the conversation between the patient and the voice could be clearly heard without the aid of special equipment.[53]

Compelling though the electromyographical data are, they do not exhaust the physiological evidence in favour of the inner speech hypothesis. Hallucinations should be accompanied, not only by activation of the speech muscles, but also by activation of the centres in the

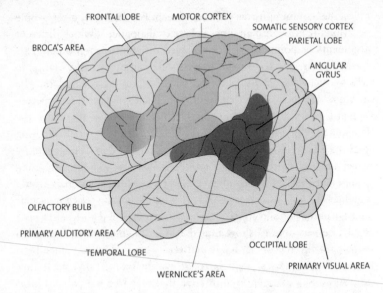

FRONTAL LOBE MOTOR CORTEX

SOMATIC SENSORY CORTEX

PARIETAL LOBE

BROCA'S AREA

ANGULAR
GYRUS

OLFACTORY BULB

PRIMARY AUDITORY AREA

OCCIPITAL LOBE

TEMPORAL LOBE

PRIMARY VISUAL AREA

WERNICKE'S AREA

Figure 14.2 The left cerebral hemisphere of the brain, showing Broca's and Wernicke's areas (from N. Gershwind (1979) 'Specializations of the human brain', in *The Brain: A Scientific American Book*. San Francisco: Freeman).

brain that control language. Since the middle years of the nineteenth century, it has been known that, in the majority of people, these centres are located on the left side of the brain. An area of the left frontal cortex, identified by the French neurologist Paul Broca in the 1860s, appears to be particularly important in speech generation, so that damage to this area causes a form of *expressive aphasia*, in which the ability to transform verbal ideas into speech patterns is impaired. A second important area, located in the left temporal lobe, was discovered by the German neurologist and psychiatrist Karl Wernicke at approximately the same time. Damage to this area causes a disorder known as *Wernicke's aphasia*, in which language comprehension is particularly disrupted.

An attempt to measure brain activations in hallucinating patients by means of EEG, reported in 1982, found that the onset of auditory hallucinations coincided with an increase in activity in the left temporal lobe.[54] This initial finding was later supplemented by evidence gathered by means of the new functional neuroimaging technologies, which allow activations in particular brain regions to be visualized with a precision that far exceeds that achievable with the best EEG equipment. Using single positron emission tomography (SPET) (a forerunner of PET) with a small group of co-operating patients, British psychiatrists Philip McGuire, G. M. Shah and Robin Murray were able to confirm that the onset of auditory hallucinations coincided with increased blood flow in the left temporal lobe, and also in Broca's area.[55]

A later study by David Silbersweig and colleagues, using PET, also found that auditory hallucinations were associated with activation of the left frontal cortex, together with structures deeper in the brain (various subcortical nuclei and paralimbic regions). They also studied a single drug-free patient who experienced combined auditory and visual hallucinations in which a disembodied head talked to him. These hallucinations were associated with activations not only in the auditory association cortex (near Wernicke's area in the temporal lobe) but also in the visual association cortex towards the rear of the brain, which is involved in processing visual imagery.[56]

Taken together, the EMG, EEG, SPET and PET findings strongly support the theory that auditory hallucinations consist of inner speech. The findings from the investigation by David Silbersweig and colleagues, which was unique in studying a patient with visual hallucinations, also imply that visual hallucinations consist of visual imagery. As Ralf Hoffman, a psychiatrist at Yale University, has pointed out, these discoveries therefore suggest that *people who experience hallucinations are mistaking their own thoughts and imaginings for things they are hearing or seeing.*[57] Hoffman attempted to explain why these errors occur, by suggesting that a difficulty in planning speech might lead hallucinating patients to experience their speech as unintended and therefore alien to themselves. According to this idea, we mentally formulate a speech plan before we speak, and we recognize our speech as self-generated because it matches the plan. The hallucinating patient, who lacks a plan, is unable to do this.

For some reason, this theory has attracted the attention of a number of professional philosophers, who have enjoyed pointing out various logical difficulties that it creates. Kathleen Akins and Daniel Dennett have objected that the idea that speech is normally preceded by a plan seems to create an infinite regress.[58] If intelligent behaviour requires a plan, the plan itself (which is evidently intelligent) must surely also require a plan, and so we go on for ever. Of course, Hoffman might escape this objection by arguing that not all speech requires a plan, and that it is only unplanned speech that is mistaken for a voice. However, as G. Lynn Stephens and George Graham have observed, when we come to consider the origins of speech plans this version of the theory still leads us into a logical dead end.[59] Presumably speech plans could themselves be intended or unintended. If they are intended, they must require a plan, and we are back in the Akins–Dennett regress. If, on the other hand, speech plans are unintended, Hoffman's theory leads us to conclude that they should be experienced as alien and, presumably therefore, the speech that follows from them would be experienced as alien also.

The answer to these conundrums is not to reject Hoffman's proposal that auditory hallucinations are inner speech, but to look more carefully at the processes involved in recognizing that thoughts and images are self-generated.

How we Recognize the Real

Most of us take for granted the process of distinguishing between our thoughts and images and the things we hear or see. The experiences of people who hallucinate remind us that the mechanisms responsible for this process are anything but self-evident. There are good philosophical and scientific reasons for supposing that we do not have *a priori* knowledge of whether a perceived event is something that we have generated by ourselves, or something that is generated by an agency or process external to the self.

The philosophical argument follows from Ludwig Wittgenstein's analysis of the difficulties involved in describing our mental states. We saw in Chapter 7 that emotional states cannot be identified by brute introspection, because they do not come with appropriate labels attached to them. Similarly, there is no reason to believe that perceptual states have the labels 'real' or 'imaginary' printed on them. We have to infer how best to describe any particular experience from whatever information there is available to us, and there is no unique source of information that we can rely on in order to make this judgement.

Scientific research on our ability to discriminate between mental events (thoughts and emotions) and events in the world (someone speaking to us or standing in front of us) has been pursued over the last two decades by American experimental psychologist Marcia Johnson.[60] Johnson calls this ability *source monitoring* and she has focused, in particular, on our ability to tell the difference between memories of things we have perceived and memories of things we have thought ourselves. As Johnson points out, professional scientists and artists often get into disputes following a failure of this kind of source monitoring. This usually results in someone claiming credit for an idea that originated from someone else, but occasionally the opposite kind of error can occur. (The songwriter Paul McCartney woke one morning with a tune that was later to be the hit song 'Yesterday' running through his mind, and spent days checking whether he had heard it from someone else.)[61]

There is not enough space here to describe Johnson's many elegant experiments. It is sufficient to say that she has shown that accurate source monitoring depends on a variety of cues. For example, we often make use of contextual information about time and location to decide whether an event has 'really happened'. The inherent plausibility of the experience may also be important – if we recall ourselves per- forming acts that violate the laws of nature we are likely to realize that we are remembering a dream. Sensory qualities also play a role, since the more vivid our memory of an event, the more likely we are to believe that it really happened. Johnson has also shown that the mental operations we use when generating a thought may provide us with useful information. Try thinking of a vehicle beginning with C – it is probably not difficult to come up with an answer. Now try thinking of a vegetable beginning with O – most people find this much more difficult.* When thinking of the vegetable, you may have been aware

* The most common and least difficult answer to the vehicle question is 'car'. Suitable answers to the vegetable question are 'onion' or 'ocra'. We know how difficult these questions are for English-speakers thanks to one of the most labori- ous studies ever carried out by psychologists, in which thousands of North Ameri- cans were asked to think of examples of each category (W. F. Battig and W. E. Montague (1969) 'Category norms for verbal items in 56 categories: a replication and extension of the Connecticut category norms', *Journal of Experimental Psy- chology Monographs*, 80: 1–46). The results of this study have proved immensely useful to other psychologists like myself, because they enable us to devise tests that vary in difficulty.

of a feeling of 'cognitive effort' as you searched your mind for an appropriate exemplar. At a later time, you will be able to remember this feeling, which will help you recognize that you were not told the name of the vegetable in question, but thought of it yourself. (The role of cognitive effort explains Paul McCartney's confusion about the authorship of 'Yesterday'. Apparently, the composition of the song had not been accompanied by the cognitive effort necessary for him to realize that the song was his.)

Marcia Johnson's research tells us that source monitoring is a skill, much like the skill of discriminating between rhinoceroses and elephants. Imagine that you are a game warden and, in order to conduct some kind of zoological research, you are required to shoot with an anaesthetic dart the former beast but not the latter. You are standing in a jungle clearing, when a large grey animal charges into view. Pulling the trigger, you discover to your dismay that you have knocked out an elephant. On asking yourself how you could have made such a bad mistake, you will discover that your judgement was undermined by the same factors that undermine the source-monitoring judgements of hallucinating patients.

Perhaps your beliefs and expectations overrode the evidence of your eyes. One of your companions may have told you that only rhinoceroses live at this particular location. You therefore assumed that you were seeing a rhinoceros and pulled the trigger without making sure. Similarly, hallucinators who mistake their inner speech or mental imagery for voices or visions of other people may be influenced by what they expect to hear or see. This is why culture has such a profound impact on hallucinations. Someone who grows up in a society that recognizes the existence of ghosts, or that values spiritual experiences, will be more likely to mistake the mental image of a deceased relative for an apparition than someone who has grown to maturity in a society that emphasizes the scientific world view.

Another possibility is that your judgement was impaired by degradation of the stimulus. You may have been stalking your prey in darkness, or your view may have been obscured by foliage, so that it was difficult to tell a rhinoceros from an elephant. Our ability to vary the level of evidence required before deciding that a stimulus is present, allows us to be flexible when making judgements about the external world. In situations in which our perception of our surroundings is degraded, it is often necessary to adopt a weak 'criterion' for deciding that an expected event has in fact occurred. (The rustle of the under-growth, and the vague perception of a bulky object moving before us, may be enough to persuade us that we are in the presence of a rhinoceros.) For similar reasons, hallucinating patients are especially likely to mistake their thoughts for voices in conditions in which there is very little external stimulation (for example, when alone at night), or when external stimulation is chaotic and unpatterned (for example, in the middle of a noisy crowd, or when bombarded by white noise during a psychology experiment).

Finally, stress and a sense of urgency may have played a role. You may have feared that a failure to anaesthetize the rhinoceros quickly would leave you vulnerable to being charged and injured. Of course, stress undermines mental efficiency. The extent to which we process the information that is available to us is reduced, and our decisions tend to be hasty and less accurate as a consequence. Just as we are more likely to pull the trigger inappropriately when adrenalin is run-ning through our veins so, too, patients under stress are especially likely to mistake their imaginings for real events.

The influence of these factors on the source-monitoring judgements of hallucinating patients is illustrated in Figure 14.3. I have laboured my analogy with hunting because the idea that source monitoring is a skill is not intuitively obvious to many people. After all, we rarely consciously think about the source of our perceptions, and source-monitoring judgements are nearly always automatic (but, then, so are many of our judgements about rhinoceroses and elephants). The analogy shows how hallucinations arise from an error of judgement rather than an error of perception. It also shows how hallucinating can be explained in terms of the same kinds of mental processes that affect normal perceptual judgements.

Testing the Source-Monitoring Hypothesis

The argument we have pursued so far states that people who halluci-nate make faulty judgements about the sources of their experiences, and it is for this reason that they mistake their inner speech or visual imagery for stimuli external to themselves. However, we have not so

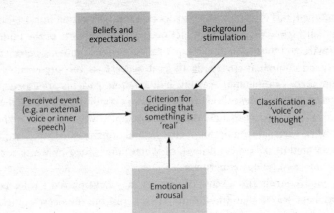

Figure 14.3 An outline model of hallucinatory experiences. Adapted from R. P. Bentall (2000) 'Hallucinatory experiences', in E. Cardena, S. J. Lynn and S. Krippner (eds.) *Varieties of Anomalous Experience: Examining the Scientific Evidence*, Washington, D.C.: American Psychological Association.

far considered direct evidence that hallucinating patients make this kind of error more frequently than other people. The experiments that have addressed this issue have been complex, and so the following account will necessarily highlight only the essential elements of key studies.

Source monitoring for memories

The earliest source-monitoring experiment with hallucinating patients was reported by psychologist Arthur Heilbrun in 1980.[62] Heilbrun, based at Emory University in Atlanta, USA, interviewed hallucinating and non-hallucinating patients and recorded their opinions about a number of topics. Their verbatim remarks were later included in a multiple-choice test alongside other statements which were similar but not identical. The hallucinators had particular difficulty when asked to recognize their own statements, and were less able to do this than the non-hallucinating patients.

Since this promising start, other source-monitoring experiments have been conducted with hallucinating patients by Heilbrun, by myself and by other investigators.[63] Rather than describing each of these experiments in detail, I will focus on a recent study reported by Liverpool-based psychologists Peter Rankin and Pierce O'Carrol, which highlights some of the complexities involved in this kind of research.[64] Rankin and O'Carrol decided not to study patients, but instead compared students who had high scores on a questionnaire measure of hallucinatory experiences with students who had low scores. Their experimental design was based on the work of Marcia Johnson. The students were asked to learn 'paired associates' (pairs of words, for example, 'vehicle–car'). Sometimes the word-pairs were presented to the students and at other times their memory was tested by presenting them with the first word in each pair and asking them to recall the second (for example, 'Which word goes with "vehicle"?'). The number of times that the words were presented and tested was cunningly varied so that, for example, some of the words were presented many times but tested on only a few occasions, whereas others were presented on only a few occasions but tested on many. At the end of this sequence of presentation and testing, the participants were asked to say how many times they thought they had been presented with each item. As Marcia Johnson had previously found, participants gave inflated estimates for those words which had been most tested, indicating that they were mistaking occasions on which they had recalled the words for occasions on which the words had been presented. In Rankin and O'Carrol's study, this effect was most evident in those students who scored high on the hallucination measure, indicating that these people were most prone to misattributing their mental events (the times they recalled the words) for events in the world (presentations).

Despite these positive results, experimental studies of source monitoring for memories with psychiatric patients, using similar methods, have produced mixed results. In one investigation, Gus Baker, Sue Havers and I found that patients who experienced hallucinations were especially likely to mistake words that they had generated themselves for words that they had heard,[65] but Mark Seal and his colleagues in Melbourne, Australia, failed to find the same result with an almost identical procedure.[66] More recently, a similar study was conducted by Gildas Brebion at the New York State Psychiatric Institute and his colleagues, who *did* find evidence that hallucinators were more likely than non-hallucinating patients to misattribute to an external source words that they had produced themselves.[67]

Monitoring current perceptions

One reason why the experiments we have considered so far may have been inconclusive is that they have focused on source monitoring for memories. However, hallucinations presumably involve errors in the source monitoring of *current* perceptions. The measurement of these kind of errors is particularly challenging, and was the focus of my first experimental study of hallucinations, which utilized a technique known as signal detection theory (SDT).

SDT is a mathematical model of perceptual judgement. When I was a psychology student, it was one of my least favourite topics in the undergraduate curriculum, partly because I found its mathematical realization hard going. It was with some dismay that I later concluded that SDT was exactly what I needed to test the source-monitoring theory of hallucinations. In order to avoid generating the same level of distress in my readers, I will try to outline the basic idea behind the theory in a non-mathematical form (see Figure 14.4 for a diagrammatic explanation).

SDT attempts to explain how we decide that we really are perceiving something. Although this is precisely the problem confronted by the person suffering from hallucinations, the theory was initially designed to account for our ability to detect weak stimuli (or 'signals' in the jargon of the theory) when working with communication devices such as telephones or radios. Imagine that you are in a darkened room. You think that you have seen a chink of light but you cannot be certain. Before the 1960s, psychologists would explain what happens in these circumstances by 'threshold theory', according to which the light is perceived only if it is above a certain magnitude. However, attempts to measure the thresholds for particular kinds of stimuli (lights or noises) failed to yield consistent results, so a different kind of approach was required.

SDT proposes that our ability to detect a signal in these kinds of circumstances depends on two factors. The first factor is *perceptual sensitivity*, which might be thought of as the efficiency of our perceptual system. The greater our perceptual sensitivity, the easier it is to detect signals. The second factor is known as *perceptual bias*, which can be thought of as our willingness to assume that the signal is present.

	Signal detection		Source monitoring	
	Judged present	Judged absent	Judged present	Judged absent
Stimulus present	HIT	MISS	'It's real'	'There's nothing there'
Stimulus absent	False alarm	Correct rejection	Hallucination	'It's my imagination'

Figure 14.4 Relationship between choices made in signal-detection experiments and source-monitoring judgements. High perceptual sensitivity results in a high proportion of hits and correct rejections and few signal-detection errors (misses and false alarms). Increasing bias towards detecting signals results in more hits and fewer misses, but at the expense of an increase in false alarms and a decrease in correct rejections (from R. P. Bentall (2000) 'Hallucinatory experiences', in E. Cardena, S. J. Lynn and S. Krippner (eds.), *Varieties of Anomolous Experience: Examining the Scientific Evidence*. Washington, DC: American Psychological Association).

Unlike perceptual sensitivity, which can only be affected by fairly gross physiological changes, perceptual bias can change from moment to moment, and is particularly affected by our beliefs and expectations.

Despite the dangers of analogy-overload, I will resort to one more in the hope of making these ideas clear. In a typical signal-detection experiment, participants listen to bursts of white noise, some of which contain a signal (for example, a brief voice). After each burst, the participant is asked to say whether the signal was present or not. In these circumstances, the participant is behaving like a Cold War radar operator whose job is to detect a possible incoming Soviet air strike. Four things can happen. The person can detect the signal (the Soviets attack, the radar operator spots them and they are intercepted), which is known as a 'hit'. The person can also correctly fail to report a signal (a 'correct rejection'). However, there are also two kinds of possible error: a 'miss' (the Soviets strike without being spotted, so that civilization as we know and love it is laid to waste) and a 'false alarm' (the radar operator incorrectly believes that the Soviet air force is on its way, and a lot of aviation fuel is wasted before the error is discovered).

Pursuing this analogy further, an improvement in perceptual sensitivity is equivalent to an upgrade of the radar system, resulting in an increase in hits and correct rejections and a decrease in misses and false alarms. However, a change in perceptual bias involves a greater willingness to believe that the signal is present without any improvement in sensitivity, as if the radar operator's haste to sound the alarm is influenced by the prevailing political climate. An increase in bias (for example, during periods of political tension such as the Cuban missile crisis) will produce an increased probability of a hit (if the Soviets come they will be detected) but also an increase in false alarms (the nervous radar operator will be more likely to scramble the intercepting aircraft unnecessarily). A decrease in bias (perhaps following a period of détente) will reduce the risk of false alarms (aviation fuel will be conserved) but increase the risk of misses (if the Soviets do attack unexpectedly, they have a better chance of getting through).

By now, it should be obvious that false alarms are the hallucinations of signal detection theory. The theory therefore provides us with a method for determining whether hallucinations are the product of perceptual problems (which would be evident as impaired perceptual sensitivity) or biased source monitoring. Peter Slade and I therefore conducted two signal-detection experiments, one comparing hallucinating and non-hallucinating patients and one comparing students who had high scores on a hallucination questionnaire with students who had low scores. Both involved participants listening to many brief episodes of white noise in order to detect occasions when a voice was also present in the background. Applying a bit of mathematics to the participants' judgements allowed us obtain separate measures for sensitivity and bias. The results, which are shown in Figure 14.5, show clearly that the hallucinating participants differed from their respective control participants in bias but not in sensitivity.[68]

This finding was later replicated by Peter Rankin and Pierce O'Carrol in their study of Liverpool students,[69] and also, using a slightly different methodology, in an experiment conducted with patients by Gildas Brebion and his colleagues.[70] Overall, these observations are consistent with our hypothesis that hallucinations arise from peculiar judgements about what is real, rather than from deficits in patients' perceptual systems.

Other researchers have devised simpler methods for measuring

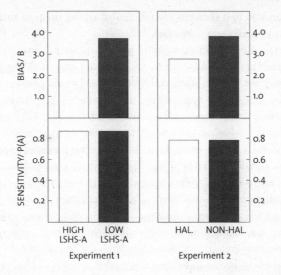

Figure 14.5 Bias (B) and sensitivity (P(A)) scores from signal-detection experiments conducted by Bentall and Slade (1985). The left panels show comparisons between students scoring high and low on the Launay–Slade Hallucination Scale (LSHS-A), and the right panels show comparisons between hallucinating and non-hallucinating schizophrenia patients. Note that low B scores indicate a strong bias towards detecting signals.

source monitoring for perceptions. My colleague Tony Morrison has carried out a series of experiments in which participants were asked to provide associations for words which were either emotionally positive (for example, 'courage'), emotionally negative (for example, 'crazy') or neutral (for example, 'bookcase'). Immediately after responding to each cue word, the participants were asked to rate their responses for 'internality' ('How much was the word that came to mind your own?'). The hallucinating patients gave much lower ratings (stating that the words that came to mind did not seem to be their own) than the other participants, especially when the cue words were either positively or negatively emotionally salient.[71] In a recent study that followed up these findings, Morrison found that these effects were more marked when patients were first encouraged to focus their thoughts on themselves (by first being required to make up a short story about themselves) and were less evident when the patients' attention was first directed elsewhere (by asking them to make up a short story about someone else).[72]

An even more direct measure of immediate source monitoring has been developed by Louise Johns and Phil McGuire at the Institute of Psychiatry in London. Johns and McGuire had participants speak into a microphone. Their speech was immediately played back to them through earphones after being distorted electronically. They were then asked to say whether the speech they were hearing was theirs or someone else's. In this experiment, hallucinating patients, in comparison with non-hallucinating patients and ordinary people, were much more likely to say that their voice belonged to someone else, especially if the content of what was being said was derogatory.[73]

This progress in establishing that hallucinating patients experience difficulty with source monitoring has been matched by progress in identifying the neural structures involved. Of course, we should not expect these to be the same structures as those involved in generating the inner speech which hallucinating people mistake for a voice. In a study carried out in Toronto, Canada, Henry Szechtman and his colleagues PET scanned ordinary people, some of whom were highly hypnotizable and had been selected for their ability to experience hypnotic hallucinations. Blood flow to different regions of the brain was measured as the participants listened to speech, imagined speech and, in the case of the hypnotizable participants, hallucinated a voice. A region in the area on the right side of the cerebral cortex known as the right anterior cingulate (also known as Brodmann area 32)* was found to be active in the hypnotizable participants when they heard or hallucinated a voice, but not when they imagined hearing it. The same conditions did not cause similar activations in the non-hypnotizable participants. Szechtman and his colleagues have concluded that the right anterior cingulate may contain neural circuits that are responsible for deciding whether experiences originate from the external world.[74]

---

* Brodmann areas are locations on the cerebral cortex defined according to a map developed by the German anatomist Korbinian Brodmann during the first decade of the twentieth century.

Unfinished Business

In this chapter I have tried to tell a story about how hallucinations have become amenable to psychological analysis. I have focused on auditory hallucinations, and have shown that they occur when people mistake their inner speech for the speech of others. This mistake seems to result from a failure of the psychological mechanisms that normally allow us to tell the difference between the things that we are thinking and the things that we are hearing. However, as a model of hallucinations, the story is obviously incomplete.

Some researchers, notably Ivan Leudar and Phil Thomas, have questioned whether it is accurate to characterize hallucinating people as poor at source monitoring, because people who hear voices usually make very clear distinctions between their hallucinations and their thoughts.[75] The implication of this observation is that the hallucinating person experiences only *some* mental events as alien, and correctly identifies others as self-generated. A related objection to the account that I have offered is that it has treated source monitoring as an 'all-or-nothing' phenomenon. The experiences of patients who have pseudohallucinations or who suffer from thought insertion suggest that source monitoring can fail to varying degrees or in different ways. As philosophers G. Lynn Stephens and George Graham have pointed out, thought insertion seems to be particularly difficult to explain, because patients having this symptom describe their experiences as thoughts but deny that the thoughts are their own.[76]

It seems likely that the selective failure of source monitoring can be partly explained by taking into account the environmental factors that are known to influence source-monitoring judgements. However, other factors almost certainly play a role. Earlier, when I discussed the work of Marcia Johnson, I pointed out that source monitoring in ordinary people is less efficient for automatic thoughts than for thoughts that require considerable cognitive effort. (When you struggle hard to think of something, you know that it is you who is doing the thinking – a modern spin on Descartes' famous dictum 'cogito ergo sum'.) It therefore follows that highly automatic thoughts are particularly likely to be misattributed to an alien source. Of course, as we discussed in the context of depression, negative thoughts about the self are usually highly automatic, so it is not surprising that psychiatric patients often mistake these kinds of thoughts for voices. Interestingly, when Tony Morrison and Caroline Baker questioned a group of hallucinating patients about their experiences, they found that they reported, in addition to their voices, many more intrusive thoughts than ordinary people. These thoughts were usually interpreted as distressing and uncontrollable.[77]

A second possibility is that people's reactions to their hallucinations help to determine which particular thoughts are misattributed in the future. Tony Morrison draws a parallel between hallucinations and intrusive thoughts that is helpful in this context.[78] People who are troubled by obsessions often struggle to suppress them, a strategy that can be counterproductive. Just as the injunction not to think of a white bear immediately evokes an image of a snow-coloured furry animal, so too, in ordinary people at least, the effort not to think of ideas that are disturbing appears to guarantee that these ideas recur.[79] As Morrison has pointed out, in hallucinating patients, this effect (another example of the reaction-maintenance principle) might well lead to further experiences of the very thoughts that the individual believes are alien.

A third possibility, suggested by G. Lynn Stephens and George Graham, is that thoughts are misattributed elsewhere when they are experienced as ego-dystonic (that is, not consistent with the individual's current beliefs about the self). As they point out, this might happen for a variety of reasons. For example, taking up a suggestion by the psychologist and philosopher Louis Sass,[80] they suggest that the hallucinating person may be unable to construct an integrated representation of his thoughts, emotions and actions, in order to make sense of his hallucinated thoughts. Alternatively, perhaps the hallucinating patient denies that she is the agent of an experience because she cannot explain it in terms of her conception of her own intentional psychology ('Someone like myself would never have a thought like this'). (The availability of an alternative explanation for an experience – for example, that it is a ghost – presumably makes this more likely.) Interesting though these speculations are, they have yet to be properly tested by researchers.

Even if one or more of these three proposals should turn out to be supported by future research, they probably fail to provide a completely satisfactory account of the hallucinating person's source-monitoring difficulties. Here are a few questions that remain unanswered: Why do some patients experience their intrusive thoughts as voices outside themselves, some experience them as voices inside their heads, and still others experience them as thoughts that have been inserted into their minds by other people? (Possibly because, once source-monitoring failures occur, different patients form different theories in order to explain their experiences.) Why do hallucinations typically begin during periods of stress or trauma? (Possibly because these periods tend to provoke a flood of intrusive, automatic thoughts about the self.) More importantly, perhaps, why is it that some people seem to be more vulnerable to source-monitoring failures than the rest of us? Could it be that they never learn to monitor efficiently in the first place, but manage to function adequately until their source-monitoring ability is further compromised by some kind of trauma? (I will discuss this idea further in Chapter 18.) Or could it be that people who later hallucinate have some kind of subtle dysfunction of the neural circuits that are responsible for source monitoring? (Henry Szechtman's findings suggest that these circuits are located in the right anterior cingulate, but do not tell us whether they are damaged in hallucinating people.)

The search for answers to these questions will probably keep psychologists busy for a few years yet.

The Language of Madness

Language is the light of the mind.   John Stuart Mill[1]

In this review of what is known about psychotic complaints I have held back until the end discussion of the symptom that has been subjected to the most extensive psychological analysis. I have done so because much of the relevant research has been misdirected by false assumptions made by the founders of modern psychiatry. We will see that even the term commonly used to describe this symptom – *thought disorder* – is fraught with difficulty.

Misunderstanding the Problem?

I have presented examples of thought disorder in earlier chapters, when discussing the work of Eugen Bleuler in Chapter 2 and when debating the boundaries of madness in Chapter 5. On the surface, at least, the speech of the thought-disordered patient seems jumbled and incoherent – in extreme cases it is sometimes described as a 'word salad'. When encountering thought-disordered patients for the first time, the neophyte clinician, like the layperson, might be forgiven for assuming that here, at last, is a symptom that unequivocally meets Karl Jaspers' criterion of unundestandability. This was certainly how Kraepelin regarded the speech of mad people, as revealed in the following case presentation to medical students:

The patient I will show you today has almost to be carried into the room, as he walks in a straddling fashion on the outside of his feet. On coming in, he throws off his slippers, sings a hymn loudly, and then cries twice (in English),

'My father, my real father!' He is eighteen years old, and a pupil of the Oberrealschule [higher-grade school], tall, and rather strongly built, but with a pale complexion, on which there is very often a transient flush. The patient sits with his eyes shut, and pays no attention to his surroundings. He does not look up even when he is spoken to, but he answers beginning in a low voice, and gradually screaming louder and louder. When asked where he is, he says, 'You want to know that too? I tell you who is being measured and is measured and shall be measured. I know all that, and could tell you, but I do not want to.' When asked his name, he screams, 'What is your name? What does he shut? He shuts his eyes. What does he hear? He does not understand; he understands not. How? Who? Where? When? What does he mean? When I tell him to look he does not look properly. You there, just look! What is it? What is the matter? Attend: he attends not. I say, what is it, then? Why do you give me no answer? Are you getting impudent again? How can you be so impudent? I'm coming! I'll show you! You don't whore for me. You mustn't be smart either; you're an impudent, lousy fellow, such an impudent lousy fellow I've never met with. Is he beginning again? You understand nothing at all, nothing at all; nothing at all does he understand. If you follow now, he won't follow, will not follow. Are you getting still more impudent? Are you getting impudent still more? How they attend, they do attend,' and so on. In the end, he scolds in quite inarticulate sounds . . .[2]

Quoting this encounter more than half a century after it was published, the British anti-psychiatrist R. D. Laing drew attention to Kraepelin's own understanding of the exchange. According to Kraepelin:

Although he understood all the questions, *he has not given us a single useful piece of useful information*. His talk was . . . *only a series of disconnected sentences having no relation whatever to the general situation*.[3]

Research into thought disorder following Kraepelin has been dominated by a set of assumptions that was made explicit by Eugen Bleuler. Recall that, according to Bleuler, loosening of the associations is one of the most important features of the disorder. Elaborating on this hypothesis, he argued that the speech of psychotic patients is difficult to understand because 'Fragments of ideas are connected in an illogical way to create a new idea', and 'New ideas crop up which neither the patient nor the observer can bring into any connection with the previous stream of thought.' Bleuler described the results of simple psychological experiments in support of this analysis. For example:

In experimental investigations of associations, we find a notable frequency of 'mediate associations'. I suspect that only the lack of sufficient observation has been responsible for our inability to demonstrate them more frequently in the thought-processes of our patients. The above mentioned example [a patient had associated the death of a relative to the word 'wood'], the association 'wood (wood-coffin) – dead cousin' may be considered as a mediate association.[4]

Although a careful reading of Bleuler reveals that he did not believe speech to be merely an overt manifestation of thought, his account suggested to many later investigators that thought disorder is literally a disorder of thinking. Because thinking was seen as a proper object of psychological inquiry by even the most hard-nosed biological psychiatrist, the thinking of psychotic patients therefore began to receive special attention from psychologists. The consequence was a plethora of studies and theories published from the 1930s onwards. Some researchers suggested, for example, that schizophrenia patients fail to follow the rules of logic.[5] Others, such as the Russian developmental psychologist Lev Vygotsky[6] and the American neurologist Kurt Goldstein,[7] argued that schizophrenia patients were incapable of dealing with abstract ideas.

A particularly influential theory was developed by the American researcher Norman Cameron in the 1940s. Cameron, who was trained both in psychology and psychiatry, observed patients as they attempted psychological tests, and proposed ways of categorizing their unusual responses. For example, some responses could be classified under the term *asyndesis*, indicating the incorrect connecting of concepts that lacked genuine causal links (as in a patient attempting to explain why the wind blows, with 'Quickness, blood, heat of deer, length; driven power, motorized cylinder, strength'). Others, in which a term is replaced by an approximately related term, were classified as *metonymic distortion* (as in a patient saying that he was alive 'because you have *menu* three times a day; that's the physical').[8] Expanding on these ideas, Cameron eventually grouped all of these deviant responses under the single heading of *over-inclusion*, which he believed was a consequence of failing to limit attention to relevant stimuli.[9]

When experiments were conducted to test these early ideas, the results were often inconclusive, or could be interpreted in many different ways. In retrospect, it is now obvious that the research conducted during this period was constrained by two major limitations. First, as University of Wisconsin psychologists Loren and Jean Chapman pointed out in a seminal review published in 1973, most investigators had failed to establish that the patients they were studying were actually thought-disordered.[10] Because 'schizophrenia' was regarded as a lump, it was often assumed that any abnormality in thinking should be observable in all schizophrenic patients, regardless of their actual symptoms.

Second, as the linguists Sherry Rochester and J. R. Martin pointed out in their book *Crazy Talk*, published in 1979,[11] Blueler's identification of thought disorder with thinking had led researchers to neglect what psychotic patients were actually saying. Flying in the face of this trend, Rochester, of the Clark Institute in Toronto, and Martin, at the University of Sydney in Australia, argued that, as the only evidence of thought disorder is peculiar speech, speech and not thinking should be the focus of the psychopathologist's inquiries (see Figure 15.1). Furthermore, they pointed out that it is the incomprehensibility of the psychotic person's speech that leads to the diagnosis of thought disorder. They therefore suggested that the question, 'What is abnormal about psychotic thinking?' should be replaced with the more useful question, 'Why do ordinary listeners find psychotic speech so difficult to understand?'

Will the real symptoms of schizophrenia please stand up?

Rochester and Martin's approach to thought disorder amounted to something of a revolution in schizophrenia research. At the same time, other investigators were questioning other assumptions about the speech of psychotic patients. Nancy Andreasen, a prominent neo-Kraepelinian who had obtained a Ph.D. in literature before training in medicine, realized that research was only likely to progress if adequate criteria could be devised for determining when speech is psychotic. Like Rochester and Martin, she noted the anomalous status of the term 'thought disorder', suggested that it might be abandoned and, after careful consideration, proposed that it be replaced by the more

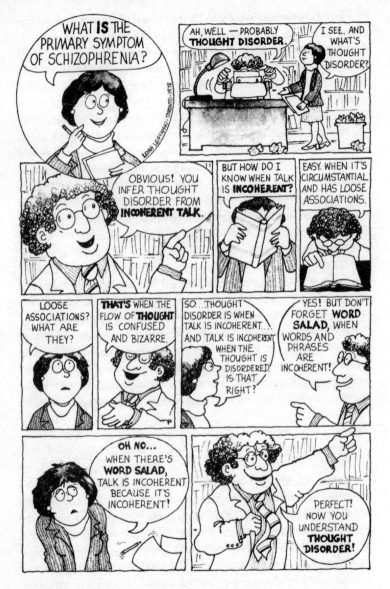

Figure 15.1 Cartoon (adapted from S. Rochester and J. R. Martin (1979). *Crazy Talk: A Study of the Discourse of Psychotic Speakers*, New York: Plenum) illustrating the problem of defining thought disorder.

precise but longer term, *disorder of thinking, language and communication*.[12]

Andreasen developed her Scale for the Assessment of Thought, Language and Communication (TLC Scale) in the hope that it would enable investigators to measure psychotic speech more precisely.[13] (In Chapter 5, p. 102 I described the use of this scale in a study of eccentrics.) On the basis of classic and modern accounts of thought disorder, and from observations of patients, she defined twenty different kinds of disordered speech, which are listed in Table 15.1. The scale provides fairly precise definitions, allowing each type of abnormality to be rated on a five-point scale. High inter-rater reliabilities can be obtained for these scores when raters are appropriately trained.

Factor analysis revealed that psychotic speech abnormalities fell into two main types. Items on the TLC Scale that reflected various kinds of speech incoherence fell into a single factor, which Andreasen labelled *positive thought, language and communication disorder*. However, some items, particularly poverty of speech (saying very little) and poverty of content of speech (speech with only vague content), fell into a second factor, which she labelled *negative thought, language and communication disorder*. (This distinction clearly maps on to the more general distinction between positive and negative symptoms of psychosis, which we considered in Chapter 4.)

When Andreasen used her scale to compare patients with different diagnoses, she found that some types of speech described in the classic literature of psychiatry – for example clanging, echolalia and neologisms – were so uncommon that they appeared to have very little practical significance. Others, for example tangentiality, derailment, incoherence, illogicality, loss of goal and perseveration, appeared to be equally common in schizophrenia and mania.[14] To Andreasen's surprise, the manic patients showed more evidence of positive thought, language and communication disorder than the schizophrenia patients, whereas the reverse was true of negative thought, language and communication disorder.[15] Positive thought, language and communication disorder, it seems, is not a specific complaint of schizophrenia patients.

Table 15.1 Main types of thought, language and communication disorder described by N. C. Andreasen (1979) 'The clinical assessment of thought, language and communication disorders', *Archives of General Psychiatry*, 36: 1315–21.

Type of disorder	Definition	Example
Poverty of speech	Restriction in the amount of spontaneous speech. Replies to questions are brief and concrete.	
Poverty of content of speech	Speech that conveys little information. Language is vague and over-abstract.	
Pressure of speech	An increase in the amount of spontaneous speech compared to what is considered customary.	
Distractible speech	During mid speech, the subject is changed in response to a stimulus.	'Then I left San Francisco and moved to . . . Where did you get that tie?'
Tangentiality	Replying to questions in an oblique, tangential or irrelevant manner.	Q: 'What city are you from?' A: 'Well, that's a hard question. I'm from Iowa. I really don't know where my relatives came from, so I don't know if I'm Irish or French.'
Derailment	Ideas slip off the track on to another which is obliquely related or unrelated.	'The next day when I'd be going out you know, I took control, like uh, I put bleach on my hair in California.'
Incoherence (word salad)	Speech that is incomprehensible at times.	Q: 'Why do people believe in God?' A: 'Because making a do in life. Isn't none of that stuff about evolution guiding isn't true any more.'

Type of disorder	Definition	Example
Illogicality	Conclusions are reached that do not follow logically (non sequiturs or faulty inductive inferences).	
Clanging	Sounds rather than meaningful relationships appear to govern words.	'I'm not trying to make noise. I'm trying to make sense. If you can make sense out of nonsense, well, have fun.'
Neologisms	New word formations.	'I got so angry I picked up a dish and threw it at the geshinker.'
Word approximations	Old words used in a new and unconventional way.	'His boss was a seeover.'
Circumstantiality	Speech that is very indirect and delayed at reaching its goal. Excessive long-windedness.	
Loss of goal	Failure to follow chain of thought to a natural conclusion.	
Perseveration	Persistent repetition of words or ideas.	'I think I'll put on my hat, my hat, my hat.'
Echolalia	Echoing of others' speech.	Q: 'Can we talk for a few minutes?' A: 'Talk for a few minutes.'
Blocking	Interruption of a train of speech before completed.	
Stilted speech	Speech excessively stilted and formal.	'The attorney comported himself indecorously.'
Self-reference	Patient repeatedly and inappropriately refers back to self.	Q: 'What's the time?' A: 'It's 7 o'clock. That's my problem.'
Phonemic paraphasia	Mispronunciation; syllables out of sequence.	'I slipped on the lice and broke my arm.'
Semantic paraphasia	Substitution of inappropriate word.	'I slipped on the coat, on the ice I mean, and broke my book.'

Meaning, Emotion and Disordered Speech

One further assumption about thought disorder has taken a tumble in the last few decades. It will be recalled that Kraepelin regarded his patient's disordered speech as merely 'a series of disconnected sentences having no relation whatever to the general situation'. Rochester and Martin's characterization of thought disorder as failed communication, in contrast, leaves open the possibility that the patient is attempting to communicate something of real importance to himself. This much was obvious to R. D. Laing, who found it is all too easy to comprehend the apparently bizarre utterances of Kraepelin's patient:

What does the patient appear to be doing? Surely he is carrying on a dialogue between his own parodied version of Kraepelin, and his own defiant rebelling self. 'You want to know that too? I tell you who is being measured and is measured and shall be measured. I know all that, and I could tell you, but I do not want to.' This seems to be plain enough talk. Presumably he deeply resents this form of interrogation, which is being carried out before a lecture room of students. He probably does not see what it has to do with the things that must be deeply distressing him. But these things would not be 'useful information' to Kraepelin except as further 'signs' of a 'disease'.

Kraepelin asks him his name. The patient replies by an exaggerated outburst in which he is now saying what he feels is the attitude implicit in Kraepelin's approach to him: What is your name? What does he shut? He shuts his eyes . . . Why do you give me no answer? Are you getting impudent again? You don't whore for me (i.e. he feels that Kraepelin is objecting because he is not prepared to prostitute himself before the whole classroom of students), and so on . . .

Now it seems clear that this patient's behaviour can be seen in at least two ways . . . One may see his behaviour as 'signs' of 'disease'; one may see his behaviour as expressive of his existence . . . What is the patient's experience of Kraepelin? He seems to be tormented and desperate. What is he 'about' in speaking and acting in this way? He is objecting to being measured and tested. He wants to be heard.[16]

Laing was correct in supposing that psychotic speech can often be accurately decoded by an empathetic clinician. Psychologist Martin Harrow and his psychiatrist colleague Mel Prosen, working in Chicago in the late 1970s, took the unusual step of asking patients to account for their apparently bizarre verbalizations.[17] Their patients were first asked to complete a few simple tests of verbal intelligence – for example, explaining the meaning of simple proverbs. Bizarre or idiosyncratic statements were then identified from the patients' tape-recorded answers. A week later, each patient was sensitively interviewed by Prosen, who said that he was interested in learning what had been in the patient's mind. Independent judges later evaluated each patient's tape-recorded explanations. It would have surprised Kraepelin to learn that the patients were often able to give coherent explanations of their incoherent speech. Their idiosyncratic statements often reflected the intrusion of personally salient ideas, for example memories from early life, a phenomenon that Harrow and Prosen described as 'intermingling'. Usually, the intermingled material centred around a variety of topics, rather than a single issue. It was as if the patient, when struggling to answer the intelligence questions, was constantly reminded of things that were more important to her, and was unable to stop herself from deviating from the task in hand.

It should therefore be no surprise that the quality of speech of thought-disordered patients depends on what they are trying to discuss. Although unequivocal evidence that this is the case has only recently become available, this possibility was considered by earlier researchers. Unfortunately, although many studies carried out during the 1950s and afterwards attempted to assess the thought and language of patients when they were presented with emotionally laden and emotionally neutral stimuli, the results were inconclusive, almost certainly because the emotionally laden material was not personally significant.[18] (For example, in a study carried out by Loren and Jean Chapman, patients were asked to solve analogy problems such as 'Vagina is to lock as penis is to . . . ?').[19] An exception was an experiment reported in 1972 by Algimantas Shimkunas, working at the University of Missouri, who interviewed patients in two conditions. In one, Shimkunas disclosed his own feelings about difficult interpersonal relationships and asked the patients to do the same; in the other, the same general themes were addressed but no pressure was put on the patients to talk about their feelings. Far more thought disorder was observed in the disclosure condition.[20]

Recent studies have supported Shimkunas' findings. In a small experiment conducted by Gill Haddock and myself, in which we used Andreasen's TLC Scale, we compared thought-disordered patients' speech when talking about emotionally neutral topics (for example, football) with their speech when talking about the circumstances leading to their admission to hospital. More thought disorder was evident in the second of these conditions.[21] Similar findings were obtained by American psychologist Nancy Docherty and her colleagues at Kent State University in Ohio, in a much more impressive and extensive series of investigations. Docherty examined the speech of schizophrenia patients when asked to talk about 'good memories of pleasant, nonstressful times' and when asked to talk about 'bad memories of stressful times'. In the different studies, communication disorder was measured in different ways, but a consistent pattern emerged – speech disturbance was markedly more evident when patients were asked to talk about negative topics.[22]

This effect of emotional arousal does not seem to be restricted to schizophrenia patients. Sara Tai, a clinical psychologist based in my own department, has recently shown that bipolar patients who are currently manic are especially sensitive to the topic of conversation.[23] Interestingly, she found that the speech of bipolar patients who are currently depressed is not affected in this way.

Drawing this evidence together, it seems that vulnerable individuals are most likely to speak in an incoherent way when they are emotionally aroused, and they are most likely to be emotionally aroused when talking about personal issues. This conclusion will probably fail to amaze any reader who has attempted to explain something complex to a friend while feeling distressed; however, the effect seems to be much more marked in psychotic patients than in ordinary people.

From Psychology to Language

Given that thought disorder appears to be primarily a disorder of communication, it is obviously important to examine the linguistic skills of affected people. In this context it is useful to distinguish between language comprehension and language production. The account I have given so far suggests that psychotic patients experience specific difficulties when generating speech, while, not surprisingly, their ability to understand the speech of others seems relatively unimpaired. William Grove and Nancy Andreasen examined the ability of schizophrenic and manic patients to understand spoken language, using a variety of measures, and also included a test of digit span (the ability to recall short sequences of numbers) in order to check that poor performance on their linguistic tests could not be attributed to global handicaps, such as poor attention or a lack of motivation. Although they expected their patients to perform poorly on the linguistic tests and not on the digit span measure, the opposite turned out to be the case.[24]

If thought-disordered patients can understand the speech of others, it might be expected that they would recognize when the speech of other patients is idiosyncratic. This prediction was supported by the results of a study carried out by Martin Harrow and Joan Miller. Patients were asked to explain the meaning of common proverbs and were then asked to judge their own answers and also the answers of other patients. Patients suffering from thought disorder failed to realize that their own incoherent answers were atypical. However, they accurately judged normal answers to be typical and the abnormal answers of other thought-disordered patients as idiosyncratic.[25]

It will be recalled that Rochester and Martin argued that researchers should attempt to find out why ordinary people find psychotic speech so difficult to understand.[26] In an early attempt to answer this question, Brendan Maher and his colleagues at Harvard University used a primitive computer program to analyse passages written* by schizophrenia patients.[27] This system worked by using a dictionary to look up and assign words to various categories. Prior to the analysis, a panel of judges divided the passages into those that were thought-disordered and those that were not. The main finding was that writing tended be judged thought-disordered when there were more objects than subjects, which usually happened at the end of sentences ('Doctor, I have pains in my chest and hope and wonder if my box is broken

---

* According to Eugen Bleuler ((1911/1950) *Dementia Praecox or the Group of Schizophrenias* (trans. E. Zinkin). New York: International Universities Press), 'The fact that the peculiarities of the associative process usually manifest themselves in an identical fashion, regardless of whether they are expressed in oral or written form, is certainly of great, if as yet unrealized, significance to the theory of associative thinking.'

and heart is beaten for my soul and salvation and heaven, Amen').[28]

Rochester and Martin's own research introduced the concept of *cohesion analysis*, which they took from the work of the linguists M. A. K. Halliday and R. Hasan. They studied three groups: thought-disordered schizophrenia patients, non-thought-disordered schizophrenia patients, and ordinary people. Speech was elicited from each of the participants using three procedures: an interview in which they were asked to speak about anything they found interesting, an experimental condition in which they were asked to talk about a series of cartoons, and a narrative task in which they had to listen to and repeat a short story.

'Cohesion', as defined by Halliday and Hasan, refers to the extent to which different parts of a spoken text are linked meaningfully together, so that they appear coherent to the listener. The links that achieve this effect are known as *cohesive ties*, and are categorized into five main types (see Table 15.2). For example, 'reference' refers to a link in which the interpretation of something said has to be sought elsewhere. An example is the use of pronomials, as in '*John* went down and later *he* returned home' (the correct interpretation of 'he' is given by 'John' earlier in the sentence). Another type of cohesion is given by ellipsis, in which part of a sentence appears to have been deleted in order to avoid repetition, as in 'He's got energy too; he's got a lot more than I do' ('energy' is implicit but missing from the second part of the construction). Lexical cohesion involves parts of the text that are linked by meaning, as in 'I got angry at my brother but I don't often get mad' ('angry' and 'mad' are synonyms in this example).

As American psychologists Phil Harvey and John Neale later observed, perhaps one of the most important findings from this study was the unexpected competence of the non-thought-disordered patients.[29] The speech of these patients appeared to be completely normal. By contrast, the thought-disordered patients produced fewer cohesive ties in the narrative condition and, during the interviews, they seemed to make excessive use of lexical cohesion. In a further analysis, Rochester and Martin classified the cohesive ties as *endophoric* and *exophoric* according to the location of the reference entailed. Endophoric ties refer to information that lies elsewhere in the text (as in, for example, 'Penny is always late. I hope she gets here soon'). Exophoric reference involves information from the context or circumstances

Table 15.2 Cohesive ties defined by Halliday and Hasan (adapted from S. Rochester and J. R. Martin (1979). *Crazy Talk: A Study of the Discourse of Psychotic Speakers*. New York: Plenum).

Type of cohesion	Example
Reference	Pronomial reference: 'We met Joy Adamson and had dinner with *her* in Nairobi.'
Substitution	Verbal substitution: 'Eastern people take it seriously, at least some of them *do*.'
Ellipsis	Nominal ellipsis: 'He's got energy too. He's got a lot more [energy] than I do.'
Conjunction	Additive conjunction: 'I read a book in the past few days *and* I liked it.'
Lexical cohesion	Synonym: 'I got *angry* at M. but I don't often get *mad*.'

surrounding the speech ('Here she comes!'). They found evidence that the thought-disordered patients made excessive use of exophoric references, and were more likely to provide unclear references than ordinary people.

The publication of Rochester and Martin's book was followed by a number of studies which mostly replicated their main findings for schizophrenia patients, although findings for manic patients were less consistent. In Britain, Til Wykes and Julian Leff conducted cohesion analyses of samples of speech from a small number of patients in both diagnostic groups. Like Rochester and Martin, they found a low number of cohesive ties in the speech of the schizophrenia patients, but more cohesive ties in the speech of the manic patients.[30] (As there were no healthy controls, this finding should not be taken to imply that manic speech is normal.) In a more ambitious study, conducted in New York, Phil Harvey divided both schizophrenia and manic patients into sub-groups according to whether they were thought-disordered or not, and compared them with ordinary people. There was no difference between the schizophrenia and manic patients overall, but there were clear differences between those patients who were thought-disordered and those who were not. The thought-disordered patients, regardless of their diagnosis, used fewer cohesive ties and more incompetent references.[31]

Although some linguists have not been persuaded by Rochester and

Martin's approach,[32] the evidence on the whole suggests that poor cohesion and abnormal references contribute to the listener's bafflement when confronted with psychotic speech. Applying these ideas, Nancy Docherty has recently developed a measure of thought, language and communication disorder that focuses specifically on these kinds of peculiarities. The Communication Disturbance Index measures six types of linguistic abnormalities observed in schizophrenia and manic patients (see Table 15.3).[33] Using this measure, Docherty was able to show that some kinds of speech disorder (overinclusive or vague references, ambiguous word meanings and confused references) increase when patients are asked to speak about emotionally negative topics, whereas others (missing referents and structural unclarities) are unaffected.[34]

And Back to Psychology

So far I have emphasized the idea that thought disorder is best considered a disorder of communication. However, our ability to speak is presumably influenced by global cognitive processes. In order to explain psychotic speech, therefore, it will be necessary to ascertain how abnormal communication is connected, if at all, to the more general psychological deficits found in psychotic patients. (Of course, this approach does not necessarily imply a return to the old idea that thought disorder is literally disordered thought.)

Discourse planning

One possibility is that psychotic people have difficulty planning what they are going to say. Consistent with this idea, Ralf Hoffman, at Yale University in the USA, inferred ineffective discourse planning in thought-disordered patients from a structural analysis of their speech, in which the links between different ideas were traced. It was found that propositions contained in the speech of ordinary people seemed to be organized into a 'strong hierarchy' of ideas whereas this was not the case for the speech of thought-disordered schizophrenia patients.[35] In a subsequent study, Hoffman claimed that his method allowed him to discriminate between the disordered speech of schizophrenia

Table 15.3 Categories of linguistic abnormality measured by the Communication Disturbance Index (Docherty, DeRosa and Andreasen, 1996).

Category	Definition	Example
Vague references	Over-inclusive words or phrases that obscure meaning because of a lack of specificity.	'Being is is, it's not bad. You can do *things* and plus you can make people afraid of you.'
Confused references	Words or phrases that refer ambiguously to one of at least two clear-cut alternative referents.	'Take the clock, for instance. You got ten, twelve on it, you got other numbers on it, you got a volume button on it, *it* go up and down.'
Missing information references	References to information not previously presented and not known to the listener.	'I like to work all right. Some of *those shops* were filthy . . . I liked *the bakeries*, some of *the shops* are clean.' (No prior mention of shops or bakeries.)
Ambiguous word meanings	Instances in which a word or phrase could have a number of different meanings, and the intended meaning is not obvious from the context.	'I had a chance to *grow* with him but I got a divorce because I couldn't.'
Wrong word references	Use of an odd or apparently inappropriate word or expression in an otherwise clear utterance.	'I was trying to *predict* them people that I need, I need to get out of there.'
Structural unclarities	Failures of meaning due to a breakdown or inadequacy of grammatical structure.	'I was socializing with friends. Girlfriends and friends *the same as male*.'

patients, and that of manic patients, which was characterized by rapid shifts from one discourse plan to another.[36] Unfortunately, Hoffman's method of analysis has been criticized by other researchers for being unreliable and subjective.[37]

Although other researchers have reported findings that have been interpreted (to my mind, unconvincingly) as consistent with Hoffman's theory,[38] it seems fatally flawed for reasons that we identified in the last chapter. The idea that speech requires a plan in order to be coherent raises the spectre of an infinite regress in which a plan is required in order to compose the discourse plan, and seems to underestimate the extent to which people can construct coherent speech 'on line'.

Speaking to the needs of the listener

A second possibility is that thought-disordered patients are somehow unable to adjust their speech to meet the needs of the listener. In principle, this might happen for one or both of two reasons. First, patients may be unable to monitor their own speech, so they fail to recognize that it is unintelligible. Second, they may be unable to understand what the needs of the listener are.

The study by Martin Harrow and Joan Miller which I discussed earlier is consistent with the first of these hypotheses; it will be recalled that thought-disordered patients failed to recognize that their own speech was unintelligible to others but could easily recognize when the speech of others was incoherent. An observation that is also consistent with the hypothesis was made by linguist Elaine Chaika when she asked psychotic patients and ordinary people to repeat a short story; when digressing or breaking off in the middle of a grammatical construction the normal participants would signal that they had done so and then return to the story, whereas the schizophrenia patients appeared unaware they were deviating from the task.[39]

A more sophisticated approach to examining the role of self-monitoring in thought-disordered patients was used in a series of studies conducted by Phil Harvey at Mount Sinai Hospital in New York. In the last chapter I introduced the concept of *source monitoring* when discussing hallucinations, focusing on difficulties that patients experience when attempting to distinguish between things that they hear and things that they think. However, there is another type of source monitoring in which we distinguish between what we have thought and what we have said. Clearly, an impairment of this skill will make individuals vulnerable to omitting important segments of information when speaking to others, making their speech appear incoherent.

Throughout the 1980s, Harvey and his colleagues carried out a number of studies in which patients were asked to read one set of words aloud, and to imagine themselves reading a second set of words (the 'think' condition). Afterwards, they were shown a list of words including those they had read aloud, those they had thought, and some which had not been presented previously, and were asked to say which of them they had read and which of them they had thought. In general, it was found that poor performance on this kind of task was associated with thought disorder in schizophrenia patients but not in manic patients.[40]

The second possible explanation for the thought-disordered patient's inability to speak to the listener's needs has also received some support. If thought-disordered patients cannot understand those needs, we should expect them to perform badly on theory-of-mind tests. This possibility has been explored in a series of studies recently undertaken at the Centre Hospitalier de Versailles in France by Yves Sarfati, Marie Christine Hardy-Bayle and others.[41] In brief, these studies have shown that patients who have high scores on Andreasen's TLC Scale perform less well on a variety of ToM tasks than patients who show no evidence of thought, language and communication disorder.

Working memory

A third possibility is that more basic cognitive processes are compromised in thought-disordered patients. We have already seen evidence that these patients suffer from deficits in working memory (the part of the memory system responsible for holding information for brief periods of time). In Chapter 8, I described a study by Tom Oltmanns and John Neale in which it was discovered that poor performance on the digit span with distraction task was associated with communication disorder.[42] The findings of Grove and Andreasen, which we considered earlier, are also consistent with this observation, as are the results of many other studies.[43]

In attempts to demonstrate a causal connection between working memory deficits and communication disorder, some investigators have experimentally impaired the working memory system in ordinary people. Deanna Barch and Howard Berenbaum of the University of Illinois at Urbana-Champaign interviewed undergraduate students in two conditions: under normal circumstances and in a 'dual-task' condition in which they also had to perform a task that was designed to keep the working memory system busy. As a consequence, the speech of the students showed less grammatical complexity and more long pauses. As Barch and Berenbaum note, these characteristics have been observed in the speech of psychotic patients. However, other well-documented features of psychotic speech (for example, incompetent references) were not observed.[44]

More dramatic impairments of working memory can be temporarily induced by administering ketamine, and a number of investigators have therefore studied the speech of healthy volunteers who have been persuaded to take this drug. A group of investigators at the US National Institute of Mental Health gave an infusion of ketamine to ten ordinary people, who, afterwards, showed evidence of thought disorder as measured by Andreasen's TLC Scale, and also poor performance on a working memory measure. Interestingly, the decrease in working memory performance experienced by the participants correlated with the severity of their communication difficulties.[45]

Terry Goldberg and Daniel Weinberger, also at NIMH, have pointed out that the relationship between working memory and communication disorder may not be as simple as these results seem to suggest. Neurological patients who have damage to their frontal lobes often suffer from impaired working memory, but almost never show evidence of thought disorder. On the other hand, thought-disordered patients often respond abnormally on simple word association tests, which do not require the use of working memory.[46]

Was Bleuler right?

A final approach to understanding the relationship between cognitive deficits and communication disorder has focused on a part of our cognitive system known as semantic memory, and bears some similarity to Bleuler's original theory. The semantic memory system – which stores meanings, knowledge and ideas – is thought to consist of complex networks of concepts, connected by *associative links*. According to this very general model (of which there are many specific versions), one concept leads to another by a process of 'spreading activation' – as a concept becomes awakened in the mind (because the individual is thinking about it) closely connected concepts are also activated or 'switched on'. In this way, one idea leads to another.

A phenomenon that demonstrates this effect is known as 'semantic priming'. In a semantic priming experiment, participants are shown words in quick succession and are asked to indicate in some way (for example, by reading aloud, or by pressing a button on a computer) when they have recognized each word. Recognition is faster (by a few tens of milliseconds) if a word is preceded by a meaningfully related word (for example, if 'black' is preceded by 'white') than if it is preceded by an unrelated word (for example, 'soft').[47] The conventional explanation for this effect is that perception of a word ('black') leads automatically to the partial activation (or 'priming') of related words ('white'), so that the brain is already 'tuned' into them, and recognition is easier.

It is believed that many of the concepts represented in semantic memory are organized hierarchically. For example, the concept of 'living things' includes 'animals', which includes 'birds', which in turn includes 'crows'. A robust finding from ordinary people is the so-called *category-relatedness effect* – it takes us less time to decide that a typical exemplar belongs to a category ('a crow is a bird') than it takes us to decide that an atypical exemplar belongs to a category ('a penguin is a bird'). Again this can be understood in terms of activation spreading from the category concept to typical exemplar concepts, but not to the atypical exemplars.

As we have already seen, some of the earliest attempts to study these processes in schizophrenia patients were made by Bleuler and Jung, who examined patients' word associations. In fact, modern research has consistently shown defective semantic memory in schizophrenia patients. For example, some studies have shown that patients often perform poorly when asked to sort objects into categories, to remember object names, or to describe the defining features of concepts such as 'animals' and 'birds'.[48] Although there is evidence that these problems cannot simply be attributed to poor motivation or more general intellectual deficits, many of these studies have been compromised by the failure to link the findings to particular complaints. Over the past few years, however, evidence has accumulated supporting Bleuler's view that abnormal semantic processes play a specific role in disordered communication.

Some of this evidence has emerged from studies of word associations. Manfred Spitzer at the University of Heidelberg in Germany replicated some of Bleuler's original experiments, and confirmed that thought-disordered schizophrenia patients show fewer typical associations and more indirect or 'mediate' associations.[49] In a study by Terry Goldberg and his colleagues in the USA, a group of schizophrenia patients and a group of normal participants were given a battery of psychological tests. Two measures discriminated those patients with severe thought disorder from those with mild or no thought disorder – a verbal fluency test (in which the individual is asked to think of as many words as possible beginning with a particular letter) and a vocabulary test – both of which depend heavily on semantic memory.[50] Goldberg and his colleagues went on to use patients' responses on a test in which they had to generate words belonging to particular categories, to 'map' the way that their semantic systems were organized. For example, by analysing the relationships between successive words generated during the task, it was possible to show that most ordinary people organize the category 'animals' along two dimensions: wild–domestic and large–small. However, when maps were generated for thought-disordered patients, they appeared to be less well organized than those of non-thought-disordered patients or ordinary people.[51]

Less consistent findings have been obtained when researchers have attempted to assess semantic functioning by measuring the kinds of priming effects I described earlier. Brendan Maher in the United States[52] and Manfred Spitzer in Germany[53] have reported that priming is *increased* in patients with communication disorder. In a particularly complex experiment, Spitzer has also observed abnormal spreading activation effects.[54] Whereas priming of direct associations (for example, priming of 'foot' by 'shoe') was found in ordinary people, communication-disordered patients also showed priming for indirect associations (for example, 'hand' by 'shoe', presumably mediated by 'foot').

Other studies, for example by Terry Goldberg and his colleagues,[55] have observed *reduced* priming in patients with thought disorder. It is possible that some of these inconsistencies are more apparent than real. Priming effects are notoriously sensitive to experimental conditions – the duration for which words are presented, and the interval between them, for example. One possible interpretation of the evidence is that reduced spreading activation to immediate associates, and increased activation of indirect associates – either as separate processes or the consequence of a single abnormality in the semantic memory system – make it more difficult for the thought-disordered patient to find appropriate words when speaking.

The Roots of Incoherence

It is possible that dysfunctions in working memory, source monitoring, theory of mind and semantic memory are all implicated in thought disorder to some degree. As American psychologists Deanna Barch and Howard Berenbaum have noted, language production processes are highly complex, and it is therefore likely that abnormalities in a number different cognitive mechanisms can influence them.[56]

A tentative model that tries to draw together some of the ideas we have considered in this chapter is shown in Figure 15.2. It suggests that semantic problems, which I assume to be long-standing, make individuals vulnerable to thought, language and communication disorder. It further assumes that, in vulnerable individuals, emotional arousal leads to working memory deficits, which in turn lead to poor source monitoring and ultimately to speech that is incomprehensible to others. However, I must emphasize that this account is *highly* speculative (and certainly not secure enough to be deemed a 'theory'), so it is possible that I have misjudged the flow of causal relationships

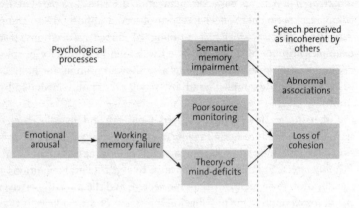

Figure 15.2 A very tentative model of positive thought, communication and language disorder.

between the different processes that appear to influence psychotic speech. More research is surely needed.*

One remaining matter of controversy is the relationship between communication disorder in schizophrenia patients and communication disorder attributed to mania. Some researchers have suggested that these are quite different, whereas others have assumed that they are similar or even identical. My own prejudice – fuelled by my earlier critique of the Kraepelinian paradigm – is to consider them similar. However, on more careful consideration it becomes obvious that 'similar' or 'different' do not exhaust the possibilities. In a thoughtful discussion of these issues, Linda Grossman and Martin Harrow remarked:

We believe that the disordered cognition that is so prominent in manic and schizophrenic patients is the product of several underlying factors acting together, rather than a single factor. Further, it is probable that there are underlying factors leading to psychopathology that are common to both manic and schizophrenic patients, and that there are also other underlying factors that differ in these two patient groups . . . Until recently, the assump-

* This is, of course, the scientist's standard lament when summarizing findings. It's true, of course, but it also gives us a nice excuse for applying for more research funds.

tion that thought disorder is found only in schizophrenia has so governed diagnostic practice as to shape routine clinical observation to such an extent that many grossly disorganized manic patients who thought and verbalized strange ideas were not seen as having disordered cognition.[57]

Part Four

Causes and their Effects

16

Things are Much More Complex than they Seem*

My own suspicion is that the universe is not only queerer than we suppose, but queerer than we can suppose.   J. B. S. Haldane[1]

In the previous parts of this book, I have attempted to show how psychological research has begun to unravel the processes involved in the various complaints of psychotic patients. In each case, these experiences and behaviours appear to be understandable when viewed in the context of what we know about the normal human mind. It is important to repeat that there is nothing 'anti-biological' in this analysis. The psychological processes that give rise to complaints are located in the brain (although whether psychosis is caused by damage to the brain is another matter, which we will return to later).

Once the various psychotic complaints have been explained in this way, no ghostly illness remains that also requires an explanation. The complaints (particular classes of behaviours and experiences that have been singled out because they sometimes cause distress) are *all* there is.

And yet, I would not be surprised if the account I have so far given seems incomplete to many readers. Although it begins to explain what happens when someone has these kinds of unusual experiences, it does not seem to explain how the complaints come into being in the first place. In short, it seems to say very little about *aetiology*. This criticism lies at the heart of Mojtabai and Rieder's objections to the symptom-orientated approach,[2] which we briefly considered at the end of Chapter 6.

* I thank Dr James McGuire of the University of Liverpool for helpful discussions about many of the issues discussed in this chapter.

In the following three chapters I will try and counter these arguments by showing how the symptom-orientated approach can be expanded to provide a richer account of aetiology than has been possible within the Kraepelinian paradigm. In doing so, I will attempt to do justice to the complexity of psychiatric problems. As we have seen, symptoms sometimes congregate together, although not in a simple way that is amenable to a categorial system of classification. Symptoms also wax and wane with time, often unpredictably. These types of complexity are difficult to explain within the Kraepelinian paradigm but I will show that they can be readily understood within the context of the symptom-orientated approach.

I would like to begin with a few words of warning. The argument I will outline in the first part of this chapter will probably seem quite abstract. I ask the reader to stick with it, because it will help us to make sense of some of the scientific findings that will be presented later on. Also, because I will sometimes have to extrapolate from limited data, some of the conclusions I will reach in this chapter and the two that follow will be fairly speculative. In these circumstances I ask the reader to focus on the general principles that I am attempting to expound (about which I feel fairly confident) rather than the details, which may have to be amended as more evidence becomes available.

Thinking Carefully about Causal Processes

Many people assume that the main aim of psychiatric research is to establish *the* cause of each psychiatric disorder. Often, psychologists and psychiatrists encourage this assumption by prejudging some kinds of causal factors as pre-eminent. (For example, Mojtabai and Rieder seem to regard genetic causes as particularly important, whereas the British historian of psychiatry German Berrios[3] seems to discount explanations unless they point to abnormalities in particular brain regions.) However, a moment's reflection will reveal that causal factors come in many different shapes and sizes. Even a simple physical event is the product of a complex network of causal effects and circumstances. Consider an example offered by the philosopher Ted Honderich.[4] In order for a match to ignite it must rub against a rough surface with a certain force. However, the match also has to be of a certain chemical composition and it must have been kept in a place that is dry for a period prior to ignition. Which of these factors should be singled out? To pursue this question further, we could choose to explain the ignition of the match in terms of its design and manufacture, or the actions of the person who strikes it. Rather than selecting one factor as pre-eminent, we need a way of classifying these different kinds of causal events and thinking about the relationships between them.

For our purposes it will help to distinguish between three general kinds of causes. (These distinctions are fairly arbitrary but will aid our thinking.) *Aetiological factors* lie somewhere in the individual's past, and will be the focus of the next two chapters. In contrast, the factors that will concern us in the present chapter play a more immediate role in determining whether complaints occur at particular points in time. These in turn can be divided into events and circumstances that appear to elicit or trigger symptoms, and those that help to keep symptoms going once they have occurred.

The former can be described as *proximate determinants* because they occur at approximately the same time as symptoms. Proximate determinants provoke or exacerbate the cognitive abnormalities that coincide with complaints. For example, unpatterned environmental noise can be thought of as a proximate determinant of auditory hallucinations, as the presence of this kind of stimulation immediately increases the likelihood that someone will misattribute their inner speech to an external source.

Events and circumstances that keep complaints going once they have become established are sometimes described as *maintenance factors*. As the reaction-maintenance principle reminds us, some maintenance factors are psychological. For example, in Chapter 10, I described research by the American psychologist Susan Nolen-Hoeksema which has shown that some ways of trying to cope with depression, particularly ruminating, tend to prolong depressive episodes. Similarly, in Chapter 12, I discussed Tony Morrison's proposal that paranoid beliefs are sometimes maintained by safety behaviours. Other maintenance factors are social or environmental. Poverty, stigmatization and unemployment all serve to keep psychotic people locked out of society and into the role of the psychiatric patient.[5] Of course, this kind of social marginalization can also be a consequence of patients' complaints. Friends, neighbours and potential employers may shun people who begin to have psychotic experiences.

Proximate determinants and maintenance factors affect the course of complaints – whether they wane so that the individual recovers, or whether they worsen so that the individual becomes more disabled. It will not be possible to provide an exhaustive account of these factors in a single chapter. Some (for example, the impact of environmental noise on hallucinations) have been described in previous chapters, so I will avoid repeating discussion of them here.

Functional Relationships

I will begin by introducing an abstract concept from mathematics that will facilitate our discussion. (Don't worry, no knowledge of maths will be required to follow my argument!) In mathematics, the association between two variables is described by a functional relationship. For example, $y = f(x)$ indicates that y is a function of x; in other words, as x changes, y changes also in some orderly fashion. The way in which y changes will, of course, reflect the precise mathematical equation that is used to express the relationship. For example, if $y = x^2$, y will increase ever more dramatically for small increases of x; the graph of this particular relationship is a parabola.

This concept of a functional relationship should not be confused with the idea that certain types of processes have a function for the individual. There is nothing wrong with this idea, which is common-place in biology (for example, we known that the function of the heart is to deliver blood to various parts of the body) and, indeed, I have resorted to it at various points in the preceding chapters (when I asserted that the human brain has evolved to sustain complex relationships, or that the function of the self-serving bias is to maintain positive beliefs about the self). However, this is not what I mean by a functional relationship in the present context.

Functional relationships provide a language for describing the inter-relations between events in nature. To take a simple example from the physical world, the laws of classical mechanics describe how the acceleration and velocity of a moving body change when a force acts on it. As this example shows, mathematical specifications of functional relationships often lead to descriptions that are more precise than those that can be given in ordinary language. Unfortunately, there have so far been few attempts to construct mathematical descriptions of the processes involved in psychotic phenomena, although there are no reasons for supposing that such descriptions will not be possible in the future.

Even in the absence of mathematical models, the idea of a functional relationship remains useful in psychopathology, and the term *functional analysis** is sometimes used to indicate the effort to describe, in general terms, those relationships that may be important in determining psychological complaints.[6] This approach has at least three strengths. First, it is relatively devoid of philosophical baggage. By describing a network of relationships between different groups of events that ultimately lead to complaints, it is not necessary to single out any particular event or class of events as *the* ultimate cause. Second, this kind of description can alert us to the possibility that many of these relationships are *non-linear*. (A linear relationship is one in which a change in one variable leads to a linear increase or decrease in another; even the simplest relationships in nature are usually more complex than this.) Third, a functional analysis can highlight reciprocal interactions in which two or more processes influence each other, either directly or indirectly. As we have already seen, these kinds of interactions can be very important.

At this point, the reader may be forgiven for wondering precisely where this argument is heading. It may help to consider whether any functional relationships have been described in the preceding chapters. In fact, the accounts I have given of the psychological processes involved in symptoms have been packed with them. A give-away is the presence of the following symbol:

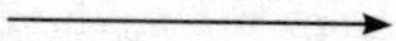

Figure 16.1 The symbol for a functional relationship.

* Most of the clinical literature on functional analysis has been written by psychologists who are sympathetic to behaviourism. However, as an organizing principle, functional analysis does not require a commitment to any particular school of psychology.

So, Figure 10.7 (p. 269) shows some functional relationships that appear to be important in depression, Figure 13.4 (p. 345) shows some that are involved in paranoid delusions, and Figure 14.3 (p. 368) shows some that seem to play a role in auditory hallucinations. These examples establish that there is nothing mysterious or magical about functional analysis. However, as I will now show, it is an approach that enables us to cut through much of the confusion that exists about the complexity of psychiatric phenomena.

At last, the problem of psychiatric classification solved (?)

First, let us return to the problem of psychiatric classification. When considering the evidence reviewed in Chapter 4 some readers may have been struck by an apparent paradox. I concluded that chapter by arguing that the Kraepelinian paradigm seems to propose at the same time too many categories of disorder and also too few. The similarities between some definitions of schizophrenia and bipolar disorder seemed to push us towards the *einheitspsychose* or unitary psychosis concept. On the other hand, the factor-analytic evidence seemed to suggest that each of these diagnostic categories could be split into a number of separate components or symptom clusters (for example, according to Peter Liddle's model, positive symptoms, negative symptoms, and symptoms of cognitive disorganization). At the same time, it is not immediately obvious why any symptoms should go with any other (for example, why someone who is suffering from delusions should have a high but less than certain probability of experiencing hallucinations). This question lies at the heart of the problem of psychiatric classification. Indeed, it is *the* problem of psychiatric classification, as a successful attempt to resolve it will make the problem go away.

Kraepelin's attempt to solve the problem can itself be expressed as a set of functional relationships. In fact, I have already done so in Figure 1.2, a part of which is reproduced below as Figure 16.2. According to this model, symptoms go together because they are functionally related to the same underlying biological abnormalities. Most people who have worked in the field of psychiatry over the last century or so have implicitly endorsed this model, even when they have disputed Kraepelin's version of it. Indeed, this model has been the driving force behind the quest to find the causes of schizophrenia and manic depression.

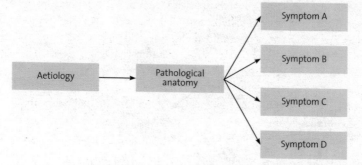

Figure 16.2 Kraepelinian paradigm expressed as a set of functional relationships.

Of course, the Kraepelinian paradigm is not the only possible model of the relationship between aetiological variables and symptoms. Symptoms could be functionally connected to several causal variables. In fact, these kinds of relationships are portrayed in many of the models outlined in previous chapters. For example, Figure 14.3 shows how hearing voices can be influenced by beliefs, environmental noise and emotional arousal.

This kind of model edges us towards an understanding of why symptoms sometimes but not invariably occur together. Perhaps they have some functional relationships in common. For example, in Chapters 12 and 13, we considered evidence that theory-of-mind deficits (the inability to understand the beliefs, thoughts and intentions of other people) may contribute to paranoid ideas. In Chapter 15 we saw that these kinds of deficits also appear to play a role in disordered communication. These relationships are portrayed together in Figure 16.3. Note that, according to this amalgamated model, we should expect paranoid delusions and disordered speech occasionally to occur together (because they are both influenced by theory-of-mind deficits). However, we should not expect this to happen very often, because theory-of-mind deficits have only an indirect influence on paranoid delusions (see Chapter 12), and because both symptoms are influenced by processes that they do not share in common.

Even this kind of model must be an oversimplification. One complication is that *complaints sometimes cause each other*. In Chapter 12, we considered Brendan Maher's anomalous perception model, which

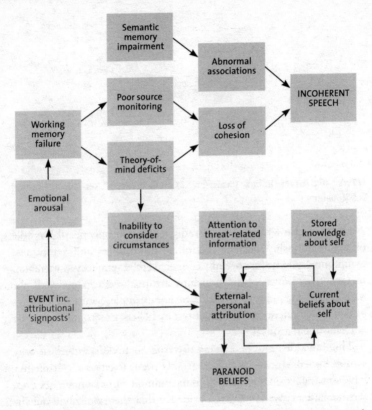

Figure 16.3 Overlapping functional relationships implicated in paranoia and incoherent speech.

suggested that delusions are sometimes rational interpretations of anomalous experiences.[7] The most obvious way that this can happen is when a patient makes a delusional interpretation of a hallucinated voice. (Recall that, in Sondra Escher and Marius Romme's prospective study of children who heard voices, some 9 per cent developed delusional interpretations of their experiences.)[8] However, in Chapter 14 we also saw that hallucinations can be facilitated by certain kinds of beliefs (for example, as demonstrated in experiments in which patients have been given various kinds of suggestions).[9] Which of these accounts of the relationship between hallucinations and delusions is correct? Given the evidence, both must be, as illustrated in Figure 16.4. If

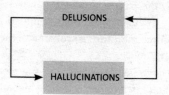

Figure 16.4 Hallucinations can influence delusions, and delusions can influence hallucinations.

delusions can provoke hallucinations and hallucinations can provoke delusions, it is no wonder that they very often occur together. However, the fact that they sometimes occur in isolation shows that this association is not inevitable. (For this reason, in order to understand the mechanisms that are responsible for these complaints it has been necessary to consider them in isolation.)

Some depressive symptoms experienced by psychotic patients may be explained in this way. As we have already seen, abnormal mood often precedes the development of hallucinations and delusions. Although, in many patients, the high levels of depression experienced during an episode reduce as they recover from their psychotic episode, about a third go on to develop a severe post-psychotic depression.[10] Max Birchwood and his colleagues at the University of Birmingham have shown that this type of depression is often a consequence of patients feeling humiliated and entrapped by their illness, and their expectation that they will be doomed to a low social status as a consequence.[11] In this case, patients' appraisals of one set of complaints (delusions and hallucinations) lead to new complaints (depression).

A final complication concerns less direct ways in which one complaint can increase the probability that another will occur. For example, there is evidence that social isolation and the absence of social support can maintain psychotic symptoms – the more that people who experience psychosis live in impoverished and unsupportive social networks, passing each day with very little contact with other people, the more likely it is that their complaints will persist or even worsen.[12] It is easy to see how psychotic people can become isolated, either because their delusions leave them in fear of others, or because they are shunned by others who are frightened of them. But it is also easy to see how isolation can further provoke difficulties. Without the company of others, the paranoid person is not able to put his fears to the test. In the absence of external stimulation in the form of conversation, the source-monitoring problems of the person who hears voices will be exacerbated.

The lessons we have just learnt can be summarized as a general *principle of functional interconnectedness*, which might be stated formally in the following way:

Psychiatric complaints are connected by a rich network of functional relationships, which may be causal, or reflect shared causal pathways. Co-occurrence of complaints depends on the strength and number of these functional relationships. The more functional relationships connecting two complaints, and the stronger they are, the more likely it is that they will occur together.

This principle gives a much richer account of the way in which symptoms cluster together than the Kraepelinian paradigm. It explains why some symptoms tend to occur together (for example, hallucinations and delusions) but also why attempts to break down psychosis into a small number of categories (schizophrenia, bipolar disorder and so on) have failed.

The Ups and Downs of Mental Health

We must now turn to the second level of complexity that I promised to address at the outset of this discussion. In ordinary language, people who suffer from psychiatric problems are sometimes said to be 'unstable'. This description reflects our common experience that psychological well-being can vary from day to day, or even from hour to hour.

In the case of those of us who have been lucky enough to avoid the psychiatric clinic, these fluctuations may be quite mild. Occasionally we 'get out on the wrong side of the bed'. We have good days and we have bad days. In contrast, day-to-day variations in the frequency and intensity of psychotic complaints may be much more marked. Sometimes superimposed on these fluctuations are changes that take place over longer intervals of weeks or months. We therefore speak of people having 'relapses' or 'episodes' – periods of time when their difficulties are quite severe – interspersed by periods of 'remission' when symptoms are attenuated, or have disappeared altogether. Unfortunately, much of the research that I reviewed in Part 3 has consisted of 'snapshots' of the relevant psychological processes. In the absence of further elaboration, these snapshots provide a rather misleading picture of what must be happening in the minds of both ordinary people and psychiatric patients. We are more like movies than still photographs.

States, traits and meaningless debates

The standard way of thinking about the relationship between psycho-pathology and time requires making a distinction between states and traits. Like many concepts widely employed by psychopathologists, this distinction seems commonsensical when first encountered but, on closer examination, appears more suspect. A *state* is said to be some characteristic of the individual (a type of cognitive organization or a facet of personality) that is present during episodes of illness. A *trait*, on the other hand, is a more enduring characteristic that seems to precede the onset of complaints, and which is often thought to be aetiologically important. This distinction is explicitly evoked in many of the theories we have encountered earlier. The models proposed by Paul Meehl[13] and Gordon Claridge[14] both suggest that schizotypal personality traits predispose people to develop schizophrenic symptoms, an idea that is mirrored in the stress-vulnerability models of psychosis developed by researchers such as Keith Nuechterlein and his colleagues in the USA.[15] The distinction between states and traits is also important in some theories of depression. For example, as we have seen, Martin Seligman, Lyn Abramson and others have argued that a pessimistic attributional style predisposes people to become depressed when they are exposed to unpleasant events.[16]

There are two problems with this distinction. First, and most obviously, it is doubtful whether states and traits are two distinct types of psychological phenomena. Psychological characteristics probably vary in their mutability from highly unstable and state-like to highly stable and trait-like. Indeed, we have already seen in Chapter 10 that individuals vary in the extent to which at least one important characteristic – global self-esteem – is trait-like. Michael Kernis found that, in some people, global self-esteem is relatively stable over time whereas, in others, it fluctuates dramatically.[17] He also found that individuals whose self-esteem fluctuated greatly tended to make extreme attributions about hassles they encountered in their lives.[18] Of course, observations of this kind are not too difficult to accommodate so long as we realize that we are talking about gradations of psychological flexibility, rather than two different kinds of processes.

A deeper and more sinister difficulty concerns the inferences that are sometimes made on the basis of this distinction. It is often assumed that state-like processes are mere epiphenomena of symptoms, and therefore causally unimportant. According to this way of thinking, unless the psychological characteristics we observe in patients can be shown to be present prior to episodes, they can play no causal role. The considerable efforts that have been directed towards determining whether psychological processes implicated in complaints are trait-like or state-like have often been motivated by this assumption.

The despair sometimes experienced by psychologists on discovering that their favoured psychological mechanisms are not trait-like may be something of an over-reaction. There is no reason why we should not attribute a causal role to psychological processes that vary alongside complaints. To see why this is the case, it will be helpful to recall the model of the attribution–self-representation cycle that I introduced in Chapter 10 (p. 254–62) According to that model, beliefs about the self influence appraisals of events, which in turn influence future beliefs about the self. We saw that one property of a non-linear system of this kind is that, under certain circumstances, the positive feedback loop between one process and another allows marked shifts in both over time. They are like neatly balanced weights that topple together when given a push of sufficient magnitude. The person making an internal attribution for a negative event feels more miserable about herself as a consequence, and this increases the probability that she will make an internal attribution for negative events in the future. Over a period of time, the psychologist observing this process sees someone whose attributions become more self-blaming at the same time as she becomes more depressed. However, this does not mean that her attributions were causally unimportant in this process.

Of course, when two people react to exactly the same event in different ways – one with stoicism and the other with distress – we can be sure that there must be something different about them to begin with. However, these differences need not be dramatic at the outset in order for them to spiral into extreme and more easily detected differences later on. Given the inherently unstable nature of psychiatric complaints, and the complex functional relationships that lie behind them, I suspect that direct or indirect feedback loops of this kind affect many of the psychological processes involved in mental illness.

Chaos and complexity

If the analysis I have just given is even half correct, fluctuations in psychotic complaints might provide a valuable source of information about the psychological processes that give rise to psychiatric problems. Unfortunately, these kinds of fluctuations, although widely recognized by clinicians, have rarely been studied in detail. A handful of studies that are exceptions to this rule are worth looking at in some detail.

American psychiatrists Allan Gottschalk, Mark Bauer and Peter Whybrow studied day-to-day fluctuations in mood in a small group of bipolar patients over periods ranging between one year and two and a half years. Using complex mathematical techniques, they searched their data for patterns but found no evidence of cyclic variations between positive and negative moods. Indeed, Gottschalk and his colleagues concluded that the mood changes in their patients appeared to be formally 'chaotic' (see Figure 16.5).[19]

Although these findings show that patients' moods do not follow a regular rhythm, they do *not* imply that mood changes are the products of random mechanisms. Although in popular language the term 'chaos' implies disorder, in the mathematical sciences it is used to describe the complex and unpatterned behaviour that often arises out of quite simple systems of interacting processes. Chaotic systems are deterministic, which is to say that each element in the system influences the others in ways that can be precisely specified as functional relationships (usually in the form of mathematical equations). Nonetheless, because of the cumulative effects of these influences, the overall behaviour of a chaotic system is highly unpredictable even over short periods of time (changes in the weather, and long-term variations in populations, tend to be chaotic in this formal sense).[20] Despite this unpredictability, chaotic systems tend to exhibit a degree of self-organization or

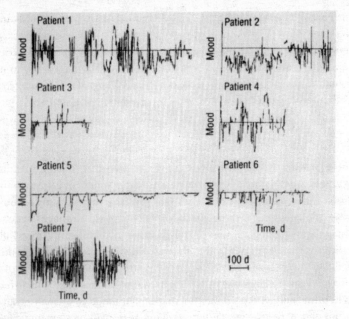

Figure 16.5 Daily mood variations (ranging from 'best I have ever felt' to 'worst I have ever felt') for seven bipolar patients (from Gottschalk et al., 1995).

homeostasis. (For example, although annual population changes in some species are chaotic, under most conditions the population levels remain between certain minimum and maximum levels; similarly the *average* rainfall in a particular region and in a particular season is reasonably predictable.)

A more recent series of studies, conducted by Inez Myin-Germeys and her colleagues at Maastricht, in Holland, has revealed something of the mechanisms involved in these kinds of mood fluctuations.[21] Myin-Germeys used portable electronic bleepers to cue participants to fill in simple questionnaires about their experiences at random points in time. (In Chapter 9 we saw that this experience-sampling method has been used to demonstrate that patients with flat affect experience subjective emotional states that are as strong as those of ordinary people.) Her participants were remitted psychotic patients, first-degree relatives of patients, and ordinary people. When the bleepers went off, the participants were asked to record their current mood, to describe the most important event that had happened to them since the last time the bleeper had sounded, and to answer a series of simple questions about how stressed they were feeling. In all of the groups, it was found that experiencing subjectively stressful events was associated with increases in negative affect and decreases in positive affect. However, the patients reported less positive affect and more negative affect than their relatives or ordinary people, made more extreme appraisals of the events they had experienced, and reacted to the experiences with more extreme shifts in mood. On Myin-Germeys's own account, these findings are evidence of extreme sensitivity to stress in psychotic patients. This, of course, is true, but they are more specifically consistent with the idea that psychotic patients make abnormal attributions for negative events, and with the model of the attribution–self-representation cycle that I developed in earlier chapters.

In an interesting further study, Myin-Germeys found that sensitivity to everyday stressors, as assessed by her experience-sampling method, was unrelated to neurocognitive functioning, as measured with the kinds of tests favoured by American neuropsychologists. She therefore argued that neurocognitive deficits and stress sensitivity separately and independently contribute towards vulnerability to psychosis.[22] Of course, this is exactly what we would expect from the research we considered earlier in this book (especially in Chapter 8, where we saw that neurocognitive deficits appear to play little or no role in positive symptoms).

Understanding relapse

The account I have just given of the ups and downs of mental health has been fairly speculative – it is more an agenda for further research than a polished theory. It also has at least two important limitations. First, I have said very little about the kinds of external events that buffet the individual, bringing about changes in mood and symptoms. Second, I have not considered the more global changes that occur as patients move from periods of remission, in which they are relatively well, to periods of illness. In the remaining part of this chapter I will attempt to show how the account I have offered can be extended still further to overcome these limitations.

Relapse is rarely a simple step-like event. Rather, the transition from remission to active psychosis is usually gradual, often taking a number of weeks, during which time the patient often shows evidence of the kind of chaotic symptom fluctuations that we have just considered.[23] Two clues suggest that social cognition may play a crucial role in this process. First, as we saw in Chapter 9, studies of the *prodromal symptoms* that precede relapses have shown that these mainly consist of depression, anxiety, irritability, tension and sleeplessness.[24] (Episodes of mania appear to be an exception to this rule, as they are usually preceded by periods of excitement, energy and sleeplessness.[25] However, we saw in Chapter 11 that fear of incipient dysphoria may nevertheless play a crucial role in the onset of manic symptoms.) Although it is possible, as some psychologists have argued,[26] that these mood symptoms are brought about by the patient's perception that another episode of illness is imminent, the absence of frank psychotic symptoms during the early stages of relapse suggests that this is usually not the case. It seems much more likely that changes in patients' attributions, their beliefs about themselves, their perceptions of other people and related processes bring about initial changes in mood, which later cascade into full-blown psychosis.

The second clue concerns the kinds of events that are known to influence the likelihood that a relapse will occur. Many types of stressors can make vulnerable individuals suffer an exacerbation of their psychotic complaints. Some, for example the taking of illicit drugs or abstaining from sleep, can be thought of as biological stressors, because they have obvious effects on the individual's physical as well as psychological well-being. However, the best-understood stressors are social, and are precisely the kinds of events that are likely to challenge the individual's social-cognitive system.

Why Stressful Relationships are Damaging to Mental Health

Most of us intuitively recognize that emotionally charged relationships, even those in which the dominant feeling is love, can make us feel miserable. The idea that such relationships can have especially adverse effects on people who are vulnerable to psychiatric symptoms has a long history. In a later chapter, we will see that theories that implicate dysfunctional family relationships in the onset of psychosis were popular in the 1950s and 1960s, but have usually been discounted in recent years. However, the idea that families can have a negative influence on the *future* well-being of people who are *already* ill is now widely accepted. Studies of this effect began with the work of a small group of investigators based at the Institute of Psychiatry in London in the late 1950s. Initially, this group consisted of Jim Birley, Morris Carstairs and Gillian Topping. However, the person who was to have most influence on how the work progressed was George Brown, an anthropology graduate who was later to become Professor of Sociology at Birkbeck College.

According to his own account, Brown arrived at the Institute knowing very little about serious mental illness:

A ... dominant memory of those days was my emotional revulsion on reading some of the standard psychiatric accounts of the condition [schizophrenia]. Was it all so clear-cut? Were the core symptoms and handicaps so clearly linked to underlying endogenous processes? My feelings were so strong that it was several years before I could force myself to finish the account of schizophrenia in Mayer-Gross, Slater and Roth's (1954) *Clinical Psychiatry*.[27]

Brown was interested in the fate of those patients who, in an era that preceded care in the community, were able to achieve discharge from psychiatric hospitals. Unlike Ronald Laing, who was beginning his work at about this time, Brown did not feel that he had any particular skill at communicating with mad people. Instead, therefore, he decided to focus on the experiences of their parents and other relatives.

An early study conducted by Brown, Carstairs and Topping published in 1958 produced an unexpected and, at the time, quite unsettling result. Following up 229 recently discharged men, most of whom had a diagnosis of schizophrenia, they found that those leaving hospital to live with wives or parents were *less* likely to remain out of hospital, and hence *more* likely to relapse, than those leaving to live in lodgings or with brothers or sisters. Among those who had been married, those who were widowed, separated or divorced were more likely to remain well than those who left hospital to live with their spouses. Among those who went to live with their parents, those who spent most of their days with their mothers were particularly likely to do badly. Although various interpretations of these findings were considered, it was impossible to escape the conclusion that close family relationships could be hazardous to patients who were recovering from a psychotic illness. This result was quite opposite to the researchers' expectations.[28]

The next step was to discover which aspects of family relationships had this toxic effect. In a prospective study in which relatives were interviewed as patients were discharged from hospital, Brown observed that patients returning to live in families characterized as having a high level of 'emotional involvement' had especially high rates of relapse. This risk was reduced in those families in which the mother worked, limiting the amount of time that she spent in face-to-face contact with her mentally ill son or daughter.[29]

Soon afterwards, Michael Rutter joined the team and an attempt was made to develop a measure of family atmosphere that would adequately capture the crucial emotional characteristics. After two years of development work, the team came up with the Camberwell Family Interview (CFI), a structured assessment in which a close relative is asked about the patient's behaviour and its impact on the household.[30] Based on the relative's responses, five scores are obtained from the interview. *Critical comments*, which are simply counted, are remarks that express a negative emotional attitude towards things that the patient has done. *Hostility*, on the other hand, is rated on a five-point scale and refers to a general negative attitude towards the patient's personality. *Emotional over-involvement*, also rated on a five-point scale, refers to extreme emotional distress experienced by the relative accompanied by self-sacrificing and over-protective behaviour towards the patient. *Positive comments*, which are counted, are remarks which praise or express a positive attitude about things the patient has done, and *warmth*, rated on a five-point scale, measures general positive attitudes towards the patient as a person.

In practice, the positive comments and warmth scales are rarely used, as they have been found to have little or no predictive value. However, scores on the critical comments, hostility and emotional over-involvement scales were found to be associated with a high risk that patients would relapse. It is easy to picture the emotional tone associated with high scores on each of these scales – anger at the patient for being ill in the case of critical comments and hostility, and guilt about the origins of the illness in the case of emotional over-involvement. In the years following Brown's work it has become commonplace to describe a relative who scores highly on any one or more of these scales as exhibiting high *expressed emotion* (or EE). It is unfortunate that the label 'high EE relative' is now occasionally used pejoratively by mental health professionals, in a way that gives the impression that there is something nasty or unpleasant about those who are so categorized. Paradoxically, perhaps, high EE parents often seem to be very caring people, who have been emotionally over-whelmed by the trauma of seeing their sons or daughters afflicted by a condition that appears to be severely disabling, but which has no obvious physical cause.

Whereas administering the Camberwell Family Interview requires no skills beyond those possessed by most competent clinicians, scoring these scales from tape-recordings of conversations between inter-viewers and relatives is very difficult indeed and requires special (and, from personal experience, very tedious) training. This is because the intonation and emotional expression of the relative are crucial. For example, a statement such as 'He wandered around town in a confused state and was picked up by the police' can be a straightforward descrip-tion of events if expressed in a level tone of voice but can be a highly critical comment if expressed with sufficient venom. Not surprisingly, some researchers have attempted to develop alternative measures to the CFI, based, for example, on questionnaires or analyses of short segments of speech, but these have never been entirely successful.[31]

The results of research on schizophrenia patients conducted in the years since Brown's initial studies have been very consistent. In 1994, Paul Bebbington and Elizabeth Kuipers of the Institute of Psychiatry in London obtained individual data from 1346 families who had been studied in twenty-five separate investigations, of which only three had yielded negative results.[32] Across the studies, about half of the families investigated were judged to include a high EE relative. The overall relapse rate during the first year after patients had returned to these families was 54.4 per cent whereas the rate for low EE families was 21.8 per cent. However, as always, other factors complicate this apparently simple picture.

Figure 16.6 shows data from a famous study of the effects of EE by

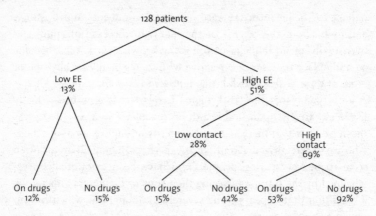

Figure 16.6 Relapse rates for schizophrenia patients living with low and high EE relatives, showing the moderating effects of face-to-face contact time with the relatives and receipt of neuroleptic medication (from Vaughn and Leff, 1976).

British researchers Christine Vaughn and Julian Leff, published in 1976, from which it is obvious that patients living with high EE relatives are especially likely to relapse if they spend a lot of time in contact with those relatives.[33] Vaughn and Leff's findings also indicate an interaction between expressed emotion and patients' medication. Over the nine months of the study, patients taking anti-psychotic drugs received some protection from their high EE relatives. Although the data seem to indicate that those living with low EE relatives received no benefit from their drugs, this finding was not supported when the patients were followed up over a longer period. Vaughn and Leff concluded that medication protected patients from all kinds of stress, and not just the stress of living with a critical or over-controlling relative.[34]

Vaughn and Leff's research led to a second important qualification about the impact of expressed emotion. Studying people who had experienced admission for depression as well as those with a diagnosis of schizophrenia, they found that the depressed patients were even more vulnerable to the adverse effects of stressful relationships than the schizophrenia patients. In fact, it is now clear that Brown's discovery was not a discovery about schizophrenia at all, but a discovery about people with psychiatric complaints in general. The impact of high EE spouses on the well-being of recovering depressed patients has since been the focus of a series of investigations by Jill Hooley, a British-trained psychologist based at Harvard University, in the USA.[35] David Miklowitz and his colleagues at the University of California in Los Angeles have extended EE research to patients with a diagnosis of bipolar disorder. Once again, it has been shown that living with a high EE relative increases the risk of future episodes of illness, in this case of depression and mania.[36]

Surprisingly, researchers have almost completely neglected the psychological mechanisms responsible for the impact of high expressed emotion. Although it seems obvious that exposure to constant criticism and over-protective (in extreme cases, infantilizing) attitudes will result in emotional distress and a loss of self-esteem, few attempts have been made to investigate these kinds of effects, or to reveal how they might lead to an exacerbation of psychotic symptoms.

A few researchers have attempted to measure the immediate emotional impact of exposure to a high EE relative. British psychologists Nick Tarrier and Graham Turpin have demonstrated that schizophrenia patients show unusually high levels of emotional arousal (as measured by changes in the electrical conductivity of their skin) when meeting a high EE relative.[37] In a study conducted by the UCLA schizophrenia research group, it was also found that high expressed emotion relatives can provoke transient increases in patients' symptoms. Patients in the study often expressed unusual thoughts immediately after hearing a critical remark from a high EE parent.[38]

Christine Barrowclough and Nick Tarrier have recently carried out the first study in which the impact of expressed emotion on self-esteem has been measured directly. They used an interview measure of self-esteem, which allowed them to distinguish between positive and negative beliefs about the self. They found that a high level of criticism by a close relative was a strong predictor of negative beliefs about the self, and that these negative beliefs in turn predicted positive symptoms.[39] This finding is, of course, consistent with other evidence about the role of the self in psychosis that we have encountered in earlier chapters.

The nature of high expressed emotion

Some investigators have wondered how the high EE attitudes translate into the actual behaviour of relatives in the presence of a patient. In an attempt to answer this question, researchers at UCLA watched schizophrenia patients and their parents as they discussed family problems. They found that high EE parents, in comparison with low EE parents, made more critical and intrusive comments to their ill sons and daughters.[40] David Miklowitz described this type of interaction as *negative affective style*. Subsequent studies have shown that, when measured as an alternative to EE, negative affective style is a strong predictor of relapse.[41]

Other researchers have wondered why some relatives exhibit high expressed emotion, whereas others do not. One approach to this problem has involved looking in more detail at the beliefs associated with high EE. In earlier chapters I have emphasized the role that patients' attributions (causal beliefs) play in their complaints, but, of course, psychotic patients are not the only people who make inferences about the causes of events. The attributions of schizophrenia patients' relatives have been investigated in studies conducted by Chris Brewin in London[42] and by Christine Barrowclough in Manchester.[43] Perhaps unsurprisingly, those relatives who were judged to be high EE, especially those who were hostile or made many critical comments, tended to explain the distressing behaviour of their mentally ill sons and daughters in terms of causes that were internal to the patient and controllable, for example, saying that they were 'lazy' or 'difficult', as if they could choose to be otherwise.

Other investigators have wondered whether parents' EE status might be related to the stress involved in caring for their mentally ill children. Of course, the experience of seeing an adult son or daughter suffering is almost always extremely distressing. This distress is often compounded by the problems involved in attempting to help the son or daughter cope with the demands of everyday life, while at the same time trying to obtain help from psychiatric services that are under-resourced and sometimes unsympathetic to parents' needs. When it is remembered that these kinds of difficulties can continue for many years, often at a time of life when most parents can expect to be released from the responsibility of caring for their children, it is not surprising that many parents in this position experience high levels of depression and anxiety.[44]

In a recent study conducted by Elizabeth Kuipers and David Raune at the Institute of Psychiatry, it was found that high EE parents experienced the burden of caring for their mentally ill sons and daughters more severely than low EE parents. However, in the same study, it was found that they often attempted to cope with this burden by 'disengaging' from it, for example by avoiding discussing problems with their children, or by using alcohol to relieve their distress.[45] This finding raises the possibility that high expressed emotion arises partly as a consequence of the parents' difficulties in coping with relationships in general.

An earlier study conducted by American psychologists Diana Diamond and Jeri Doane provides some support for this idea.[46] Parents of severely disturbed adolescents and young adults (some of whom were psychotic) were interviewed about their relationships with their children, and also about their relationships with their own mothers and fathers. The more inadequate the attachment relationship between the mothers in the study and their own mothers, the more likely they were to show a negative affective style towards their children. As a consequence of not receiving adequate emotional support in childhood, it seemed that they did not have the emotional resources necessary to offer effective support to their own distressed children. This finding has since been replicated by a group of British investigators.[47]

Further caveats

Overall, studies of expressed emotion add up to one of the few unequivocally successful stories in modern psychiatric research. The findings from these studies clearly demonstrate that the behaviour of psychotic patients cannot be fully understood without understanding the social environment in which they live. However, two further qualifications about the expressed emotion findings are warranted. First, we must recognize that interactions between patients and their relatives are determined in part by both parties. It is dangerous to assume that high EE parents are somehow exclusively 'to blame' for the adverse affects that they have on their children. Patients themselves contribute to these kinds of negative emotional interactions. This was demonstrated in the UCLA study that examined the immediate impact of criticism on patients' symptoms. Careful analysis revealed that critical comments by parents were often triggered by unusual or psychotic comments made by their children. Indeed, high EE behaviour appears to be part of a cycle of escalating negative emotion, in which the bizarre or unusual behaviour of the patient triggers critical comments, which in turn lead to more bizarre and unusual behaviour.

The second qualification concerns researchers' focus on stressful relationships with *parents*. Jill Hooley's work with people suffering from depression has mostly examined expressed emotion in spouses, so it is clear that husbands and wives can also have a negative impact on the well-being of people who are recovering from a psychiatric crisis. More recently, researchers have wondered whether mental health professionals can also be capable of high expressed emotion attitudes.

Studies carried out by Elizabeth Kuipers and Estelle Moore at the Institute of Psychiatry in London have demonstrated that expressed emotion can be reliably measured in psychiatric care staff.[48] In a comparison of two hostels for recovering patients, one of which was staffed by high EE carers, it was found that patients were more likely to leave the high EE hostel, presumably because it did not provide a comfortable living environment.[49] A similar study in Los Angeles found that patients living in a residential care home staffed by high EE carers had a poorer quality of life and worse symptoms than patients living in a low EE environment.[50] Clearly, mental health professionals cannot afford to be complacent about their therapeutic impact on their patients. Indeed, it seems likely that there are high EE psychiatrists, high EE nurses and (although I do not like to admit it) high EE clinical psychologists who would probably be better employed doing something different.

The Slings and Arrows of Outrageous Fortune

When recovering patients live with a high EE relative, spouse or care worker they are exposed to a constant and persisting form of stress. Other stressful events, which occur more suddenly and unpredictably, are known as *life events* in the jargon of modern psychiatric research. These may include separation from a loved one, losing a job, being forced to move home, being arrested by the police, or any number of other calamities. Again, the idea that such events can have a negative impact on mental health is hardly new – Kraepelin noted that periods in which his patients' symptoms remitted often came to an end when they experienced major life changes. However, despite the intuitive appeal of this observation, it has been surprisingly difficult to establish a clear link between specific life events and episodes of illness.

Part of the problem lies in the formidable challenges facing researchers. For practical reasons, most studies have been retrospective, and have attempted to assess what has happened to patients in the weeks or months preceding a breakdown. However, memories are not always reliable, patients' interpretations of events may be affected by their difficulties and, in any case, the importance of different kinds of events may vary between individuals. In practice, researchers have attempted to overcome these problems in one of two ways.[51] Some have attempted to draw up questionnaires listing life events that have previously been judged as stressful by a panel of ordinary people. Participants have then been asked to indicate those events on the questionnaire that they have experienced within a particular period. The second, more sophisticated approach was developed by George Brown and his colleagues in London and involves interviewing patients, using a Life Events and Difficulties Schedule (LEDS), to obtain a detailed account of their recent experiences. The patients' descriptions of events are then presented to a panel of independent judges who score them on various rating scales, for example measuring their severity from the standpoint of the patient.

A further difficulty has been that of teasing out the causal relationship between an event and the emergence of symptoms. Although it is easy to assume that stressful life events must precipitate complaints, sometimes the relationship is the other way round. For example, a patient may become so paranoid that she falls out with her employers and loses her job. George Brown and his colleague Tirril Harris therefore argued that life events should be rated according to whether or not they appear to be independent of symptoms. This is usually done by assigning each recorded event to one of three categories: *independent*, *possibly independent* and *dependent*. In general, researchers have only counted the first two of these categories when exploring the link between life events and increases in episodes of illness.

Using this approach, in 1978 Brown and Harris reported the results of a landmark study, which they had carried out in Camberwell, an economically deprived suburb of London. In by far the majority of cases of depression they detected in a group of women living in the community, they found that significant life events preceded the onset of symptoms by only a few weeks. However, they found that many women who experienced life events did not become depressed, so other factors were obviously important. Women who were living in stressful social circumstances (who were unemployed, had small children at home or lacked supportive relationships), or who had lost their mothers at an early age, were especially vulnerable to reacting badly to an adverse event.[52] In general, later studies have confirmed Brown and Harris's finding of a clear link between negative life events and depression. Indeed, in twenty studies using Brown's Life Events and Difficulties Schedule, estimates of the number of depressive episodes closely preceded by negative life events have varied between 67 per cent and 90 per cent.[53] These studies have also shown that the kinds of social factors that leave people vulnerable to the impact of life events may vary with location. (In a study conducted in the Outer Hebrides, for example, Brown found that people who were poorly integrated with the local community were especially vulnerable.)[54]

Not surprisingly, some researchers have tried to discover whether there is a similar association between life events and episodes of psychosis. The earliest study of this kind was conducted by Brown and his colleague Jim Birley, which was published in 1968.[55] They reported that 46 per cent of a group of schizophrenia patients had suffered a life event in the three weeks preceding a relapse, and therefore concluded that life events could trigger the onset of psychotic symptoms. However, the results of subsequent studies have not always been consistent with these findings. Whereas some found a similar link between life events and relapse, others did not. A study by Paul Bebbington, conducted in Camberwell in the early 1990s, compared the life events of fifty-one patients who had experienced a relapse with the life events experienced by a group of ordinary people living in the community, and found that the patients had experienced an excess of independent life events in the three months prior to becoming ill.[56] Another recent study, carried out by Steven Hirsch and his colleagues, also in London, involved the regular assessment of patients who received either anti-psychotic medication or a placebo. In this study, no effect of life events was observed when the four weeks preceding a relapse were examined, but an effect was found when life events over the previous year were calculated.[57] One possible implication of this finding is that psychotic breakdowns sometimes occur after stressful experiences have accumulated over a long period of time.

In a 1995 review of similar studies conducted with bipolar patients, American psychologists Sheri Johnson and John Roberts were able to identify fifteen studies that had used questionnaire measures and ten that had used interview methods (usually the LEDS).[58] Although the findings were not entirely consistent, the overall picture suggested that life events can trigger episodes of mania as well as depression. Johnson's own study of sixty-seven bipolar patients, published two years later, found that those whose episodes had been triggered by negative life events took, on average, three times longer to recover than those whose episodes began without severe life events.[59]

It would obviously be very useful to know whether different kinds of life events tend to provoke different complaints. Unfortunately, this question (which is much more complex than the question of whether life events, in general, provoke episodes of psychosis) has rarely been studied. In one investigation, Brown and his colleague Robert Finlay-Jones found that events associated with loss (broadly defined to include not only the loss of a person but also the loss of a role, goal or cherished idea) were especially likely to lead to depression, whereas events associated with long-term threat were more likely to lead to anxiety.[60] In later studies it was found that depression was also likely to follow humiliating events (for example, being deserted by a partner) or events that created a sense of entrapment (for example, the onset of a debilitating physical illness). It was also found that life events were particularly likely to have an emotional impact if they matched an ongoing difficulty (for example, a mother's discovery that her son has been arrested, matching her ongoing concerns about their difficult relationship and his delinquent behaviour).[61]

As we saw in Chapter 12, Brown's colleague Tirril Harris has suggested that the events most likely to lead to psychotic and especially paranoid symptoms can be characterized as intrusive, because they involve unwanted experiences being forced on the patient (examples include threats, burglaries and police investigations).[62] This suggestion has been partially supported by research conducted by other investigators.[63] In the case of mania, as we saw in Chapter 11, it appears that episodes of illness are often precipitated by events that disrupt social rhythms[64] or which involve goal attainment.[65] Each of these effects seems to be relatively easy to understand in the context of our knowledge of the psychological mechanisms involved in these kinds of symptoms. Those which bring to mind a sense of loss or failure are most dangerous to people who already doubt their self-worth; those with a persecutory element appear to bring out pre-existing fears about others' intentions; and those which exacerbate subjective feelings of energy and excitement are particularly hazardous to people who are vulnerable to mania.

Despite these findings, some researchers have been sceptical about the link between life events and psychotic episodes. In part, this has been because they have been influenced by genetic evidence, which has suggested to them that there is little room for environmental influences on patients' symptoms (a prejudice that I will address in the next chapter). Whereas I have tried to point to the overall pattern of the findings from many research projects, critics have focused on the methodological inadequacies of some investigations and some inconsistencies in the results from different studies. As a counter to these kinds of arguments, it is worth pointing out that there are at least two reasons to think that existing findings *underestimate* the role of life events in psychosis.

First, as Paul Bebbington has noted, some of the apparent inconsistencies in the research findings may reflect the *extreme sensitivity* of psychotic patients.[66] Perhaps they are so easily affected by adverse experiences that even relatively trivial events affect them. Consistent with this suggestion, studies have shown a clearer link between life events and psychosis in patients who take anti-psychotic drugs or who live in low EE households, than in patients who refuse drugs or live in high EE environments. The implication of these findings is that even very minor events – which would not be picked up by the methods developed by Brown and Harris – may be capable of triggering symptoms in patients who refuse medication or are embroiled in stressful relationships.

Second, because most researchers have deliberately ignored life events that could be the consequence of symptoms, they have failed to record circumstances in which life events and symptoms exacerbate each other in an escalating spiral of psychopathology. Imagine a remitted patient who is not coping well with life, becomes depressed and, as a consequence, loses his job. Later, the patient becomes floridly psychotic. In this case, the loss of the job is clearly not independent of the patient's prodromal symptoms, so it would not be counted in a study of life events. Nonetheless, sudden unemployment will almost certainly have been a further source of distress and may well have played a role in moving the patient from a prodromal phase into frank psychosis.

The Process of Relapse

Stressful relationships and life events do not exhaust the factors that can increase the likelihood that a person will once again experience psychotic complaints. There is evidence that the excessive use of either legal or street drugs, such as alcohol, amphetamine, cannabis or the hallucinogens, can increase the probability of relapse in both schizophrenia patients[67] and patients with a diagnosis of bipolar disorder.[68] Unfortunately, in Europe and North America at least, psychotic patients very commonly abuse alcohol or take drugs, partly because these substances often make them feel better in the short term.[69]

Keith Nuechterlein and his colleagues at UCLA have proposed an influential model of schizophrenic relapse, which is shown in Figure 16.7.[70] Although at first glance it appears very complex, it encompasses just a few simple ideas. Nuechterlein argues that the risk of a psychotic episode is affected by a combination of personal and environmental factors. The personal factors include those (such as schizotypal personality traits and putative abnormalities in the dopamine system) that increase an individual's likelihood of experiencing complaints, and also protective factors (such as coping skills and taking medication), which have the opposite effect. The environmental factors are similarly divided into those that protect (a supportive family, for example) and those that increase the risk of symptoms (stressful life events, for example). According to the model, some interactions between these factors can exacerbate existing cognitive deficits, leading the patient's cognitive system to become overloaded and also to increased emotional arousal. These in turn are thought to lead to prodromal symptoms and then, eventually, to the full symptoms of a psychotic episode. Importantly, the UCLA group propose that the experience of an episode can feed back to change the earlier personal and environmental factors, so that further episodes are more likely (a sort of kindling effect).

The UCLA group has marshalled a lot of evidence for some of the core assumptions of their model. As I explained in Chapter 7, they have carried out experiments to show that working memory deficits become more severe as patients become ill. However, notice that, despite its apparent complexity, the model remains very general in its scope. In fact, although it is proposed as a theory of schizophrenic relapse, with a few modifications it could equally well serve as an account of relapse in depression or mania. This is because the main weakness of the model is that it does not explain how cognitive changes lead to specific complaints such as hallucinations, delusions or mania. What appears to be missing is any reference to the social-cognitive processes that play a role in prodromal dysphoria, and which we have directly implicated in these symptoms.

It is easy to see how the model might be tinkered with to overcome some of these limitations, and I will leave this task to the reader. Of course, as different cognitive processes are implicated in different complaints, the protective and vulnerability factors associated with them are also likely to differ. If this is the case, a truly comprehensive model of psychotic relapse will consist of a series of inter-related and more specific models, each specifying pathways involved in the exacerbation of one particular type of psychotic behaviour or experience.

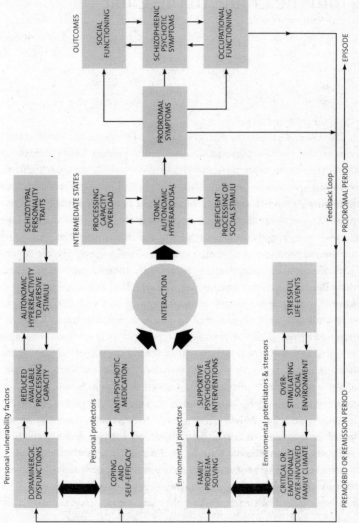

Figure 16.7 The UCLA model of psychotic relapse (from Nuechterlein et al., 1992).

17

From the Cradle to the Clinic

The childhood shows the man,
As morning shows the day.
John Milton[1]

Any attempt to explain the origins of madness must address an important puzzle. Since Kraepelin's time, it has been known that schizophrenia symptoms most often appear for the first time during late adolescence or early adulthood. It was for this reason that Kraepelin christened his disorder *dementia praecox*. Modern studies have generally supported this observation. Figure 17.1 shows a fairly typical age distribution for the onset of psychosis, which I have obtained from a sample of 254 first-episode schizophrenia or schizoaffective patients who took part in a clinical trial of psychological treatment for early psychosis carried out at my own University.[2] It is obvious from the graph that most people became ill in their early twenties; the age of maximum risk seems to be about 22 years. However, notice also that a few patients were in their sixties when they were first affected, so that the mean (average) age of onset was exactly 29 years. However, a better indication of the *typical* age of onset is the median (the age at which half of the patients are younger and half are older), which is 26.5 years. When the data are broken down by sex, we find that the median age of onset for women (29.3 years) is a few years older than that for men (25.6 years). This earlier onset for men than for women has been found in nearly every other study that has examined this issue.[3]

It is sometimes forgotten that diagnoses of bipolar disorder follow similar age trends. The period of peak risk for developing bipolar

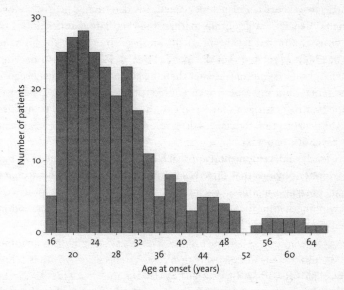

Figure 17.1 Ages of onset of illness for 254 first-episode schizophrenia and schizoaffective patients recruited to the SoCRATES (Study of Cognitive-Realignment Therapy in Early Schizophrenia) project.

symptoms is during adolescence and early adulthood and the distribution of ages of onset is very similar to that of schizophrenia patients; interestingly, there is evidence that those who first show symptoms early in life are especially likely to become floridly psychotic.[4] There is also some evidence that women are slightly more likely than men to develop bipolar symptoms later in life, although the data pertaining to this difference are relatively sparse and not entirely consistent.[5]

These observations raise the possibility that psychosis is the end-point of a developmental process. But what kind of process? Once again, the ground has been staked out by biological researchers, who have proposed various versions of what I term the *biological time-bomb hypothesis*. According to this theory, schizophrenia and bipolar disorder are consequences of defects in the developing brain, which only 'explode' into frank illness as or after the afflicted person reaches maturity. The exact nature of the hypothesized time-bomb varies from theorist to theorist, and includes genetically determined neurodevelopmental deficits,[6] faulty brain maturation,[7] and late manifestations of a virus contracted by the pregnant mother.[8] In a twist to this tale, it has been suggested that the average age at which women develop schizophrenia symptoms is later than the average age for men because the female hormone oestrogen confers protection against psychosis (apparently, oestrogen shares some of the pharmacological properties of the neuroleptics, the class of drugs most widely used in the treatment of psychotic patients).[9]

Clearly, a developmental approach has much to recommend it, but it is pretty obvious that there is something missing from any account that portrays madness exclusively as the product of processes unwinding within the individual. What is missing is any recognition that psychosis might be influenced by the trials of life.

Rethinking the Genetics of Psychosis

Writing in 1939, Robert Gaupp, one-time Professor of Psychiatry at the University of Tübingen, made the following comment:

We are, of course, clearly aware of the fact, which we don't deny even for a second, that the greater part of all genetic work in psychiatry would immediately collapse like a house of cards if Kraepelin's theory was shown to be altogether mistaken.[10]

In Chapter 4, I discussed family, twin and adoption studies that have pointed to the role of genetic factors in the origins of psychosis. I suggested that genetic researchers have often exaggerated the weight of the evidence obtained from these kinds of studies, and have tended to ignore serious methodological weaknesses in their own work. I think this observation would be widely accepted by many fellow psychologists and psychiatrists who are familiar with the data. However, what is less widely recognized is that even if (and it is a big if) *very substantial* genetic contributions to psychosis could be proven, this proof would not preclude the possibility that the environment also plays a major role in the development of symptoms.

Geneticists commonly use the data from their studies to calculate *heritability estimates*, which describe the amount of variability in some phenomenon (say, intelligence or mental illness) that can be attributed to genes.* Typically, researchers investigating schizophrenia or bipolar symptoms obtain estimates that are very high – as much as 80 or 90 per cent. Values of this sort *seem* to leave little room for environmental influences. However, this conclusion is based on the assumption that the amount of variability attributed to genes and that attributed to the environment are independent of each other, and therefore can be simply added to total 100 per cent. In real life, genes and environments are almost always correlated, so that genetic and environmental influences cannot be separated out in this way. This happens because individuals (not only human beings, but even plants and small animals)[11] influence their environments in ways that depend on their genetic endowment. When this happens, environmental influences can bring about dramatic changes in behaviours or abilities, even when the behaviours and abilities are under strong genetic control.

A formal mathematical analysis of this kind of interaction† has recently been published by William Dickins of Harvard University and James Flynn of the University of Otago.[12] However, rather than attempting to summarize their difficult proof here, I will offer a hypothetical case study that may help the reader to understand how gene–environment correlations can have this effect. Imagine that a young man, who is destined to become psychotic by virtue of inheriting genes that make him vulnerable to negative symptoms, has poor social skills. Such a person might be more likely than most to be rejected when

---

* To be more precise, these estimates give the proportion of variance in a characteristic which can be attributed to genetic variation as compared with the proportion attributed to environmental variation in a given population. This definition assumes a simple additive model of the two sources of variation, such that

$$\text{heritability} = \frac{\text{variance due to genes}}{\text{variance due to genes} + \text{variance due to environment}}$$

† Nowhere has the debate between heredity versus environment been more contentious than in relation to measured IQ and its implications for racial differences. While this debate has raged, research has demonstrated massive IQ gains in different countries (an increase in the average IQ of as much as 20 points in 40 years). This phenomenon is known as the Flynn effect, after James Flynn, the New Zealand political scientist who first identified it. Accepting, for the sake of argument, heritability estimates of 75 per cent or more, Dickins and Flynn's mathematical analysis demonstrates that there remains room for the very strong environmental influences on IQ that are necessary to explain the Flynn effect.

asking a potential girlfriend for a date. Moreover, because he does not know how to seek emotional support from friends, or because his parents (who also have poor social skills) do not know how to reassure him, he may become more socially anxious and self-conscious afterwards. Consequently, he may become withdrawn, making him more likely to be ridiculed by unkind peers. As time goes by, he may become progressively more isolated until, perhaps reacting to some further difficulties, he becomes psychotic. In this imaginary, but not implausible, scenario, genes have predisposed the unlucky young man to an environmental trauma (being rejected by a potential girlfriend), but the trauma has had a major impact on his future life. Had he decided to approach the one girl in his neighbourhood who was attracted to quiet young men, the outcome might have been very different.

Evidence that gene–environment interactions of this sort happen in psychiatric conditions has emerged from genetic studies of depression, which have shown that the close relatives of depressed patients experience a higher rate of unpleasant life events than the general population.[13] Presumably because of their genetically determined characteristics they are more likely to find themselves in circumstances in which these kinds of events are likely to occur. If these kinds of effects occur across the spectrum of patients suffering from severe psychiatric disorders (and I would be amazed if they did not) environmental events may have a much greater ability to influence psychosis than most psychiatric geneticists have supposed.

From genes to madness

Perhaps the central argument of this book is that the problems involved in explaining 'schizophrenia' and 'bipolar disorder' will disappear once we have adequately explained the complaints that lead to these diagnoses. An implication of this argument is that we must consider genetic influences on particular kinds of psychotic behaviours and experiences. This task is especially important because, in their critique of the symptom-orientated approach, Ramin Mojtabai and Ronald Rieder have argued that no such influences can be discerned.[14]

According to Mojtabai and Rieder, twin and family studies show that a diagnosis of schizophrenia is more heritable than any of the symptoms that contribute to the diagnosis. American psychologists

Howard Berenbaum, Tom Oltmanns and Irving Gottesman analysed data from a twin study to show that the concordance rates for positive or negative symptoms were lower than the concordance rate calculated for a global diagnosis.[15] In a more recent study of 'high density schizophrenia families' living in Ireland, conducted by American researcher Kenneth Kendler and his colleagues, sibling pairs in which both had received a diagnosis of schizophrenia were examined to see whether they experienced similar symptoms; in general the concordance between the symptoms of the affected pairs were low.[16] According to Mojtabai and Rieder, these observations are impossible to square with a symptom-orientated approach.

It is worth unpacking Mojtabai and Rieder's argument, using the functional analysis framework that I introduced in the last chapter. They have implicitly contrasted two models, which I have shown in Figure 17.2. According to their preferred model (which is a version of the Kraepelinian paradigm), genes influence the development of a disease, which in turn causes the affected individual to experience symptoms. The alternative model supposes that genes influence symptoms, without the mediating disease step. Mojtabai and Rieder argue that this alternative model must be rejected because the empirical evidence shows that genes have only a relatively weak effect on each of the symptoms but a strong impact on the overall diagnosis.

In fact, there is evidence of a specific genetic contribution to at least one psychotic symptom. It has been known for some time that thought disorder runs in families. In the 1960s, American researchers Margaret Singer and Lyman Wynne carried out a series of studies in an attempt to show that this happened because thought-disordered parents communicate inadequately with their children. (In essence, they proposed that thought disorder is learnt.)[17] The comments of patients' parents were recorded as they completed a series of psychological tests, which were also administered to the patients.[18] A detailed rating procedure was then used to analyse the comments for unusual styles of communication (particularly, abnormal ways of handling attention and meaning which might 'impair a growing child's capacity for selective attention, purposive behaviour, and subjectively meaningful experiences'). They also rated unusual ways of talking about relationships, abnormal emotional responses (especially comments thought to reflect 'underlying feelings of pervasive meaninglessness'), and statements suggesting that

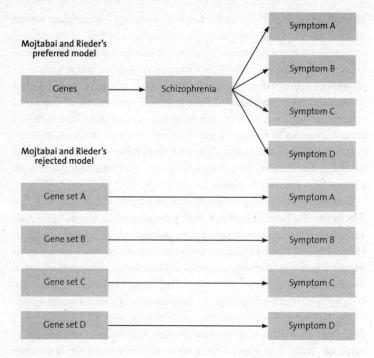

Figure 17.2 Two models of genetic influences contrasted by Mojtabai and Rieder (1998).

the overall structure of the family was poorly organized to cope with stress. Singer then attempted to predict the patient's ratings from the ratings taken from the parent, and found that she could do so with a high degree of success. When given transcripts from the parents and the patients without knowing which transcript went with which, she was able to match them together, again with a high degree of accuracy.

Most subsequent studies have supported Singer and Wynne's conclusion that *communication deviance* (to use their terminology) is found in the families of thought-disordered patients.[19] For example, in two recent studies Nancy Docherty (whose work I discussed in some detail in Chapter 15) found that the speech of the parents of thought-disordered patients contains frequent referential failures.[20] However, whereas the speech of patients becomes more incoherent as they become emotionally aroused, Docherty found their parents' speech was not affected in this way.[21]

Communication deviance appears to be completely unrelated to expressed emotion, the type of critical or over-controlling behaviour sometimes observed in the families of psychotic patients, which I described in the last chapter.[22] There is some evidence that it reflects, in part, genetic factors. For example, Orsola Gambini and colleagues at the University of Milan recently studied the speech of normal monozygotic and dizygotic twins. When they rated the speech for thought disorder, they found higher concordance rates in the MZ twins than in the DZ twins.[23] In another recent study, Dennis Kinney and colleagues at Harvard University used an adoption study strategy to investigate the heritability of thought disorder, which they measured in Danish adoptees who had developed schizophrenia symptoms and adoptees not diagnosed as schizophrenic, before then tracing their biological parents through Denmark's comprehensive adoption records. They found high levels of thought disorder in the parents of the schizophrenia patients, but not in the parents of the healthy adoptees.[24]

Of course, as we have already seen, strong genetic influences do not exclude the role of environmental factors. That such factors may play a decisive role in the case of thought disorder was revealed in another adoption study, this time carried out in Finland by a large team that included Lyman Wynne and Pekka Tienari, a respected psychiatric geneticist.[25] The team used a refined version of Singer and Wynne's methodology to assess disordered communication both in the adopted-away children of schizophrenia patients and in their adopting relatives. Adoptees who were regarded as being at high risk because their biological parents had been diagnosed as schizophrenic showed high levels of communication deviance *only* if their adopting parents showed evidence of communication deviance. Adoptees who were not at genetic risk of developing a psychotic illness did not develop thought disorder, even if their adopting parents showed evidence of communication deviance. These findings show that *thought disorder results from an interaction between genes and the environment*.

In contrast to these findings, genetic evidence on paranoid symptoms suggests that these are very little influenced by heredity. For example, studies of patients diagnosed as suffering from personality disorders have consistently yielded lower heritability estimates for the diagnosis of paranoid personality disorder than for any other DSM axis-2 diagnoses.[26] Furthermore, it also appears that, even if genes make a minor contribution, they are unlikely to be the same genes as those involved in other complaints attributed to schizophrenia. In a series of studies carried out in the 1980s, Kenneth Kendler found that the relatives of patients given a diagnosis of delusional disorder rarely showed evidence of schizotypal traits,[27] a finding that has been replicated many times in subsequent investigations.[28]

On this evidence at least, different psychotic complaints seem to be differentially influenced by genes. Of course, this still leaves us with Mojtabai and Rieder's paradox that diagnoses seem to be more heritable than individual symptoms, to which I will return later.

What the new genetics tells us

In order to understand further the relationship between genes and symptoms it will be helpful to think about the mechanisms by which genes influence behaviour. This takes us into the complex territory of molecular genetics, where we will find evidence that will further discomfort neoKraepelinians. I will begin with a very brief primer covering some of the most important scientific concepts in this area.

Even when strong genetic effects can be demonstrated by family, twin or adoption studies, many intermediate steps must lie between genes and madness. Genes consist of sequences of chemical elements, known as nucleotides, joined together in long molecules of DNA, which in turn are contained in the chromosomes held in the nucleus of every cell. In humans there are twenty-three chromosomes, which together comprise the genetic material known as the human *genome*. However, most cells contain a double set, so that there are twenty-three *pairs*, with one member of each pair drawn from one parent and one from the other. The gametes – sperm and egg cells – are exceptions to this rule, as they contain only one version of each chromosome. During the initial formation of these cells, DNA may be swapped between corresponding sections of each pair of chromosomes, and one chromosome from each pair is then selected at random to enter each gamete. Of course, when sperm from the father and egg cells from the mother combine at fertilization the single sets of chromosomes in each gamete pair together, so that the resultant embryo contains twenty-three new chromosome pairs.

There are four types of nucleotides, labelled A (for adenine), G (guanine), C (cytosine) and T (thymine). The order in which these are arranged (sometimes described as the genetic code) determines the synthesis of proteins in each cell. Some sequences of nucleotides are involved directly in protein synthesis in co-operation with other bio-chemical systems; some sequences switch on or off the production of different proteins during different developmental periods and in different parts of the body. Genetic variation occurs because genes (sequences of nucleotides in particular regions – loci – on the chromo-somes that are responsible for particular proteins) come in different varieties (differences in the sequence), known as *alleles*. Strictly speak-ing, therefore, rather than saying that someone has inherited the gene for a particular characteristic, we should say that they have inherited (one or two copies of) the relevant allele of that gene. For some characteristics, inheriting one crucial allele is sufficient, in which case the allele is said to be *dominant*. For others, the characteristic does not appear unless both of the corresponding alleles on a pair of chromosomes are of a particular type, in which case the allele is said to be *recessive*. The precise composition of alleles in the chromosomes is known as the individual's *genotype*.

Ultimately, the synthesis of proteins controls the structure of the developing body. Thoughtful biologists have pointed out that unravelling this process of development is a task that will dwarf in complexity the much-vaunted efforts to map the human genome (that is, to determine the exact sequence of nucleotides on the DNA in the twenty-three chromosome pairs).[29] Of course, it has long been recognized that single genes rarely exclusively determine character-istics in the adult person, either because interactions between different genes are involved, or because of environmental influences. When only a small proportion of individuals carrying crucial alleles develop a trait, the alleles are said to have low *penetrance*. In fact, the penetrance of an allele can be expressed as a simple percentage describing the proportion of carriers who are affected. Alleles also vary in their *expressivity*, which refers to the extent to which genetic traits, when present, vary in magnitude. The alleles responsible for some physical disorders, for example Marfan's syndrome, which is characterized by various abnormalities in the skeleton and connective tissues, are 100 per cent penetrant (everyone carrying the crucial allele gets it to some degree) but variable in their expression (some people suffer from life-threatening defects in the wall of the aorta, whereas some people just look odd).[30] Not surprisingly, given the evidence from twin and adoption studies reviewed earlier in this book, most psychiatric geneticists assume that alleles responsible for schizophrenia and bipolar disorder must be less than completely penetrant and variable in their expression. Geneticists sometimes use complex mathematical analyses of data from family, twin and adoption studies to derive estimates of the number of genes contributing to a particular disorder, whether the alleles are dominant or recessive, and the extent to which they are penetrant and variable in their expression. However, despite considerable efforts, no widely accepted model of the genetic contribution to psychosis has been generated this way.

In the case of the brain, some genes that cause undifferentiated cells in the embryo to become brain cells have been identified, together with genes that control the segmentation of the developing nervous system into different regions containing different kinds of neurones utilizing different chemical transmitter systems.[31] However, although genes help to determine the broad structure of the nervous system, it is clear that they do not precisely determine the final 'wiring diagram' of the adult brain. It has been estimated that about 30,000 genes play a role in determining the structure of the human body, a number that is remarkably invariant across mammalian species that differ dramatically in the complexity of their nervous systems. By contrast, it has been estimated that the adult human brain contains about 100 trillion synapses, and that more than a quarter of a million of these are formed *every second* during the very early stages of development.[32] Animals raised in impoverished environments compared to animals raised in enriched environments develop fewer synapses, and a lower density of blood capillaries (which supply neurones with nutrients),[33] confirming that this process is influenced by experience. In a recent attempt to draw together evidence about this process, a group of distinguished researchers from Britain and the United States, led by Jeffrey Elman of the University of California at San Diego, concluded that brain development is determined by interactions with the environment at every stage, leading them to ponder whether the idea of 'innate' behaviour should be dispensed with altogether.[34] Unfortunately, these advances in the understanding of the genetic control of neurodevelopment appear to have largely escaped the attention of psychiatric researchers.

Following the development of techniques for mapping DNA,[35] psychiatric geneticists have hoped to identify genes, and eventually alleles of those genes, that determine the major psychiatric disorders. The most widely explored approach is known as *linkage analysis*, which capitalizes on existing knowledge about the location of certain genes (known as markers) on particular chromosomes. Linkage analysis is usually carried out on data collected from small numbers of families in which there are many affected cases, as this increases the probability that specific alleles are involved in the affected individuals' psychiatric problems. The closer the physical location on a chromosome of a marker gene to a psychosis gene, the more likely the marker gene will be shuffled together with the psychosis gene during the interchange of DNA between chromosomes prior to conception. Therefore, if marker genes are found mostly in those family members who are affected by the illness, the gene responsible for the illness is likely to be located close to the marker gene on the relevant chromosome. Most linkage studies utilize a small number of markers located along a single chromosome. However, in some recent studies, markers spread evenly across all the chromosomes have been examined together, a technique known as *genome scanning*.[36]

There are several points to note about this approach. First, these techniques assume that researchers can accurately diagnose affected individuals. As most genetic researchers have accepted the validity of the neoKraepelinian system, it is not surprising that they have come unstuck on this very problem. Second, linkage analysis not only requires the use of complex biochemical techniques, but also sophisticated mathematical checks to ensure that any observed association between an illness and a marker is not the result of chance. Third, even if it is possible to locate psychosis genes in affected families, it is possible that the genes play no or little role in non-familial forms of psychosis (that is, in psychotic illnesses that appear sporadically, without a history of illness in the family). Finally, for reasons that should now be obvious, discovering the location of a psychosis gene is a long way from understanding how that gene plays some part in the genesis of psychotic behaviours and experiences. To make further progress, it will be necessary to understand how the implicated gene is involved in the synthesis of proteins, or how it influences the activity of other genes which do this. We would need to know the difference that the aberrant allele makes to that process, the role of the relevant proteins in brain development, the final consequences of any developmental abnormalities for the structure and function of different brain systems in adulthood, the cognitive processes that are supported by those brain systems and, last but not least, the role of those processes in patients' complaints.

The earliest linkage studies of psychosis were hailed as major breakthroughs but soon turned out to be a source of embarrassment to biological psychiatrists. Janice Egeland and her colleagues in the United States chose to study a population with a restricted gene pool, the Old Order Amish living in southeastern Pennsylvania. The Amish (familiar to many people from their portrayal in Peter Weir's film *The Witness*) are a religious sect that has shunned the trappings of modern life, has pursued a rural existence with the minimum use of mechanical aids, and whose members have rarely married outsiders. Psychiatric interviews were conducted and hospital records examined for a pedigree of 120 related individuals. Using the RDC, 19 received a diagnosis of major depression, 14 received a diagnosis of bipolar disorder, and 5 received a diagnosis of unipolar depression. In 1987, Egeland and her co-workers reported strong linkage between bipolar disorder and two markers on chromosome 11, indicating that a gene for bipolar disorder lay somewhere on this chromosome.[37] Only two years later, the investigators reported a second analysis of the pedigree, adding data from a further 37 members.[38] These new data, on their own, had little impact on the findings. However, in the period between the two analyses, two individuals who had been considered unaffected in the original analysis developed bipolar symptoms. When these individuals were taken into account in their mathematical analysis, Egeland and her colleagues discovered that the association between bipolar disorder and their markers disappeared. The earlier finding had been spurious.

Reflecting on similar efforts to find genes for schizophrenia, American geneticist Cathy Barr described waking up one morning in 1988 to hear a radio news bulletin announcing that researchers had found linkage for the diagnosis. 'The significance of such a finding caused me to bolt straight up from bed', she recalled.[39] She immediately reviewed her career plans and, soon afterwards, was carrying out her own research in psychiatric genetics. Most British researchers similarly learned of the first apparently successful linkage study of schizophrenia from a news bulletin. Returning home from work one night in 1988, I turned on my television set, to be greeted by a headline informing me that researchers had discovered *the* gene for schizophrenia on chromosome 5. The news bulletin announced that the results of a study conducted by investigators at the Middlesex Hospital would shortly appear in the prestigious journal *Nature*. When David Hill, a sceptical clinical psychologist, rang *Nature* on behalf of a British news magazine to inquire about the status of the report, he was told that it had not yet been considered by the journal.[40] Presumably, the researchers' enthusiasm to win the race to find a schizophrenia gene led them to assume that the journal would accept their report when it was eventually submitted for publication. In this respect, at least, they showed sound judgement, as their paper eventually appeared in *Nature* later in the year,[41] alongside a report from a group of US and Swedish researchers claiming that a gene for schizophrenia did *not* exist on chromosome 5.[42]

The Middlesex group had obtained data from 104 people in five Icelandic and two British pedigrees whereas the US–Swedish team had obtained data from 81 people from a single Swedish pedigree but had used more powerful mapping techniques. An examination of the Middlesex report reveals causes for concern that should have been obvious to any competent reviewer (raising important questions about why *Nature* accepted the paper). For example, the researchers compared various different definitions of schizophrenia in order to maximize their linkage findings. Maximum linkage was achieved by including as 'schizophrenic' individuals who were diagnosed as suffering from depression, phobias, alcoholism and drug addiction. Although these individuals would not be considered remotely schizophrenic according to any definition of the disorder promulgated in the last 100 years, the researchers described them as 'fringe phenotypes' (that is, as individuals who were assumed to be genetically schizophrenic, but whose symptoms differed from the prototype because of presumed environmental influences). A subsequent study published by a group of researchers in Edinburgh used markers similar to those employed by the Middlesex group but obtained negative findings.[43] After several further failures to replicate their findings, the Middlesex group reanalysed their data with an expanded sample and withdrew their original conclusions.[44]

Linkage research has been pursued vigorously in the decade or so since these first reports. However, consistent findings have been elusive. In the case of bipolar disorder, efforts have focused not only on chromosome 11, but also on chromosomes 4, 5, 6, 9, 10, 13, 16, 18, 21, 22 and the X chromosome, but without consistent results.[45] In the case of schizophrenia, numerous gene sites have been investigated, and special efforts have been made to study loci known to influence the structure and distribution of dopamine receptors in the brain.[46] Sites on chromosomes 10, 13, 18 and 22, which have been tentatively linked to schizophrenia, appear to overlap those that have been tentatively linked to bipolar disorder,[47] an observation that has special significance in the light of the persisting doubts about the distinction between the two diagnoses. Again, however, findings have been almost entirely inconsistent.[48]

In a particularly challenging review of this kind of research, Tim Crow reflected on his own participation in a multinational collaborative project that aimed to replicate previously observed associations between schizophrenia and ten genetic markers.[49] Although the main authors of the collaborative group's research report stated that they had found evidence of linkage with genes on chromosomes 6 and 8,[50] Crow disputed these findings on statistical grounds. In an accompanying table, he listed no fewer than twelve genetic loci that had been associated with schizophrenia by linkage analysis. At the time that he was writing in 1997, other researchers had failed to replicate these findings for eleven of the twelve gene sites. As I complete the final draft of this chapter in late 2002, it is still the case that replicable linkage results for major psychiatric disorders have remained elusive.[51]

Frustrated by this 'maddening hunt for madness genes',[52] many commentators have begun to reflect on the limitations of the molecular genetic approach.[53] No doubt, the disappointing findings partly reflect the obstacles that must be overcome by investigators (the difficulty of diagnosing a homogeneous group of affected individuals; the difficulties involved in statistically evaluating the results). In the face of these obstacles, some researchers have even begun to search for genes that influence particular complaints. For example, a research group at the University of Milan reported a study of over 400 psychotic patients with a range of diagnoses, in which they attempted to determine which symptoms were associated with different alleles of a gene known to influence the structure of the dopamine D4 receptor in the brain. The gene is highly polymorphic (that is, there are many different alleles of it) and there is evidence that different variants produce different proteins in the receptor. It was found that patients with some of these alleles were much more likely to be deluded than patients with others.[54]

If we do not entirely reject the findings of the molecular geneticists, it is reasonable to reach three conclusions. First, the findings, such as they are, seem surprisingly consistent with critical reviews of the family, twin and adoption study data, which have argued that genetic investigators have almost always overstated the evidence that psychosis is inherited.[55] Second, it seems likely that psychotic disorders are heterogeneous at the molecular level (that is, genes that predispose some people to become psychotic may play no role in the psychotic experiences of other people).[56] Third – and this is perhaps the most important conclusion – it seems likely that *any genetic contribution to psychosis is caused by many genes of minor effect*. Despite the limitations of existing methods, if just one or two genes played a major role, they would almost certainly have been identified by now. For this reason, it seems much more likely that many genes each make a small contribution towards vulnerability to symptoms.

On the inheritance of symptoms: a genetic footnote

Before leaving genetic studies of psychosis behind us, I would like to return briefly to the apparent paradox raised by Mojtabai and Rieder in their critique of the symptom-orientated approach. Recall their claim that diagnoses such as schizophrenia and manic depression are more heritable than individual symptoms. Although they argued that this observation is inconsistent with an analysis of madness that focuses on particular complaints, we can now see why this is not necessarily the case.

Let us take the molecular geneticists' observations seriously and suppose that there are no major genes for psychosis. Instead, let us suppose that there are many minor genes, and that each gene influences a particular complaint by means of a complex causal chain. As the heritability of complaints, in general, appears to be quite small, we can also assume that many other (perhaps environmental) factors play a role in determining whether a complaint is experienced by a person who inherits the relevant gene. (In other words, we can assume that the relevant alleles have low expressivity and/or low penetrance.)

Mojtabai and Rieder's paradox is resolved when we note that psychiatric studies mainly focus on people with many complaints. This is because the rules embodied in the DSM and similar systems require several complaints to be present before a diagnosis can be made, and also because people with many complaints are especially likely to experience distress and seek psychiatric treatment. The more complaints people have, the more psychosis genes they are likely to have inherited, and the more likely it will be that some of those genes will be shared by close relatives. Because of the role that other factors play in each complaint, an affected person's close relatives may not experience the same complaint. However, if they have a sufficient number of psychosis genes, enough may be expressed as complaints to enable them to meet the criteria for a global diagnosis. As a consequence, the diagnosis will appear to be more heritable than each of the complaints.

I offer this argument merely to establish that Mojtabai and Rieder's genetic objection to the approach I am advocating is not as compelling as it at first appears. Although admittedly highly speculative, it probably understates the weakness of Mojtabai and Rieder's position. As we have seen, genes do not directly cause particular kinds of experiences and behaviours but instead influence the development of the brain, which in turn affects the cognitive resources available to the individual. Furthermore, as I described in the last chapter, complaints may be functionally interconnected to each other in complex ways. When these added levels of complexity are taken into account, the Kraepelinian paradigm seems even less buttressed by the genetic evidence.

Is There a Biological Time-Bomb?

Earlier in this chapter, I introduced the biological time-bomb hypothesis, the idea that some kind of neurodevelopmental defect is responsible for psychotic breakdowns that occur in late adolescence. Theories of this kind have been stimulated by the recent discovery that the normal brain undergoes major structural changes throughout the second decade of life. This process was first detected in electro-encephalographic (brain-wave) studies, which revealed that the kind of electrical activity generated by the brain changes during this period.[57] Anatomical studies subsequently revealed that these changes coincide with a decrease in the density of synapses (connections between neurones) in the human cortex,[58] a process now known as 'neural pruning'. Whereas early brain development is accompanied by a rapid increase in the brain's connectivity, it now appears that late development is accompanied by some kind of 'weeding out' of connections that serve no purpose. (Not surprisingly, some brain scientists have drawn analogies between this process and the process of natural selection.)[59]

Although there are several different versions of the biological time-bomb hypothesis, it is usual to distinguish between 'early' and 'late' theories. According to the former, damage to the brain or abnormal development very early in life (perhaps before birth) only leads to symptoms when the brain reaches a particular developmental stage; on this view, the primary cause of the psychotic patient's neurodevelopmental deficits is the early insult experienced by the brain.[60] According to late versions of the hypothesis, excessive neural pruning in the second decade of life leads directly to symptoms.[61]

Arduous research

The best way to test developmental theories of psychosis is to study children who later become psychotic. Of course, the practical difficulties inherent in this kind of research are formidable.

It is possible to collect some developmental data retrospectively, for example by asking parents to recall milestones or by examining school reports or other kinds of archives. A recent study of this kind examined psychological tests routinely administered to all Israeli adolescents in preparation for their induction into the military, and matched them against a national register of psychiatric patients. It was found that adolescents who were diagnosed as schizophrenic between four and ten years after their military assessment functioned more poorly socially, and scored considerably lower on intellectual tests, than peers who remained well.[62]

American psychologist Elaine Walker at Emory University has reported a particularly interesting series of archive investigations, in which she analysed home movies taken by the parents of children who developed schizophrenia symptoms in later life. In one study, evidence of abnormal or clumsy movements was observed in seven future patients but not in their brothers or sisters who later remained well.[63] A similar analysis of film clips of a larger group of future patients and their siblings revealed emotional problems in the future patients.[64] In film clips taken between birth and adolescence, there was more evidence of negative emotion and, in the case of girls, less evidence of positive emotion in the future patients in comparison with their brothers and sisters.

Other retrospective investigations have used educational records to show that children who later develop negative symptoms function poorly at school,[65] and child-guidance records to show that unhappy adolescents who later develop positive symptoms are abnormally suspicious of other people.[66] Although these findings suggest that social, cognitive and emotional problems may precede the onset of psychosis by decades, retrospectively collected information is rarely entirely reliable, limiting the conclusions that can be drawn from this kind of research.

Prospective investigations are of greater scientific value but are inevitably more difficult. Because they require children to be followed up over many years, a single investigation may take up a researcher's entire career. Studies of this kind require considerable forethought about the kinds of measures to be employed, as decades of effort can be wasted if the wrong kind of information is collected during the early stages of the project.

The most common type of longitudinal investigation is the *high-risk study*, in which children who are believed to have a high risk of developing a future psychiatric disorder (usually because one or both of their parents have been diagnosed as suffering from a mental illness) are examined at regular intervals, together with comparison children who are believed to be at low risk. These studies aim to discover whether or not the high-risk children are especially likely to become psychotic in adulthood, and whether any indications of future illness can be detected in early life. One of the earliest studies of this kind was initiated by psychologist Sarnoff Mednick and psychiatrist Fini Schulsinger in Copenhagen in 1962 and has involved 207 children of schizophrenic mothers and 104 children of normal parents.[67] The New York High-Risk Project, which commenced in 1971 under the direction of geneticist L. Erlenmeyer-Kimling and psychologist Barbara Cornblatt, has followed up two separate cohorts, each including some children whose parents had been diagnosed as schizophrenic, some whose parents suffered from affective disorders, and some whose parents were psychiatrically normal.[68]

Although these studies might appear relatively simple in conception, interpretation of the findings has not always been straightforward, as important factors have often been confounded. For example, many of the children of schizophrenia patients recruited to the Copenhagen study had been given up for adoption or raised in institutions. It was therefore decided to compare them with children who had similar histories. It later transpired that the biological parents of many of the children in the control group were recidivist criminals. (In an effort to overcome these kinds of difficulties, a study was set up in Israel in which some high-risk and control children were recruited from kibbutzim.[69] In the kibbutz system of communal living, which is unique to that country, children are raised collectively, live in dormitories, and spend comparatively little time in the exclusive presence of their parents.)

Because of these kinds of confounds, researchers have usually employed complex statistical techniques (especially a group of procedures known collectively as *path analysis*) to try to tease out the way in which different possible predictor variables interact to influence the future development of psychotic complaints.[70] However, these efforts have sometimes been undermined by the unexpectedly low rates of psychiatric disorder observed in many of the high-risk children as they have matured. For example, in the Copenhagen study, only 13 of the high-risk group had met the ICD-8 criteria for schizophrenia by the age of 25 years, although many more were said to show evidence of neurosis, personality disorder or 'borderline states'.[71] In the New York study, only 36 out of 208 individuals had shown evidence of any psychiatric disturbance by the time they reached the age of 20 years, most of these having come from the high-risk group. Of these, only 13 appeared to be psychotic, and they were drawn in equal proportions from the disturbed children in all three groups.[72] Clearer evidence of the emergence of psychotic symptoms was reported when the children had reached 25 years of age, by which time 13 per cent of the children of parents diagnosed as suffering from schizophrenia had themselves met the criteria for the disorder.[73]

In total, more than twenty high-risk studies designed to detect the developmental precursors of psychosis have been carried out, mostly focusing on schizophrenia. (Oddly, there have been no high-risk studies that have specifically focused on the children of bipolar parents, even though, as we saw in Chapter 4, family and twin studies have generally yielded stronger genetic effects for bipolar symptoms.) The results of these studies are not entirely consistent, but the broad picture that emerges has been drawn together by American psychologist Joan Asarnow[74] and more recently by British psychiatrists Chris Hollis and Eric Taylor.[75] Some studies have detected evidence of motor abnormalities in the first few years of life. During middle childhood, many future schizophrenia patients show evidence of poor social adjustment, and poor performance on attentional and other cognitive tests, and these differences from children who do not later become psychotic become more evident during adolescence. Overall, the balance of this evidence points to the role of early brain abnormalities in children who will later become psychotic, although a contribution from later maturational processes such as neural pruning cannot be ruled out.

More detailed analyses of the data from the individual studies point to complex interactions between biological and environmental factors and suggest that different pathways may lead to different complaints. For example, the Copenhagen researchers identified those in their sample who had predominately positive or negative symptoms.[76] In the positive group there was strong evidence of inadequate parenting (six out of eight had been separated from their mothers for more than one and a half years during early childhood, one had been separated from her mother for more than five years, and one had been physically abused by her father). Similar evidence of inadequate parenting was absent in the negative symptom group, many of whom had suffered complicated births and showed enlarged cerebral ventricles on CT scans. In the New York study, poor social adjustment in adulthood (suspicious solitude, social insecurity or a lack of empathy) was associated with physical anhedonia and attentional impairments in childhood.[77]

Almost certainly, the children recruited to high-risk studies are an unrepresentative sample of pre-psychotic children. After all, by far the majority of people who receive a diagnosis of schizophrenia or bipolar disorder do not have psychotic parents. This potential source of bias is avoided in a second type of longitudinal approach, in which individuals from the general population are followed up from birth. These kinds of investigations, known as *cohort studies*, are usually set up with broad aims in mind, and so measures of specific interest to psychiatrists and clinical psychologists are often not included at the outset. Two such studies carried out in the UK are the National Survey of Health and Development (NSHD) and the National Child Development Study (NCDS). The NSHD was originally a survey of all children born in England, Scotland and Wales between 3 and 9 March 1946, and was carried out to assess the need for maternity services in the planned National Health Service. Multiple and illegitimate births were excluded, and 13,687 births were studied in total. Regular contact has been maintained with a subset of 5362 individuals, who receive a birthday card from the project every year. As time has passed, various assessments have been made and additional data have been collected from educational and health services. The NCDS is a similar study, set up in 1958, designed to monitor the physical, social and educational development of children through to adulthood.

British psychiatrists Peter Jones, Robin Murray and their colleagues have exploited these studies by identifying participants who had been admitted to psychiatric hospitals.[78] Diagnoses were obtained by scrutinizing hospital case notes. From the data collected at an NSHD assessment at 2 years of age, it was found that the future psychotic patients were later to walk than their peers by an average of 1.2 months. Evidence of higher levels of clumsiness at 7 years in the pre-psychotic children was observed in the NCDS. In both studies, the future patients had, on average, slightly lower scores on IQ or similar tests when assessed between the ages of 7 and 16 years. However, perhaps the most interesting findings concerned speech. In the NCDS, qualitative reports of speech difficulties by mothers and teachers at 7 and 11 years discriminated between pre-psychotic and normal children, and a similar association between future psychosis and non-specific speech difficulties assessed by school doctors emerged from the NSHD. It would be interesting to know whether speech problems early in life are specifically associated with later thought disorder, but the NSHD and NCDS studies do not provide sufficient clinical information to answer this question.

Unfortunately, most of the high-risk or cohort studies have not included measures of the kinds of social-cognitive processes which, I have argued, play a crucial role in depression, mania and paranoia. In fact, so far as I am aware, only the Israeli High-Risk Study has included a measure of this sort.[79] In that study, the adolescent children of schizophrenia patients were administered a questionnaire measure of *locus of control*, a construct that is similar to but predates the concept of attributional style. Individuals are said to have an external locus of control if they believe that important facets of their life, including their own behaviour, are controlled by external influences, whereas they are said to have an internal locus of control if they believe that they control their own destinies. In the Israeli study, high-risk adolescents who later became psychotic were found to have a more external locus of control than those who did not later become psychotic. If verified by future studies, this finding suggests that the attributional abnormalities observed in some psychotic patients may be present, to some degree, well before the onset of their delusional ideas.

The role of early brain damage

Many investigators have assumed that the neurodevelopmental abnormalities found in pre-psychotic children must be genetically determined. However, others have argued that other kinds of influences on the developing nervous system may affect a person's vulnerability to psychosis. In the Copenhagen study it was found that high-risk children who were later to become ill were more likely to have experienced difficult births than children who stayed well.[80] As complications during birth can cause the brain to be temporarily starved of oxygen, this observation is consistent with early versions of the biological time-bomb hypothesis. Although some studies have replicated this finding,[81] others have not,[82] or have found that the association between birth complication and psychosis exists only for males.[83] For these reasons, the contribution of birth complications to psychosis remains uncertain.

A more recent hypothesis suggests that foetal exposure to a virus contracted by the expectant mother might be the cause of early neuro-developmental abnormalities responsible for psychosis. This sugges-tion was originally made to explain the much repeated observation of a very slightly increased risk of psychosis in people born in the late winter or early spring (and who were therefore second trimester foetuses during the winter, when viral infections are most common).[84]* A bizarre version of this theory, proposed by American psychiatrists E. F. Torrey and Robert Yolken, holds that the 'schizovirus' can be caught by expectant mothers from domestic house cats, which tend to spend more time indoors during the winter. (Fuller and Yolken claim that schizophrenia is especially common in countries where people keep cats as pets.)[85] However, most researchers have focused on the influenza virus. Although some retrospective studies have reported evidence that mothers of psychotic patients suffered from influenza during pregnancy more often than mothers of non-psychotic people,[86] many others have failed to find this association.[87]

Even if the influenza virus is not the culprit, one piece of evidence suggests that the role of maternal infections in conferring vulnerability to psychosis should not be dismissed entirely. Several studies have found that the season-of-birth effect is especially evident in patients born in urban areas characterized by high population density and crowded housing but is absent or almost absent in patients born in rural areas.[88] Of course, the importance of this observation can be debated. In one study the combined effect of season of birth and urban birth was only evident in females.[89] However, in another, more recent, study, it was calculated that the population risk (number of cases) attributable to place and season of birth exceeded the risk associated with having a first-degree relative suffering from psychosis.[90]

* Of course, other interpretations of this finding are possible. The astrologically minded might want to note that the star signs associated with a high-risk of psychosis are Capricorn, Aquarius and Pisces.

Of course, the urban environment probably contains a number of psychological hazards to the developing child, as we will see in the next chapter. Nonetheless, one explanation for the greater evidence of the season-of-birth effect in urban environments is infections; in crowded conditions viruses and other infectious agents are easily passed from one person to another.

Viral infections are not the only conceivable cause of the season-of-birth effect. As there is no seasonal bias in the births of brothers and sisters of psychotic patients, the hypothesis that the effect is caused by the seasonal reproductive enthusiasms of parents can probably be ruled out.[91] However, the possibility that poor maternal nutrition in the winter months plays a role is raised by a study that found that a higher than expected number of future schizophrenia patients were born during the Dutch 'hunger winter' of 1944 to 1945, when a Nazi blockade precipitated a severe famine in western Holland.[92]

Unfortunately the interactions between these kinds of factors and others that appear to contribute to psychosis are not understood. Attempts to determine whether birth complications play a greater role in patients with or without a family history of mental illness have yielded almost entirely inconsistent results,[93] so it is not clear whether early brain damage and genetic vulnerability represent separate or interacting contributions to later psychosis. Attempts to demonstrate an association between birth complications and the kinds of structural brain abnormalities sometimes observed in brain scans of adult patients have also been inconclusive.[94] Nor can interactions with psychological and social factors be excluded. The authors of a recent study, which found an association between schizophrenia and maternal bleeding during pregnancy,[95] speculate that some aspects of maternal lifestyle (for example, smoking during pregnancy, failure to comply with routines of antenatal care) may partially explain their observations. As some of these lifestyle characteristics are especially evident in mothers who suffer from psychiatric problems, this hypothesis suggests a *non-genetic* mechanism that might explain why psychosis sometimes runs in families.

What can we Conclude from Neurodevelopmental Studies?

Overall, the findings from developmental studies consistently show that unusual characteristics are present in at least some future psychotic patients many years before they become obviously ill. The findings on birth complications and prenatal exposure to viruses or malnutrition lend further support to the theory that early brain damage can make individuals more vulnerable to becoming psychotic in later life. However, it is important not to leap from these observations to simple conclusions. Other types of challenges to the developing brain, for example prenatal exposure to high levels of alcohol,[96] have been proposed as potential causes of vulnerability to psychosis. Perhaps any kind of early brain damage can have this effect.

Nor are these effects specific to people who later receive a particular diagnosis. Although most of the relevant studies have been conducted by investigators who have been searching for the origins of schizophrenia, whenever comparable data have been collected, similar observations have been made for children who later develop psychotic mood disorders.[97] For example, in one study it was found that the average IQ scores of future schizophrenia and future bipolar patients were both slightly lower than normal during middle childhood.[98] In the NSHD, there was evidence that those who later developed severe depression, on average, showed poor performance on IQ measures, together with speech irregularities.[99] Retrospective reports by parents suggest that future bipolar patients, like future schizophrenia patients, show impaired social functioning in adolescence.[100] The season-of-birth effect has also been found for bipolar patients[101] who, like future schizophrenia patients, may have experienced higher than expected rates of obstetric birth complications.[102] Unexpectedly high rates of depression and bipolar disorder, as well as schizophrenia, have been found in children born in the Dutch 'hunger winter'.[103] It is pretty clear from this evidence that non-specific kinds of early brain damage cause a non-specific vulnerability to psychotic symptoms later in life (a conclusion that could obviously be interpreted as consistent with a unitary psychosis model).

The magnitude of this effect is drawn into question by the low

e of psychotic illness. As we have seen, studies of birth compli-
nd prenatal influenza reveal, at best, a very modest increase
ure to these phenomena in future patients in comparison to
ordinary people. In this context it is important to remember that, for
every person who receives a diagnosis of schizophrenia or bipolar disorder, there are about 100 people who do not. Simple arithmetic reveals
that, even if exposure to these challenges to the nervous system were
three times more common in future patients than in others (which would
certainly be more than a modest increase), the number of people who
suffer these insults *without* becoming psychotic would still be more than
thirty times greater than the number who do so and later become ill. *

A final, and very important, qualification about the evidence we have
examined concerns the logic of the neurodevelopmental time-bomb
hypothesis. Whether theories of this kind implicate processes early or
late in development, their main strength is that they explain the age of
onset data discussed at the beginning of this chapter. Herein also lies
their fundamental weakness. Whereas adolescents and young adults
are more vulnerable to developing psychotic symptoms than any other
age group, symptoms can appear as early as the age of 10 or as late as
the age of 70 or afterwards. In fact, despite the over-representation of
adolescents among people experiencing their first episode of psychosis,
*it seems likely that the number of non-adolescents experiencing psy-
chotic symptoms for the first time exceeds the number of adolescents.*†

* Readers who are confused on this point might like to carry out a few simple
calculations based on hypothetical data. Suppose 10 per cent of the normal
population experience birth complications and that this increases to 30 per cent
in the case of future patients. Also suppose that, out of a population of 1000
people, 10 (1 per cent) become psychotic. It follows that 3 of the future psychotic
patients (30 per cent of the 10) will have experienced birth complications. However, out of the 990 non-psychotic members of the population, 99 (10 per cent of
the 990) will also have experienced birth complications – 33 times more than
patients with birth complications. Even if we assume that psychotic symptoms are
experienced by, say, 10 per cent of the population on the basis of the evidence we
considered in Chapter 5, ordinary people with a history of birth complications
would outnumber the number of psychotic patients with birth complications by a
factor of 3:1.

† For example, consider the data on the onset of schizophrenia symptoms shown
in Figure 17.1. Half of the males in the sample first became ill after the age of 25
years and half of all females became ill after the age of 29. Similar proportions of
'older' patients can be calculated from nearly all comparable studies.

Because biological researchers have attempted to explain the typical age of onset exclusively in terms of some kind of endogenous process – the biological time-bomb that 'explodes' during a critical period of development – they struggle to explain the very wide *range* of ages at which psychotic symptoms first appear. In order to explain this range, it will be necessary to take into account factors external to the individual, in particular the life-experiences of those who become psychotic.

The Trials of Life

There is but one truly serious philosophical problem and that is
suicide. Judging whether life is or is not worth living amounts to
answering the fundamental problem of philosophy. Albert Camus[1]

Life's a bitch, and then you die . . .   Common saying

My mother telephoned me on a Sunday evening to tell me that my
brother had killed himself. It was a brief conversation, muted by
shock. Afterwards, the fact of Andrew's death seemed so big and
difficult to absorb that I sat silently on my living-room couch, searching
my brain for appropriate thoughts but finding none. The coldness of
my home – the small house I had retreated to after the break-up of my
marriage – suddenly became more evident. As minutes passed into
hours, guilt began to lay siege to my defences. I had visited my mother
earlier in the day. She had telephoned me only an hour after my return.
Andrew had also planned to visit her but for some reason, probably
because he and I did not get on very well, she had asked him not to
come until the following weekend. He had killed himself that morning
by leaping from the fourteenth floor of the tower block in which he
lived.

Visiting a police station early the next day, my sister and I were
relieved to discover that our brother's body had already been identified
by one of his friends. However, other grim tasks fell to us later in the
week – clearing out the shabby flat in which he had lived in his final
years; sitting in an empty courtroom to hear the coroner open and
then adjourn the inquest; organizing the funeral, which was attended
by a surprising number of his friends, most of whom were previously
unknown to us. In the middle of the week, a local priest called on my

mother and, knowing my profession, remarked that Andrew's suicide must have been especially difficult for me to cope with.

Tragedy always unleashes an immediate search for explanations. We launch into attributional overdrive. However, as the priest who had visited my mother had shrewdly observed, it was unlikely that the concepts I had absorbed during my training would adequately satisfy my need to understand my brother's final and most decisive act. Of course, Andrew had always been different. At school, he had constantly been at loggerheads with his teachers and his peers. He had dropped out from formal education without achieving qualifications, and had drifted into a life of drug-taking and unemployment. From the comfortable perspective of a professional clinical psychologist, some of his behaviour could be described as schizotypal. He complained of flashback hallucinatory experiences that he attributed to his experiments with LSD. He sometimes professed strange and magical beliefs, at one time telling my mother's elderly neighbour of his ambition to absorb all the knowledge in the universe. And yet, this kind of diagnostic labelling does not seem to do justice to the story of my brother's life. He might have been 'schizotypal', for want of any better word, but he was not schizotypal in a vacuum. The more he became disengaged from his roots, and the middle-class values of his family, the more his relationships with us came under stress. We became angry and distant from him and ultimately, for my own part, quite rejecting. At his funeral, the friend who had identified his body told me that all Andrew had wanted from us was to be treated as 'an acceptable failure'.

Yet Another Interminable Debate

They fuck you up, your mum and dad.
They may not mean to, but they do.
They fill you with the faults they had
And add some extra, just for you.

But they were fucked up in their turn
By fools in old-style hats and coats,
Who half the time were soppy-stern
And half at one another's throats.

> Man hands on misery to man,
> It deepens like a coastal shelf.
> Get out as early as you can,
> And don't have any kids yourself.   Philip Larkin[2]

The idea that environmental factors, and especially family relationships, contribute to madness is so difficult for many patients and their relatives that many professionals treat it as taboo.[3] Most of those who have worked on the concept of expressed emotion, in particular, have been at pains to argue that, although families may influence the course of illness, 'We consider that families do not exert a *causal* influence.'[4] In making this kind of assertion, psychologists and psychiatrists have attempted to distance themselves from the equally extreme viewpoint of an earlier era, in which the causes of madness were exclusively laid at the door of 'schizogenic' parents. In the late 1950s, for example, the American anthropologist Geoffrey Bateson argued that the parents of future schizophrenia patients drove their children mad by giving them simultaneous but logically contradictory messages (known as 'double-binds').[5] A few years later, the British anti-psychiatrists R. D. Laing and Aaron Esterson suggested that young schizophrenia patients were victimized and scapegoated by family members who wished to avoid dwelling on their own inadequacies.[6] One consequence of characterizing the parents of psychiatric patients as evil in this way was described by the philosopher Peter Sedgwick, who witnessed a meeting between trainee social workers and a group of parents in the late 1970s, in which the former greeted the latter with undisguised hostility.[7]

The taboo against considering the role of environmental influences on psychosis has bolstered exclusively biological accounts of madness, particularly genetic accounts that portray the close relatives of patients as passive victims of a preordained tragedy. However, prejudicial assumptions of any sort are a poor basis for a scientific analysis. As we have seen in previous chapters, debates about the origins of madness have tended to focus exclusively on single causes that are either biological or environmental, as if the two were mutually exclusive. Advocates of both positions have often naively assumed that a focus on family relationships amounts to holding parents morally culpable for the troubles of their children.

In the last chapter we saw some evidence that environmental factors play a role in the development of psychosis. For example, in the adoption study reported by Tienari and his colleagues, an interaction was observed between genetic and environmental influences on thought disorder. In the Copenhagen high-risk study, patients with positive symptoms were especially likely to have suffered separation from their parents at an early age. Of course, many different kinds of environmental factors might, in theory, help to determine whether or not an individual eventually becomes mad. In this chapter I will consider what these factors might be, focusing on three broad types of influences: family relationships, the general social environment, and traumatic experiences. Wherever possible, I will try to indicate how specific environmental influences contribute to specific complaints.

Family Influences

We begin with the difficult question of whether family relationships play a role in the aetiology of psychosis. One impediment to thinking clearly about this issue has been some over-simplistic ideas about how family relationships can go awry. The early family causation theories of schizophrenia created an image of the 'schizogenic' parent as a kind of monster. However, we do not need to assume that the parents of future psychotic patients are wilfully neglectful, deranged or cruel in order to accept that they have some influence on their children's mental health.

Psychopathologists have studied three different kinds of non-optimal relationships between children and their families. The first involves some kind of disruption of the emotional bond that is usually formed between parent and infant at the beginning of the infant's life. This kind of bond, known as an *attachment relationship*, has been the subject of intense investigation by psychoanalysts, psychologists and animal behaviourists. The second kind concerns the emotional climate that develops in families as the child grows older, and is reflected in the concepts of *expressed emotion* and *affective style*, which we encountered in Chapter 16. Finally, as we have already seen, some research has focused on the concept of *communication deviance*, the idea that persistently vague, fragmented or contradictory communications from parents can lead to cognitive confusion in the child, increasing the probability that he will eventually become thought-disordered.

Attachment relationships

Following the British psychiatrist John Bowlby's claim that secure attachment to a parental figure is necessary for healthy psychological development,[8] opinions about the impact of early relationships have varied widely. In part, this reflects the difficulty of studying influences across the human life span. Sceptics have argued that emotional deprivation at an early age can be compensated for by adequate emotional care later in childhood. Certainly, some highly resilient children survive appalling mistreatment by their parents and emerge relatively unscathed as adults. However, studies in which attachment relationships have been deliberately disrupted in young animals suggest that negative consequences often ensue. Infant rhesus monkeys who are separated from their parents and raised with their peers, even if nurtured adequately in other ways, develop quite marked behavioural and emotional difficulties in adolescence, and these difficulties are accompanied by biochemical changes in the brain (decreased levels of 5-hydroxyindolacetic acid, the primary metabolite of the neurotransmitter serotonin).[9] Moreover, recent studies of insecurely attached human children have revealed that they are handicapped by subtle social-cognitive deficits that may not be obvious to the casual observer. Although intellectually the equal of securely attached children, at 2 years of age they are less persistent and enthusiastic when solving problems.[10] At the age of 11 years, they are less able to recall specific incidents from earlier in life, and are less able to reflect on their own mental processes.[11] Perhaps more importantly for our purposes, studies conducted by Peter Fonagy and his colleagues at University College London[12] and by Elizabeth Meins at Durham University[13] have shown that children between 4 and 6 years of age who are insecurely attached perform less well than securely attached children on tests designed to measure their ability to understand the mental states of other people ('theory-of-mind' skills).

The suspicion that insecure attachment relationships confer vulnerability to psychosis is fuelled by the results of the Copenhagen high-risk study, which found an association between positive symptoms and early separation from parents. However, more powerful prospective evidence of this effect has emerged from a large cohort study carried out in Northern Finland, which was initiated in 1966. Before the birth of the 11,000 children who were entered into the study, their mothers were questioned about whether their pregnancies had been planned and whether they had considered an abortion. Examining outcome data twenty-eight years later, a team of British and Finnish investigators found that unwanted pregnancies resulted in a four-fold increase in later psychosis, even when possible confounding socio-demographic and medical factors were taken into account.[14] Although the researchers did not offer a psychological interpretation of their findings, the obvious implication is that parents' emotional ambivalence towards their children increases the risk that they will grow up to suffer from positive symptoms.

If this idea is correct, we should be able to detect evidence of insecure attachment styles in adult patients who have become psychotic. The definition and measurement of attachment styles is a complex field, and there is not enough space here to describe this kind of work in detail.[15] Suffice it to say that several different styles are commonly observed in normal children and adults. Furthermore, there is evidence of inter-generational transmission of these styles. Children who have secure relationships with their parents typically but not always grow up to form secure relationships with adult partners, and later become parents of securely attached children. Insecurely attached children, on the other hand, often encounter problems when attempting to form relationships in later life, and sometimes fail to bond adequately with their own children.

In a series of studies carried out in the USA, Mary Dozier used questionnaires and interviews to assess psychiatric patients' attachments to their parents. It is important to note that Dozier's aim was to study *attachment representations* – the patients' understanding of their relationships with their parents, rather than actual relationships. She accepted that her participants' accounts might not be an accurate reflection of what actually happened in their families many years before. In an initial study, she found that patients with a diagnosis of schizophrenia, in comparison with patients with affective disorders, often had the kind of insecure attachment style that is described as *dismissing* or *avoidant*.[16] Most people feel that their relationships are very important to them, however troublesome they may be. However, the dismissing-avoidant person devalues the importance of attachments and often fails to recall specific details about his relationship with his parents during childhood. It is as if, as a consequence of early emotional disappointment, the growing child develops a strategy that allows him to avoid the emotional hazards of mature relationships. In a later study, Dozier found that patients with this attachment style were especially likely to be deluded, hallucinated and suspicious.[17] Perhaps this is unsurprising, as the emotional theme underlying the dismissing style is lack of trust.

Evidence supporting Dozier's findings has emerged from community surveys of attachment styles undertaken by social psychologist Philip Shaver and his colleagues in the USA. In two studies, large representative samples of adults and adolescents were administered questionnaires measuring attachments to others. Several measures of psychopathology were also administered. In the adult sample of over 8000 people, schizophrenia as defined by DSM-III-R criteria was associated with an insecure and especially dismissing attachment style.[18] In the adolescent sample of over 1500 individuals, high levels of psychoticism and paranoia were associated with both the dismissing style and a second type of insecure style, known as *anxious-ambivalent*.[19] As the name suggests, people with this attachment style desperately want to have relationships, but feel in their hearts that no one will ever want to get close to them.

Of course, it might be argued that these styles are *consequences* rather than causes of paranoid thinking. If this were so, we might expect recovered paranoid patients to report warm and supportive relationships with their families. However, in a recent study conducted by Peter Rankin, myself and former colleagues at the University of Liverpool, we found that both currently ill and recovered paranoid patients report extremely difficult relationships with their parents.[20]

The idea that negative attitudes towards parents is a consequence of psychosis is also difficult to square with some of the prospective evidence we considered earlier – for example, from the Finnish cohort study and the Copenhagen high-risk study. In fact, early in the Copenhagen high-risk study, the high-risk children were interviewed about their relationships with their parents. Many years later, it was found that those who reported a negative relationship with their parents were especially likely to develop schizophrenia symptoms.[21]

Expressed emotion and communication deviance

We have already considered evidence that communication deviance in parents can contribute to the later development of thought disorder in their children. Perhaps the best indication that this is partly an environmental effect has emerged from Pekka Tienari's adoption study, which found that both a genetic predisposition and exposure to vague and fragmented parental communications are necessary conditions for the development of this complaint.[22]

The possible causal role of expressed emotion in psychosis has hardly been investigated, perhaps because most researchers have decided to reject this possibility from the outset. In support of this prejudice, some have pointed out that studies of the relatives of patients experiencing their first episode of psychosis have usually found lower rates of high expressed emotion than studies carried out with the families of patients who have been ill for some time.[23] This observation certainly supports the idea that expressed emotion grows during interactions between psychotic people and their parents, so that the emotional climate in families tends to deteriorate as patients become more disturbed and less able to look after themselves. However, it does not preclude the possibility that excessive criticism and parental overcontrol can play a role in causing symptoms in the first place. The only adequate way of addressing this possibility is by studying the effects of expressed emotion prospectively.

The University of California at Los Angeles (UCLA) Family Project was initiated by psychologist Michael Goldstein and his colleagues in 1965.[24] The sixty-five families who agreed to participate had all sought help from the UCLA Psychology Department's outpatient clinic because of difficulties they were experiencing with an adolescent child. At the time at which the project started, none of these adolescents had experienced psychotic symptoms. Two measures of family relationships were employed: a measure of communication deviance derived from the work of Singer and Wynne, and a measure of emotional climate (the Affective Style Index, based on the concept of expressed emotion, but derived from observations of the family members attempting to discuss a problem). Five and fifteen years later, the children were graded on a seven-point scale of psychopathology ranging from normal, through neuroses, more severe personality problems, to borderline, probable and definite schizophrenia. As in the other high-risk studies we have considered, the proportion of children developing frank psychotic symptoms was quite small (only four out of the fifty-two followed up met the criteria for probable or definite schizophrenia). Nonetheless, there was evidence that both communication deviance and affective style predicted future psychosis. These two types of interactions between parents and their children appeared to be independent influences, so that the combination of high communication deviance and a negative affective style appeared to be particularly dangerous to the children's mental health. Moreover, there was evidence that the harmful effects of communication deviance were most marked in families with a high genetic risk of psychosis (that is, with other psychotic people in the family).[25] This finding of an interaction between family processes and genetic risk is, of course, consistent with the results from Tienari's adoption study.

How families affect their children

A complete account of the way that families affect the development of madness would explain how different family characteristics influence the psychological processes responsible for particular complaints. Fortunately, clues about these influences can be discerned from research carried out by developmental psychologists, whose efforts to map out the pathways to *ordinary* adulthood have too often been ignored by psychopathologists. For example, we have already seen that secure attachment relationships facilitate the development of 'theory-of-mind' skills, an observation of some importance given that these skills seem to be compromised in some psychotic patients.

Similar progress has been made in mapping the ways in which parents influence children's beliefs about themselves, and the kinds of explanations that they make for important events. Martin Seligman found that the attributional styles of 11-year-old children correlate strongly with the styles of their mothers but not their fathers.[26] Although this observation seems to indicate that children somehow 'copy' their mothers' characteristic way of explaining things, other

studies have shown that parents can influence their children's attributions in less direct ways.[27] For example, if a parent makes
attributions for a child's poor academic performance that are *internal*
to herself ('It's my fault because I did not bring up my child properly'),
the child is likely to make attributions for the failure that are *external*
to himself ('It's not my fault that I keep failing my exams'). Conversely,
if a parent criticizes a child's performance, the criticism may be-
embraced by the child and later repeated as an internal attribution ('I
failed because I'm stupid'). These kinds of influences may be important
even in adolescence and early adulthood. In a recent study, Judy Garber
at Vanderbilt University in Nashville found that explanations for
positive and negative events given by adolescents tend to match the
explanations given by their mothers.[28]

Comparable findings have been obtained from studies of children
and young adults judged to be at high risk of depression. Constance
Hammen at the University of California found that the children of
depressed mothers have more pessimistic styles of thinking, and more
negative beliefs about themselves, than the children of non-depressed
mothers.[29] In the recent Temple–Wisconsin Cognitive Vulnerability to
Depression (CVD) Project (see Chapter 10, pp. 245–6), interviews
conducted with parents of students participating in the study revealed
that the parents of the high-risk students were less accepting of their
children and more likely to be 'negatively controlling' or emotionally
abusive than the parents of the low-risk students.[30] Moreover, the
parents of the high-risk students were especially prone to explain
hypothetical negative events happening to their children in terms of
causes that were internal to the child (for example, deciding that a
child was not invited to a party because she was unpopular).[31]

These findings strongly suggest that parents may inadvertently teach
their children a depressive style of thinking. As attributions also play
an important role in persecutory delusions, it is reasonable to ask
whether paranoid thinking is similarly influenced by early relationships with caregivers. Studies have yet to be carried out to test this
possibility..

To summarize, there seems to be quite good evidence that family
relationships affect the risk that the developing child will eventually
become psychotic. Families have this effect because they influence the
child's beliefs about himself, his thoughts about the causes of things

that happen to him, and his ability to understand the behaviour of other people. At the risk of being tedious, it is worth repeating that this conclusion does *not* imply that every psychotic patient is a victim of an inadequate family, that parents choose to confuse or criticize their vulnerable children, or that the child plays no role in influencing these processes. It is also important to remember, as attachment theorists have been at pains to note, that parents are products of their relationships with their own parents. As we saw in Chapter 16, parents who are unable to provide an optimal emotional environment for their children have often themselves been raised by parents who were unable to provide them with adequate emotional support.[32]

This intergenerational spiral of affects was brilliantly captured by the poet Philip Larkin. The less remembered second verse of his most famous and irreverent poem, which I quoted earlier in this chapter, encourages us not judge our parents too harshly.

A World not of our own Making

The research literature contains several hints that long-term exposure to a stressful social environment can contribute to the development of madness. One hint comes from the over-representation of people with paranoid or manic symptoms among immigrant populations. As I explained in Chapter 6, this has been most extensively investigated in black Afro-Caribbean immigrants to Britain.[33] Although the reasons for this over-representation have been the subject of much debate, careful epidemiological studies indicate that the increased risk is real, and cannot be explained away as just the product of culturally insensitive diagnostic practices. Moreover, obvious biological factors (for example, genetic influences) appear to be ruled out, or at least diminished in likelihood, by the finding that incidence rates of psychosis in the Caribbean are no higher than in other countries,[34] by the observation that the children of Afro-Caribbean immigrants are especially vulnerable,[35] and by the recent discovery that immigrant groups in other parts of the world are similarly affected – for example, Surinamese immigrants to Holland,[36] East African immigrants to Sweden,[37] migrants to Germany,[38] and even Afro-Caribbeans returning to Jamaica after a period of living in Britain.[39] Further evidence that the critical factor is something to do with different ethnic groups mixing closely has emerged from a recent study carried out in London, in which the researchers analysed the incidence of psychotic illnesses in different neighbourhoods. It was found that non-white people living in white neighbourhoods are more likely to become psychotic than non-white people living in predominantly non-white neighbourhoods.[40] Exposure to racial tension, it seems, can drive people mad.

It is easy to see how exposure to overt discrimination and institutional racism, perhaps coupled with experiences of alienation and isolation, might affect psychological processes (especially attributions and self-representations) that appear to play an important role in paranoia and mania. It is perhaps less obvious why the children of immigrants should be particularly affected in this way. One possibility is that the practical and economic problems associated with migration make it difficult for families to provide their children with optimum child-rearing experiences that would protect them from these influences. Evidence that this might be the case was found in a study of Afro-Caribbean schizophrenia patients living in London carried out by psychiatrist Dinesh Bhugra and his colleagues. Of 38 Afro-Caribbean patients studied, 12 (34 per cent) had suffered separation from their mothers for a period of four years or longer during childhood, and 19 (53 per cent) had suffered a similar period of separation from their fathers.[41]

Another possibility is that problems of cultural identity are especially troublesome for second-generation members of immigrant families. Cross-cultural researchers use the term *acculturation* to describe the process of psychological transition that occurs when people move from one culture to another.[42] According to one influential theory, proposed by Canadian psychologist John Berry, the outcome of this process can be of four kinds, depending on whether an individual chooses to identify with her culture of origin or with the host culture (see Table 18.1).[43] *Integration* occurs when the individual identifies with and exhibits some characteristics of both cultures. *Assimilation* occurs when the host culture is embraced and the culture of origin is disowned. *Separation* is the outcome when the individual retains the identity of her culture of origin and rejects the host culture. Finally, *marginalization* occurs when the individual feels uncommitted to either culture. Because the children of immigrants may be at special

Table 18.1 The four types of acculturation identified by John Berry (1988).

| | | *Identification with host culture* | |
		Yes	No
Identification with culture of origin	Yes	Integration	Separation
	No	Assimilation	Marginalization

risk of becoming trapped between two identity groups and rejected by both, it is possible that they will be especially likely to experience this last outcome, which, according to Berry, is the most stressful of the four.

Cultural stressors and ethnic tension are not the only features of the social environment that seem to confer an increased risk of psychosis. In 1939, during the Great Depression, two American sociologists, Robert Faris and Warren Dunham, reported a survey carried out in Chicago, in which they attempted to identify areas with a high prevalence of schizophrenia patients. They found the highest rates in a slum area surrounding the centre of the city, which was occupied mainly by unskilled workers with low incomes. In areas further out from the centre, occupied by skilled workers, the rates were lower, and they were lower still in commuter areas occupied by middle-class professionals.[44] This apparent relationship between the prevalence of schizophrenia and socio-economic status has since been observed in many other studies, and appears to be most evident in the largest cities.

The explanation of this phenomenon has been a matter of some debate. Although Faris and Dunham concluded that the stress associated with living in poor economic circumstances plays a causal role in schizophrenic symptoms, other researchers have suggested that the association between psychosis and poverty might be accounted for by *downwards social drift*.[45] According to this theory, psychotic people are often unable to work, and so are forced to move to the poorer areas, where accommodation is cheaper.

The reality of social drift has been documented in a number of studies. A recent survey of psychiatric patients living in Inner London found that a large number of patients had moved into the area from outside the city.[46] However, clear evidence that exposure to an urban environment can play a *causal* role in psychosis has recently emerged from a very large Danish study, in which data on childhood living circumstances and psychiatric difficulties in adulthood were collated for nearly 2 million people.[47] The researchers found of a *dose–response* relationship between exposure to an urban environment in childhood and the development of psychosis in later life. It seems that the greater the proportion of childhood spent living in urban environments the greater the risk of madness, with those who spend their entire childhood in cities being most at risk in later life.

A recent World Health Organization study found that psychotic patients living in urban and rural environments tend to have different types of complaints.[48] In rural areas, negative symptoms such as a loss of interest in appearance and cleanliness are most often observed, whereas urban patients are more likely to hear voices and to feel persecuted. These observations are quite easy to understand from a psychological perspective. Intrusive life events of the kind that are likely to induce paranoid thinking are especially likely to occur in city environments. On the other hand, social isolation, leading to the absence of the kind of social reinforcement that is necessary to maintain self-care skills, is more likely the occur in a rural environment.

Trauma

In this discussion of environmental influences on psychosis, I have left the contribution of trauma until last because, for many psychologists and psychiatrists at least, even to raise this issue is to court controversy. For this reason, I am going to outline the available evidence in quite a lot of detail.

Of course, many different kinds of disasters may befall us if we are unlucky. As children we may suffer physical or sexual abuse at the hands of our parents or other people. In adulthood, we may lose loved ones in sudden tragedies, find ourselves in conflict with the law, or suffer sudden reversals of our financial fortunes. If we are extremely unfortunate, we may become involved in civil unrest, warfare or other kinds of violent conflict. After Vietnam veterans persuaded American psychiatrists to include the diagnosis of post-traumatic stress disorder (PTSD) in the DSM, the effects of these kinds of experiences on mental health became the subject of vigorous research. The DSM-IV definition of PTSD points to three groups of symptoms commonly experienced by trauma victims. First, many complain that they persistently re-experience their traumatic experiences (for example, as intrusive and distressing memories or dreams). Second, many avoid stimuli associated with their trauma (for example, by never returning to the scene of an accident) or, alternatively, become emotionally numb (believed to be a form of psychological detachment that acts as a defence against intolerable feelings). Finally, many victims show symptoms of persistent physiological arousal (for example, insomnia and irritability).[49] Although hallucinations and delusions do not fall within this definition, a few researchers have not been deterred from asking whether trauma can lead to psychotic breakdowns.

Some studies have examined the relationship between psychosis and sexual and physical abuse. Investigations of this sort are quite difficult to carry out. To begin with, there is considerable disagreement about the best way of defining abuse. Depending on the definition used, a larger or smaller proportion of the population can be said to be victims of assaults. Moreover, evidence of assault is usually obtained from descriptions given by patients during interviews. Recent debates about whether patients ever experience false memories of abuse testify to widespread suspicions that these kinds of descriptions are sometimes unreliable. However, it is also worth remembering that victims sometimes have powerful motives for *not* reporting this kind of trauma. They may be embarrassed or ashamed about what has happened to them, or expect others to blame them for allowing themselves to be victimized.

Despite these difficulties, there is consistent evidence that a history of physical or sexual abuse is unusually common in psychotic women. In a review of the research on this topic, American psychologists Linda Goodman, Kim Mueser and their colleagues were able to identify thirteen adequately conducted studies.[50] For the purpose of their review, they defined physical abuse as acts, 'intended to produce severe pain or injury, including repeated slapping, kicking, biting, choking, burning, beating, or threatening with or using a weapon'. They defined sexual abuse as, 'forcible touching of breasts or genitals or forcible intercourse, including anal, oral or vaginal sex'. The highest estimates of abuse were obtained in those studies that Goodman and her colleagues judged to be most meticulously executed. Across the thirteen studies, between 51 and 97 per cent of women reported some form of physical or sexual abuse in their lifetime, suggesting that perhaps the majority of mentally ill women have been victimized in this way.

Although most studies have focused on abuse during childhood, high levels of assaults during adulthood have also been reported. In a study published several years after they completed their review, Mueser and Goodman estimated that 52 per cent of 153 severely ill female patients they interviewed had experienced sexual abuse during childhood, but nearly 64 per cent had suffered sexual abuse in later life.[51] These figures suggest that many psychotic women have been victimized on more than one occasion. As Mueser and Goodman's figures are so much higher than even the highest estimates for the general population (between 14 and 34 per cent for abuse in adulthood, and between 15 and 33 per cent for childhood sexual abuse, according to their own figures) I do not think they can be easily dismissed. Nor is this association restricted to schizophrenia patients; higher than expected rates of abuse have recently been reported for patients diagnosed as suffering from bipolar disorder.[52]

Comparable evidence of an association between trauma and psychosis has emerged from studies of men. In Mueser and Goodman's research, 35.5 per cent of male patients reported being sexually assaulted in childhood, and 25.9 per cent reported that they had been sexually assaulted as adults. Seventeen per cent had witnessed an attack leading to the killing or serious injury of another person during childhood, and the comparable figure for adult life was nearly 47 per cent. These findings are supported by the results of studies that have focused on the psychological impact of armed conflict. Follow-up investigations of American soldiers taken prisoner by the Japanese during the Pacific campaign of the Second World War, carried out in the 1970s, found higher than expected rates of schizophrenia in the most severely traumatized, although elevated rates were not found in prisoners taken by the Germans.[53] (This difference may reflect the comparative harshness of the treatment given to the POWs in the two theatres. A survey of POWs living in Minnesota, USA, found that, overall, 1.9 per cent met the DSM-III criteria for schizophrenia whereas, among those who had lost more than 35 per cent of their body weight while in captivity, the rate was 4.2 per cent, about four times the expected rate in the general population.)[54] Similarly, in two studies conducted by Kim Mueser, high levels of auditory hallucinations and delusions were found in Vietnam veterans diagnosed as suffering from PTSD.[55] The severity of these symptoms correlated with the severity of their combat experience. (Of course, combatants are not the only psychological casualties of warfare or political conflict. Psychotic reactions have also been reported in Nazi concentration camp victims[56] and, more recently, in survivors of Pol Pot's regime in Cambodia.)[57]

It might be argued that the high level of trauma reported by patients sometimes reflects events that have befallen them after they have become ill. On this view, patients whose judgement is impaired may be especially likely to place themselves in situations of risk, may be unable to take adequate avoiding actions if attacked, or may be forced by economic necessity to live in unsafe environments. At a push, the findings from veterans might even be interpreted this way (a sceptic might argue that a mentally unstable soldier is especially likely to be captured by an enemy). However, a recent large-scale survey of patients experiencing their first admission for psychosis carried out in the United States found very high levels of trauma that were comparable to those reported by patients who had been ill for some time. When the researchers took steps to exclude from their analyses any traumatic events that could be a consequence of psychotic behaviour, only 5 per cent of incidents could be accounted for in this way.[58]

If trauma does play an important role in the development of psychosis, many psychotic patients should also suffer from post-traumatic symptoms. Mueser and Goodman found that, although fewer than 3 per cent of the patients they surveyed had a PTSD diagnosis recorded in their medical notes, 40 per cent of those with a primary diagnosis of bipolar disorder, 37 per cent of those with a diagnosis of schizoaffective disorder and 28 per cent of those with a diagnosis of schizophrenia also met the DSM criteria for PTSD. By comparison, they estimated the risk of developing PTSD in the lifetime of an average member of the population to be less than 9 per cent.

By now the reader might be wondering whether crises more mundane than assaults or warfare can lead to madness. In fact, one particular type of commonplace trauma has long been known to trigger psychotic episodes. This trauma is, of course, the experience of giving birth to a child. In the nineteenth century, Esquirol carried out the first quantitative studies of *puerperal psychosis*, describing a series of 92 cases.[59] He noted that unmarried mothers seemed to be at special risk, presumably because, at that time, they suffered from many additional stresses and disadvantages. Modern studies – such as those by Robert Kendell in Edinburgh,[60] and by Ian Brockington in Manchester[61] – suggest that about 1 in every 1000 births is followed within three months by a psychotic reaction in the mother. Consistent with Esquirol's much earlier observations, these studies have also shown that additional stressors contribute to the risk of breakdown. For example, both separation from a husband and a stillbirth seem to increase the risk of psychosis.

In a detailed (and fascinating) historical review of research on puerperal psychosis, Ian Brockington has noted that some clinicians have assumed it to be a disease entity in its own right, whereas others have argued that it is a variant of one of the diagnostic categories defined within the Kraepelinian system. Brockington's own preference is to regard puerperal psychosis as a form of manic depression, because manic features are often evident. However, he notes that a minority of cases appear more schizophrenic, according to conventional definitions.[62]

The similarity between puerperal psychosis and mania is perhaps understandable when it is remembered that new mothers frequently experience sleep loss in the months following the birth of a child. However, in the case of other types of trauma, delusions and especially hallucinations have been more frequently recorded. For example, in two studies carried out by Colin Ross and his colleagues in Canada, the number of Schneiderian first-rank symptoms experienced by female inpatients correlated strongly with measures of how severely they had been sexually abused.[63] In a more recent study carried out by University of Auckland psychologist John Read, the case notes of 92 patients with a documented history of sexual and physical abuse were compared with the case notes of 108 who had not, and hallucinations stood out as the symptom most strongly predicted by a history of trauma.[64] To test whether this specific association is confined to schizophrenia patients, Paul Hammersley, in my own department, recently examined therapists' reports on nearly 100 bipolar disorder patients participating in a clinical trial of a new form of psychological treatment.[65] As part of the trial procedure, a group of research assistants had independently interviewed the patients about their lifetime history of symptoms. Although only a minority of the patients reported hallucinations, Paul found that these patients were especially likely to have disclosed to their therapists that they had been sexually abused.[66]

Overall, then, and contrary to received wisdom, the evidence that trauma can play a causal role in psychosis appears to be surprisingly *strong*. However, we are still left with a couple of unresolved questions. First, it is difficult to explain why (with the possible exception of the trauma of childbirth) there should be a specific association between trauma and hallucinations. Second, it is also difficult to explain why the effects of adverse experiences are sometimes delayed (so that, for example, sexual abuse in early life increases the risk of psychosis in adulthood).

We will not be able to answer these questions properly until we have an adequate understanding of how the cognitive processes responsible for hallucinations develop during childhood and afterwards. However, once again child psychologists have provided us with a few clues, which may point us in roughly the right direction. Recall, first of all, that hallucinations are the consequence of failing to monitor accurately the source of thoughts and images. It is therefore especially interesting that British developmental psychologists Charles Fernyhough and James Russell have recently found an association between efficiency at source monitoring in early childhood and the use of private speech in social settings – children who speak a lot to themselves when other people are present tend to be good at discriminating between their thoughts and other people's voices.[67] Perhaps children learn to tell the difference between the external ('real') and the cognitive ('imaginary') relatively easily in circumstances in which both types of events can readily be contrasted. Opportunities for this kind of learning might include not only private speech in social settings but also, for example, waking from vivid dreams, or situations in which the child learns to use mental imagery to solve complex visual problems. Speculating, as I would hardly dare to when writing a paper in a psychiatric journal, it is possible that some children who (for whatever reason) are relatively deprived of these kinds of experiences never become completely efficient at source monitoring.

On this account, it becomes possible to see why trauma might later lead to hallucinatory experiences. In Chapter 14 we saw that source-monitoring failures tend to occur when we experience intrusive or automatic thoughts. (This is because the effort taken to generate a thought acts as a cue telling us that the thought is self-generated.) It follows that a person who has poor source-monitoring skills will be most vulnerable to hallucinations when experiencing a flood of intrusive thoughts and images. Trauma (we know from the research literature on post-traumatic stress disorder) often has exactly this effect.

It is less easy to explain the delay that often occurs between trauma and the onset of hallucinations. One possibility is that this happens when there is a delay in the production of intrusive thoughts and images. This might happen, for example, when an individual initially copes well with a traumatic experience but is later reminded of it by a further trauma or period of severe stress. Many of the patients interviewed by Marius Romme and his colleagues in Holland reported being retraumatized in this way.[68] (I can think of several of my own patients whose life stories fit this picture; for example a young man who was sexually abused by his stepfather, who coped very well until his long-term girlfriend suddenly deserted him for another man, and who then became very depressed and lost his job, after which he began to hear threatening voices.) Another possibility is that stressful events some time after a trauma lead to a further reduction in the individual's already compromised source-monitoring ability, so that mental events that are initially experienced as intrusive thoughts are later experienced as hallucinations. (Again, I can think of patients who have complained of progressing from intrusive thoughts to hallucinations, but I have no evidence that this happens very often.)

If required to bet that these ideas about the mechanisms linking trauma to hallucinations will turn out to be correct, I would not offer more than a very small portion of my salary as a stake. However, they at least offer plenty of opportunities for further research.

Dialogue with a Sceptical Voice

Experience tells me that, for many of my colleagues, the account I have just given of environmental contributions to psychosis is likely to be seen as very controversial. (When I recently gave a talk about my research on paranoid patients' perceptions of their parents, a much respected psychologist – ironically, a researcher who studies expressed emotion – became very heated and said that she thought my ideas were 'dangerous'.) Indeed, the suggestion that environmental influences could be important has been so effectively censored over the last few decades that these kinds of effects are scarcely mentioned in most textbooks of psychiatry or clinical psychology.

It seems a good idea, therefore, to anticipate some of the objections that might be made to the ideas I have introduced in this chapter. For example, an advocate of an exclusively neoKraepelinian approach to psychiatry might argue that the biological findings we have considered in the previous chapter are somehow more *fundamental* or *tangible* than the findings on environmental influences.

Perhaps the idea behind this objection is that biological variables, such as sequences of DNA, brain scans or chemical assays, are more easily defined, more objective phenomena than traumas or emotional maltreatment. However, when making this claim, our sceptical friend surely cannot doubt that traumas and frosty relationships really happen. Moreover, he seems to forget that biological observations usually require many inferential steps. Geneticists routinely manipulate their data, inflating observed concordance rates to estimate the number of participants in their studies who have not yet become psychotic but who will do so in the future. Homovanillic acid is measured in the cerebrospinal fluid instead of making more difficult measurements of dopamine in the brain. The areas of the brain that appear to be activated during a functional neuroimaging experiment depend on the choice of the 'off-task' used as a comparison condition. Neither biologist nor psychologist, it seems, has unfiltered access to the world.

Perhaps what my sceptical friend really means is that biological abnormalities create the *necessary* conditions for psychosis, whereas specific environmental factors merely increase the risk of symptoms. This assumption lies behind stress-vulnerability theories of schizophrenia such as Paul Meehl's schizotypy model or the model of relapse proposed by the UCLA research group. My reply is that this is an assumption, rather than a fact. However strong the overall influence of heredity on psychosis, no one has yet proven that everyone who becomes psychotic must carry particular genes. When we look at other biological correlates of psychosis, in all cases we find people who go mad but who do not show the relevant characteristics. Some schizophrenia patients do not have enlarged cerebral ventricles, some do not perform poorly on neurocognitive tests, and so on.

A deeper problem with my sceptical friend's attempt to prioritize biological causes over environmental factors is that it assumes that these two types of influences are independent of each other and can be easily distinguished. However, in Chapter 7, I pointed to evidence that environmental influences literally shape the brain. For example, I cited evidence that some brain structures change in volume following the experience of trauma or sexual abuse. We have also seen that disruption to attachment relationships can have long-term effects on the chemistry of the brain. As neuroscience progresses, it seems likely that many more of these kinds of relationships between behavioural and biological variables will be uncovered by researchers. Perhaps eventually the distinction between what is psychological and what is biological will cease to be important. Reviewing the evidence for these kinds of relationships that has been gathered so far, University of Auckland psychologist John Read has argued that many of the biological abnormalities apparent in psychotic patients are similar to those demonstrated in the victims of trauma.[69] These abnormalities therefore might be seen as evidence supporting the hypothesis that adverse experiences contribute to psychosis, rather than as evidence that is inconsistent with it.

A related argument that my sceptical friend might make is that environmental factors are simply not strong or specific enough to be considered major determinants of psychosis. Dealing with the strength issue first, it is now possible to calculate a single value, known as an *effect size*, which can be used to compare the magnitudes of different kinds of influences. The larger the effect size, the greater the magnitude of the effect being measured, with effect sizes over 0.50 usually being considered quite large. Walter Heinrichs of York University in Toronto, Canada, has recently calculated effect sizes for comparisons between schizophrenia patients and ordinary people on a wide range of neurocognitive and biological measures.[70] For example, for the Continuous Performance Test (see Chapter 8), the average effect size was 0.67, whereas, for the backward masking test (also described in Chapter 8), it was 1.27. For levels of homovanillic acid (a metabolite of dopamine) in the cerebrospinal fluid of medication-free patients, the effect size was not only small but in the wrong direction (−0.11). For the density of dopamine D2 receptors, the average effect size was 0.93 but the effect sizes obtained in individual experiments varied between large in the expected direction (2.44) and moderately large in the wrong direction (−0.57). For structural neuroimaging studies comparing the size of the prefrontal brain in schizophrenia patients and ordinary people, the average effect size was 0.33. From the review of the literature on sexual abuse in psychotic women carried out by Goodman and her colleagues, I have calculated effect sizes for the influence of childhood sexual abuse varying between 0.70 and 2.04, depending on various assumptions about the rate of abuse in the general population. These values compare well with those found for more widely recognized factors influencing psychosis.

The question of whether the environmental effects I have identified are specific enough to be counted as major determinants of psychosis cannot be answered quite so simply. It is true, for example, that a very sizeable minority of the population is insecurely attached whereas, my sceptical friend would surely point out, only about 1 per cent of the population receives treatment for a psychotic illness. However, it is worth recalling that more people have psychotic experiences than receive psychiatric treatment. For this reason, we might really be trying to explain the experiences of 10 per cent of the population, rather than 1 per cent. Moreover, given the difficulty in defining effects such as family relationships and trauma, it is possible that any apparent lack of specificity reflects the limitations of our current measures. (Perhaps attachment relationships have to be disrupted in a specific, as yet undefined way. Although this counter-argument may sound weak, it is worth remembering that it has taken forty years to progress from George Brown's original studies to our current knowledge about expressed emotion.) We must also consider the importance of inter-actions between different risk factors for psychosis. These interactions may be between different environmental factors. (For example, someone who is securely attached might cope reasonably well with a violent or sexual assault, whereas someone who has a dismissing-avoidant attachment style, and who has grown to maturity in a stressful and threatening environment, might respond by developing paranoid ideas.) There may also be interactions between environmental and biological variables, for example between attachment style and genes, or between trauma and early brain damage. (In the last chapter, I described how gene–environment correlations can inflate the impact of environmental influences on psychosis.)

The Origins of Psychosis

This brings me nearly to the end of my outline of an alternative to Kraepelin's paradigm. The findings we have considered in the last three parts of this book are summarized in Table 18.2, which draws together what is known about the developmental pathways and psychological processes that lead to specific kinds of madness. Of course, many pieces of these parallel and overlapping jigsaws remain missing. Nonetheless, in the case of each type of complaint we can see a tentative outline of the steps that lead from the cradle to the psychiatric clinic.

For the last thirty years, neoKraepelinian psychiatrists, like their predecessors in the first era of biological psychiatry, have promoted the idea that madness is a brain disease. In an earlier chapter, I described this paradigm as a cultural system, because it reflects the starting assumptions made by researchers, rather than conclusions drawn from scientific evidence. Recent neurodevelopmental models of schizophrenia and bipolar disorder are the latest manifestation of this cultural system. In making this claim, I am not attempting to deny that there is value in the neurodevelopmental approach. However, the grip of the Kraepelinian paradigm on the minds of researchers has been so great that many have ignored the evidence on psychological or social influences, denied that they are important, or treated them as peripheral to the problem of explaining madness, by diagnosing traumatized psychotic patients as suffering from an atypical form of PTSD.[71]

Despite the enormous efforts made by biological researchers, the effects that have been detected (for example, on the influence of foetal

Table 18.2 Probable pathways to different kinds of madness.

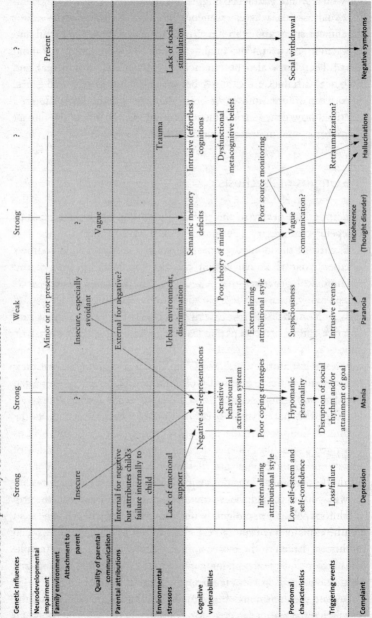

exposure to the influenza virus or on obstetric complications) have usually been small in magnitude, and the findings have often been inconsistent. Moreover, the link between these factors and the positive symptoms appears to be especially tenuous. This observation parallels the results obtained from the psychological studies I reviewed in Chapter 7, which have found only modest relationships between the severity of cognitive deficits and negative symptoms, and almost no relationship at all between deficits and hallucinations and delusions.

In contrast, although much less effort has been made to unravel the psychological and social origins of psychosis, the evidence that is available is consistent and points to effects that are at least as strong as those measured by biological investigators. Moreover, this evidence suggests that a socially stressful environment, attachment and other family difficulties, and trauma, all have an impact on positive symptoms, especially persecutory delusions and hallucinations.

It seems that we are presented with something of a paradox. Although there can be no doubt that early brain damage confers vulnerability to madness, it seems to have very little impact on those symptoms which, since Schneider, have been considered the hallmark of psychosis. Perhaps Bleuler[72] and Michael Foster Green[73] are right in concluding that muted cognitive and emotional signs lie at the core of madness, and that the more flamboyant symptoms that have perplexed modern researchers are merely the individual's reaction to these subtle deficits. Or perhaps cognitive deficits impede the individual's ability to cope in times of crisis, creating challenges that the individual's social reasoning skills are unable to meet.

Why adolescence is a high-risk period

With this possibility in mind, let us now return briefly to the question of why psychotic symptoms so often appear in adolescence and early adulthood. NeoKraepelinians would have us believe that this age trend can be explained entirely in terms of biological processes unwinding within the person – the biological time-bomb theory. But, of course, this high-risk period is a part of the life cycle that places special demands on the developing person's social and cognitive skills. The American psychologist G. Stanley Hall, author of the first considered psychological theory of adolescence, famously borrowed the German phrase *Sturm und Drang* (storm and stress) to characterize it.[74] This view of the transition to adulthood as a period of emotional turmoil has since been assimilated by popular culture, so that most people, at least in Western countries, accept it as self-evident. If someone calls you an adolescent you are unlikely to feel flattered.

Unfortunately, adolescence is perhaps the least understood developmental stage. There are not even agreed conventions for defining where it begins and ends. (Hall's view was that it extended from puberty to when full adult status was attained, which he took to be around the age of 25.) Nor is it clear that it really is a time of storm and stress, at least for the majority of young people. It has been estimated that only 15 per cent of adolescents report severe emotional disturbance.[75]

Nonetheless, the time between puberty and settled adulthood clearly involves a number of developmental tasks, each of which may be seen as a hurdle at which the weak or ill-prepared may fall. In the ten years after puberty, the emerging adult must remodel her relationship with her parents, begin to explore sexual and emotional relationships with potential partners, and decide on a career path. Overarching these tasks, there is the need to establish an identity, a process that the developmental psychologist and psychoanalyst Eric Erikson portrayed as the central problem of adolescence in his famous book *Childhood and Society*.[76]

British psychologists Chris Harrop and Peter Trower note that these challenges seem to provoke in adolescents traits that are reminiscent of characteristics often seen in psychotic patients: marked shifts of mood coupled with equally dramatic shifts in self-esteem; self-consciousness, egocentricity and grandiosity; magical thinking and a preoccupation with powerful role models and the fable of one's own life.[77] In a study of normal adolescents carried out by Patrick McGorry and his colleagues in Melbourne, Australia, it was found that these kinds of characteristics are extremely difficult to distinguish from the typical prodromal symptoms of psychosis.[78]

It seems unlikely that the high risk of psychosis experienced by adolescents and young adults is unrelated to these experiences. As American psychologist Barbara Cornblatt has pointed out, children who suffer from the kinds of subtle social and cognitive difficulties that have sometimes been found in pre-psychotic children may be poorly equipped to face the developmental tasks of adolescence.[79]

Although she based this hypothesis on American psychological research that has emphasized the role of cognitive deficits in psychosis (described in Chapter 7 of this book), her proposal seems even more plausible when what we know about social-cognitive processes is added into the equation. Children who reason abnormally about the causes of important events in their lives, or who are unable to guess accurately the thoughts of others, will be especially handicapped when faced with the demands of complex social situations. It is therefore quite unnecessary to assume that, in every case, disasters must trip up the child on his pathway to adulthood (although, as we have seen, this sometimes happens). The mere inability to adapt to new demands, to cross hurdles which brothers, sisters, friends and neighbours stride over with relative ease, may be sufficient to instil a sense of failure and personal inadequacy, magnify pre-existing social-cognitive peculiarities, and provoke thoughts that are increasingly psychotic.

Of course, the mere appearance of psychotic experiences is not enough to turn a troubled adolescent into a *patient*. For this to happen the experiences must be negatively valued and perceived as at odds with the individual's culture. This suspicion may arise suddenly, or may develop over a long period of time. Often people wrestle with a variety of explanations of what is happening, sometimes entertaining several contradictory hypotheses at the same time ('Maybe I'm special? Maybe I'm going insane? Maybe this is just a phase I'm going through?'). My colleague Tony Morrison has argued that the outcome of this process often depends partly on the person's metacognitive belief system (for example, a person who has unrealistic views about the efficiency of the human mind may be especially troubled by the discovery that his own mind is playing tricks on him).[80] Often, the decision that 'something is seriously wrong' is reached with the help or persuasion of other people: typically, a combination of parents, friends and diagnostic experts.

As I look back, I can remember many patients who, at the end of this process, have seemed stranded in the no man's land between childhood and the adult world. Often very sensitive individuals, most have seemed aware, at least at some level, of the nature of their predicament. Sometimes, the pain of being stuck and forced to watch as peers have moved on to get jobs, marry and buy cars and houses has been almost palpable. The task of helping young psychotic people to liberate themselves from this state of frozen development is one of the greatest challenges that a psychologist can face.

A Final Caveat

Over forty years ago, the philosopher Karl Popper pointed out that complex chains of interacting processes can rarely be reduced to simple causal laws:

The crucial point is this: although we may assume that any actual succession of phenomena proceeds according to the laws of nature, it is important to realize that practically no sequence of, say, three or more causally connected concrete events proceeds according to any single law of nature. If the wind shakes a tree and Newton's apple falls to the ground, nobody would deny that these events can be described in terms of causal laws. But, there is no single law, such as that of gravity, nor even a single definite set of laws, to describe the actual or concrete succession of causally connected events; apart from gravity, we would have to consider the laws explaining wind pressure; jerking movements of the branch; the tension in the apple's stalk; the bruise suffered by the apple on impact; all of which is succeeded by chemical processes resulting from the bruise, etc. The idea that any concrete sequence or succession of events (apart from such examples as the movement of a pendulum or a solar system) can be described by any one law, or even by a definite set of laws, is simply mistaken.[81]

This is precisely the situation that we find ourselves in when we try and understand the origins of madness. No doubt this conclusion will seem disappointing – perhaps even nihilistic – to many readers. It implies that we should abandon hope of a quick scientific breakthrough that will curtail madness in the way that antibiotics have curtailed infections. The Nobel Prize that awaits the scientist who discovers *the* cause of schizophrenia will never be claimed (or worse, it will be awarded to someone who does not deserve it). However, a positive implication can be drawn. Despite the tragedies that we encounter in the psychiatric clinic, most children do not grow up to be disabled by delusions, hallucinations, manic episodes or disordered thinking. In fact, because psychotic complaints seem to require a combination of many factors, even the majority of children of psychotic parents grow up to lead healthy and rewarding lives. Adaptation and triumph over adversity are the norm. Lives that are blighted by insanity are the exception.

Madness and Society

Any man who goes to see a psychiatrist should have his head examined.
Samuel Goldwyn[1]

The first principle in the psychic treatment of mental patients is frankness and unconditional love of the truth. It is just in this point where laymen and doctors make such serious mistakes.
Emil Kraepelin[2]

The main purpose of this book has been to present a new way of thinking about madness. This has necessitated, first of all, showing that the traditional way of explaining psychosis is fatally flawed, and then bringing together a (hopefully) novel synthesis of research from a wide range of disciplines. Along the way, I have attempted to explain relevant concepts from psychology and the neurosciences in a manner that will allow the layperson to follow my arguments, while at the same time covering relevant findings in sufficient detail to satisfy the curiosity of sceptical psychiatrists and psychologists. Inevitably, this has been a lengthy process and, yet, even at the end, I am aware of so much that I have left out in my attempt to avoid producing a book that (in the nicely ambiguous terminology of my editor) is too 'monumental'.

It is worth reiterating, in just a few sentences, what I see to be the main benefits of this new way of thinking. Its greatest advantage is that it does not require us to make three dubious assumptions that were central to Kraepelin's paradigm and its most recent manifestation as the neoKraepelinian project – that there is an unambiguous dividing line between the psychologically healthy and the psychologically disturbed, that there is a finite and countable number of different mental illnesses, and that these types of illness must be explained primarily in terms of aberrant biology. Second, it allows us to make sense of (in Jaspers' terminology, both explain *and* understand) the actual experiences of men and women who receive diagnoses such as schizo-phrenia and bipolar disorder. (In contrast, Kraepelinian psychiatry had almost nothing to say about why people hear voices, make strange inferences about the actions of other people, become frighteningly excitable or just sit around all day doing nothing.) Third, the account links the experience of madness to processes that are important in ordinary life, and which are reasonably well understood by psychol-ogists (this is in contrast to the old assumption that 'however much is known about the psychology of the normal individual, in the patho-logical field new laws will be found to operate').[3] Fourth, I hope the vision I have offered is of a truly 'joined-up' psychopathology, in which the findings from various disciplines (anthropology, sociology, developmental and cognitive psychology, developmental biology, gen-etics and the neurosciences) are linked together in a meaningful way, and in which no single level of explanation (genetic or neurobiological) is seen as somehow 'trumping' all the others.

It is also worth emphasizing, for one last time, that the approach I have outlined is genuinely scientific, in the sense that it is evidence-based, so that most of the hypotheses that are components of the framework have been tested by observation or experiment. Critics have very occasionally attempted to dismiss my approach as emotional, self-serving (because I am a psychologist criticizing theories mostly but not exclusively put forwards by psychiatrists), or some kind of throwback to 1960s style anti-psychiatry (as if all criticisms of con-ventional psychiatry are equivalent). As it is clearly unscientific to cling to the Kraepelinian paradigm, which enjoys almost no evidential support, these kinds of criticisms amount to what Freudians sometimes term *projection* (the tendency to attribute one's own faults to other people).

When planning this book, I had originally hoped to discuss at length the many practical implications of the post-Kraepelinian approach. In the end it proved to be impossible to provide a detailed treatment of these implications while, at the same time, keeping this book to a reasonable length. However, I will spend a few pages indicating what I think they are.

Us and Them

The Kraepelinian paradigm encouraged an 'us' and 'them' distinction between the mad and the sane, whereas the evidence I have described (especially in Chapters 5 and 6) shows that we are mad to varying degrees, that the boundaries of madness are subject to negotiation, and that some of us get on very well despite being (in psychiatric terms) quite psychotic for much of the time.

The 'us' and 'them' distinction has had a number of very serious negative consequences for those living at the mad end of this spectrum. Most importantly, it has denied them a voice. In the clinical and research literature, this is most evident in discussions of the concept of *insight*, an absence of which has often been seen to be a cardinal feature of psychosis.

In a famous paper published in 1934, British psychiatrist Aubrey Lewis defined insight as: 'The *correct* attitude to morbid change in oneself, and moreover, the realisation that the illness is mental' (italics mine).[4] Elaborating on this idea, Xavier Amador and Henry Kronengold, psychologists working at the New York State Psychiatric Institute, have recently suggested that lack of insight has two separate components: unawareness of illness and 'incorrect attributions' about the causes of illness.[5] Armed with these kinds of definitions, researchers have laboured mightily to discover how common lack of insight really is in psychotic patients (very common, apparently),[6] and whether it is related to other variables of interest such as the patient's neurocognitive abilities or a willingness to take psychiatric drugs. Most of this research has been inconclusive.[7] However, the real problem with this kind of approach is that it assumes that psychologists and psychiatrists are privileged possessors of a correct theory of psychosis, which patients are foolish to dispute. It fails to recognize that patients may have good reasons to form hypotheses about their difficulties that are at variance with those accepted by mental health professionals. It also places patients in a terrible double bind, in which their objections to unsatisfactory aspects of psychiatric care are seen by the clinician as further evidence that treatment is imperative. Indeed, the notion that patients lack insight is routinely used to justify cajoling, threatening or misleading patients about their rights in the hope that these strategies will pressure patients into accepting treatment. Recent surveys in Europe and North America have confirmed that, even in these enlightened times, coercion is widely regarded as an acceptable and routine strategy in the clinical management of madness.[8]

Because patients have been denied a voice, they have often been subjected to cruel and ineffective treatments. In the past, these have included insulin coma (which involved patients being injected with the hormone insulin, causing them to fall into a comatose state perilously close to death, whereupon they were revived and the process was repeated), and electroconvulsive therapy (which, before the introduction of muscle-relaxing drugs, sometimes caused patients to suffer spinal fractures). Even more drastic was the prefrontal leucotomy, which was pioneered by the Portuguese neurosurgeon Egas Moniz in the 1930s and practised throughout the developed world until well after the introduction of chlorpromazine.[9] This crude brain operation was championed in North America by the manically enthusiastic neurosurgeon Walter Freeman, who, travelling throughout the USA and Canada in the summer of 1951 in a car loaded with equipment, visited mental hospitals to demonstrate his chillingly efficient technique for carrying it out. After administering a jolt of ECT, Freeman would insert an ice-pick-like instrument above the eye of the dazed and convulsing patient, smashing it through the bone of the orbit and into the brain behind. This procedure was cheap and quick; Freeman estimated that he could complete as many as twenty-five operations in a single day, and claimed to have carried out over 5000 during his professional career.[10]

These ghastly practices were, of course, exceeded in Germany during the Nazi period, when doctors introduced extermination as a treatment for severe mental illness.[11] Inspired by genetic theories which suggested that madness, unless checked, would gradually weaken the Aryan gene-pool, they did not require great encouragement from the state first to compulsorily sterilize and then to kill the most vulnerable members of their society. Gas chambers were constructed in psychiatric hospitals, where tens of thousands of psychotic adults (and many more children said to be suffering from genetic illnesses) were put to death, usually with carbon monoxide, but sometimes by deliberate starvation. As historian Robert Proctor has noted:

It is important to recognise the banality of the operation. In 1941 the psychi-atric institution at Hadamar celebrated the cremation of its ten-thousandth patient in a special ceremony, where everyone in attendance – secretaries, nurses, and psychiatrists – received a bottle of beer for the occasion.[12]

At the beginning of the twenty-first century, it is easy to dismiss these excesses as products of more primitive times. However, the abuses that were perpetrated against psychiatric patients in every country in the West, and which reached a crescendo in Nazi Germany, were made possible by assumptions about psychosis that are the main elements of the Kraepelinian paradigm. Without regarding madness as merely the product of a damaged brain, it would not have been possible to devise a therapeutic system that relied exclusively on physi-cal treatments at the expense of treating people with warmth and humanity. Without the hypothesis that this brain damage is genetically determined, killing would not have been regarded as a rational treat-ment by a generation of well-trained nurses and physicians in Ger-many. Above all, without regarding psychosis as *ununderstandable* (to use Jaspers' terminology), it would not have been possible to deny psychiatric patients a voice, which might otherwise have been raised in protest against these horrors.

(Of course, I am not suggesting that it was inevitable that Kraepelin's work would have these consequences. Cruel treatments preceded Kraepelin and, in any case, judgements about what *ought* to be done to other people are never exclusively determined by beliefs about what *is* the case. It is perfectly possible to believe that schizophrenia is a genetically determined brain disease while at the same time acting compassionately towards people who receive the diagnosis. But factual beliefs are often used to justify moral intuitions, and the beliefs about psychosis promulgated by Kraepelin and his followers were peculiarly suited to justifying the worst excesses of twentieth-century psychiatric care. In this sense, these excesses were a legacy of the paradigm, a legacy that, in human terms, has been much more costly than the stifling effect that it has had on research.)

Medicines for Madness

Today the assumption that psychosis is a form of brain disease is translated into clinical reality by psychiatric services that rely exclusively on
neuroleptic medication, and which make little or no effort to respond to
patients' psychological needs. This bias in the kinds of therapies that are
made available to patients reflects systematic misunderstandings about
the relative effectiveness of medical and psychological treatments that
mirror the misunderstandings about biological and environmental
causes of psychosis which I addressed in the previous chapter.

I do not doubt that the accidental discovery of the therapeutic effects
of chlorpromazine was a major breakthrough in the treatment of severe
mental illness. (It has recently been described as one of twelve defining
moments in the history of modern medicine.)[13] Clinical trials have
consistently demonstrated that patients who take chlorpromazine, or
any of the other widely used neuroleptic drugs, experience fewer
psychotic complaints and, if they continue to take them when well,
fewer relapses than patients who do not take them.[14] However, this
obvious good news must be qualified by considering the disadvantages
of this kind of treatment.

Long-term outcome studies suggest that today's psychiatric patients
do not do much better than the patients of Kraepelin's era.[15] Although
most modern recipients of psychiatric care find that neuroleptics to
some extent control their symptoms, it is doubtful whether any are
cured by this kind of treatment, and a substantial minority obtain no
benefit whatsoever. Despite extensive research, no one has found a
way of predicting in advance which patients will respond to neuroleptic treatment.[16] However, there is very good evidence that patients
who fail to benefit from one type of neuroleptic will fail to respond
to any other.[17] These persistent 'neuroleptic non-responders' would
almost certainly do better if given no neuroleptic treatment whatsoever, yet drug-free strategies for managing symptoms are almost never
considered by modern psychiatric services.

The distressing and sometimes dangerous side effects caused by
conventional neuroleptics add to the difficulty in forming a balanced
opinion about their value. The most obvious of these are the 'extrapyramidal'[18] side effects, which include Parkinsonian symptoms (the

patient becomes stiff or suffers from uncontrollable tremors, experienced by about 25 per cent of patients), akathisia (a very unpleasant subjective feeling of restlessness and agitation) and tardive dyskinesia (spasmodic movements of the jaw and tongue, which are unsightly and, once established, are sometimes irreversible even after the medication has been discontinued; now thankfully very rare). Side effects that are less obvious to the observer but which cause considerable distress to patients include sexual dysfunction[19] (experienced by over a third of patients)[20] and severe weight gain (probably the consequence of an increased craving for carbohydrates;[21] experienced by about 50 per cent of patients).[22]

The psychological side effects of neuroleptics can be very distressing.* Akathisia is often accompanied by a type of depression sometimes described as *neuroleptic dysphoria*,[23] which can persist for many years.[24] In the long term, taking neuroleptics can also lead to a profound lack of motivation, known as the *neuroleptic induced deficit syndrome*, which is almost impossible to distinguish from negative symptoms.[25] In one clinical trial it was found that patients treated with neuroleptics, although less symptomatic, achieved fewer life goals than patients treated with a placebo.[26]

---

* One way in which sceptical clinicians might overcome any doubts they might have about the subjective effects of neuroleptics is to take one. Two British psychiatrists, R. H. Belmaker and D. Wald ('Haloperidol in normals', *British Journal of Psychiatry*, 131: 222–3, 1977), long ago reported the effects of taking 5 mg of haloperidol: 'The effect was marked and very similar in both of us: within ten minutes a marked slowing of thinking and movement developed, along with a profound inner restlessness. Neither subject could continue work, and each left work for over 36 hours. Each subject complained of paralysis of volition, a lack of physical and psychic energy. The subjects were unable to read, telephone or perform household tasks of their own will, but could perform these tasks if demanded to do so.'

I was a participant in a similar experiment conducted by my friend and colleague David Healy, in which I received 5 mg of droperidol, and became restless and dysphoric to the point of being very distressed (I burst into tears and, for some reason, I felt compelled to tell David everything I had ever felt guilty about). I had a hangover for several days. Similar effects were recorded from the other volunteers in the study (D. Healy and G. Farquhar (1998) 'Immediate effects of droperidol', *Human Psychopharmacology: Clinical and Experimental*, 13: 113–20).

The doses in these experiments were far lower than those typically given to patients.

Effects that are life-threatening but fortunately less common include sudden heart failure (psychotic patients are about twice as likely to die this way than ordinary people);[27] the *neuroleptic malignant syndrome* (a disorder characterized by muscular rigidity, fever and fluctuating consciousness, which is often mistaken for a bacterial infection, and which is fatal if drugs are not promptly discontinued);[28] and agranulocytosis (a loss of white blood cells, which is also fatal unless treated promptly).[29] There are also hidden risks of death associated with neuroleptic medication that are difficult to calculate. For example, because obesity increases the risk of myocardial infarction and stroke, patients who experience neuroleptic-induced weight gain presumably suffer an increased risk of dying from these illnesses, but such deaths are never recorded as drug reactions.[30] Similarly, there is evidence that severe akathisia can provoke patients to attempt suicide,[31] but patients' suicides are rarely regarded as drug-induced.

Because of these many adverse effects, neuroleptics, if used indiscriminately, can cause more harm than good. Biological psychiatrists should therefore have been strongly motivated to establish the safest and most effective dose of this kind of treatment. It is therefore all the more remarkable that the first experiments to address this question were not published until 1990 – *approximately 40 years after the drugs were first introduced*.[32] The results of these studies surprised many psychiatrists, because they showed that no additional clinical benefits were obtained for doses equivalent to more than about 350 milligrams of chlorpromazine a day, a much lower dose than was commonly used in routine practice. The same studies provided clear evidence of a simple linear relationship between dose and side effects – the higher the dose the more likely it is that patients will experience side effects that are severe and very distressing.[33] The inescapable conclusion that follows from these findings is that the overzealous use of neuroleptic medication has led to a worldwide epidemic of avoidable iatrogenic illness, causing unnecessary distress to countless vulnerable people, and no doubt sending some to early graves. Astonishingly, this problem continues at the time of writing. Despite advice to the contrary from organizations such as the Royal College of Psychiatrists in Britain[34] and the US National Institute of Mental Health,[35] surveys show that psychiatrists continue to treat many of their patients with bizarrely high doses of neuroleptic drugs.[36]

The recent development of a new group of *atypical neuroleptics* adds a final twist to this unfortunate story. The first of these drugs, clozapine, was synthesized in the 1960s[37] but was quickly discontinued when it was discovered that about one in 200 patients receiving it suffered from agranulocitosis (as a consequence, eight elderly patients in Finland died during an early clinical trial). However, interest in the drug was revived when it was realized that its low profile of extrapyramidal side effects made it an attractive treatment for patients suffering from tardive dyskinesia. Procedures were therefore developed to allow patients to be closely monitored so that they could be quickly withdrawn from the drug if signs of agranulocitosis became evident. A clinical trial conducted by John Kane, Herbert Meltzer and their colleagues in the United States, published in 1988, seemed to confirm that clozapine could be taken safely, caused fewer extrapyramidal side effects than chlorpromazine and was an effective treatment for patients who failed to respond to conventional drugs.[38]

Pharmaceutical companies quickly realized that drugs such as clozapine might provide an opportunity to increase dramatically the profits they made from selling their products to psychiatric services. (As most of the conventional neuroleptics are out of patent, they can be manufactured as 'generic drugs' by any company, keeping profit margins very tight.) In the last few years, therefore, several more atypical neuroleptics have been licensed and marketed as being kinder and more effective than conventional anti-psychotic medication. Given that these drugs are extremely expensive to taxpayers (in the UK) and insurance companies (in the USA) it is obviously important to establish whether these claims are justified. A good starting point is John Kane's 1988 trial.

In order to select patients who had failed to respond to typical neuroleptics, Kane and his colleagues required that anyone entering their study had experienced at least three attempts at conventional treatment with doses equivalent to one gram of chlorpromazine a day or higher. Of the 268 patients who eventually took part, half were randomly assigned to treatment with clozapine. The remaining patients were assigned to treatment with doses of chlorpromazine up to a (literally) staggering 1.8 grams per day. The patients were then followed up for six weeks, during which time their psychotic symptoms and side effects were monitored. The researchers claimed that those treated with clozapine experienced less severe psychotic symptoms, and also fewer extrapyramidal side effects, than those treated with chlorpromazine (although statistically significant differences were only observed on one of the two side-effect measures used in the study).

Considerable effort was required in order to carry out the experiment. Herbert Meltzer has estimated that, because of the difficulty in finding suitable patients and in monitoring them adequately, it cost the pharmaceutical company Sandoz over $5 million to complete.[39] However, despite this investment, the results of the study are almost impossible to interpret because the comparison drug, chlorpromazine, was given at a dose that was much too high to be optimally therapeutic. It has been shown that patients treated with unnecessarily high doses of conventional neuroleptics sometimes improve when their drug doses are reduced.[40] It is therefore possible that the patients in the control group would have done as well as those patients given clozapine had they been given a more sensible amount of chlorpromazine. Furthermore, given the dose they actually received, it is astonishing that much larger differences in side effects were not observed.

A recent analysis of data from clinical trials of the atypicals, published in the *British Medical Journal*, has confirmed that the effectiveness of the new drugs has been systematically exaggerated by studies that have compared them to inappropriate doses of conventional medication. British psychiatrist John Geddes and his colleagues analysed data from fifty-two studies involving a total of 12,649 patients, in which the experimental medication was either clozapine or one of four other recently introduced atypicals (risperidone, olanzapine, quetiapine, or sertindole).[41] When the trials were divided into those in which control patients had received a daily dose equivalent to 12 milligrams or less of haloperidol (equivalent to about 300 milligrams of chlorpromazine), and those in which the comparison dose was greater, no differences in outcome were observed in the former studies, but the atypicals appeared more effective and more acceptable to patients in the latter. The only evidence of superiority for the atypicals that remained when the dose of the comparison drug was optimal was in extrapyramidal effects, which remained less frequent and less severe in those receiving the new medications. However, even this benefit seems less than impressive when it is realized that the atypical medications can cause other types of side effects in abundance (olanzapine, for example, is notorious for causing weight gain).

Addressing Patients' Psychological Needs

I expect that some psychiatrists will react to the account I have given of neuroleptic treatment by assuming that I am motivated by some kind of ideological hostility to medical treatment. Certainly, there are some mental health professionals – usually psychologists, but sometimes nurses or even psychiatrists – who believe that the use of psychiatric drugs is always wrong, and that neuroleptics are mere 'chemical straitjackets'.[42] This is not my position. What I am arguing for is a balanced appraisal of the benefits and costs of neuroleptic treatment, based on scientific evidence. There is no doubt that neuroleptics are a useful therapeutic tool if prescribed to the right patients in sensible doses, but there is equally no doubt that they can be harmful if used in excess. The failure to recognize the very real limitations of this kind of treatment is just as shortsighted as the blanket rejection of drug treatment of any kind.

The way forward in the drug treatment of psychosis is therefore to find ways of targeting medication more accurately to meet the needs of patients. As it is not possible to predict neuroleptic response in advance of treatment, the only way that this can be achieved is by adopting a systematic policy of 'suck it and see'. To do this effectively, prescribers will have to work closely with patients in order to monitor therapeutic benefits and side effects, and will also need the courage to withdraw patients completely from their drugs if they are obviously failing to benefit. Without proper research into drug-free treatment (which is almost impossible in medically dominated psychiatric services) it is difficult to know how many patients are best treated without drugs of any kind, but the number is likely to be many more than are treated this way at present. (In the only study so far conducted to address this question, carried out by Loren Mosher in the USA in the 1970s, it was found that most first-episode patients treated without drugs but given very intensive psychological support did just as well as drug-treated patients at two-year follow-up.[43] However, this important study has never been properly replicated and, given the dominance of Kraepelinian thinking in psychiatry, is not likely to be repeated in the foreseeable future.)

Just as the Kraepelinian paradigm has encouraged clinicians to rely on neuroleptic drugs, it has discouraged the provision of psychological treatments. Further discouragement has been provided by the results of clinical trials of intensive psychoanalytic treatment (based on the ideas of Freud and his followers). This type of psychotherapy encourages patients to explore difficult emotional issues with therapists who offer interpretations of their thoughts and feelings, but little in the way of concrete advice. Although Freud himself was sceptical about the value of this approach in the treatment of psychosis, it was adapted for this use by a number of American psychoanalysts, most notably Harry Stack Sullivan,[44] a charismatic psychiatrist who was influential in the 1930s and 1940s, and whose theories of mental illness were a blend of ideas garnered from Freud and social psychology.[45]

Unfortunately, when clinical trials have been conducted to assess the effects of psychoanalytic treatment on positive symptoms the results have been almost universally negative.[46] The most rigorous study of this kind was carried out in the early 1980s by Alfred Stanton, John Gunderson and their colleagues in Boston, USA.[47] One hundred and sixty-five patients were offered therapy by highly experienced clinicians twice a week for up to two years. By six months, all but sixty-nine had dropped out, itself an indication that the therapy failed to meet the needs of the majority of patients. After two years, a control group of patients who had received simple supportive counselling (emotional support and advice about practical difficulties) were no more symptomatic, and had spent less time in hospital and more time in employment, than those psychoanalytically treated patients who had persisted to the end. Naturalistic long-term follow-up studies of patients who had received intensive psychoanalytic therapy in specialist hospitals, published at about the same time, yielded equally discouraging results.[48]

Although psychoanalytic theory has at times led to useful insights into the behaviour and experience of patients, analysts have been reluctant to integrate their ideas with equally important insights gained from scientific research. As a consequence, the theory has not led to a coherent understanding of the origins of psychosis, or experimentally testable theories about the psychological processes responsible for complaints such as delusions and hallucinations. Perhaps we therefore should not be surprised that treatment based on psychoanalytic principles offers few benefits for psychotic patients. By contrast, the psychological models discussed throughout this book have been based on studies that have followed the normal conventions of scientific investigation. They should therefore be robust enough to guide the development of novel interventions. In fact, two types of treatment that are consistent with these models seem to offer tangible benefits for patients and their families.

In Chapter 16 I described evidence that family relationships can affect the long-term course of psychotic difficulties. Patients returning from hospital to live with relatives who are either critical and hostile or emotionally over-controlling are more likely to relapse than patients living in less stressful circumstances. It did not take long for the researchers who made this discovery to realize that providing assistance to patients' families might therefore benefit both the families and patients. In a paper published in 1982, Julian Leff and his colleagues reported the effects of a nine-month treatment programme, in which the relatives of schizophrenia patients were educated about psychosis, took part in support groups, and met with therapists who tried to help them improve their ability to resolve family conflicts.[49] Twenty-four patients were followed up, initially for nine months and then, in a subsequent report, two years after treatment had begun.[50] Patients whose families had received the intervention had a much lower rate of relapse than patients in the control group (8 per cent versus 50 per cent at nine months and 20 per cent versus 78 per cent at two years).

This finding has since been repeated many times, for example by Ian Falloon and his colleagues in southern California,[51] by Gerry Hogarty and others in Pittsburgh,[52] and by my colleagues Nick Tarrier and Christine Barrowclough in Salford, near Manchester.[53] A recent systematic review identified twenty-five clinical trials published in English- and German-language journals in which relatives had been included in treatments for schizophrenia patients.[54] In some of these studies, benefits were maintained many years after treatment had ended.[55] Overall, the patients whose relatives participated in these programmes benefited from a 20 per cent reduction in relapses during the first year after treatment commenced, a benefit similar in magnitude to that observed in trials comparing neuroleptic medication with placebos. Much less effort has been made to investigate the value of this kind of treatment for bipolar patients and their families, but at least one study has reported encouraging results.[56]

Whereas family interventions attempt to ameliorate the kind of stress that makes psychotic symptoms worse, more recently developed cognitive behaviour therapy (CBT) interventions are designed to influence the cognitive processes that give rise to symptoms. These interventions have been modified from earlier techniques that were developed for the treatment of depression by Aaron Beck and others in the USA.[57] Unlike psychoanalytic therapy, CBT is targeted at precisely specified difficulties that are identified by the patient and the therapist together. (Often, the first thing that they do together is draw up a 'problem list'.) It involves the patient and therapist collaborating in a very practical way to find solutions to the patient's problems. (At the end of each session, patients usually take away homework assignments so that they can test out new ideas or try out novel solutions to their problems that emerge during the course of discussion with the therapist.) The core idea of CBT is that patients can learn to reflect on their own thoughts and beliefs, find ways of testing their validity, and, if necessary, substitute more helpful thoughts and beliefs. Patients receiving CBT for depression, for example, learn to recognize when their attributions for events are unnecessarily pessimistic, to replace them with more realistic appraisals of events, and to find proactive ways of solving their problems.

Many of the psychologists who first began to experiment with CBT for psychosis were also involved in some of the basic research that I have described earlier in this book. For some reason (probably because they were relatively uncommitted to the neoKraepelinian dogma) nearly all were British. Paul Chadwick, whose ideas about paranoia were briefly considered in Chapter 13, reported some early case studies of deluded patients who had been successfully encouraged to reconsider their abnormal beliefs.[58] Gill Haddock, whose work we briefly touched on in Chapter 14, investigated different methods of helping hallucinating patients to identify the source of their inner speech.[59] Max Birchwood, working with Paul Chadwick, studied the effects of encouraging hallucinating patients to question their beliefs about their voices.[60] However, psychiatrists David Kingdon (now at the University of Southampton) and Douglas Turkington (now at the University of Newcastle) and clinical psychologist Nick Tarrier (at the University of Manchester) probably deserve most credit for integrating these ideas into comprehensive therapeutic strategies.

Kingdon and Turkington proposed a general framework for working with psychotic patients, which they described as a *normalizing strategy*.[61] The idea behind this approach is to demystify psychotic experiences and make them seem less frightening, for example by pointing out the similarities between hallucinations or paranoia and more mundane mental states, or by explaining to patients that these experiences are much more common than is often realized. Nick Tarrier's approach was initially named *coping skills enhancement*, because it aimed to help patients learn better ways of coping with their experiences, but was soon expanded to incorporate various strategies for addressing patients' delusional ideas or beliefs about their voices.[62]

Nick Tarrier published the first randomized controlled clinical trial of cognitive behaviour therapy for schizophrenia patients. At six-month follow-up, patients whose delusions and hallucinations had not responded to neuroleptic medication, and who had been offered CBT, had shown a greater improvement in their complaints compared to patients who were taught simpler problem-solving skills.[63] The trial was soon followed by another small-scale study, carried out by Philippa Garety and her colleagues at the Institute of Psychiatry in London, who found greater improvements in delusional beliefs in chronically ill patients treated with CBT than in patients who did not receive this kind of therapy.[64] In the last few years, larger trials have begun to appear in scientific and medical journals, nearly all of which have supported these initial results. At the time of writing, seven trials have appeared, including further studies by David Kingdon, Douglas Turkington and their colleagues,[65] by investigators at the Institute of Psychiatry,[66] and by Nick Tarrier and his colleagues.[67] Several others have been completed and are awaiting publication. One of these is the SoCRATES (Study of Cognitive-Realignment Therapy in Early Schizophrenia) trial conducted by Shôn Lewis, Nick Tarrier, Gill Haddock, myself and others, in which we have found that a very brief (five-week) intervention offered to patients when they become acutely ill for the very first time results in modest benefits at eighteen-month follow-up.[68] Another is a study conducted by Andrew Gumley and his colleagues in Scotland, who have found that a very brief intervention with patients who have been ill for some time can dramatically reduce the likelihood that they will relapse.[69] Although bipolar patients have, again, been largely overlooked in these developments, three small-scale studies have provided preliminary evidence that CBT may be an effective method of reducing the risk of manic episodes.[70]

None of these findings suggests that CBT or family therapy is a panacea for madness. Despite our best efforts, some patients fail to respond to psychological treatment and it is often forgotten that less glamorous interventions, for example providing opportunities for marginalized and isolated patients to find work, or solving their accommodation problems, can have effects on quality of life that are just as dramatic as any that can be achieved by psychologists or psychiatrists.

Nonetheless, very real progress has been made in the psychological treatment of madness over the last decade or so. Furthermore, it is unlikely that the best that can be accomplished today is the last word on what is possible. Just as pharmaceutical companies do not assume that today's medications cannot be bettered, we should not assume that existing results represent some kind of limit on what psychological interventions can do for people afflicted with madness.

Can Psychosis be Prevented?

Increasing optimism about both drug and psychological treatments for psychosis, whether or not justified, has led to a debate about *when* treatment should be offered. Recently, clinicians and researchers have begun to consider the possibility of intervening very early in the development of an illness.[71] One impetus for this has been the emerging understanding, discussed in the last two chapters, that psychosis is the end point of a long developmental pathway. Another has been the discovery that many psychotic patients experience distressing symptoms for long periods before either seeking or being offered psychiatric help, and that a long delay in receiving treatment can lead to a poor outcome.[72] This discovery suggests that the early detection of psychosis might substantially benefit patients.

A team of investigators in Melbourne, Australia, which includes Patrick McGorry, Henry Jackson and Alison Yung among others, deserves particular credit for pushing this idea to its logical conclusion. In one of their studies, they reported that they could use a combination of methods to identify an ultra high-risk group who were very likely to become ill in the near future.[73] An amazing 40 per cent of their sample, who either had experienced subclinical or transient psychotic complaints, or who were suffering from non-psychotic distress and had a first-degree relative with psychosis, became floridly ill within six months of being identified. Clearly, at this rate of transition to psychosis, *preventative intervention* becomes a real possibility.

Several prevention studies are ongoing at the time of writing. The first, carried out by the Melbourne team, has already found evidence that a combination of psychotherapy and low-dose drug treatment for people at very high risk can at least delay madness in some people.[74] In another trial, currently being conducted in the United States, a similar high-risk group is being offered olanzapine, one of the new atypical neuroleptics.[75] However, giving drug treatments to people who have not yet become ill raises some very real ethical problems.[76] From the experience of the Melbourne investigators, it seems that this strategy will expose a large number of people who would never make the transition to psychosis to a risk of very severe side effects. It is for this reason that Tony Morrison, Shôn Lewis and I are now conducting a small trial of CBT without medication for a high-risk group of people identified using the methods developed in Melbourne.[77]

Even the use of purely psychological interventions in this way is not without danger. There is a risk of stigmatizing people by entrapping them into psychiatric services that they might otherwise have managed to avoid (for this reason, in our ongoing trial, we offer treatment separately from already established psychiatric clinics). There is also the risk of inflicting unwanted treatment on people who are quite happily living with psychosis, or the prospect of becoming psychotic (which is why we ask our patients to decide which difficulties should be prioritized in therapy, and focus on problems other than psychosis if they so wish).

Liberation or Cure?

In Chapters 6 and 7 of this book I argued that diagnostic judgements in psychiatry always involve implicit reference to broader human values.[78] It is therefore important to recognize that psychotic people may value their experiences differently from people such as friends, family or mental health professionals, who are observing the experiences at second hand. They may also appraise the effects of treatment differently. For some the hazards of psychiatric care may far outweigh any disadvantages conferred by madness itself, whereas, for others, the opposite may be the case. Whether for or against treatment, there is no obvious reason why patients' own opinions should not be respected, especially if (as is usually the case)[79] they present no danger to other people. Ironically, I have found myself supporting the wishes of psychotic patients who want to receive neuroleptic drugs (on one memorable occasion attracting considerable hostility from many of the delegates at a conference of psychotherapists) almost as often as I have found myself defending their right to refuse them.

Some years ago, Marius Romme invited me to give a talk at a conference at Maastricht, in Holland. Romme, it will be recalled, is the psychiatrist who discovered that large numbers of Dutch citizens (and presumably citizens of other countries also) hear voices without needing psychiatric treatment. His conference had been planned as an opportunity for sympathetic professionals like myself to exchange ideas with members of Resonance, his organization for voice-hearers. As we walked through the pristine white corridors of the brand-new conference centre one morning, Romme and I discussed our different approaches and, in the middle of this conversation, he said something that I will never forget:

'I really like your research on hallucinations, Richard. But the trouble is, you want to *cure* hallucinators, whereas I want to *liberate* them. I think they are like homosexuals in the 1950s – in need of liberation, not cure.'

It took me a little time to recognize the power of this simple idea. If people can sometimes live healthy, productive lives while experiencing some degree of psychosis (and the evidence we considered in Chapter 5 suggests that they can), if the boundaries between madness and normality are open to negotiation (and the cross-cultural evidence we considered in Chapter 6 suggests that they are), and if (as we have seen in this chapter) our psychiatric services are imperfect and sometimes damaging to patients, why not help some psychotic people just to *accept* that they are different from the rest of us? *Fear of madness* may be a much bigger problem than madness itself.

Of course, this suggestion does not imply that people in distress should not be offered the most effective treatment that is available (drug or psychotherapeutic). It also does not imply that steps should not be taken to protect society from the very small number of patients who behave dangerously towards others. However, it acknowledges that, for many people experiencing psychosis, treatment may not be the most helpful way forward in their lives.

Putting this idea into practice would require a fairly major shift in society's attitude towards eccentricity and madness. It would involve giving mad people some control over our asylums. It would probably win no support from drug companies or politicians. But it would almost certainly make the world a better place for mad and ordinary people alike.

Appendix: A Glossary of Technical and Scientific Terms

Unless otherwise stated, the following definitions are my own.

Adoption study A type of study designed to tease out genetic and environmental influences, by examining what happens to children who are reared by adoptive parents to whom they are not biologically related. One method involves examining adopted-away children of parents who have a disease, and comparing them with adopted-away children whose biological parents do not have the disease. The alternative approach involves identifying adoptees who have a disease, and comparing their biological parents with the biological parents of adoptees who do not have the disease.

Affective blunting See Flat affect

Affective reactivity The extent to which symptoms are reactive to emotional stimulation. Affectively reactive symptoms, for example some types of communication disorders, become more severe when the individual is reminded of unpleasant events.

Affective style The style of interaction between relatives or significant others and psychiatric patients, as observed in actual interactions. Relatives with a negative affective style make many critical and intrusive comments to patients, and also tend to score highly on measures of expressed emotion.

Akathisia An extrapyramidal side effect of neuroleptic medication. The patient experiences a very unpleasant subjective feeling of restlessness, often accompanied by profound feelings of depression. There is some evidence that akathisia may be associated with suicide attempts in patients receiving neuroleptics.

Alleles Different variations of the same gene. Thus, strictly speaking, all human beings have the same genes and genetic variation is a consequence of our having different alleles of those genes.

Ambivalent attachment A type of insecure attachment. In young children, it is manifest in distress on separation from the caregiver, and an inability to be comforted on the caregiver's return. In adulthood, ambivalent attachment is associated with emotional over-responsiveness towards potential partners, often leading to clingy behaviours or even jealousy, often culminating in rejection.

Anhedonia An inability to experience pleasure. It is sometimes subdivided into physical anhedonia (the inability to experience physical pleasures) and social anhedonia (the inability to experience social pleasures). Although anhedonia has been recognized as a negative symptom of schizophrenia, it is found in a wide range of other conditions, especially depression.

Anti-cholinergic drugs Drugs that affect neural pathways that utilize the neurotransmitter acetylcholine; used to control the extrapyramidal side effects of antipsychotic (neuroleptic) drugs.

Attachment relationships The kind of close emotional bond formed with a parent figure early in life, which serves as a model for emotional relationships in adulthood.

Attention The psychological processes involved in responding only to important environmental stimuli. Often a distinction is made between selective attention (the filtering out of irrelevant stimuli) measured by tests such as the digit span with distraction task, and sustained attention (or vigilance, involving maintaining a focus on one task over a period of time) measured by tests such as the continuous performance test.

Attribution A causal statement; a statement that either includes or implies the word 'because'. It has been estimated that, on average, ordinary speech contains an attribution in every few hundred words. The types of attributions that people make are thought to have an important impact on mental health, and play a role in depression, mania and paranoia.

Attributional (explanatory) style An individual's characteristic style of making attributions. Attributional style is often assumed to be a stable personality trait, and is thought to play a role in a variety of symptoms, especially dysphoria, paranoia and mania.

Atypical neuroleptics A new class of antipsychotic drugs, which are said to have a kinder side-effect profile, and possibly to be more effective, than traditional neuroleptic medication. The evidence for these claims is equivocal, but these drugs are certainly much more expensive than the typical drugs.

Autonomy A type of self-schema, by which the individual evaluates his or her worth according to freedom of choice and the achievement of goals.

Avoidant attachment A type of insecure attachment. Avoidantly attached children are unmoved by the departure of a caregiver, and ignore the caregiver on her return. In adulthood, the avoidantly attached person avoids emotional closeness with others. This type of attachment style is associated with the positive symptoms of psychosis, especially paranoid delusions.

Backward masking Visual information processed by the brain is first held in a brief store, sometimes known as 'the iconic memory'. The immediate presentation of an unpatterned stimulus after an initial stimulus can displace information about the initial stimulus held in the store, preventing it from being passed on to other parts of the cognitive system for further processing. In these circumstances the individual does not have a conscious experience of the initial stimulus. This phenomenon is known as backward masking, and has been exploited to investigate information processing in psychotic patients.

Basic emotions (theory of) The idea that there are a small number of distinct emotions.

Behavioural activation system (BAS) A hypothesized neural system thought to be responsible for determining response to reinforcement (reward). According to some theorists, the BAS is overactive in bipolar disorder.

Behaviourism A much misunderstood approach to psychology pioneered by the American psychologist John Watson, who argued that psychology should be the scientific study of observable behaviour. According to Watson (*Behaviorism*, New York: W. W. Norton, 1924), 'Let us limit ourselves to things that can be observed, and formulate laws concerning only those things. Now what can we observe? We can observe *behavior – what the organism does or says*. And let us point out at once: that *saying* is doing – that is, *behaving*. Speaking overtly or to ourselves (thinking) is just as objective a type of behavior as baseball.'

Bias See Cognitive bias

Bipolar disorder Modern term for manic depression; a psychiatric illness in which the individual experiences episodes of depression and also of either mania or hypomania.

Blood-oxygen-level-dependent (BOLD) response Areas of the brain that become active when we attempt some kind of task demand increased oxygen. Several seconds after we start to perform the task, there is therefore a surge of oxygenated haemoglobin (oxygen enriched blood) to those areas. This can be detected by the latest fMRI scanning techniques, which thereby reveal which parts of the brain are most active at any point in time. This technique can therefore be used to determine which areas of the brain are most involved in different types of tasks.

Capgras syndrome A delusional system in which the individual believes that someone (usually a loved one) has been replaced by an imposter or *doppelgänger*.

Cerebral lateralization The tendency for the left and right hemispheres of the brain to take on different functions. In most people, the left side of the brain is much more involved in generating and understanding language than the right, although some people are exceptions to this rule.

Cerebral ventricles Fluid-filled cavities inside the brain; it is thought that these are enlarged in some psychiatric conditions.

Circadian dysrhythmia Desynchronization of the circadian rhythm with the natural 24-hour light–dark cycle, brought about by a severe disruption of routine, which may play an important role in mood symptoms.

Circadian rhythm The daily rhythm of bodily changes accompanying waking, sleeping and regular changes in activity.

Circumplex model of emotions See Emotional circumplex

Clinical psychologist A psychologist who has specialized in using psychological methods to assess and treat clinical problems. Training begins with the basic degree in psychology, followed by a postgraduate programme lasting at least three years which includes a large amount of supervised clinical work. In North America this has always led to the degree of Ph.D. (doctor of philosophy) or D.Psy. (doctor of psychology). Until recently, trainee clinical psychologists in Britain graduated with a masters degree, but in the early 1990s all universities offering training in clinical psychology upgraded the basic qualification to a doctorate (usually D.Psy. or D.Clin.Psy.) on the American model.

After qualifying, clinical psychologists can learn to specialize in a number of areas, including child clinical psychology, adult mental health, learning disabilities, clinical neuropsychology and forensic clinical psychology. Clinical psychologists in Britain cannot prescribe psychiatric drugs. However, a small number in the United States have been trained to do so, and the question of whether this should become a routine part of the psychologist's role is being extensively debated in that country.

Not surprisingly, the American Psychiatric Association is not keen on the idea.

Cognitive behaviour therapy A type of individual psychological therapy that is problem-focused and usually time-limited. The patient and the therapist work together collaboratively to define goals, to identify dysfunctional thinking processes that may prevent the patient from achieving those goals, and to find better ways of coping with life stresses.

Cognitive bias A bias towards preferentially processing (attending to, remembering or thinking about) some kinds of information as opposed to others. For example, depressed patients tend to recall more easily negative than positive information. Because patients with abnormal cognitive biases can process some kinds of information perfectly well (for example, negative information in the case of depressed patients) biases must be distinguished from more general cognitive deficits.

Cognitive deficit A gross, content-independent deficiency of a fundamental cognitive process, such as attention or memory. Often attributed to brain damage, cognitive deficits may also reflect general motivational deficits.

Cohesive ties Parts of speech that serve the function of informing the listener that different segments of speech are meaningfully related. There is evidence that these are to some degree absent in thought-disordered speech.

Cohort study A study in which an entire (unselected) cohort of the population (for example, all children born in a particular week) is followed up, often over decades.

Communication deviance An unusual style of parental communication involving abnormal ways of handling attention and meaning, unusual ways of talking about relationships, and abnormal emotional responses.

Comorbidity The occurrence of more than one illness in the same person. Neo-Kraepelinian researchers have often assumed that comorbidity reflects the fact that individuals, through some misfortune, really do suffer from more than one illness. Of course, apparent comorbidity often reflects the fact that two illnesses are not really separate and independent entities.

Computer tomography (CT; sometimes known as computed axial tomography or CAT) A type of structural imaging, in which information from X-rays taken at different angles is integrated to produce a picture of a cross-sectional slice of the body.

Concordance Agreement. In twin studies, this term is used to indicate the proportion of twins in which, if one is affected by a disease (say schizophrenia), the other is also affected. Confusingly, there are several different methods of calculating concordance rates, some of which give higher values than others (and hence are favoured by geneticists). See Chapter 4 for an explanation.

Continuous performance test (CPT) A type of psychological test used to measure vigilance; participants sit at a computer screen and watch stimuli being flashed up before them, perhaps at a rate of one every second, and are required to press a key when seeing a particular target.

Coping skills enhancement A type of cognitive behaviour therapy for psychosis which has the primary aim of improving a patient's coping skills.

Cotard syndrome A delusional syndrome in which extremely nihilistic delusions (for example, 'I am dead') predominate.

Culture-bound syndromes Psychiatric conditions which appear to be specific to one culture. Examples include *koro* (an illness suffered by Chinese people, usually males, who believe that their sexual organs are shrinking), *latah* (experienced by Indonesians, who develop an exaggerated startle response, which includes shouting rude words and mimicking the behaviour of those nearby) and witiko psychosis (a rare disorder in which Algonquian-speaking Indians of Canada believe themselves to be possessed by vampires). It has been argued that anorexia nervosa and chronic fatigue syndromes are Western culture-bound syndromes.

Deficit See Cognitive deficit

Delusion A bizarre or irrational belief. It has been difficult to find a definition of delusions that clearly distinguishes them from normal beliefs and attitudes. According to Karl Jaspers, delusions are held with extraordinary conviction, are not amenable to counter-argument, and have a bizarre or impossible content. However, Jaspers held that true delusions were also ununderstandable, in the sense that they cannot be understood as arising meaningfully from the individual's personality and experiences.

Delusional disorder The term introduced in DSM-III-R to replace 'paranoia', and which indicates a psychotic illness in which delusions are present but other psychotic symptoms are absent.

Dementia praecox Literally, senility of the young. The term was used by Kraepelin to describe psychiatric disorders characterized by progressive intellectual deterioration. Later replaced by the term 'schizophrenia'.

Dismissing or avoidant attachment style See Avoidant attachment style.

Distracting response (coping) style A response to dysphoric mood, in which the individual seeks out activities that distract attention from the mood. It has been shown that this kind of response reduces the duration and severity of dysphoria.

Dizygotic (DZ) twins Non-identical (fraternal) twins. DZ twins develop when two separate eggs are fertilized by two separate sperm and grow into two foetuses. In effect, they are sibs born at the same time. They have approximately 50 per cent of their DNA in common and may be either the same sex or of opposite sexes. A gene for psychiatric disorder inherited by one DZ twin need not necessarily be inherited by the other.

Dopamine One of the neurotransmitters found in the brain. Some theories of schizophrenia and manic depression propose that neural pathways that utilize dopamine are abnormal in these conditions.

Downward social drift The tendency for people with severe mental illness to live in poor social circumstances, usually because they are unable to work.

Dualism The belief that mental processes and brain processes are separate and consist of different substances: a non-material mind in the case of the former, and physical matter in the case of the latter. Although few scientists and philosophers claim to support this doctrine today, it has been surprisingly difficult to shake it from our heads. Many psychiatric theories are implicitly dualist.

Dysphoria Negative mood state

Electrodermal response A brief change in the electrical conductivity of the skin that occurs during exposure to a stressful event. Caused by sweating, the response can be easily measured using electrodes placed on the back of the hand.

Electroencephalography The technique of measuring changes in electrical potential ('brain waves') generated by neuronal activity from electrodes placed on the scalp.

Electromyography The technique of measuring changes in electrical potential in muscles as they become more or less active. This technique can be used to measure the subvocalization that accompanies inner speech.

Emotional circumplex A model of subjective emotional states, which proposes that these can all be accounted for by two dimensions of emotion. According to one version of this theory, the two fundamental dimensions of subjective emotion are pleasantness versus unpleasantness and the degree to which the individual is physiologically aroused. According to another, the two fundamental dimensions are positive affect and negative affect (this model has the implication that individuals can experience both positive and negative emotion at the same time).

Expressed emotion A term describing the emotional attitude of relatives or significant others towards patients suffering from mental illness. High expressed emotion is reflected in a high rate of critical comments, hostility, and/or emotional involvement (as indicated by extreme emotional responses and over-protective behaviour towards the patient). High expressed emotion relatives or significant others tend to score highly on measures of negative affective style. Low expressed emotion relatives or significant others, in contrast, might be described as very laid back.

Expressivity The extent to which genetic traits vary in the degree to which they are expressed by those carrying the relevant genes.

Extrapyramidal side effects The most obvious side effects of conventional neuroleptic medication, including Parkinsonian symptoms such as stiffness and tremor, dystonias (uncontrollable muscle spasms), akathisia and tardive dyskinesia.

Factor analysis A method of analysing correlations between many different measures, often used to assess which symptoms cluster together. Factor analysis reduces the matrix of correlations between the measures to a small number of factors or dimensions. Symptoms appearing together in the same factor often (although not invariably) 'go together'. The number of factors corresponds to the number of different clusters of symptoms that occur in the patients studied.

There are many different methods of factor analysis, and the choice between them is often arbitrary. Therefore, although the technique looks highly objective, some degree of subjectivity sneaks in when researchers decide which method to use.

Family therapy A type of psychological treatment that involves the entire family. In the case of patients suffering from psychosis, this approach is used to reduce stress in the family, which is known to make the course of psychosis worse. Family members are educated about psychosis so that they do not criticize the member who is experiencing symptoms. The family is also taught ways of managing family conflicts. This approach does not imply that families are responsible for mental illness experienced by their members. Effective treatment usually takes at least nine months.

Flat affect An apparent absence of emotion; one of the negative symptoms of psychosis. In fact, the subjective emotional life of patients with flat affect appears to be normal, and the problem seems to be a difficulty in expressing emotion.

Functional imaging/scanning Any scanning method that is used to detect changing physiological functioning.

Functional magnetic resonance imaging (fMRI) A form of MRI scan that uses the BOLD response to measure the flow of oxygenated blood to different regions of the brain, thereby allowing the areas that are most active at any particular time to be identified.

Genome The entire genetic code contained in the strands of DNA in the twenty-three human chromosomes. Most cells in the human body have two sets, one derived from the mother and the other from the father, forming twenty-three pairs of chromosomes.

Hallucination Usually defined as a perception in the absence of an appropriate stimulus. The most common example is hearing a voice when no one is present to account for it.

Heritability The proportion of variance in a trait that can be attributed to genes. Usually expressed as a percentage, so that a heritability of 100 per cent implies that the trait is completely genetic. Psychiatric geneticists often assume that high heritability values for psychiatric disorders leave little room for environmental influences. However, this assumption is incorrect (see Chapter 17 for an explanation).

High-risk study A type of study in which individuals thought to be at special risk of developing a disorder are followed up over a period of time to see if they actually become ill, and to identify factors that predict the development of illness. The most common variant of this type of research starts with young people known to be at genetic risk because they have a first-degree relative who is suffering from the disorder. However, high-risk groups can also be identified using psychological or behavioural indicators, for example by selecting individuals who score highly on questionnaire measures of schizotypal personality traits.

Homovanillic acid A metabolite of dopamine that can be measured in the cerebrospinal fluid.

Hypofrontality Reduced activation of the frontal lobes of the brain in response to demanding tasks. Normally, when we try to solve certain types of problems, the frontal lobes become engaged and demand more oxygenated blood. In hypofrontal individuals this effect is less marked. Some biological psychiatrists have argued that hypofrontality is a feature of schizophrenia.

Hypomania A subclinical form of manic symptomatology, defined in DSM-IV as a distinct period of 'abnormally and persistently elevated, irritable or expansive mood' accompanied by at least three additional symptoms such as inflated self-esteem, non-delusional grandiosity, decreased need for sleep, flight of ideas, distractibility or 'excessive involvement in pleasurable activities that have a high potential for painful consequences'.

Hypomanic personality A personality type, in which hypomanic traits are a persistent feature.

Incidence The number of new cases of a disorder appearing within a particular population in a particular period.

Inner or private speech Speech that is addressed to the self, which occurs internally and which cannot be heard by other people. In other words, verbal thought. It is believed that children first learn to talk to themselves out loud, before internalizing this process. As the reader will be aware, most adults still talk to themselves out loud under some circumstances (a phenomenon which, by convention, is known as private speech), especially when stressed or alone.

Insight According to British psychiatrist Aubrey Lewis, 'The correct attitude to morbid change in oneself, and moreover, the realization that the illness is mental' ('The psychopathology of insight', *British Journal of Medical Psychology*, 14: 332–48, 1934). Psychotic patients who do not believe that they have an illness requiring treatment are therefore said to lack insight. Conversely, patients are said to have insight when they agree with their doctor.

Internality–externality An important dimension along which attributions can be categorized. Internal attributions locate the cause of an event with the individual (for example, 'I failed the exam because I'm not very bright') whereas external attributions locate the cause of the event with other people ('The examiner had it in for me') or with circumstances ('I was unable to revise because I had to go to my sister's wedding').

Linkage analysis A method for attempting to identify particular sites on particular chromosomes where genes responsible for a trait or illness reside.

Magnetic resonance imaging (MRI) A technique for constructing detailed images of the body, by placing the body in a very strong magnetic field in order to trick it to emit radio waves when the field is turned off. This approach can be used to generate spectacularly beautiful pictures of the structure of soft tissues, for example the brain.

Mania A state of very intense emotional, cognitive and behavioural disturbance, in which the individual may feel highly energetic, may act impulsively, and may be both euphoric and irritable. Although sometimes regarded as the opposite of depression, dysphoric (depressive) symptoms commonly occur during manic episodes. Mania is often accompanied by psychotic symptoms such as grandiose delusions and thought disorder.

Manic depression A term used by Kraepe-lin to describe any disorder in which abnormal mood is the main symptom. However, in recent years the term has been used to describe an illness in which the patient suffers from recurrent episodes of depression and mania. Now often (and misleadingly) called 'bipolar disorder' to distinguish it from 'unipolar depression' in which only episodes of depression occur.

Mentalizing Understanding the mental states (beliefs, desires and intentions) of other people.

Metacognition Cognition about cognition; in other words, one's beliefs about one's own mental processes.

Monozygotic (MZ) twins Identical twins formed when a fertilized egg splits in the uterus and grows into two separate foetuses. MZ twins have identical DNA and are always the same sex. Therefore, any genes for mental illness inherited by one MZ twin must be inherited by the other.

Negative symptoms Symptoms characterized by the absence of desirable behaviours or experiences; for example social withdrawal, flat affect, anhedonia and apathy (avolition).

Neuroleptic induced deficit syndrome (NIDS) Lack of motivation necessary to achieve even modest goals, an undesirable consequence of long-term neuroleptic treatment.

Neuroleptic malignant syndrome A side effect of neuroleptic medication, characterized by muscular rigidity, fever and fluctuating consciousness, which is often mistaken for a bacterial infection, and which is fatal if drugs are not promptly discontinued.

Neuroleptic (antipsychotic) medication The class of drugs, first identified in the late 1940s and early 1950s, which are known to have an ameliorative effect on positive symptoms, and to reduce the risk of psychotic relapse. They have numerous side effects.

Neuropsychological tests Psychological tests devised to detect different types of brain damage. Test designers administer a large number of tests to patients with different kinds of brain damage and select items on which patients suffering from the type of brain damage of interest perform poorly. In the case of certain types of diffuse damage, neuropsychological tests may be more sensitive than brain scans.

Normalizing strategy A strategy employed by therapists practising cognitive behaviour therapy with psychotic clients. Efforts are made to demystify psychosis and make it seem more 'normal'. Patients may be educated about the prevalence of psychotic complaints in the population, and about similarities between psychotic experiences and normal mental states.

Operational definition A definition that specifies the method or rule used to measure a concept. For example, an operational definition of length would be something like 'the number obtained when a ruler is laid alongside an object'. Operationalism was proposed as a philosophy of science by the physicist Percy Bridgeman in the 1930s. It was later embraced by some psychologists, especially behaviourists such as B. F. Skinner, as a way of making psychology more objective. It was the philosopher Carl Hempel who first suggested that some of the diagnostic arguments in psychiatry could be resolved by agreeing on operational definitions of different disorders. DSM-III (and subsequent revisions of the manual) took this route by attempting to specify precisely which symptoms are required for a diagnosis to be made.

Paranoia and paranoid These terms have a confusing history. First used by the Ancient Greeks to mean crazy or mad,

they were reintroduced in the nineteenth century to describe a type of delusional disorder, a usage embraced by Kraepelin. During the era after the Second World War, when psychiatric diagnoses briefly became unfashionable among US psychiatrists, the term 'paranoid' was often used to describe persecutory beliefs that were not necessarily delusional; hence the ordinary-language definition given in the *Shorter Oxford English Dictionary*, 'A tendency to suspect or distrust others or to believe oneself unfairly used'. DSM-III used the term *paranoia* to refer to a pure delusional psychosis (Kraepelin's concept) but the term *delusional disorder* was used in its place in DSM-III-R and DSM-IV. However, *paranoid personality disorder* remains in DSM-IV as an axis-2 disorder, and is defined in a way that closely matches the ordinary-language definition given in the *OED*. In this book, the term 'paranoid delusion' is used to describe any delusional system in which themes of persecution are prominent.

Penetrance The extent to which people in possession of a particular allele or set of alleles are likely to have particular characteristics determined by those alleles. If penetrance is low, only a fraction of those carrying the crucial alleles will show the relevant traits. Not to be confused with expressivity.

Personality disorder Defined in the DSM system as 'enduring patterns of perceiving, relating to, and thinking about the environment and oneself'. They are considered to be distinct from illnesses because they are present throughout adulthood, whereas the illnesses are episodic. In the DSM system, they are listed on a separate axis (axis 2) from psychiatric illnesses (axis 1).

Positive symptoms Symptoms that consist of experiences and behaviours that would preferably be absent, such as hallucinations and delusions.

Positron emission tomography (PET) A technique used to image activity in the brain, in which radio-labelled substances are injected into the body. On reaching the brain, the substances release positrons which almost immediately decay, releasing photons that travel in opposite directions and which are then detected by a scanner.

Post-traumatic stress disorder A cluster of symptoms often experienced by survivors of life-threatening events. These include constant re-experiencing of the traumatic event (in the form of intrusive memories, flashbacks or dreams), avoidance of stimuli associated with the event, and persistent emotional over-arousal (for example, as indicated by irritability).

Prefrontal leucotomy A crude brain operation devised by the Portuguese neurosurgeon Egas Moniz and inflicted on many psychotic patients, especially in the 1950s. It involves severing neural pathways from the frontal regions of the brain to the anterior regions. Often performed quickly under local anaesthetic, by inserting a knife in a hole drilled towards rear of the forehead, with little care about the precise location of the lesions created. A version developed by Walter Freeman involved displacing the eyeball downwards and thrusting an ice-pick-like instrument through the bone of the orbit behind the eyes. There is no evidence that this operation affects symptoms, but it may leave patients more passive and easier to manage.

Prevalence The proportion of a population suffering from a condition at a particular point in time. Not to be confused with incidence (the number of new cases in a particular period).

Prodromal symptoms Symptoms that precede the appearance of full-blown psychosis. Typically, these include disturbances of mood, but may also include subtle cognitive (thinking) and perceptual abnormalities.

Psychiatrist A medical doctor who specializes in the treatment of psychiatric problems. After receiving the basic medical qualification, the doctor receives a further four or more years of training which mostly consists of supervised clinical work. Psychiatrists often use psychiatric drugs as their main line of treatment, but many also acquire training in psychological techniques. Because psychiatrists have important legal responsibilities (they can have patients compulsorily admitted to hospital), because they are the only profession currently allowed to prescribe psychiatric drugs, and because doctors have a long history of telling other health professionals what to do, they are usually the leaders of multidisciplinary psychiatric teams.

Psychoanalysis This has two meanings: the theory about the mind and the origins of mental illness developed by Sigmund Freud, and the particular type of psychotherapy that he invented. Psychoanalysis as a theory has often been criticized as woolly and untestable by modern scientific psychologists, but there is no doubt that Freud was an astute observer whose sometimes bizarre ideas are peppered with acute insights into human nature. Psychoanalysis as a treatment is long (often several years), intensive (often several times a week), extremely expensive, and has never been shown to be of benefit to psychotic patients. However, it remains fashionable and is even regarded as a gold-standard therapy in some intellectual quarters. More recent brief psychodynamic therapies, which draw on Freud's ideas to some extent, have been shown to be effective for some non-psychotic conditions.

Psychoanalyst 'Analyst' for short. One who practises psychoanalysis. Although Freud was a doctor, he came to believe that medicine was a bad initial training for those wishing to be psychoanalysts. However, this did not stop the American Psychoanalytic Association from restricting training to doctors until they were successfully sued by a group of disgruntled psychologists in 1965. Now psychoanalytic associations in most countries will take on trainees from a wide range of backgrounds. The training includes a personal analysis, in which the trainee is analysed by a qualified analyst. The length of training is usually long and indeterminate and is completed when the supervisor and his/her colleagues think the trainee is ready. Why anyone would wish to undertake an expensive training in this old-fashioned and ineffective treatment is another matter.

Psychopharmacology The scientific study of the effects of drugs (including psychiatric drugs) on the brain, behaviour and experience.

Psychosis A term which has undergone dramatic changes of meaning since the end of the nineteenth century, when it was used to describe mild psychiatric problems with presumed psychological causes. It now refers to the most *severe* psychiatric disorders, in which the individual to some extent can be said to be out of touch with reality, which many psychiatrists and psychologists have presumed to be biological diseases. In practice, this means disorders in which the individual suffers from delusions and/or hallucinations.

Puerperal psychosis A psychotic reaction experienced by a mother soon after (usually within three months of) the birth of her child.

Reinforcement and reinforcers Technically, stimuli that, when consequent on a behaviour, increase the likelihood that the behaviour will occur again in the future. In lay terms, a reward (although it is important to recognize that some things which we think are rewarding may not actually be powerful reinforcers). Primary reinforcers reflect basic biological needs and include food, contact with an attachment figure (caregiver) and sex. Secondary reinforcers acquire their power by virtue of our learning history, and include social reinforcement (praise for our achievements) and, of course, money.

Reliability The first test that must be passed by a diagnostic concept if we are to say that it is scientifically valid. Reliability refers to the consistency with which diagnoses are made, either by different clinicians or on different occasions. Reliability can be measured by having independent clinicians attempt to diagnose the same patients and then measuring their level of agreement with the kappa statistic, which varies between 0 (agreement at chance level) and 1 (perfect agreement). It can also be measured by making diagnoses at one point in time and then repeating the procedure at a later date, again using the kappa statistic to assess agreement between the two time points. (Obviously this kind of *test–retest reliability* is only meaningful in the case of measurements which we expect to remain fairly stable across time.)

Although a diagnosis must be reliable to be scientifically valid, reliability is no guarantee of validity. For this purpose, additional validity tests must be passed.

Ruminative response (coping) style A response to dysphoric mood, in which the individual focuses excessively on the mood and its causes, asking questions such as, 'How did I get in this mess?'

and 'Will I ever feel better?' This response seems to prolong dysphoric episodes.

Self Cognitive representation of who you are; roughly what is meant when saying 'I'. It has been argued that the self consists of many domains (for example, the self as it actually is, the ideal self, the self as it ought to be, the self that might be possible in the future) and also different perspectives on the self (for example, my beliefs about what sort of person my mother thinks I am, and so on).

Self-discrepancy Discrepancy between one domain or perspective on the self and another. So, for example, an actual–ideal discrepancy is a discrepancy between beliefs about the self as it actually is, and the ideal self.

Self-esteem Global evaluation of the self. Typically regarded as a unidimensional scale running from self-loathing to self-satisfaction. However, this is an over-simplification, and there may be several different types of self-esteem. For example positive self-esteem (positive beliefs about the self) may be relatively independent of negative self-esteem (negative beliefs about the self).

Self-guides Self-representations that have motivational properties, for example the ideal self and the ought self, which are two different kinds of standards for self-evaluation.

Self-schema Core assumptions or beliefs about the self, often barely articulated, including enduring standards of self-evaluation.

Self-serving bias The tendency to attribute positive events or experiences to one's own actions and characteristics and negative events to causes external to the self. This bias is found in ordinary people, is exaggerated in paranoid patients and is absent or even reversed in depressed people.

Signal detection theory (SDT) As much an experimental method as a theory. SDT presumes that an individual's decision that he or she has detected a stimulus – or signal – is a function of two separate factors: the sensitivity of the individual's perceptual system (the more sensitive, the more likely that the signal will be accurately detected, or that the individual will correctly realize that it is not present) and perceptual bias, which can be roughly understood as the individual's willingness to guess that a signal is present under conditions of uncertainty (the greater the bias, the more likely that the individual will correctly detect stimuli, but this gain is made at the risk of falsely detecting signals which are in fact absent).

SDT experimental methodology allows these two factors to be measured separately. This has been useful in the study of hallucinations.

Social brain hypothesis The hypothesis that the brain has evolved specific mechanisms for dealing with the demands of complex social relationships.

Sociotropy A type of self-schema in which there is a tendency to judge one's value in terms of relationships with other people. People high in sociotropy tend to be very sensitive to rejection or relationship problems.

Source monitoring The process of determining the likely source of a cognition. One type of source monitoring involves discriminating between cognitions (thought, image or memories) and perceptions (especially things heard). It is believed that this skill may be compromised in people who hear voices. Another involves telling the difference between things one has thought, and things one has said. It is believed that people with thought, language and communication disorder have difficulty with this skill.

State-dependent memory Material which is memorized while in a particular state (physiological condition or context) is more likely to be recalled when the individual is in the same state than when the individual is in some other state. This state-dependent memory effect has been shown to be true for a variety of circumstances, for example, when material in learned under conditions of intoxication (in which case, re-intoxication may improve recall) or when the individual is scuba-diving (in which case, recall is better in the water than on dry land). These observations show that even cognitive psychologists can devise fun experiments.

Stress-vulnerability models Models of psychopathology that assume that some people are especially vulnerable to developing psychiatric symptoms by dint of possessing particular biological or psychological characteristics, but that exposure to stressful experiences is required for a full-blown psychiatric disorder to develop. It follows from these assumptions that many people who are vulnerable to psychiatric disorder may be spared as a consequence of living in a stress-free environment.

Stroop effect The tendency to experience difficulty when naming the ink colours of words that grab attention. The effect is particularly evident when colour words are printed in incongruent ink colours (for example, 'RED' printed in green, or 'BLUE' printed in pink). Under these conditions, the individual experiences competition between the urge to name the word ('Red') and saying the ink colour ('Green'), which slows down the latter response. A similar but slightly less strong effect is found for any emotionally salient words and, under these circumstances, is known as the emotional Stroop effect.

Psychologists can use the emotional Stroop effect to show that certain themes are troubling to patients. The effect is strongest (that is, colour-naming is slowest) for the most troubling words.

Structural imaging/scanning A type of neuroimaging (using, for example, CAT or MRI) that reveals the structure of the brain. Used to make anatomical comparisons between psychotic patients and ordinary people.

Subvocalization Microactivations of the speech muscles that occur during inner speech. These can be recorded by means of electromyography. Subvocalization typically occurs when we are thinking about demanding or emotionally challenging problems.

Tardive dyskinesia An extrapyramidal side effect of neuroleptic medication, now thankfully rare. The patient experiences spasmodic movements of the jaw and tongue, which are unsightly and, once established, are sometimes irreversible even after the medication has been discontinued.

Theory of mind (skills) A misleading term for the ability to understand the mental states (beliefs, desires, wishes and intentions) of other people. People who can do this are said to possess a theory of mind, in contrast to autistic children, who seem unaware that others have mental states. Theory-of-mind (perhaps better called mentalizing) skills are often tested using problems that can only be solved by understanding that others have false beliefs.

A typical example used with children concerns two individuals, Sally and Ann, who watch something (perhaps a sweet or toy) being placed in one of two boxes. Sally leaves the room and Ann moves the object to the other box before she returns. The child is asked which box Sally looks in when attempting to find the object. To answer correctly, the child must know that Sally believes the object is in the wrong box.

Psychotic patients tend to be impaired on more complex theory-of-mind tests. It has been argued that their inability to understand the mental states of others contributes both to paranoia and to speech and communication disorders. However, the evidence on this is not clear cut.

Thought disorder A misleading term for psychotic speech, which is incoherent to the listener and, in extreme cases, forms a kind of 'word salad'. The term was introduced by early psychiatrists and psychologists who assumed that incoherent speech reflected incoherent thinking. However, modern research has established that this is generally not the case.

Thought, language and communication disorder A rather unwieldy term introduced by Nancy Andreasen as an alternative to 'thought disorder'.

Unipolar depression A mood disorder in which only episodes of depression occur (i.e. mania is absent).

Validity The extent to which a set of measurements or a diagnostic system fulfils the purpose for which it is designed. Not to be confused with reliability. There is no single test of validity. For example, the validity of a diagnostic concept might be assessed by seeing whether it corresponds to a naturally occurring cluster of symptoms, by seeing whether the diagnosis runs in families or is associated with any particular type of pathology, or by seeing whether it usefully predicts what happens to the patient in the future or which types of treatment are likely to be effective.

Ventricular enlargement Enlargement of the cerebral ventricles, reported in some psychiatric conditions.

Verbal community The community of competent language-users.

Working memory A relatively brief (tens of seconds) memory store, used in everyday tasks such as comprehending speech. When we repeat telephone numbers to ourselves when walking from the telephone directory to the telephone, we are continually refreshing the working memory store.

Zeitgeber A clock-setting stimulus. Any regular event (for example, dawn) or activity (for example, eating breakfast) that has the effect of resetting the circadian clock, and thereby keeping circadian rhythms in step with the natural 24-hour light–dark cycle.

Notes

Chapter 1   Emil Kraepelin's Big Idea

1. L. Wittgenstein (1980) *Culture and Value* (trans. P. Winch). Oxford: Blackwell.
2. A few years before I arrived at Denbigh, a series of articles in the *Guardian* newspaper (reprinted in T. S. Szasz (ed.) (1975) *The Age of Madness*. London: Routledge & Kegan Paul) had revealed that many elderly female psychiatric patients in Britain had been incarcerated in their youth after giving birth to illegitimate children, a form of behaviour deemed to be evidence of psychiatric disorder in the 1920s and 1930s. Although there was speculation that this might be true of some of the elderly women in Denbigh, no evidence was uncovered to suggest that any of the patients on the ward fell into this category.
3. The experiment, together with some further work, actually appeared in a paper that I wrote up, partly out of bloody-mindedness, many years later. The full reference is: R. P. Bentall, P. Higson and C. F. Lowe (1987) 'Teaching self-instructions to chronic schizophrenic patients: efficacy and generalisation', *Behavioural Psychotherapy*, 15: 58–76.
4. See Richard Warner (1988) *Recovery from Schizophrenia: Psychiatry and Political Economy*. New York: Routledge & Kegan Paul.
5. Quoted in E. J. Engstrom (1991) 'Emil Kraepelin: psychiatry and public affairs in Wilhelmine Germany', *History of Psychiatry*, 2: 111–32. The mission referred to in the poem was apparently Kraepelin's fight against the evils of alcoholism.
6. E. Shorter (1997) *A History of Psychiatry*. New York: Wiley.
7. The English-language literature on the life of Emil Kraepelin is relatively limited. I have used the following as the basis for my own account: E. Kraepelin (1987) *Memoirs* (trans. H. Hippius, G. Peters and D. Ploog). New York: Springer-Verlag; Franz G. Alexander and Sheldon T. Selesnick (1966) *The History of Psychiatry: An Evaluation of Psychiatric Thought from Prehistoric Times to the Present*. New York: Harper & Row; Edward Shorter (1992) *From Paralysis to Fatigue: a History of Psychosomatic Illness in the Modern Era*. New York: Free Press; and also *A History of Psychiatry*. op. cit.

In addition, the following sources have provided useful information about specific aspects of Kraepelin's work: G. E. Berrios and R. Hauser (1988) 'The early development of Kraepelin's ideas on classification: a conceptual history', *Psychological Medicine*, 18: 813–21 (on Kraepelin's scientific ideas); G. E. Berrios and R. Hauser (1995) 'Kraepelin', in G. E. Berrios and R. Porter (eds.), *A History of Clinical Psychiatry*. London: Athlone Press (on Kraepelin's scientific ideas); E. J. Engstrom (1991) 'Emil Kraepelin: psychiatry and public affairs in Wilhelmine Germany', *History of Psychiatry*, 2: 111–32 (on Kraepelin's attitudes towards alcohol, syphilis and nationalism); E. J. Engstrom (1995) 'Kraepelin', in Berrios and Porter (eds.), *A History*, op. cit. (on Kraepelin's battles with bureaucracy while at Heidelberg); P. Hoff (1995) 'Kraepelin', in Berrios and Porter (eds.), *A History*, op. cit. (on Kraepelin's scientific ideas); S. E. Jelliffe (1932) 'Emil Kraepelin, the man and his work', *Archives of Neurology and Psychiatry*, 27: 761–75 (an admiring account of Kraepelin's character and achievements); M. Shepherd (1995) 'Two faces of Emil Kraepelin', *British Journal of Psychiatry*, 167: 174–83 (on Kraepelin's nationalism).

8. My account of Kraepelin's fall-out with Flechsig is based on Kraepelin's memoirs, and also on the account of Flechsig's life given in Z. Lothane (1992) *In Defense of Schreber: Soul Murder and Psychiatry*. Hillsdale, NJ: Analytic Press.

9. See Engstrom, 'Kraepelin', in Berrios and Porter (eds.), *A History*, op. cit.

10. See Engstrom, 'Emil Kraepelin', op. cit.

11. Jelliffe, 'Emil Kraepelin, the man and his work', op. cit.: 762.

12. Quoted in Shorter *From Paralysis to Fatigue*, op cit., p. 243.

13. F. Heynick (1993) *Language and its Disturbances in Dreams: The Pioneering Work of Freud and Kraepelin Updated*. London: Wiley.

14. See E. Kraepelin (1904/1974) 'Comparative psychiatry', reprinted in S. R. Hirsch and M. Shepherd (eds.), *Themes and Variations in European Psychiatry*. Bristol: Wright.

15. Engstrom, 'Emil Kraepelin', op. cit.

16. Kraepelin (1907) quoted in O. Reider (1974) 'The origin of our confusion about schizophrenia', *Psychiatry*, 37: 197–208. The italics are mine.

17. His thinking about this approach was influenced by Karl Ludwig Kahlbaum, a psychiatrist who owned a private hospital in the German town of Görlitz. Kahlbaum had written extensively on problems of psychiatric classification and had noted that 'snapshot' observations of patients' symptoms could be misleading because the presentation of an illness could vary over time. According to Kahlbaum: 'We do not see the forms of the various disease entities, but only the forms of their various stadia or better still the forms of various symptom complexes any one of which the illness can adopt during different periods of its course . . .' (quoted in J. Hoenig (1995) 'Schizophrenia', in Berrios and Porter (eds.), *A History*, op. cit.).

18. The eighth edition of the *Textbook*, quoted in Hoenig, 'Schizophrenia', in Berrios and Porter (eds.), *A History*, op. cit.

19. See G. E. Berrios (1995) 'Mood disorders', in Berrios and Porter (eds.), *A History*, op. cit.

20. E. Kraepelin (1921) *Manic-Depressive Insanity and Paranoia* (trans. R. M.

Barclay). Edinburgh: Livingstone. See also F. K. Goodwin and K. R. Jamison (1990) *Manic-Depressive Illness*. Oxford: Oxford University Press.

21. E. Kraepelin (1920/1992) 'Clinical manifestations of mental illness', *History of Psychiatry*, 3: 499–529. All the remaining quotations in this chapter are from this paper. In the third of these, I have substituted Kraepelin's original term 'dementia praecox' for 'schizophrenia', a new name for the disorder introduced by Eugen Bleuler, and which Kraepelin used sometimes in his later publications (see next chapter).

22. Victor Parant (1905) quoted in G. E. Berrios and R. Hauser (1995) 'Kraepelin', in Berrios and Porter (eds.), *A History*, op. cit.

Chapter 2   After Kraepelin

1. O. Wilde (1891) *Intentions*. London: J. R. Osgood, McIlvaine.

2. My account of Eugen Bleuler's life is based mainly on the following two sources: M. Bleuler and R. Bleuler (1986) 'Books reconsidered: *Dementia praecox oder die gruppe der schizophrenien* by Eugen Bleuler', *British Journal of Psychiatry*, 149: 661–4; H. F. Ellenberger (1970) *The Discovery of the Unconscious: The History and Evolution of Dynamic Psychiatry*. New York: Basic Books.

For my account of Bleuler's rift with Freud I have relied on the following sources: F. G. Alexander and S. T. Selesnick (1966) *The History of Psychiatry: An Evaluation of Psychiatric Thought from Prehistoric Times to the Present*. New York: Harper & Row; E. Jones (1962) *The Life and Work of Sigmund Freud* (abridged edn). London: Hogarth Press.

My account of Bleuler's concept of schizophrenia is mainly from his own work, *Dementia Praecox or the Group of Schizophrenias* (trans. E. Zinkin), New York: International Universities Press, from the same historical sources I have used in writing my account of Kraepelin's work, and also from J. K. Wing (1995) 'Concepts of schizophrenia', in S. R. Hirsch and D. R. Weinberger (eds.), *Schizophrenia*. Oxford: Blackwell.

3. Ellenberger, *The Discovery of the Unconscious*, op. cit.

4. Bleuler and Bleuler, 'Books reconsidered', op. cit.

5. See C. G. Jung (1907/1960) *The Psychology of Dementia Praecox*, vol. 3, in H. Read, M. Fordham, G. Adler and W. McGuire (eds.), *The Collected Works of C. G. Jung*. London: Routledge.

6. Quoted in Alexander and Selesnick, *The History of Psychiatry*, op. cit.

7. Quoted in Alexander and Selesnick, *The History of Psychiatry*, op. cit.

8. Quoted in L. J. Chapman and J. P. Chapman (1973) *Disordered Thought in Schizophrenia*. Englewood Cliffs, NJ: Prentice-Hall.

9. Bleuler, *Dementia Praecox*, op. cit., p. 236.

10. Bleuler, *Dementia Praecox*, op. cit.

11. See F. K. Goodwin and K. R. Jamison (1990) *Manic-Depressive Illness*. Oxford: Oxford University Press.

12. My account of Jaspers' life is based largely on his *Philosophical Autobiography*, in P. A. Schilpp (ed.) (1981) *The Philosophy of Karl Jaspers*. Illinois: Open Court Publishing Company.

13. Unless indicated otherwise, all the following quotations from Jaspers are from his *Philosophical Autobiography*.

14. See K. Kolle (1981) 'Karl Jaspers as Psychopathologist', in Schilpp (ed.), *The Philosophy of Karl Jaspers*, op. cit.

15. ibid.

16. In raising this distinction, Jaspers anticipated later arguments between philosophers about the relationship between everyday and scientific explanations of human behaviour. The term *folk psychology*, introduced by the Austrian-born philosopher Paul Feyerabend in 1963 ('Materialism and the mind–body problem', *Review of Metaphysics*, 17: 49–65), refers to the ordinary system of explaining human behaviour in terms of causal mental states such as beliefs, desires and intentions. (Such states are sometimes called intentional states. This convention follows the work of the German philosopher Franz Brentano (*Psychology from an Empirical Standpoint*. London: Routledge, 1874/1973), who argued that the hallmark of all mental states was the property he called 'intentionality', by which he meant the 'aboutness' that linked the mental state to the world. On this view it is impossible to have a mental state which is not about something.) According to self-styled *eliminative materialists*, for example the American philosophers Paul and Patricia Churchland (e.g. Paul M. Churchland, *Matter and Consciousness*. Cambridge, MA: MIT Press, 1984), folk psychology is a pre-scientific approach to explaining human behaviour, and must be replaced by accounts that emphasize specific brain mechanisms; after all, the Churchlands argue, examination of the brain reveals nothing corresponding to beliefs, desires and intentions. On this view, psychology must eventually give way to neuroscience. Jaspers' position, however, is closer to that of another American philosopher, Dan Dennett (*The Intentional Stance*, Cambridge, MA: MIT Press, 1987), who argues that we can choose between taking an intentional stance (in which we explain behaviour in terms of the elements of folk psychology; for example, explaining my writing of this book in terms of my desire for fame, money and career enhancement) and the design stance (in which we explain behaviour in terms of the biological machinery of the brain; for example, explaining my writing of this book in terms of the various neurobiological processes which sustain my memory of previous research, allow me to generate sentences, and control the movement of my fingers across my Macintosh keyboard). Dennett argues that both stances have distinct advantages and that, for most purposes, the intentional stance provides us with a powerful way of explaining and predicting the behaviour of our fellows (for example, from my belief that my editor at Penguin is a nice fellow I can predict that he will not be angry if this manuscript is many months overdue). Like Jaspers, Dennett notes that we tend to be thrown on to design stance explanations ('there's something wrong with the brain') when intentional stance explanations fail us (that is, when we say that the behaviour we are observing is 'mad', 'crazy', 'loco' or, in Jaspers' terminology, ununderstandable).

17. I have managed to find few English-language sources on Schneider's career. The account here is based largely on the following papers by J. Hoenig: 'Kurt Schneider and anglophone psychiatry', *Comprehensive Psychiatry*, 23: 391–400, 1982; 'The concept of schizophrenia: Kraepelin–Bleuler–Schneider', *British Journal of Psychiatry*, 142: 547–56, 1983; 'Schneider's first rank symptoms and the tabulators', *Comprehensive Psychiatry*, 25: 77–87, 1984.

18. Understandably, psychiatrists have not advertised this part of their history. However, much has been made of the association between Nazism and genetic research by critics of institutional psychiatry, for example radical psychiatrist Peter Breggin (*Toxic Psychiatry*. London: Fontana, 1993) and the scientology movement (see, for example, T. Roder, V. Kubillus and A. Burwell (1995) *Psychiatrists: The Men behind Hitler*. Los Angeles: Freedom Publications). For a less partisan but nonetheless disturbing account see J.-E. Meyer (1988) 'The fate of the mentally ill in Germany during the Third Reich', *Psychological Medicine*, 18: 575–81.

19. Quoted in Hoenig, 'Kurt Schneider', op. cit.

20. K. Schneider (1959) *Clinical Psychopathology*. New York: Grune & Stratton, p. 135.

21. R. E. Bourdillon, C. A. Clark and A. P. Ridges (1965) ' "Pink spot" in the urine of schizophrenics', *Nature*, 208: 453–5.

22. J. K. Wing, J. E. Cooper and N. Sartorius (1974) *The Measurement and Classification of Psychiatric Symptoms*. Cambridge: Cambridge University Press.

23. Quoted in Hoenig, 'Kurt Schneider', op. cit.

24. J. Kasanin (1933) 'The acute schizoaffective psychoses', *American Journal of Psychiatry*, 90: 97–126. See also F. K. Goodwin and K. R. Jamison (1990) *Manic-Depressive Illness*. Oxford: Oxford University Press.

25. B. T. Carroll (1998) 'Karl Leonhard, 1904–1988', *American Journal of Psychiatry*, 155: 1309.

26. See C. Perris (1995) 'Leonhard and the cycloid psychoses', in G. E. Berrios and R. Porter (eds.), *A History of Clinical Psychiatry*, London: Athlone Press.

27. K. Leonhard (1957/1979) *The Classification of the Endogenous Psychoses* (trans. R. Berman). New York: Irvington.

28. See Goodwin and Jamison, *Manic-Depressive Illness*, op. cit.

29. S. Kety (1980) 'The syndrome of schizophrenia: unresolved questions and opportunities for research', *British Journal of Psychiatry*, 136: 421–36.

30. M. Boyle (1990) *Schizophrenia: A Scientific Delusion*. London: Routledge.

31. For vivid descriptions of the disorder, see O. Sacks (1973) *Awakenings*. London: Duckworth.

32. See R. Porter (1995) 'Parkinson's disease (paralysis agitans)', in Berrios and Porter (eds.), *A History*, op. cit.

Chapter 3 The Great Classification Crisis

1. R. E. Kendell (1975) *The Role of Diagnosis in Psychiatry*. Oxford: Blackwell.

2. T. Kuhn (1970) *The Structure of Scientific Revolutions* (2nd edn). Chicago: Chicago University Press.

3. A. F. Chalmers (1976) *What is This Thing Called Science?* Milton Keynes: Open University Press.

4. World Health Organization (1992) *ICD-10: International Statistical Classification of Diseases and Related Health Problems* (10th revised edn). Geneva: World Health Organization.

5. American Psychiatric Association (1994) *Diagnostic and Statistical Manual of Mental Disorders* (4th edn). Washington, DC: APA.

6. My account of developments in standardized classification is largely drawn from Kendell, *The Role of Diagnosis*, op. cit. Other useful sources have been R. K. Blashfield (1984) *The Classification of Psychopathology: NeoKraepelinian and Quantitative Approaches*. New York: Plenum, and E. Shorter (1997) *A History of Psychiatry*. New York: Wiley.

7. Shorter, *A History of Psychiatry*, op. cit.

8. Blashfield, *The Classification of Psychopathology*, op. cit.

9. J. H. Masserman and H. T. Carmichael (1938) 'Diagnosis and prognosis in psychiatry: with a follow-up study of the results of short term general hospital therapy in psychiatric cases', *Journal of Mental Science*, 84: 893–946.

10. W. A. Hunt, C. L. Wittson and E. B. Hunt (1953) 'A theoretical and practical analysis of the diagnostic process', in P. H. Hoch and J. Zubin (eds.), *Current Problems of Psychiatric Diagnosis*. New York: Grune & Stratton.

11. P. Ash (1949) 'The reliability of psychiatric diagnosis', *Journal of Abnormal and Social Psychology*, 44: 272–6.

12. Detailed accounts are given in Blashfield, *The Classification of Psychopathology*, op. cit. and Kendell, *The Role of Diagnosis*, op. cit.

13. M. G. Sandifer, C. Pettus and D. Quade (1964) 'A study of psychiatric diagnosis', *Journal of Nervous and Mental Disease*, 139: 350–6.

14. M. Kramer (1961) 'Some problems of international research suggested by observations on differences in first admission rates to the mental hospitals of England and Wales and of the United States', in *Proceedings of the Third World Congress of Psychiatry*, 3. Montreal: Toronto University Press, pp. 153–60.

15. J. E. Cooper, R. E. Kendell, B. J. Gurland, L. Sharpe, J. R. M. Copeland and R. Simon (1972) *Psychiatric Diagnosis in New York and London: Maudsley Monograph No. 20*. Oxford: Oxford University Press.

16. World Health Organization (1973) *International Pilot Study of Schizophrenia*. Geneva: WHO.

17. See S. Bloch (1984) 'The political misuse of psychiatry in the Soviet Union', in S. Bloch and P. Chodoff (eds.), *Psychiatric Ethics*. Oxford: Oxford University

Press, and S. Bloch and P. Reddaway (1977) *Russia's Political Hospitals: The Abuse of Psychiatry in the Soviet Union*. New York: Basic Books.

Bloch seems to have assumed that psychiatric diagnosis is a relatively uncontroversial procedure, so that the Russians were simply wrong to assume that dissidents were mentally ill. For alternative perspectives, see: R. P. Bentall (1990) 'Compulsory care', in D. Evans (ed.), *Why Should we Care?* London: Macmillan; K. W. M. Fulford, A. Y. U. Smirnov and E. Snow (1993) 'Concepts of disease and the abuse of psychiatry in the USSR', *British Journal of Psychiatry*, 162; 801–10.

18. W. Reich (1984) 'Psychiatric diagnosis as an ethical problem', in Bloch and Chodoff (eds.), *Psychiatric Ethics*, op. cit. The italics are Reich's.

19. This brief account of Spitzer's career is taken from Blashfield, *The Classification of Psychopathology*, op. cit.

20. This brief biography of Spitzer is taken from Blashfield, op. cit. The article on DSM-II was R. L. Spitzer and P. T. Wilson (1968) 'A guide to the American Psychiatric Association's new diagnostic nomenclature', *American Journal of Psychiatry*, 124: 1619–29.

21. R. L. Spitzer and J. L. Fliess (1974) 'A reanalysis of the reliability of psychiatric diagnosis', *British Journal of Psychiatry*, 123: 341–7.

22. Sandifer, Pettus and Quade, 'A study of psychiatric diagnosis', op. cit.

23. H. Kutchins and S. A. Kirk (1997) *Making us Crazy: DSM – the Psychiatric Bible and the Creation of Mental Disorders*. New York: Free Press.

24. D. Healy (1997) *The Anti-depressant Era*. Cambridge, MA: Harvard University Press.

25. G. L. Klerman (1978) 'The evolution of a scientific nosology', in J. C. Shershow (ed.), *Schizophrenia: Science and Practice*. Cambridge, MA: Harvard University Press.

26. J. P. Feighner, E. Robins, S. B. Guze, R. A. Woodruff, G. Winokur and R. Munoz (1972) 'Diagnostic criteria for use in psychiatric research', *Archives of General Psychiatry*, 26: 57–63.

27. American Psychiatric Association (1980). *Diagnostic and Statistical Manual of Mental Disorders* (3rd edn). Washington, DC: APA.

28. . American Psychiatric Association (1987) *Diagnostic and Statistical Manual of Mental Disorders* (revised 3rd edn). Washington, DC: APA.

29. R. E. Kendell (1991) 'Relationship between DSM-IV and ICD-10', *Journal of Abnormal Psychology*, 100: 297–301.

30. American Psychiatric Association (1994) *Diagnostic and Statistical Manual of Mental Disorders* (4th edn). Washington, DC: APA.

31. M. B. First (2002) 'The DSM series and experience with DSM-IV', *Psychopathology*, 35: 67–71.

32. R. K. Blashfield (1996) 'Predicting DSM-V', *Journal of Nervous and Mental Disease*, 184: 4–7.

33. S. Hyler, J. Williams and R. Spitzer (1982) 'Reliability in the DSM-III field trials', *Archives of General Psychiatry*, 39: 1275–8.

34. G. Klerman (1986) 'Historical perspectives on contemporary schools of psy-

chopathology', in T. Millon and G. Klerman (eds.), *Contemporary Directions in Psychopathology: Towards DSM-IV*. New York: Guilford Press.

35. Kutchins and Kirk, *Making us Crazy*, op. cit.

36. J. B. Williams, M. Gibbon, M. B. First, R. L. Spitzer, M. Davies, J. Borus, M. Howes, J. Kane, H. G. Pope, B. Rounsaville and H.-U. Wittchen (1992) 'The Structured Clinical Interview for DSM-III-R (SCID): II. Multi-site test–retest reliability', *Archives of General Psychiatry*, 49: 630–6.

37. P. D. McGorry, C. Mihalopoulos, L. Henry, J. Dakis, H. J. Jackson, M. Flaum, S. Harrigan, D. McKenzie, J. Kulkarni and R. Karoly (1995) 'Spurious precision: procedural validity of diagnostic assessment in psychotic disorders', *American Journal of Psychiatry*, 152: 220–3.

38. M. A. Taylor and R. Abrams (1978) 'The prevalence of schizophrenia: a reassessment using modern criteria', *American Journal of Psychiatry*, 135: 945–8.

39. W. T. Carpenter, J. S. Strauss and J. J. Bartko (1973) 'Flexible system for the diagnosis of schizophrenia', *Science*, 182: 1275–8.

40. I. Brockington (1992) 'Schizophrenia: yesterday's concept', *European Psychiatry*, 7: 203–7.

41. J. van Os, C. Gilvarry, R. Bale, E. van Horn, T. Tattan, I. White and R. Murray (1999) 'A comparison of the utility of dimensional and categorical representations of psychosis', *Psychological Medicine*, 29: 595–606.

42. P. McGuffin, A. Farmer and I. Harvey (1991) 'A polydiagnostic application of operational criteria in studies of psychotic illness', *Archives of General Psychiatry*, 48: 764–70.

Chapter 4   Fool's Gold

1. From J. Borges (1960) 'El idioma analitico de John Wilkins', in *Otras inquisiciones*, Buenos Aires: Emece. I am indebted to Michael Dewey for translating this quotation and drawing it to my attention.

2. G. H. Gallup and F. Newport (1991) 'Belief in paranormal phenomena among adult Americans', *Sceptical Inquirer*, 15: 137–46.

3. R. E. Kendell (1975) *The Role of Diagnosis in Psychiatry*. Oxford: Blackwell.

4. For a review of research on comorbidity, and other defects of the DSM system, see L. A. Clark, D. Watson and S. Reynolds (1995) 'Diagnosis and classification of psychopathology: challenges to the current system and future directions', *Annual Review of Psychology*, 46: 121–53.

5. L. N. Robins, B. Z. Locke and D. A. Reiger (1991) 'An overview of psychiatric disorders in America', in L. N. Robins and B. Z. Locke (eds.), *Psychiatric Disorders in America*. New York: Free Press.

6. ibid.

7. Although mathematically complex, the principles behind the technique are not difficult to understand. Symptom data from patients who have already been diagnosed as suffering from either schizophrenia or manic depression are fed into

a computer. The computer program is also 'told' the diagnosis assigned to each patient. The program then attempts to determine which symptoms best discriminate between the two groups of patients, calculating a mathematical weight for each symptom according to how well it does this. (Symptoms assigned high values are found in only one diagnostic group whereas those with weights close to zero are found in both groups. Arbitrarily, positive weights are given to those symptoms found mostly in one of the groups whereas negative weights are given to the symptoms present mostly in the other group.) In this way, the program attempts to discover the symptoms that most influenced the clinicians to give one diagnosis or the other.

In a second phase of the analysis the computer constructs an equation, which it uses to measure the balance of symptoms in each patient. This equation, known as a discriminant function, consists of the sum of the weights assigned to the symptoms experienced by the patient. A patient's score on this function indicates the extent to which he or she is more or less schizophrenic, more or less manic-depressive, or somewhere in between. If the distinction between schizophrenia and manic depression is a real one, most patients should fall at the two ends of this scale (patients should have either mostly schizophrenia symptoms or mostly the symptoms of manic depression) and few patients should have scores close to zero. If, on the other hand, schizophrenia and manic depression are not separate disorders, most patients should have near zero scores, and should be located towards the centre of the scale.

For a more detailed but remarkably clear non-mathematical account of this and other statistical methods I describe in this chapter, together with their advantages and disadvantages, see R. K. Blashfield (1984) *The Classification of Psychopathology: NeoKraepelinian and Quantitative Approaches*. New York: Plenum. For simplicity, I have not discussed a third technique, known as cluster analysis, also described by Blashfield. However, readers of Blashfield will discover that this technique has yielded results that are even less supportive of Kraepelin's paradigm than the two approaches discussed in this book.

8. R. E. Kendell and J. A. Gourlay (1970) 'The clinical distinction between the affective psychoses and schizophrenia', *British Journal of Psychiatry*, 117: 261–6.
9. A study by Robert Cloninger and colleagues ('Diagnosis and prognosis in schizophrenia', *Archives of General Psychiatry*, 42: 15–25, 1985) claimed to have identified a separation between patients with four schizophrenic features (persecutory delusions, delusions of control, mood-incongruent delusions and auditory hallucinations) and other psychotic patients, but this group was so tightly defined that many patients meeting most definitions of schizophrenia would be excluded from it.

Ian Brockington and his colleagues ('Bipolar disorder, cycloid psychosis and schizophrenia: a study using "lifetime" psychopathology ratings, factor analysis and canonical variate analysis', *European Psychiatry*, 6: 223–36, 1991) found some evidence of a separation between schizophrenia and mania, but not of a separation between schizophrenia and depression. Indeed, the patients diagnosed as suffering from schizophrenia according to DSM-III criteria appeared to belong to a clinical spectrum in which schizophrenia merged with schizoaffective disorder and schizoaffective disorder merged with non-psychotic depression.

10. For a history of factor analysis which focuses on its use in studies of intelligence, see S. J. Gould (1984) *The Mismeasure of Man*. London: Penguin.

11. T. V. Moore (1930) 'The empirical determination of certain syndromes underlying praecox and manic-depressive psychoses', *American Journal of Psychiatry*, 86: 719–38.

12. Extensive studies of psychotic symptoms were undertaken between the early 1940s and the late 1960s, notably by American psychologists John Wittenbourne, Maurice Lorr and John Overall (see R. K. Blashfield (1984) *The Classification of Psychopathology: NeoKraepelinian and Quantitative Approaches*. New York: Plenum). The work conducted by Overall culminated in the creation of a standard instrument for measuring the severity of psychotic illnesses, known as the Brief Psychiatric Rating Scale, which provided detailed rules for rating symptoms, and which remains popular among researchers today because it is reliable and relatively simple to use. Factor analyses of BPRS ratings consistently revealed four main symptom clusters. Overall and his colleagues ('Major psychiatric disorders: a four-dimensional model', *Archives of General Psychiatry*, 16: 146–51, 1967) named these thinking disorder (consisting of conceptual disorganization, hallucinations and unusual thought content), anxious depression (anxiety, depression and guilt), hostile suspiciousness (hostility, suspiciousness and uncooperativeness) and withdrawal-retardation (emotional withdrawal, motor retardation and blunted emotions).

13. T. J. Crow (1980) 'Molecular pathology of schizophrenia: more than one disease process?' *British Medical Journal*, 280: 66–8.

14. P. F. Liddle (1987) 'The symptoms of chronic schizophrenia: a reexamination of the positive–negative dichotomy', *British Journal of Psychiatry*, 151: 145–51.

15. See N. C. Andreasen, M.-A. Roy and M. Flaum (1995) 'Positive and negative symptoms', in S. R. Hirsch and D. R. Weinberger (eds.), *Schizophrenia*, Oxford: Blackwell, pp. 28–45.

An Australian group has re-analysed previous studies of schizophrenia symptoms, also finding the three-factor solution. See S. Klimidis, G. W. Stuart, I. H. Minas, D. L. Copolov and B. S. Singh (1993) 'Positive and negative symptoms in psychoses: re-analysis of published SAPS and SANS global ratings', *Schizophrenia Research*, 9: 11–18.

16. P. D. McGorry, R. C. Bell, P. L. Dudgeon and H. J. Jackson (1998) 'The dimensional structure of first episode psychosis: an exploratory factor analysis', *Psychological Medicine*, 28: 935–47; V. Peralta, J. de Leon and M. J. Cuesta (1992) 'Are there more than two syndromes in schizophrenia? A critique of the positive–negative dichotomy', *British Journal of Psychiatry*, 161: 335–43; J. van Os, C. Gilvarry, R. Bale, E. van Horn, T. Tattan, I. White and R. Murray (1999) 'A comparison of the utility of dimensional and categorical representations of psychosis', *Psychological Medicine*, 29: 595–606.

17. R. Toomey, S. V. Faraone, J. C. Simpson and M. T. Tsuang (1998) 'Negative, positive and disorganized symptom dimensions in schizophrenia, major depression and bipolar disorder', *Journal of Nervous and Mental Disease*, 186: 470–76.

For other studies finding that the three-factor solution applies to non-schizophrenia patients see: S. Klimidis, G. W. Stuart, I. H. Minas, D. L. Copolov and B. S. Singh (1993) 'Positive and negative symptoms in psychoses: re-analysis of published SAPS and SANS global ratings', *Schizophrenia Research*, 9: 11–18; M. Maziade, M. Roy, M. Martinez, D. Cliche, J. Fournier, Y. Garveneau, L. Nicole, N. Montgrain, C. Dion, A. Ponton, A. Potvin, J. Lavallee, A. Pires, S. Bouchard, P. Boutin, F. Brisebois and C. Merette (1995) 'Negative, psychoticism, and disorganized dimensions in patients with familial schizophrenia or bipolar disorder: continuity and discontinuity between the major psychoses', *American Journal of Psychiatry*, 152: 1458–63.

18. S. S. Kety (1974) 'From rationalization to reason', *American Journal of Psychiatry*, 131: 957–63.

19. S. Rose, L. J. Kamin and R. C. Lewontin (1985) *Not in Our Genes*. Harmondsworth: Penguin.

20. See ibid. Detailed discussions of the limitations of genetic research into schizophrenia can be found in the following sources also: M. Boyle (1990) *Schizophrenia: A Scientific Delusion*. London: Routledge; R. Marshall (1990) 'The genetics of schizophrenia: axiom or hypothesis?' in R. P. Bentall (ed.), *Reconstructing Schizophrenia*. London: Routledge.

21. S. Kety, D. Rosenthal, P. H. Wender, F. Schulsinger and B. Jacobsen (1975) 'Mental illness in the biological and adoptive families of adopted individuals who have become schizophrenic: a preliminary report based on psychiatric interviews', in R. Fieve, D. Rosenthal and H. Brill (eds.), *Genetic Research in Psychiatry*. Baltimore, MD: Johns Hopkins University Press; D. Rosenthal, P. H. Wender, S. S. Kety, J. Welner and F. Schulsinger (1974) 'The adopted away offspring of schizophrenics', in S. A. Mednick, F. Schulsinger, J. Higgins and B. Bell (eds.), *Genetics, Environment and Psychopathology*. Amsterdam: North Holland Publishing Co.

22. Rose et al., *Not in Our Genes*, op. cit.

23. For a collection of essays addressing these findings and their implications, see A. C. Sandbank (ed.) (1999) *Twin and Triplet Psychology: A Professional Guide to Working with Multiples*. London: Routledge.

24. Rose et al., *Not in Our Genes*, op. cit.

25. K. S. Kendler, N. L. Pederesen, B. Y. Farahmand, and P.-G. Persson (1996) 'The treated incidence of psychotic and affective illness in twins compared with population expectation: a study in the Swedish twin and psychiatric registries', *Archives of General Psychiatry*, 26: 1135–44; C. M. Hultman, P. Sparen, N. Takei, R. M. Murray and S. Cnattingius (1999) 'Prenatal and perinatal risk factors for schizophrenia, affective psychosis, and reactive psychosis of early onset: case control study', *British Medical Journal*, 318: 421–6.

26. Rosenthal and his colleagues published many accounts of the Genain quadruplets. The account given here is based on D. Rosenthal and O. W. Quinn (1977) 'Quadruplet hallucinations: phenotypic variations of a schizophrenic genotype', *Archives of General Psychiatry*, 34: 817–27. All quotations about the Genains are from this paper.

27. A. F. Mirsky and O. W. Quinn (1988) 'The Genain quadruplets', *Schizophrenia Bulletin*, 14: 595–611.

28. A. F. Mirsky, L. A. Bieliauskas, L. M. French, D. P. van Kammen, E. Jonsson and G. Sedvall (2000) 'A 39-year follow-up of the Genain quadruplets', *Schizophrenia Bulletin*, 26: 699–708.

29. Rosenthal and Quinn, 'Quadruplet hallucinations', op. cit.

30. E. F. Torrey, A. E. Bowler, E. H. Taylor and I. I. Gottesman (1994) *Schizophrenia and Manic-Depressive Disorder*. New York: Basic Books.

31. T. J. Crow (1986) 'The continuum of psychosis and its implications for the structure of the gene', *British Journal of Psychiatry*, 149: 419–29; T. Crow (1991) 'The failure of the binary concept and the psychosis gene', in A. Kerr and H. McClelland (eds.), *Concepts of Mental Disorder: A Continuing Debate*. London: Gaskell.

32. M. A. Taylor (1992) 'Are schizophrenia and affective disorders related? A selective literature review', *American Journal of Psychiatry*, 149: 22–32.

33. For example, K. S. Kendler, A. M. Gruenberg and M. T. Tsuang (1985) 'Psychiatric illness in first-degree relatives of schizophrenic and surgical control patients: a family study using DSM-III criteria', *Archives of General Psychiatry*, 42: 770–9. See review by Taylor, 'Are schizophrenia and affective disorders related?' op. cit., for further examples.

34. For example, M. T. Tsuang, G. Winokur and R. R. Crowe (1980) 'Morbid risk of schizophrenia and affective disorders among first-degree relatives of patients with schizophrenia, mania, depression and surgical conditions', *British Journal of Psychiatry*, 137: 497–504.

For a recent study finding the same result, see V. Valles, J. van Os, R. Guillamat, B. Gutierrez, M. Campillo, P. Gento and L. Fananas (2000) 'Increased morbid risk for schizophrenia in families of in-patients with bipolar illness', *Schizophrenia Research*, 42: 83–90.

35. J. Angst and C. Scharfetter (1990) 'Schizoaffective psychosen', in E. Lungershausen, W. P. Kascha and R. J. Witkowski (eds.), *Affective Psychosen Kongress Band DGPN*. Stuttgart: Schattauer Verlag. Cited in Crow, 'The failure of the binary concept', op. cit.

36. J. T. Dalby, D. Morgan and M. L. Lee (1986) 'Schizophrenia and mania in identical twin brothers', *Journal of Nervous and Mental Disease*, 174: 304–8; J. B. Lohr and H. S. Bracha (1992) 'A monozygotic mirror-image twin pair with discordant psychiatric illness: a neuropsychiatric and neurodevelopmental evaluation', *American Journal of Psychiatry*, 149: 1091–5; P. McGuffin, A. Reveley and A. Holland (1982) 'Identical triplets: non-identical psychosis', *British Journal of Psychiatry*, 140: 1–6.

37. A. E. Farmer, P. McGuffin and I. I. Gottesman (1987) 'Twin concordance for

DSM-III schizophrenia: scrutinizing the validity of the definition', *Archives of General Psychiatry*, 44: 634–41.

38. J. S. Strauss and W. T. Carpenter (1974) 'The prediction of outcome in schizophrenia: II. Relationships between predictor and outcome variables', *Archives of General Psychiatry*, 31: 37–42.

39. J. S. Strauss (1992) 'The person – key to understanding mental illness: towards a new dynamic psychiatry III', *British Journal of Psychiatry*, 161: 19–26.

40. M. Harrow, J. F. Goldberg, L. S. Grossman and H. Y. Meltzer (1990) 'Outcome in manic disorders: a naturalistic follow-up study', *Archives of General Psychiatry*, 47: 665–71.

41. F. K. Goodwin and K. R. Jamison (1990) *Manic-Depressive Illness*. Oxford: Oxford University Press.

42. M. Maj, R. Priozzi and F. Starace (1989) 'Previous pattern of course of illness as a predictor of response to lithium prophylaxis in bipolar patients', *Journal of Affective Disorders*, 17: 237–41.

43. R. M. Post, D. R. Rubinow and J. C. Ballenger (1986) 'Conditioning and sensitization in the longitudinal course of affective illness', *British Journal of Psychiatry*, 149: 191–201.

44. L. Ciompi (1984) 'Is there really a schizophrenia? The long term course of psychotic phenomena', *British Journal of Psychiatry*, 145: 636–40.

45. M. Bleuler (1978) *The Schizophrenic Disorders*. New Haven, CT: Yale University Press.

46. Goodwin and Jamison, *Manic-Depressive Illness*, op. cit.

47. M. Tsuang, R. F. Woolson and J. A. Fleming (1979) 'Long-term outcome of major psychoses: I. Schizophrenia and affective disorders compared with psychiatrically symptom-free surgical conditions', *Archives of General Psychiatry*, 36: 1295–1301.

48. World Health Organization (1979) *Schizophrenia: An International Follow-up Study*. New York: Wiley.

49. Crow, 'The failure of the binary concept', op. cit.

50. R. E. Kendell and I. F. Brockington (1980) 'The identification of disease entities and the relationship between schizophrenic and affective psychoses', *British Journal of Psychiatry*, 137: 324–31. See also R. E. Kendell (1991) 'The major functional psychoses: are they independent entities or part of a continuum? Philosophical and conceptual issues underlying the debate', in Kerr and McClelland (eds.), *Concepts of Mental Disorder*, op. cit.

51. For fascinating accounts of the history of psychopharmacology, see David Healy's books *The Psychopharmacologists: Interviews with David Healy* (London: Chapman and Hall, 1996) and *The Anti-Depressant Era* (Cambridge, MA: Harvard University Press, 1997).

52. E. Shorter (1997) *A History of Psychiatry*. New York: Wiley.

53. E. Kraepelin (1899/1990) *Psychiatry: A Textbook for Students and Physicians*, vol. 1: *General Psychiatry*. Canton, MA: Watson Publishing International.

54. A. D. Smith, 'Henri Laborit: in humanity's laboratory', *Guardian*, 14 June 1995.

55. E. C. Johnstone, T. J. Crow, C. D. Frith and D. G. C. Owens (1988) 'The Northwick Park "functional" psychosis study: diagnosis and treatment response', *Lancet*, ii: 119–25.

56. G. E. Berrios and D. Beer (1995) 'Unitary psychosis concept', in G. E. Berrios and R. Porter (eds.), *A History of Clinical Psychiatry*. London: Athlone Press.

57. Crow, 'The failure of the binary concept', op. cit.

58. L. A. Clark, D. Watson and S. Reynolds (1995) 'Diagnosis and classification of psychopathology: challenges to the current system and future directions', *Annual Review of Psychology*, 46: 121–53.

59. American Psychiatric Association (1994) *Diagnostic and Statistical Manual for Mental Disorders* (4th edition). Washington, DC: APA.

60. J. van Os, C. Gilvarry, R. Bale, E. van Horn, T. Tattan, I. White and R. Murray (1999) 'A comparison of the utility of dimensional and categorical representations of psychosis', *Psychological Medicine*, 29, 595–606.

Chapter 5   The Boundaries of Madness

1. L. Wittgenstein (1980) *Culture and Value* (trans. P. Winch). Oxford: Blackwell.

2. G. E. Berrios (1996) *The History of Mental Symptoms: Descriptive Psychopathology since the Nineteenth Century*. Cambridge: Cambridge University Press.

3. H. A. Sidgewick (1894) 'Report of the census on hallucinations', *Proceedings of the Society for Psychical Research*, 26: 259–394.

4. D. J. West (1948) 'A mass observation questionnaire on hallucinations', *Journal of the Society for Psychical Research*, 34: 187–96.

5. T. B. Posey and M. E. Losch (1983) 'Auditory hallucinations of hearing voices in 375 normal subjects', *Imagination, Cognition and Personality*, 2: 99–113.

6. R. P. Bentall and P. D. Slade (1985) 'Reliability of a measure of disposition towards hallucinations', *Personality and Individual Differences*, 6: 527–9; H. F. Young, R. P. Bentall, P. D. Slade and M. E. Dewey (1986) 'Disposition towards hallucinations, gender and IQ score', *Personality and Individual Differences*, 7: 247–9.

7. T. R. Barrett and J. B. Etheridge (1992) 'Verbal hallucinations in normals: I. People who hear voices', *Applied Cognitive Psychology*, 6: 379–87; T. R. Barrett and J. B. Etheridge (1993) 'Verbal hallucinations in normals: II. Self-reported imagery vividness', *Personality and Individual Differences*, 15: 61–7; T. R. Barrett and J. B. Etheridge (1994) 'Verbal hallucinations in normals: III. Dysfunctional personality correlates', *Personality and Individual Differences*, 16: 57–62.

8. A. Y. Tien (1991) 'Distribution of hallucinations in the population', *Social Psychiatry and Psychiatric Epidemiology*, 26: 287–92.

9. J. van Os, M. Hanssen, R. V. Bijl and A. Ravelli (2000) 'Strauss (1969) revisited: a psychosis continuum in the normal population?' *Schizophrenia Research*, 45: 11–20.

10. R. Poulton, A. Caspi, T. E. Moffitt, M. Cannon, R. Murray and H. Harrington

(2000) 'Children's self-reported psychotic symptoms and adult schizophreniform disorder: a 15-year longitudinal study', *Archives of General Psychiatry*, 57: 1053–8.

11. A. Jablensky (1995) 'Schizophrenia: the epidemiological horizon', in S. R. Hirsch and D. R. Weinberger (eds.), *Schizophrenia*, Oxford: Blackwell.

12. G. H. Gallup and F. Newport (1991) 'Belief in paranormal phenomena among adult Americans', *Sceptical Inquirer*, 15: 137–46.

13. C. A. Ross and S. Joshi (1992) 'Paranormal experiences in the general population', *The Journal of Nervous and Mental Disease*, 180: 357–61.

14. A. Greeley (1975) *The Sociology of the Paranormal: A Reconnaissance*. Beverly Hills: Sage.

15. Group for the Advancement of Psychiatry (1976) *Mysticism: Spiritual Quest or Psychotic Disorder?* New York: GAP Publications.

16. D. Lyons (2001) 'Soviet-style psychiatry is alive and well in the People's Republic', *British Journal of Psychiatry*, 178: 380–1.

17. M. Jackson and K. W. M. Fulford (1997) 'Spiritual experience and psychopathology', *Philosophy, Psychiatry and Psychology*, 1: 41–65.

18. G. Roberts (1991) 'Delusional belief systems and meaning in life: a preferred reality?' *British Journal of Psychiatry*, 159, Supplement 14: 19–28.

19. E. Peters, S. Day, J. McKenna and G. Orbach (1999) 'Delusional ideation in religious and psychotic populations', *British Journal of Clinical Psychology*, 38: 83–96.

20. See L. S. Newman and R. F. Baumeister (1996) 'Towards an explanation of the UFO abduction phenomenon: hypnotic elaboration, extraterrestrial sadomasochism, and spurious memories', *Psychological Inquiry*, 7: 99–126.

21. J. E. Mack (1994) *Abduction: Human Encounters with Aliens*. New York: Macmillan.

22. S. Appelle, S. J. Lynn and L. Newman (2000) 'Alien abduction experiences', in E. Cardena, S. J. Lynn and S. Krippner (eds.), *Varieties of Anomalous Experience: Examining the Scientific Evidence*. Washington, DC: American Psychological Association, pp. 253–82.

23. N. P. Spanos, P. A. Cross, K. Dickson and S. C. DuBreuil (1993) 'Close encounters: an examination of UFO experiences', *Journal of Personality and Social Psychology*, 102: 624–32.

24. J. Chequers, S. Joseph and D. Diduca (1997) 'Belief in extraterrestrial life, UFO-related beliefs, and schizotypal personality', *Personality and Individual Differences*, 23: 519–21.

25. van Os et al., 'Strauss (1969) revisited', op. cit.

26. Poulton et al., 'Children's self-reported psychotic symptoms', op. cit.

27. H. Verdoux, S. Maurice-Tison, B. Gay, J. van Os, R. Salamon and M. L. Bourgeois (1998) 'A survey of delusional ideation in primary-care patients', *Psychological Medicine*, 28: 127–34.

28. N. C. Andreasen (1979) 'Thought, language and communication disorders: diagnostic significance', *Archives of General Psychiatry*, 36: 1325–30.

29. This study is reported in two books: D. J. Weeks and K. Ward (1988) *Eccentrics: The Scientific Investigation*. Stirling: Stirling University Press; and D. J. Weeks and J. James (1995) *Eccentrics*. London: Weidenfeld & Nicolson.

30. Quoted in Weeks and James, *Eccentrics*, op. cit.

31. T. S. Szasz (1993) 'Crazy talk: thought disorder or psychiatric arrogance?', *British Journal of Medical Psychology*, 66: 61–7.

32. J. Leff (1993) '"Crazy talk: thought disorder or psychiatric arrogance?": Comment', *British Journal of Medical Psychology*, 66: 77–8.

33. R. Littlewood and M. Lipsedge (1989) *Aliens and Alienists: Ethnic Minorities and Psychiatry* (2nd edn). London: Unwin Hyman.

34. Poulton et al., 'Children's self-reported psychotic symptoms', op. cit.

35. R. A. Depue, J. F. Slater, H. Wolfstetter-Kausch, D. Klein, E. Goplerud and D. Farr (1981) 'A behavioral paradigm for identifying persons at risk for bipolar depressive disorder: a conceptual framework and five validation studies', *Journal of Abnormal Psychology*, 90: 381–437.

36. W. Wicki and J. Angst (1991) 'The Zurich study. X: Hypomania in a 28- to 30-year-old cohort', *European Archives of Psychiatry and Clinical Neuroscience*, 240: 339–48.

37. J. Angst (1998) 'The emerging epidemiology of hypomania and bipolar II disorder', *Journal of Affective Disorders*, 50: 143–51.

38. H. S. Akiskal (1994) 'The temperamental borders of affective disorders', *Acta Psychiatrica Scandinavica*, 89 (suppl. 379): 32–7. See also H. S. Akiskal, M. L. Bourgeois, J. Angst, R. Post, H.-J. Moller and R. Hirschfeld (2000) 'Re-evaluating the prevalence of and diagnostic composition within the broad clinical spectrum of bipolar disorders', *Journal of Affective Disorders*, 59: S5–S30.

39. E. Kretschmer (1925) *Physique and Character* (trans. W. J. H. Sprott). London: Kegan, Trench & Trubner.

40. L. Rees (1973) 'Constitutional factors and abnormal behaviour', in H. J. Eysenck (ed.), *Handbook of Abnormal Psychology*. San Diego, CA: Edits Publishers.

41. One researcher who was influenced by Kretschmer was Hans Eysenck, one of the most controversial psychologists of the twentieth century, who was born in Germany but moved to Britain in the early 1930s in order to escape Nazism. After working as a psychologist at the Mill Hill Emergency Hospital during the Second World War, he became head of the Department of Psychology at the University of London Institute of Psychiatry. His controversial status arose from his views about racial differences in innate intelligence. However, he was at least as well known for his less contentious ideas about human personality.

It is impossible to do full justice to Eysenck's theory of personality in a few paragraphs. Suffice it to say that, in his early work, he proposed that ordinary people varied along two independent dimensions which he believed to be largely influenced by genetic factors: *neuroticism* (roughly, the extent to which the individual is easily emotionally aroused) and *introversion–extroversion* (roughly, the extent to which the individual is comfortable with and seeks out the company of others). However, building on Kretschmer's ideas, in his later work with his wife Sybil (H. J. Eysenck and S. B. G. Eysenck (1976) *Psychoticism as a Dimension of Personality*. London: Hodder & Stoughton) he argued that he had identified a third dimension, which he called *psychoticism*. Eysenck believed that, as the name implied, psychotic illness lay at the extreme end of this dimension.

Eysenck was able to develop questionnaire measures of his three dimensions, which became known as the N, E and P scales. Although his theory became one of the standard models of personality, his concept of psychoticism has been criticized by clinicians for several reasons. Inspection of items from the P scale (for example, 'Would being in debt worry you?', 'Do you sometimes like teasing animals?', 'Do you enjoy hurting people you love?') reveals that they assess impulsiveness and indifference to the needs of others, rather than the kinds of experiences reported by psychotic patients. Criminals often score at least as high on P as psychotic patients. More importantly perhaps, and consistent with the idea that emotional arousal plays an important role in psychosis, recent studies suggest that psychotic patients score highly on N rather than P (R. J. Gurrera, P. G. Nestor and B. F. O'Donnell (2000) 'Personality traits in schizophrenia: comparison with a community sample', *Journal of Nervous and Mental Disease*, 188: 31–5). In short, it seems doubtful that Eysenck's concept of psychoticism, however valid as a measure of personality, measures traits that are directly related to psychotic illness.

42. P. Meehl (1962) 'Schizotaxia, schizotypia, schizophrenia', *American Psychologist*, 17: 827–38. For an updated version of the theory, see P. Meehl (1989) 'Schizotaxia revisited', *Archives of General Psychiatry*, 46: 935–44.

43. S. Kety, D. Rosenthal, P. H. Wender, F. Schulsinger and B. Jacobsen (1975) 'Mental illness in the biological and adoptive families of adopted individuals who have become schizophrenic: a preliminary report based on psychiatric interviews', in R. Fieve, D. Rosenthal and H. Brill (eds.), *Genetic Research in Psychiatry*. Baltimore, MD: Johns Hopkins University Press.

44. R. L. Spitzer, J. Endicott and M. Gibbon (1979) 'Crossing the border into borderline personality and borderline schizophrenia', *Archives of General Psychiatry*, 36: 17–24.

45. G. Mellsop, F. Varghese, S. Joshua and A. Hicks (1982) 'The reliability of Axis II of DSM-III', *American Journal of Psychiatry*, 139: 1360–61.

46. For a review of this work, see W. M. Grove (1982) 'Psychometric detection of schizotypy', *Psychological Bulletin*, 92: 27–38.

47. L. J. Chapman, J. P. Chapman and M. L. Raulin (1976) 'Scales for physical and social anhedonia', *Journal of Abnormal Psychology*, 85: 374–82; L. J. Chapman, E. W. Edell and J. P. Chapman (1980) 'Physical anhedonia, perceptual aberration and psychosis proneness', *Schizophrenia Bulletin*, 6: 639–53; M. Eckblad and L. J. Chapman (1983) 'Magical ideation as an indicator of schizotypy', *Journal of Consulting and Clinical Psychology*, 51: 215–25; M. Eckblad and L. J. Chapman (1986) 'Development and validation of a scale for hypomanic personality', *Journal of Abnormal Psychology*, 95: 214–22.

48. G. S. Claridge and P. Brocks (1984) 'Schizotypy and hemisphere function – I. Theoretical considerations and the measurement of schizotypy', *Personality and Individual Differences*, 5: 633–48.

49. G. S. Claridge (1990) 'Can a disease model of schizophrenia survive?' in R. P. Bentall (ed.), *Reconstructing Schizophrenia*. London: Routledge, pp. 157–83.

50. L. J. Chapman, J. P. Chapman, T. R. Kwapil, M. Eckblad and M. C. Zinser (1994) 'Putatively psychosis-prone subjects 10 years later', *Journal of Abnormal Psychology*, 103: 171–83.

51. Akiskal, 'The temperamental borders of affective disorders', op. cit.

52. Spitzer et al., 'Crossing the border', op. cit.

53. R. P. Bentall, G. S. Claridge and P. D. Slade (1989) 'The multidimensional nature of schizotypal traits: a factor-analytic study with normal subjects', *British Journal of Clinical Psychology*, 28: 363–75.

54. G. S. Claridge and T. Beech (1995) 'Fully and quasi-dimensional constructions of schizotypy', in A. Raine, T. Lencz and S. A. Mednick (eds.), *Schizotypal Personality*. Cambridge: Cambridge University Press; M. G. Vollema and R. J. van den Bosch (1995) 'The multidimensionality of schizotypy', *Schizophrenia Bulletin*, 21: 19–31.

55. G. Claridge, C. McCreery, O. Mason, R. P. Bentall, G. Boyle, P. D. Slade and D. Popplewell (1996) 'The factor structure of "schizotypal" traits: a large replication study', *British Journal of Clinical Psychology*, 35: 103–15.

56. C. A. Reynolds, A. Raine, K. Mellingen, P. H. Venables and S. A. Mednick (2000) 'Three-factor model of schizotypal personality: invariance across culture, gender, religious affiliation, family adversity, and psychopathology', *Schizophrenia Bulletin*, 26: 603–18.

57. S. Nasar (1998) *A Beautiful Mind*. London: Faber & Faber.

58. For a review of suicide in schizophrenia patients, see C. B. Caldwell and I. I. Gottesman (1990) 'Schizophrenics kill themselves too: a review of risk factors for suicide', *Schizophrenia Bulletin*, 16: 571–89. For similar data on bipolar patients, see F. K. Goodwin and K. R. Jamison (1990) *Manic-Depressive Illness*. Oxford: Oxford University Press.

59. Ö. Ödegaard (1980) 'Fertility of psychiatric first admissions in Norway, 1936–75', *Acta Psychiatrica Scandinavica*, 62: 212–20; G. Hutchinson, D. Bhugra, R. Mallett, R. Burnett, B. Corridan and J. P. Leff (1999) 'Fertility and marital rates in first-onset schizophrenia', *Social Psychiatry and Psychiatric Epidemiology*, 34: 617–21.

60. J. Huxley, E. Mayr, H. Osmond and A. Hoffer (1964) 'Schizophrenia as a genetic morphism', *Nature*, 204: 220–1.

61. L. F. Jarvik and S. B. Chadwick (1972) 'Schizophrenia and survival', in S. B. Hammer, K. Salzinger and A. Sutton (eds.), *Psychopathology*. New York: Wiley.

62. A. Stevens and J. Price (1996) *Evolutionary Psychiatry*. London: Routledge.

63. J. H. Brod (1997) 'Creativity and schizotypy, in G. S. Claridge (ed.), *Schizotypy: Implications for Illness and Health*. Oxford: Oxford University Press.

64. D. K. Simonton (1994) *Greatness: Who Makes History and Why*. New York: Guilford.

65. E. Regis (1989) *Who Got Einstein's Office?: Eccentricity and Genius at the Princeton Institute of Advanced Study*. London: Penguin.

66. Nasar, *A Beautiful Mind*, op. cit.

67. See for example: A. M. Ludwig (1995) *The Price of Greatness: Resolving the Creativity and Madness Controversy*. New York: Guilford; F. Post (1996) 'Verbal creativity, depression and alcoholism: an investigation of 100 American and British writers', *British Journal of Psychiatry*, 168: 545–55; G. S. Claridge (1998) 'Creativity and madness: clues from modern psychiatric diagnosis', in A. Steptoe (ed.), *Genius and the Mind*. Oxford: Oxford University Press.

68. N. C. Andreasen (1987) 'Creativity and mental illness: prevalence rates in writers and their first-degree relatives', *American Journal of Psychiatry*, 144: 1288–92.

69. K. R. Jamison (1989) 'Mood disorders and patterns of creativity in British writers and artists', *British Journal of Psychiatry*, 52: 125–34.

70. J. L. Karlsson (1984) 'Creative intelligence in relatives of mental patients', *Hereditas*, 100: 83–6.

71. R. Richards, D. Kinney, I. Lundy and M. Benet (1988) 'Creativity in manic-depressives, cyclothymes, and their normal first-degree relatives', *Journal of Abnormal Psychology*, 97: 281–8.

72. Some studies have attempted to demonstrate similar styles of reasoning in psychotic patients and creative people. See, for example: N. J. C. Andreasen and P. S. Powers (1975) 'Creativity and psychosis: an examination of conceptual style', *Archives of General Psychiatry*, 32: 70–3; M. Dykes and A. McGhie (1976) 'A comparative study of attentional strategies in schizophrenic and highly creative normal subjects', *British Journal of Psychiatry*, 128: 50–56; J. A. Keefe and P. A. Magaro (1980) 'Creativity and schizophrenia: an equivalence of cognitive processing', *Journal of Abnormal Psychology*, 89: 390–98; H. J. Eysenck (1993) 'Creativity and personality: suggestions for a theory', *Psychological Inquiry*, 4: 147–78.

Other studies have demonstrated, in psychiatrically healthy individuals, a positive correlation between scores on questionnaire measures of schizotypy and psychological measures of creative thinking. Examples of this kind of research can be found in: P. K. Chadwick (1997) *Schizophrenia: A Positive Perspective*. London: Routledge; D. Schuldberg (1990) 'Schizotypal and hypomanic traits, creativity and psychological health', *Creativity Research Journal*, 3: 218–30; T. O'Reilly, R. Dunbar and R. P. Bentall (2001) 'Schizotypy and creativity: an evolutionary connection?', *Personality and Individual Differences*, 31: 1067–78.

73. Claridge, 'Creativity and madness', op. cit.

74. S. Freud (1926/1959) 'The question of lay analysis: conversations with an impartial person', in *Collected Works*. London: Hogarth Press. See also B. Bettelheim (1983) *Freud and Man's Soul*. London: Hogarth Press.

75. E. Shorter (1997) *A History of Psychiatry*. New York: Wiley.

76. R. D. Laing (1960) *The Divided Self.* London: Tavistock Press; R. D. Laing (1961) *The Self and Others.* London: Tavistock.

77. R. D. Laing and A. Esterson (1964) *Sanity, Madness and the Family: Families of Schizophrenics.* London: Tavistock; R. D. Laing (1967) *The Politics of Experience and the Bird of Paradise.* London: Penguin Press.

78. For an account of Laing's life, see J. Clay (1996) *R. D. Laing: A Divided Self.* London: Hodder & Stoughton.

79. T. S. Szasz (1960) 'The myth of mental illness', *American Psychologist,* 15: 564–80; T. S. Szasz (1979) *Schizophrenia: The Sacred Symbol of Psychiatry.* Oxford: Oxford University Press.

Chapter 6   Them and Us

1. 'We and They', from *Rudyard Kipling: The Complete Verse*, London: Kyle Cathie Ltd.

2. S. Butler (1872/1970) *Erewhon, Or Over the Range.* London: Penguin. For a discussion of the social context of Butler's utopian fiction, see A. L. Morton (1969) *The English Utopia.* London: Lawrence & Wishart.

3. H. Fabrega (1993) 'A cultural analysis of human behavioral breakdowns: an approach to the ontology and epistemology of psychiatric phenomena', *Culture, Medicine and Psychiatry,* 17: 99–132.

4. J. H. Orley (1970) *Culture and Mental Illness.* Kampala: Makerere Institute of Social Research.

5. E. Kraepelin (1904/1974) 'Comparative psychiatry', in S. R. Hirsch and M. Shepherd (eds.), *Themes and Variations in European Psychiatry.* Bristol: Wright, pp. 3–6.

6. Quoted in H. Fabrega (1989) 'On the significance of the anthropological approach to schizophrenia', *Psychiatry,* 52: 45–65.

7. My account of the work of Carothers is drawn from Jock McCulloch's fascinating book *Colonial Psychiatry and 'the African Mind'.* Cambridge: Cambridge University Press, 1995.

8. World Health Organization (1973) *International Pilot Study of Schizophrenia.* Geneva: WHO.

9. World Health Organization (1979) *Schizophrenia: An International Follow-up Study.* New York: Wiley.

10. A. Kleinman (1980) *Patients and Healers in the Context of Culture.* Berkeley: University of California Press.

11. A. Jablensky, N. Sartorius, G. Ernberg, M. Anker, A. Korten, J. E. Cooper, R. Day and A. Bertelsen (1992) 'Schizophrenia: manifestations, incidence and course in different cultures', *Psychological Medicine,* Supplement 20: 1–97.

12. To appreciate this point it is necessary to consider briefly the purpose of statistical testing in studies of this sort. Such tests are used to decide whether the differences observed between the sites could be caused by random variations in the data. For example, a very small difference (say, an annual incidence rate of 0.80 per 10,000 population at one site and a rate of 0.81 per 10,000 at another) would not be interesting, because it would probably be the result of chance processes (for example, random fluctuations in the number of people becoming ill in different periods and at different places). If statistical calculations show the probability that an observed difference is due to chance is less than 1 in 20 (probability = 0.05) the convention is to assume that the difference is a real one. However, this strategy creates a risk that a true difference will be rejected as statistically non-significant. Studies that have insufficient sample sizes to distinguish between large differences that are genuine and similar sized differences that are due to chance factors are said to be 'underpowered'. This is most likely to happen when, as in the DOSMD, many different sites are compared, as the number of participants required per site to achieve adequate power increases as the number of sites increases.

13. A. Kleinman (1987) 'Anthropology and psychiatry: the role of culture in cross-cultural research on illness', *British Journal of Psychiatry*, 151: 447–54.

14. See E. F. Torrey (1987) 'Prevalence studies in schizophrenia', *British Journal of Psychiatry*, 150: 598–608; and also J. Thakker and T. Ward (1998) 'Culture and classification: the cross-cultural application of the DSM-IV', *Clinical Psychology Review*, 18: 501–29.

15. J. S. Allen (1997) 'At issue: are traditional societies schizophrenogenic?' *Schizophrenia Bulletin*, 23: 357–64.

16. L. Hemsi (1971) 'Psychiatric morbidity in West Indian immigrants', *Social Psychiatry*, 2: 95–100; I. Carpenter and I. Brockington (1980) 'A study of mental illness in Asians, West Indians and Africans living in Manchester', *British Journal of Psychiatry*, 137: 201–5.

17. G. Kirov and R. M. Murray (1999) 'Ethnic differences in the presentation of bipolar affective disorder', *European Psychiatry*, 14: 199–204; J. van Os, N. Takei, D. J. Castle and S. Wessely (1996) 'The incidence of mania: time trends in relation to gender and ethnicity', *Social Psychiatry and Psychiatric Epidemiology*, 31: 129–36.

18. R. Littlewood and M. Lipsedge (1989) *Aliens and Alienists: Ethnic Minorities and Psychiatry* (2nd edn). London: Unwin Hyman.

19. F. W. Hickling, K. McKenzie, R. Mullen and R. Murray (1999) 'A Jamaican psychiatrist evaluates diagnoses at a London psychiatric hospital', *British Journal of Psychiatry*, 175: 283–5.

20. D. Pilgrim and A. Rogers (1993) *A Sociology of Mental Health and Illness*. Buckingham: Open University Press.

21. G. Harrison, D. Owens, A. Holton, D. Neilson and D. Boot (1988) 'A prospective study of severe mental disorder in Afro-Caribbean patients', *Psychological Medicine*, 18: 643–57.

22. D. Bhugra, J. Leff, R. Mallett, G. Der, B. Corridan and S. Rudge (1997) 'Incidence and outcome of schizophrenia in Whites, African-Caribbeans and Asians in London', *Psychological Medicine*, 27: 791–8.

23. D. Bhugra, M. Hilwig, B. Hossein, H. Marceau, J. Neehall, J. P. Leff, R. Mallett and G. Der (1996) 'First contact incidence rates of schizophrenia in Trinidad and one-year follow-up', *British Journal of Psychiatry*, 169: 587–92.

24. D. Bhugra, J. Leff, R. Mallett and G. E. Mahy (1999) 'First-contact incidence rate of schizophrenia on Barbados', *British Journal of Psychiatry*, 175: 28–33.

25. Harrison et al., 'A prospective study', op. cit.; G. Hutchinson, N. Takei, T. A. Fahy, D. Bhugra, C. Gilvarry, O. Moran, R. Mallett, P. Sham, J. Leff and R. M. Murray (1996) 'Morbid risk of schizophrenia in first-degree relatives of white and Afro-Caribbean patients with psychosis', *British Journal of Psychiatry*, 171: 776–80; P. A. Sugarman and D. Crawford (1994) 'Schizophrenia in the Afro-Caribbean community', *British Journal of Psychiatry*, 164: 474–80.

26. World Health Organization, *Schizophrenia: An International Follow-up Study*, op. cit.

27. K. M. Lin and A. M. Kleinman (1988) 'Psychopathology and clinical course of schizophrenia', *Schizophrenia Bulletin*, 14: 555–67.

28. E. Susser and J. Wanderling (1994) 'Epidemiology of nonaffective acute remitting psychosis vs schizophrenia: sex and sociocultural setting', *Archives of General Psychiatry*, 51: 294–301.

29. R. B. Edgerton and A. Cohen (1994) 'Culture and schizophrenia: the DOSMD challenge', *British Journal of Psychiatry*, 164: 222–31.

30. Fabrega, 'On the significance of the anthropological approach', op. cit.

31. I. Al-Issa (1978) 'Sociocultural factors in hallucinations', *International Journal of Social Psychiatry*, 24: 167–76; I. Al-Issa (1995) 'The illusion of reality or the reality of an illusion?: hallucinations and culture', *British Journal of Psychiatry*, 166: 368–73.

32. D. M. Ndetei and A. Vadher (1984) 'Frequency and clinical significance of delusions across cultures', *Acta Psychiatrica Scandinavica*, 70: 73–6.

33. J. Mitchell and A. D. Vierkant (1989) 'Delusions and hallucinations as a reflection of the subcultural milieu among psychotic patients of the 1930s and 1980s', *Journal of Psychology*, 123: 269–74.

34. For discussions of culture-bound syndromes, see C. Helman (1994) *Culture, Health and Illness*. London: Butterworth & Heinemann; and M. MacLachlan (1997) *Culture and Health*. London: Wiley.

35. For example, see A. Kiev (1972) *Transcultural Psychiatry*. Harmondsworth: Penguin.

36. R. Littlewood (1986) 'Russian dolls and Chinese boxes: an anthropological approach to the implicit models of comparative psychiatry', in J. L. Cox (ed.), *Transcultural Psychiatry*. Beckenham: Croom-Helm.

37. D. Sperber (1982) *On Anthropological Knowledge: Three Essays*. Cambridge: Cambridge University Press.

38. Littlewood, 'Russian dolls and Chinese boxes', op. cit.

39. Sperber, *On Anthropological Knowledge*, op. cit.

40. L. A. Sass (1994) *The Paradoxes of Delusion: Wittgenstein, Schreber and the Schizophrenic Mind*. Ithaca, NY: Cornell University Press.

41. American Psychiatric Association (1994) *Diagnostic and Statistical Manual for Mental Disorders*, 4th edn. Washington, DC: APA.

42. Littlewood and Lipsedge, *Aliens and Alienists*, op. cit.

43. E. Bourguignon (1970) 'Hallucinations and trance: an anthropologist's perspective', in W. Keup (ed.), *Origins and Mechanisms of Hallucinations*. New York: Plenum.

44. Al-Issa, 'The illusion of reality', op. cit.

45. W. S. McDonald and C. W. Oden (1977) 'Aumakua: behavior direction visions in Hawaiians', *Journal of Abnormal Psychology*, 86: 189–94.

46. Helman, *Culture, Health and Illness*, op. cit.

47. R. B. Edgerton (1971) 'A traditional African psychiatrist', *Southwestern Journal of Anthropology*, 27: 259–78.

48. A. Honig, M. A. J. Romme, B. J. Ensink, S. Escher, M. H. A. Pennings and M. W. DeVries (1998) 'Auditory hallucinations: a comparison between patients and nonpatients', *Journal of Nervous and Mental Disease*, 186: 646–51.

49. S. Krippner and J. Achterberg (2000) 'Anomalous healing experiences', in E. Cardena, S. J. Lynn and S. Krippner (eds.), *Varieties of Anomalous Experience: Examining the Scientific Evidence*. Washington, DC: American Psychological Association, pp. 353–95.

50. J. M. Murphy (1976) 'Psychiatric labelling in cross-cultural perspective', *Science*, 191: 1019–28.

51. R. Noll (1983) 'Shamanism and schizophrenia', *American Ethnologist*, 10: 443–59.

52. Fabrega, 'A cultural analysis', op. cit.

53. K. Kutchins and S. A. Kirk (1997) *Making us Crazy: DSM – the Psychiatric Bible and the Creation of Mental Disorders*. New York: Free Press.

54. K. Hyams, F. S. Wignall and R. Roswell (1996) 'War syndromes and their evaluation: from the U.S. Civil War to the Persian Gulf War', *Annals of Internal Medicine*, 125: 402. See also P. Bracken (1998) 'Hidden agenda: deconstructing post traumatic stress disorder', in P. J. Bracken and C. Petty (eds.), *Rethinking the Trauma of War*. London: Free Association Books.

55. Kutchins and Kirk, *Making us Crazy*, op. cit.

56. See M. Romme and S. Escher (eds.) (1993) *Accepting Voices*. London: MIND Publications.

57. J. Jaynes (1979) *The Origins of Consciousness in the Breakdown of the Bicameral Mind*. London: Penguin.

58. The main evidence that Jaynes cites to support this unlikely hypothesis is from the language of the Ancient Greeks as revealed in the *Iliad*. Apparently, the Ancient Greeks made no reference to mental states as we would think of them today. The late Professor Henry Blumenthal, a distinguished classicist at the University of Liverpool, confirmed to me that Jaynes' observation is correct, but doubted his explanation for it. However, my colleague Ivan Leudar and his collaborator Phil Thomas (*Voices of Reason, Voices of Insanity: Studies of Verbal Hallucinations*. London: Routledge, 2000) have suggested that Jaynes may have misread the *Iliad*,

and that indirect evidence that the Greeks knew of their own mental states can be inferred from the text.

In this context, it is helpful to note that some modern languages represent mental states in ways which differ strikingly from English (see K. Wilkes, '_____, yishi, duh, um, and consciousness', in A. J. Marcel and E. Bisiach (eds.), *Consciousness in Contemporary Society*. Oxford: Oxford University Press, 1988).

59. M. Romme and A. Escher (1989) 'Hearing voices', *Schizophrenia Bulletin*, 15: 209–16; M. Romme and A. Escher (1996) 'Empowering people who hear voices', in G. Haddock and P. D. Slade (eds.), *Cognitive Behavioural Interventions with Psychotic Disorders*. London: Routledge; Honig et al., 'Auditory hallucinations', op. cit.

60. J. E. Mezzich, H. Fabrega and A. Kleinman (1992) 'Cultural validity and DSM-IV', *Journal of Nervous and Mental Disease*, 180: 4.

61. S. R. Lopez and P. J. J. Guarnaccia (2000) 'Cultural psychopathology', *Annual Review of Psychology*, 51: 571–98.

62. A. Kleinman (1978) 'Concepts and a model for the comparison of medical systems as cultural systems', *Social Science and Medicine*, 12: 85–93.

63. Social constructionists (sometimes called postmodernists) argue that there is no such thing as a 'reality' beyond the descriptions made by the observer. Scientific knowledge is thereby seen as *nothing more than* a product of a particular cultural stance, and hence no more valid than witchcraft. For an example of this kind of approach to psychopathology, see I. Parker, E. Georgaca, D. Harper, T. McLaughlin and M. Stowell-Smith (1995) *Deconstructing Psychopathology*. London: Sage.

A thoughtful philosophical critique of social constructionist approaches to psychology can be found in J. D. Greenwood's book *Realism, Identity and Emotion* (London: Sage, 1994). Greenwood agrees with social constructionists that it is important to examine the way that cultural and historical forces have misshapen our scientific theories, but argues that we should use the insights gained to improve our scientific knowledge and develop better theories. The approach taken in this book is consistent with his *critical realist* approach.

64. H. D. Ellis and K. W. de Pauw (1994) 'The cognitive neuropsychiatric origins of the Capgras delusion', in A. S. David and J. C. Cutting (eds.), *The Neuropsychology of Schizophrenia*. Hove: Erlbaum, pp. 317–35.

65. G. L. Klerman (1978) 'The evolution of a scientific nosology', in J. C. Shershow (ed.), *Schizophrenia: Science and Practice*. Cambridge, MA: Harvard University Press.

66. D. Bannister (1968) 'The logical requirements of research into schizophrenia', *British Journal of Psychiatry*, 114: 181–8.

More recent papers and books advocating this approach include: C. G. Costello (1992) 'Research on symptoms versus research on syndromes: arguments in favour of allocating more research time to the study of symptoms', *British Journal of Psychiatry*, 160: 304–8; C. D. Frith (1992) *The Cognitive Neuropsychology of Schizophrenia*. Hillsdale, NJ: Lawrence Erlbaum; J. Persons (1986) 'The advantages of studying psychological phenomena rather than psychiatric diagnoses',

American Psychologist, 41: 1252–60; P. D. Slade and R. Cooper (1979) 'Some conceptual difficulties with the term "schizophrenia": an alternative model', *British Journal of Social and Clinical Psychology*, 18: 309–17.

Earlier attempts by myself to outline the symptom-orientated strategy include: R. P. Bentall, H. F. Jackson and D. Pilgrim (1988) 'Abandoning the concept of schizophrenia: some implications of validity arguments for psychological research into psychotic phenomena', *British Journal of Clinical Psychology*, 27: 303–24.

R. P. Bentall (1990) 'The syndromes and symptoms of psychosis: or why you can't play 20 questions with the concept of schizophrenia and hope to win', in R. P. Bentall (ed.), *Reconstructing Schizophrenia*. London: Routledge.

67. R. Mojtabai and R. O. Rieder (1998) 'Limitations of the symptom-orientated approach to psychiatric research', *British Journal of Psychiatry*, 173: 198–202.

68. M. J. Muller and H. Wetzel (1998) 'Improvement of inter-rater reliability of PANSS items and subscales by a standardized rater training', *Acta Psychiatrica Scandinavica*, 98: 135–9.

69. D. M. Carter, A. Mackinnon, S. Howard, T. Zeegers and D. L. Copolov (1995) 'The development and reliability of the Mental Health Research Institute Unusual Perceptions Schedule (MUPS): an instrument to record auditory hallucinatory experiences', *Schizophrenia Research*, 16: 157–65.

70. G. Haddock, J. McCarron and N. Tarrier (1999) 'Scales to measure dimensions of hallucinations and delusions: the Psychotic Symptom Rating Scale (PSYRATS)', *Psychological Medicine*, 29: 879–89.

71. N. C. Andreasen (1979) 'The clinical assessment of thought, language and communication disorders', *Archives of General Psychiatry*, 36: 1315–21.

72. N. M. Docherty, J. P. Rhinewine, R. P. Labhart and S. Gordinier (1998) 'Communication disturbance and family psychiatric history in parents of schizophrenic patients', *Journal of Nervous and Mental Disease*, 186: 761–8.

Chapter 7   The Significance of Biology

1. Quoted in A. Hodges (1983) *Alan Turing: The Enigma of Intelligence*. London: Burnette Books.

2. Quoted in E. Shorter (1997) *A History of Psychiatry*. New York: Wiley.

3. R. Hunter and I. MacAlpine (1963) *Three Hundred Years of Psychiatry*. London: Hogarth Press.

4. W. Mayer-Gross, E. Slater and M. Roth (1975) *Clinical Psychiatry*. London: Cassell.

5. S. Guze (1989) 'Biological psychiatry: is there any other kind?', *Psychological Medicine*, 19: 315–23.

6. T. S. Szasz (1960) 'The myth of mental illness', *American Psychologist*, 15: 564–80.

7. T. S. Szasz (1992) 'The United States v. drugs', in J. K. Zeig (ed.), *The Evolution*

of Psychotherapy: The Second Conference. New York: Brunner/Mazel Inc., pp. 300–12.

8. T. S. Szasz (1999) *Fatal Freedom: The Ethics and Politics of Suicide.* Westport, CT: Praeger.

9. This quote is from Thomas Szasz's summary statement and manifesto, which can be found on the website of the Thomas S. Szasz MD Cybercenter for Liberty and Responsibility.

10. T. S. Szasz (1979) *Schizophrenia: The Sacred Symbol of Psychiatry.* Oxford: Oxford University Press.

11. F. G. Glaser (1965) 'The dichotomy game: a further consideration of the writings of Dr Thomas Szasz', *American Journal of Psychiatry*, 121: 1069–74.

12. M. Roth (1973) 'Psychiatry and its critics', *British Journal of Psychiatry*, 122: 374.

13. S. Finger (2000) *Minds Behind the Brain: A History of the Pioneers and their Discoveries.* Oxford: Oxford University Press.

14. D. Healy (1997) *The Anti-Depressant Era.* Cambridge, MA: Harvard University Press.

15. E. Kraepelin (1907) *Textbook of Psychiatry*, 7th edn (trans. A. R. Diefendorf) London: Macmillan.

16. P. J. McKenna (1994) *Schizophrenia and Related Syndromes.* Oxford: Oxford University Press.

17. G. W. Roberts (1991) 'Schizophrenia: a neuropathological perspective', *British Journal of Psychiatry*, 158: 8–17.

18. P. J. Harrison (1999) 'The neuropathology of schizophrenia: a critical review of the data and their interpretation', *Brain and Language*, 122: 593–624.

19. See E. H. Burrows (1996) 'A brief history of brain imaging', in S. Lewis and N. Higgins (eds.), *Brain Imaging in Psychiatry.* Oxford: Blackwell, pp. 1–13.

20. E. C. Johnstone, T. J. Crow, C. D. Frith, J. Husband and L. Kreel (1976) 'Cerebral ventricular size and cognitive impairment in chronic schizophrenia', *Lancet*, ii: 924–6.

21. P. W. R. Woodruff and S. Lewis (1996) 'Structural brain imaging in schizophrenia', in Lewis and Higgins (eds.), *Brain Imaging in Psychiatry*, op. cit., pp. 188–214.

22. See, for example, D. Fannon, X. Chitnis, V. Doku, L. Tennakoon, S. O'Ceallaigh, W. Soni, A. Sumich, J. Lowe, M. Santamaria and T. Sharma (2000) 'Features of structural brain abnormality detected in first-episode psychosis', *American Journal of Psychiatry*, 157: 1829–34.

23. Harrison, 'The neuropathology of schizophrenia', op. cit.

24. For systematic reviews of CT and structural MRI studies of schizophrenia, see: S. W. Lewis (1990) 'Computed tomography in schizophrenia, 15 years on', *British Journal of Psychiatry*, 157 (Supplement 9): 16–24 (in this review, significant ventricular enlargement was reported in only nine out of twenty-one studies, and enlargement was marginal in a further three); Woodruff and Lewis, 'Structural brain imaging in schizophrenia', op. cit., pp. 188–214 (in this review, it is reported

that ventricular enlargement was observed in the majority of studies, although the differences between the schizophrenia patients and the controls was statistically significant in only the minority).

25. R. J. Dolan and G. M. Goodwin (1996) 'Brain imaging in affective disorders', in Lewis and Higgins (eds.), *Brain Imaging in Psychiatry*, op. cit., pp. 227–43.

26. S. Raz and N. Raz (1990) 'Structural brain abnormalities in the major psychoses: a quantitative review of the evidence', *Psychological Bulletin*, 108: 93–108.

For two recent studies which have compared and failed to find a difference between schizophrenia and bipolar patients, one using CT and the other using MRI, see: J. Danckert, D. Velakoulis, P. McGorry, N. Bridle, A. Kelman, A. Hoberton and P. Pantelis (1998) 'A CT study of ventricular size in first episode psychosis', *Schizophrenia Research*, 29: 75; S. C. Schulz, L. Friedman, R. Findling, J. Kenny, T. Swales and A. Wise (1998) 'Both schizophrenic and bipolar adolescents differ from controls on MRI measures', *Schizophrenia Research*, 29: 81.

27. G. N. Smith and W. G. Iacano (1986) 'Lateral ventricular enlargement in schizophrenia and choice of control group', *Lancet*, i: 1450.

28. J. D. van Horn and I. C. McManus (1992) 'Ventricular enlargement in schizophrenia: a meta-analysis of studies of ventricular:brain ratio', *British Journal of Psychiatry*, 160: 687–97; P. J. McKenna (1994) *Schizophrenia and Related Syndromes*. Oxford: Oxford University Press.

29. Woodruff and Lewis, 'Structural brain imaging in schizophrenia', op. cit., pp. 188–214.

30. B. K. Piri, N. Saeed, A. Oatridge, J. V. Hajnal, S. B. Hutton, L.-J. Duncan, M. J. Chapman, T. R. E. Barnes, G. M. Bydder and E. M. Joyce (1998) 'A longitudinal MRI study of first-episode schizophrenia: assessment of cerebral changes and quantification of ventricular changes', *Schizophrenia Research*, 29: 76.

31. For example, in most people the two cerebral hemispheres are not quite symmetrical, and the left frontal and right temporal lobes are slightly larger than their opposing anatomical structures. In a recent study (T. M. Sharma, E. Lancaster, T. Sigmundsson et al. (1999) 'Lack of cerebral asymmetry in familial schizophrenic patients and their relatives: the Maudsley family study', *Schizophrenia Research*, 40: 111–20) it was observed that this skew is less marked or is even absent in some schizophrenia patients.

A number of studies have also revealed evidence that the area of the corpus callosum – the large bundle of nerve fibres that connects the two hemispheres – is reduced in schizophrenia patients compared with normal controls (see P. W. R. Woodruff, I. C. McManus and A. S. David (1995) 'Meta-analysis of corpus callosum size in schizophrenia', *Journal of Neurology, Neurosurgery and Psychiatry*, 58: 457–61).

32. See S. Rose (1993) *The Making of Memory: From Molecules to Mind*. London: Bantam.

33. See J. D. Bremner, P. Randall, T. M. Scott, R. A. Bronen, J. P. Seibyl, S. M.

Southwick, R. C. Delaney, G. McCarthy, D. S. Charney and R. D. Innis (1995) 'MRI-based measurement of hippocampal volume in patients with combat-related posttraumatic stress disorder', *American Journal of Psychiatry*, 152: 973–81; and also M. B. Stein, C. Koverola, C. Hanna, M. G. Torchia and B. McClarty (1997) 'Hippocampal volume in women victimized by child sexual abuse', *Psychological Medicine*, 27: 951–9.

34. M. H. Teicher (2000) 'Brain abnormalities common in survivors of childhood abuse', *Cerebrum*, 2: 50–67.

35. E. A. Maguire, D. G. Gadian, I. S. Johnsrude, C. D. Good, J. Ashburner, R. S. J. Frackowiak and C. D. Frith (2000) 'Navigation-related structural changes in the hippocampi of taxi drivers', *Proceedings of the National Academy of Science*.

36. My account of the work by Mosso is taken from M. Posner and M. E. Raichle (1994) *Images of Mind*. New York: Scientific American Library.

37. S. W. Lewis (1996) 'Functional brain imaging', in Lewis and Higgins (eds.), *Brain Imaging in Psychiatry*, op. cit., pp. 108–15.

38. M. S. Keshavan and J. D. Cohen (1996) 'Magnetic resonance spectroscopy and functional MRI', in Lewis and Higgins (eds.), *Brain Imaging in Psychiatry*, op. cit., pp. 116–37.

39. P. Flor-Henry (1969) 'Psychosis and temporal lobe epilepsy: a controlled investigation', *Epilepsia*, 10: 365–95.

40. P. Green (1978) 'Interhemispheric transfer in schizophrenia: recent developments', *Behavioural Psychotherapy*, 6: 105–10.

41. T. Crow (1991) 'The origins of psychosis and "The descent of man"', *British Journal of Psychiatry*, 159 (Supplement 14): 76–82; T. Crow (1995) 'A Darwinian approach to the origins of psychosis', *British Journal of Psychiatry*, 167: 12–25.

42. T. J. Crow (1998) 'Nuclear schizophrenic symptoms as the key to the evolution of modern homo sapiens', in S. Rose (ed.), *From Brains to Consciousness: Essays on the New Sciences of the Mind*. London: Penguin, pp. 137–53.

43. P. Satz and M. F. Green (1999) 'Atypical handedness in schizophrenia: some methodological and theoretical issues', *Schizophrenia Bulletin*, 25: 63–78.

44. Sharma et al., 'Lack of cerebral asymmetry', op. cit.

45. R. E. Gur (1999) 'Is schizophrenia a lateralized brain disorder?: Editor's introduction', *Schizophrenia Bulletin*, 25: 7–9.

46. J. H. Gruzelier (1999) 'Functional neuropsychological asymmetry in schizophrenia: a review and reorientation', *Schizophrenia Bulletin*, 25: 91–120.

47. D. H. Ingvar and G. Franzen (1974) 'Abnormalities of cerebral blood flow distribution in patients with chronic schizophrenia', *Acta Psychiatrica Scandinavica*, 50: 425–62.

48. P. F. Liddle (1996) 'Functional imaging in schizophrenia', in Lewis and Higgins (eds.), *Brain Imaging in Psychiatry*, op. cit., pp. 215–26.

49. D. R. Weinberger, K. F. Berman and R. F. Zec (1986) 'Physiologic dysfunction of dorsolateral prefrontal cortex in schizophrenia: I. Regional blood flow evidence', *Archives of General Psychiatry*, 45: 609–15.

50. R. Erkwoh, O. Sabri, K. Willmes, E. M. Steinmeyer, U. Buell and H. Sass

(1999) 'Active and remitted schizophrenia: psychopathological and regional cerebral blood flow findings', *Psychiatry Research: Neuroimaging*, 90: 17–30; S. A. Spence, S. R. Hirsch, D. J. Brooks and P. M. Grasby (1998) 'Prefrontal cortex activity in people with schizophrenia and control subjects: evidence from positron emission tomography for remission of "hypofrontality" with recovery from acute schizophrenia', *British Journal of Psychiatry*, 172: 316–23.

51. G. D. Pearlson (1999) 'Structural and functional brain changes in bipolar disorder: a selective review', *Schizophrenia Research*, 39: 133–40.

52. R. Penades, T. Boget, F. Lomena, M. Bernardo, J. J. Mateos, C. Laterza, J. Pavia and M. Salamero (2000) 'Brain perfusion and neuropsychological changes in schizophrenia patients after cognitive rehabilitation', *Psychiatry Research: Neuroimaging*, 98: 127–32.

53. M. H. Teicher (2000) 'Brain abnormalities common in survivors of childhood abuse', *Cerebrum*, 2: 50–67.

54. M. Trimble (1996) *Biological Psychiatry* (2nd edn). Chichester: Wiley.

55. Quoted in R. M. Julien (1975) *A Primer of Drug Action*. San Francisco, CA: Freeman.

56. D. E. Wooley and E. Shaw (1954) 'A biochemical and pharmacological suggestion about certain mental disorders', *Proceedings of the National Academy of Sciences USA*, 40: 228–31.

57. A. Friedhoff and E. van Winkle (1962) 'The characteristics of an amine found in the urine of schizophrenic patients', *Journal of Nervous and Mental Disease*, 135: 550.

58. G. S. Claridge (1978) 'Animal models of schizophrenia: the case for LSD-25', *Schizophrenia Bulletin*, 4: 186–209. Interestingly, there has recently been a revival of interest in the role of serotonin in the symptoms of schizophrenia, probably because of persisting lack of evidence in favour of the dopamine hypothesis. For example, it has been reported that there is an unusual distribution of serotonin receptors in the frontal cortex of some psychotic patients (see F. Owen and M. D. C. Simpson (1995) 'The neurochemistry of schizophrenia', in S. R. Hirsch and D. R. Weinberger (eds.), *Schizophrenia*. Oxford: Blackwell, pp. 358–78).

59. R. K. Siegel and M. E. Jarvick (1975) 'Drug-induced hallucinations in animals and man', in R. K. Siegel and L. J. West (eds.), *Hallucinations: Behavior, Experience and Theory*. New York: Wiley.

60. A. Carlsson and M. Lindqvist (1963) 'Effect of chlorpromazine or haloperidol on formation of 3-methoxytyramine and normetanephrine in mouse brain', *Acta Pharmacologica et Toxicologica*, 20: 140–4.

61. For details of these and other milestones in the development of the dopamine hypothesis, see P. J. McKenna (1994) *Schizophrenia and Related Syndromes*. Oxford: Oxford University Press.

62. P. Connell (1958) *Amphetamine Psychosis*. London: Chapman & Hall. For a recent study which has reported similar observations, see D. Harris and S. L. Bakti (2000) 'Stimulant psychosis: symptom profile and acute clinical course', *American Journal of Addictions*, 9: 28–37.

63. B. M. Angrist and S. Gershon (1970) 'The phenomenology of experimentally induced amphetamine psychosis: preliminary observations', *Biological Psychiatry*, 2: 95–107.

64. A. Carlsson (1995) 'The dopamine theory revisited', in Hirsch and Weinberger (eds.), *Schizophrenia*, op. cit.

65. Trimble, *Biological Psychiatry*, op. cit.

66. W. A. Brown and L. R. Herz (1989) 'Response to neuroleptic drugs as a device for classifying schizophrenia', *Schizophrenia Bulletin*, 15: 123–8.

67. H. J. Coppens, C. J. Sloof, A. M. J. Paans, T. Wiegman, W. Vaalburg and J. Korf (1991) 'High central D2-dopamine receptor occupancy as assessed with positron emission tomography in medicated but therapy-resistant patients', *Biological Psychiatry*, 29: 629–34.

68. The first and most extensively researched of these is clozapine, which is thought to have a low affinity for the DA_2 receptor. Whether or not it has sufficient affinity to account for its anti-psychotic effects is a matter of controversy, and is discussed in McKenna, *Schizophrenia and Related Syndromes*, op. cit.

For a recent study demonstrating low DA_2 receptor affinity of another atypical neuroleptic, quetiapine, see S. Kapur, R. Zipursky, C. Jones, C. S. Shammi, G. Remington and P. Seeman (2000) 'A positron emission tomography study of quetiapine in schizophrenia: a preliminary finding of an antipsychotic effect with only transiently high dopamine D-sub-2 receptor occupancy', *Archives of General Psychiatry*, 57: 553–9.

69. McKenna, *Schizophrenia and Related Syndromes*, op. cit.

70. A. Clow, P. Jenner, A. Theodorou and C. D. Marsden (1979) 'Neuroleptic drugs and the dopamine hypothesis', *Lancet*, i: 934.

71. McKenna, *Schizophrenia and Related Syndromes*, op. cit.

72. D. F. Wong, H. N. Wagner, L. E. Tune, R. F. Dannals, G. D. Pearlson and J. M. Links (1986) 'Positron emission tomography reveals elevated D2 dopamine receptors in drug-naive schizophrenics', *Science*, 234: 1558–63.

73. L. Fadre, F. A. Wiesel, H. Hall, C. Halldin, S. Stone-Elander and G. Sedvall (1987) 'No D2 receptor increase in PET study of schizophrenia', *Archives of General Psychiatry*, 44: 671–2.

74. G. D. Pearlson, D. F. Wong, L. E. Tune, C. A. Ross, G. A. Chase, J. M. Links, R. F. Dannals, A. A. Wilson, H. Ravert, H. N. Wagner and J. R. DePaulo (1995) 'In vivo D-sub-2 dopamine receptor density in psychotic and nonpsychotic patients with bipolar disorder', *Archives of General Psychiatry*, 52: 471–7.

75. E. K. G. Syvaelahti, V. Raekkoelaeinen, J. Aaltonen, V. Lehtinen and J. Hietala (2000) 'Striatal D-sub-2 dopamine receptor density and psychotic symptoms in schizophrenia: a longitudinal study', *Schizophrenia Research*, 43: 159–61.

76. Trimble, *Biological Psychiatry*, op. cit.

77. S. Rose (1984) 'Disordered molecules and diseased minds', *Journal of Psychiatric Research*, 18: 351–60.

78. M. Laruelle and A. Abi-Dargham (1999) 'Dopamine as the wind in the psychotic fire: new evidence from brain imaging studies', *Journal of Psycho-*

pharmacology, 13: 358–71; M. Laruelle, A. Abi-Dargham, R. Gil, L. Kegeles and R. Innis (1999) 'Increased dopamine transmission in schizophrenia: relationship to illness phases', *Biological Psychiatry*, 46: 56–72.

79. M. B. Hamner and P. B. Gold (1998) 'Plasma dopamine beta-hydroxylase activity in psychotic and non-psychotic post-traumatic stress disorder', *Psychiatry Research*, 77: 175–81.

80. P. Sedgwick (1982) *Psychopolitics*. London: Pluto Press.

81. K. W. M. Fulford (2002) 'Values in psychiatric diagnosis: executive summary of a report to the chair of the ICD-12/DSM-VI coordination taskforce (dateline 2010)', *Psychopathology*, 35: 132–8.

82. T. L. Beauchamp and J. F. Childress (1979) *Principles of Biomedical Ethics*. Oxford: Oxford University Press; R. Gillon (1985) *Philsophical Medical Ethics*. London: Wiley.

Chapter 8   Mental Life and Human Nature

1. L. Wittgenstein (1980) *Culture and Value* (trans. P. Winch). Oxford: Blackwell.

2. D. Shakow and P. E. Huston (1936) 'Studies of motor function in schizophrenia: I. Speed of tapping', *Journal of General Psychology*, 15: 63–108.

3. A. J. W. van der Does and R. J. van den Bosch (1992) 'What determines Wisconsin Card Sorting performance in schizophrenia?', *Clinical Psychology Review*, 12: 567–83.

4. W.-C. C. Tam, K. W. Sewell and H.-W. Deng (1998) 'Information processing in schizophrenia and bipolar disorder: a discriminant analysis', *Journal of Nervous and Mental Disease*, 186: 597–603.

5. A. S. Bellack, K. T. Mueser, R. L. Morrison, A. Tierney and K. Podell (1990) 'Remediation of cognitive deficits in schizophrenia', *American Journal of Psychiatry*, 147: 1650–5; M. F. Green, P. Satz, S. Ganzell and J. F. Vaclav (1992) 'Wisconsin Card Sorting Test performance in schizophrenia: remediation of a stubborn deficit', *American Journal of Psychiatry*, 149: 62–7; H. Nisbet, R. Siegert, M. Hunt and N. Fairley (1996) 'Improving schizophrenic in-patients' Wisconsin card-sorting performance', *British Journal of Clinical Psychology*, 35: 631–3.

6. H. E. Spohn and M. E. Strauss (1989) 'Relation of neuroleptic and anticholinergic medication to cognitive functions in schizophrenia', *Journal of Abnormal Psychology*, 98: 367–80.

7. L. J. Chapman and J. P. Chapman (1973) *Disordered Thought in Schizophrenia*. Englewood Cliffs, NJ: Prentice-Hall.

8. R. P. Bentall (1992) 'Psychological deficits and biases in psychiatric disorders', *Current Opinion in Psychiatry*, 5: 825–30.

9. E. Kraepelin (1899/1990) *Psychiatry: A Textbook for Students and Physicians*. Vol. 1: *General Psychiatry*. Canton, MA: Watson Publishing International, p. 89.

10. A. McGhie and J. Chapman (1961) 'Disorders of attention and perception in early schizophrenia', *British Journal of Medical Psychology*, 34: 103–16.

11. See, for example, Chapman and Chapman, *Disordered Thought*, op. cit.

12. T. F. Oltmanns and J. M. Neale (1978) 'Distractability in relation to other aspects of schizophrenic disorder', in S. Schwartz (ed.), *Language and Cognition in Schizophrenia*. Hillsdale, NJ: Erlbaum.

13. M. R. Serper, M. Davidson and P. Harvey (1994) 'Attentional predictors of clinical change during neuroleptic treatment in schizophrenia', *Schizophrenia Research*, 13: 65–71.

14. M. F. Green (1992) 'Information processing in schizophrenia', in D. J. Kavanagh (ed.), *Schizophrenia: An Overview and Practical Handbook*. London: Chapman and Hall.

15. K. H. Nuechterlein, R. Parasuraman and Q. Jiang (1983) 'Visual sustained attention: image degradation produces rapid sensitivity decrement over time', *Science*, 220: 327–9. See also K. H. Nuechterlein (1991) 'Vigilance in schizophrenia and related disorders', in S. R. Steinhauer, J. H. Gruzelier and J. Zubin (eds.), *Handbook of Schizophrenia*, Vol. 5: *Neuropsychology, Psychophysiology, and Information Processing*. Amsterdam: Elsevier.

16. K. H. Nuechterlein, W. S. Edell, M. Norris and M. E. Dawson (1986) 'Attentional vulnerability indicators, thought disorder and negative symptoms', *Schizophrenia Bulletin*, 12: 408–26; R. W. Buchanan, M. E. Strauss, A. Breier, B. Kirkpatrick and W. T. Carpenter (1997) 'Attentional impairments in deficit and nondeficit forms of schizophrenia', *American Journal of Psychiatry*, 154: 363–70.

17. Green, 'Information processing in schizophrenia', op. cit.

18. D. P. Saccuzzo and D. L. Braff (1981) 'Early information processing deficit in schizophrenia', *Archives of General Psychiatry*, 38: 175–9.

19. D. L. Braff and D. P. Saccuzzo (1982) 'Effect of antipsychotic medication on speed of information processing in schizophrenia patients', *American Journal of Psychiatry*, 139: 1127–30.

20. K. H. Nuechterlein and K. L. Subotnik (1998) 'The cognitive origins of schizophrenia and prospects for intervention', in T. Wykes, N. Tarrier and S. Lewis (eds.), *Outcome and Innovation in Psychological Treatment of Schizophrenia*. Chichester: Wiley.

21. T. F. Oltmanns (1978) 'Selective attention in schizophrenic and manic psychoses: the effect of distraction on information processing', *Journal of Abnormal Psychology*, 87: 212–25.

22. K. Fleming and M. F. Green (1995) 'Backward masking performance during and after manic episodes', *Journal of Abnormal Psychology*, 104: 63–8.

23. M. R. Serper (1993) 'Visual controlled information processing resources and formal thought disorder in schizophrenia and mania', *Schizophrenia Research*, 9: 59–66; J. McGrath, B. Chapple and M. Wright (1998) 'Working memory in schizophrenia and mania: acute and subacute phases', *Schizophrenia Research*, 29: 48.

24. K. Nuechterlein, M. Dawson, J. Ventura, D. Miklowitz and G. Konishi (1991) 'Information processing abnormalities in the early course of schizophrenia and

bipolar disorder', *Schizophrenia Research*, 5: 195–6; K. W. Sax, S. M. Strakowski, S. L. McElroy, P. E. Keck and S. A. West (1995) 'Attention and formal thought disorder in mixed and pure mania', *Biological Psychiatry*, 37: 420–23.

25. E. B. Nelson, K. W. Sax and S. M. Strakowski (1998) 'Attentional performance in patients with psychotic and nonpsychotic major depression and schizophrenia', *American Journal of Psychiatry*, 155: 137–9.

26. M. F. Green (1998) *Schizophrenia from a Neurocognitive Perspective: Probing the Impenetrable Darkness*. Boston: Allyn & Bacon.

27. H. J. Jerison (1985) 'On the evolution of mind', in D. A. Oakley (ed.), *Brain and Mind*. London: Methuen.

28. R. I. M. Dunbar (1993) 'Coevolution of neocortical size, group size and language in humans', *Behavioral and Brain Sciences*, 16: 681–735.

29. L. Brothers (1997) *Friday's Footprint: How Society Shapes the Human Mind*. Oxford: Oxford University Press.

30. J. Le Doux (1996) *The Emotional Brain: The Mysterious Underpinnings of Emotional Life*. New York: Simon & Schuster.

31. J. Piaget and B. Inhelder (1956) *The Child's Conception of Space*. London: Routledge & Kegan Paul.

32. M. Donaldson (1978) *Children's Minds*. London: Fontana.

33. F. Happé (1994) *Autism: An Introduction to Psychological Theory*. London: University College London Press.

34. S. Baron-Cohen, H. Tager-Flusberg and D. J. Cohen (1993) *Understanding Other Minds: Perspectives from Autism*. Oxford: Oxford University Press.

35. P. Hobson (2002) *The Cradle of Thought*. London: Macmillan.

36. M. Boyes, R. Giorano and M. Pool (1997) 'Internalization of social discourse: a Vygotskian account of the development of young children's theories of mind', in B. D. Cox and C. Lightfoot (eds.), *Sociogenetic Perspectives on Internalization*. Mahwah, NJ: Erlbaum.

37. Happé, *Autism*, op. cit.

38. S. Baron-Cohen (1995) *Mindblindness: An Essay on Autism and Theory of Mind*. Cambridge, MA: MIT Press.

39. J. A. Fodor (1983) *The Modularity of Mind: An Essay on Faculty Psychology*. Cambridge, MA: MIT Press.

40. P. Nichelli, J. Grafman, P. Pietrini, D. Alway, J. C. Carton and R. Miletich (1994) 'Brain activity in chess playing', *Nature*, 369: 191.

41. J. L. Elman, E. A. Bates, M. H. Johnson, A. Karmiloff-Smith, D. Parisi and K. Plunkett (1999) *Rethinking Innateness: A Connectionist Perspective on Development*. Cambridge, MA: MIT Press.

42. D. Bickerton (1995) *Language and Human Behaviour*. Seattle, WA: University of Washington Press.

43. E. Hoff (2000) *Language Development* (2nd edn). London: Wadsworth.

44. S. Pinker (1994) *The Language Instinct*. London: Penguin.

45. R. I. M. Dunbar (1997) *Grooming, Gossip and the Evolution of Language*. London: Faber & Faber.

46. S. Pinker and P. Bloom (1990) 'Natural language and natural selection', *Behavioral and Brain Sciences*, 13: 707–84.

47. L. S. V. Vygotsky (1962) *Thought and Language*. Cambridge, MA: MIT Press.

48. J. V. Wetsch and C. A. Stone (1985) 'The concept of internalization in Vygotsky's account of the genesis of internal mental functions', in J. V. Wertsch (ed.), *Culture, Communication and Cognition: Vygotskyian Perspectives*. Cambridge: Cambridge University Press, pp. 162–79.

49. J. Piaget (1926) *The Language and Thought of the Child*. London: Routledge & Kegan Paul.

50. R. M. Diaz and L. E. Berk (eds.) (1992) *Private Speech: From Social Integration to Self-Regulation*. Hillsdale, NJ: Erlbaum.

51. L. E. Berk (1994) 'Why children talk to themselves', *Scientific American*, November: 61–5.

52. K. A. Ericsson and H. A. Simon (1998) 'How to study thinking in everyday life: contrasting think-aloud protocols with descriptions and explanations of thinking', *Mind, Culture and Activity*, 5: 178–86.

53. R. J. Korba (1990) 'The rate of inner speech', *Perceptual and Motor Skills*, 71: 1043–52.

54. A. Morin and J. Everett (1990) 'Inner speech as a mediator of self-awareness, self-consciousness and self-knowledge: an hypothesis', *New Ideas in Psychology*, 8: 337–56.

55. I have been unable to find recent reviews of the subvocalization literature, which has been largely ignored by modern cognitive psychologists. However, for a detailed account of the large volume of research conducted on this topic before the mid-1970s, see F. J. McGuigan (1978) *Cognitive Psychophysiology: Principles of Covert Behavior*. Englewood Cliffs, NJ: Prentice-Hall.

56. F. J. McGuigan (1971) 'Covert linguistic behavior in deaf subjects during thinking', *Journal of Comparative and Physiological Psychology*, 75: 417–20.

57. J. T. Cacioppo (1982) 'Social psychophysiology: a classic perspective and contemporary approach', *Psychophysiology*, 19: 241–51; J. T. Cacioppo and R. E. Petty (1981) 'Electromyograms as measures of extent of affectivity and information processing', *American Psychologist*, 36: 441–56.

58. R. F. Baumeister (1999) 'The nature and structure of the self: an overview', in R. F. Baumeister (ed.), *The Self in Social Psychology*. Philadelphia, PA: Psychology Press, pp. 1–20.

59. D. C. Dennett (1991) *Consciousness Explained*. London: Allen Lane.

60. S. T. Fiske and S. E. Taylor (1991). *Social Cognition*. New York: McGraw-Hill.

61. C. Trevarthen (1993) 'The self born in intersubjectivity: the psychology of an infant communicating', in U. Neisser (ed.), *The Perceived Self: Ecological and Interpersonal Sources of Self-Knowledge*. Cambridge: Cambridge University Press.

62. R. F. Baumeister (1987) 'How the self became a problem: a psychological review of historical research', *Journal of Personality and Social Psychology*, 52: 163–76.

63. A. P. Cohen (1994) *Self-Conscious: An Alternative Anthropology of Identity*. London: Routledge.

64. H. Markus and S. Kitayama (1991) 'Culture and the self: implications for cognition, emotion, and motivation', *Psychological Review*, 98: 224–53.

65. T. T. J. Kircher, C. Senior, M. Phillips, P. J. Benson, E. T. Bullmore, M. Brammer, A. Simmons, S. C. R. Williams and A. S. David (2000) 'Towards a functional neuroanatomy of self-processing effects of faces and words', *Cognition and Brain Research*, 10: 133–44; T. T. J. Kircher, C. Senior, M. Phillips, S. Rabe-Hesketh, P. J. Benson, E. T. Bullmore, M. Brammer, A. Simmons, M. Bartels and A. S. David (2000) 'Recognizing one's own face', *Cognition*, 78: B1–B15.

66. T. J. Crow (1998) 'Nuclear schizophrenic symptoms as the key to the evolution of modern homo sapiens', in S. Rose (ed.), *From Brains to Consciousness: Essays on the New Sciences of the Mind*. London: Penguin, pp. 137–53.

67. For a review, see D. L. Penn, P. W. Corrigan, R. P. Bentall, J. M. Racenstein and L. Newman (1997) 'Social cognition in schizophrenia', *Psychological Bulletin*, 121: 114–32.

68. M. Musalek, P. Berner and H. Katschnig (1989) 'Delusional theme, sex and age', *Psychopathology*, 22: 260–7.

Chapter 9 Madness and Emotion

1. D. Hume (1739–40/1888) *A Treatise of Human Nature*. Oxford: Oxford University Press.

2. D. Goldberg and P. Huxley (1992) *Common Mental Disorders: A Bio-social Model*. London: Routledge.

3. S. G. Siris (1995) 'Depression and schizophrenia', in S. R. Hirsch and D. R. Weinberger (eds.), *Schizophrenia*. Oxford: Blackwell.

4. J. D. Huppert and T. E. Smith (2001) 'Longitudinal analysis of subjective quality of life in schizophrenia: anxiety as the best symptom predictor', *Journal of Nervous and Mental Disease*, 189: 669–75; R. Emsley, P. Oosthuizen, D. Niehaus and D. Stein (2001) 'Anxiety symptoms in schizophrenia: the need for heightened clinical awareness', *Primary Care Psychiatry*, 7: 25–9.

5. R. M. G. Norman and A. K. Malla (1991) 'Dysphoric mood and symptomatology in schizophrenia', *Psychological Medicine*, 21: 897–903.

6. M. I. Herz and C. Melville (1980) 'Relapse in schizophrenia', *American Journal of Psychiatry*, 127: 801–12.

7. M. Birchwood, J. Smith, F. Macmillan, B. Hogg, R. Prasad, C. Harvey and S. Bering (1989) 'Predicting relapse in schizophrenia: the development and implementation of an early signs monitoring system using patients and families as observers', *Psychological Medicine*, 19: 649–56.

8. N. M. Docherty (1996) 'Affective reactivity of symptoms as a process discriminator in schizophrenia', *Journal of Nervous and Mental Disease*, 184: 535–41.

9. M. Power and T. Dalgleish (1996) *Cognition and Emotion: From Order to Disorder*. London: Psychology Press.

10. R. Zajonc (1980) 'Feeling and thinking: preferences need no inferences', *American Psychologist*, 35: 151–75.

11. R. S. Lazarus (1984) 'On the primacy of cognition', *American Psychologist*, 39: 124–9.

12. A. Sloman (1987) 'Motives, mechanisms and emotions', *Cognition and Emotion*, 1: 217–33.

13. A. Mellers, A. Schwartz, K. Ho and I. Ritov (1997) 'Decision affect theory: emotional reactions to outcomes of risky options', *Psychological Science*, 8: 423–9.

14. L. C. Charland (1998) 'Is Mr. Spock mentally competent?' *Philosophy, Psychiatry and Psychology*, 5: 67–80.

15. J. Tooby and L. Cosmides (1990) 'The past explains the present: emotional adaptations and the structure of ancestral environments', *Ethology and Sociobiology*, 11: 375–424.

16. P. Gilbert (1992) *Depression: The Evolution of Powerlessness*. Hove: Erlbaum.

17. See, for example, I. Eibl-Eibesfeldt (1970) *Ethology: The Biology of Behavior*. New York: Holt, Rinehart & Winston; or P. Ekman (1992) 'An argument for basic emotions', *Cognition and Emotion*, 6: 169–200.

18. See, for example, Ekman, 'An argument for basic emotions', op. cit.; and also P. Ekman (1994) 'Strong evidence for universals in facial expression: a reply to Russell's mistaken critique', *Psychological Bulletin*, 115: 268–87.

19. J. A. Russell (1994) 'Is there universal recognition of emotion from facial expression? A review of the cross-cultural studies', *Psychological Bulletin*, 115: 102–41.

20. B. F. Skinner (1945) 'The operational analysis of psychological terms', *Psychological Review*, 52: 270–7.

21. W. James (1890) *The Principles of Psychology* (2 vols). New York: George Holt.

22. D. Zillman, R. C. Johnson and K. D. Day (1974) 'Attribution of apparent arousal and proficiency of recovery from sympathetic activation affecting excitation transfer to aggressive behavior', *Journal of Experimental Social Psychology*, 10: 503–15.

23. W. Winton (1986) 'The role of facial response in self-reports of emotion: a critique of Laird', *Journal of Personality and Social Psychology*, 50: 808–12.

24. R. B. Zajonc, S. T. Murphy and M. Ingelhart (1989) 'Feeling and facial efference: implications of the vascular feeling of emotion', *Psychological Review*, 96: 395–416.

25. See, for example, Power and Dalgleish, *Cognition and Emotion*, op. cit.

26. L. Wittgenstein (1953) *Philosophical Investigations*. London: Blackwell. See also D. Bloor (1983) *Wittgenstein: A Social Theory of Knowledge*. London: Macmillan (especially Chapter 4) for a very clear exposition of Wittgenstein's approach to private stimuli.

27. Skinner, 'The operational analysis of psychological terms', op. cit.

28. G. Richards (1989) *On Psychological Language and the Physiomorphic Basis of Human Nature*. London: Routledge.

29. G. E. Berrios (1995) 'Mood disorders', in G. E. Berrios and R. Porter (eds.), *A History of Clinical Psychiatry*. London: Athlone Press.

30. J. A. Russell (1991) 'Culture and categorization of emotions', *Psychological Bulletin*, 110: 426–50.

31. J. A. Russell and J. M. Carroll (1999) 'On the bipolarity of positive and negative affect', *Psychological Bulletin*, 125: 3–30.

32. D. Watson and A. Tellegren (1985) 'Towards a consensual structure of mood', *Psychological Bulletin*, 98: 219–35.

33. J. T. Cacioppo and W. L. Gardner (1999) 'Emotion', *Annual Review of Psychology*, 50: 191–214.

34. B. Parkinson, P. Totterdell, R. B. Briner and S. Reynolds (1996) *Changing Moods: The Psychology of Mood and Mood Regulation*. Harlow: Longman.

35. J. T. Larsen, A. P. McGraw and J. T. Cacioppo (2001) 'Can people feel happy and sad at the same time?' *Journal of Personality and Social Psychology*, 81: 684–96.

36. See, for example, L. A. Clark, D. Watson and S. Reynolds (1995) 'Diagnosis and classification of psychopathology: challenges to the current system and future directions', *Annual Review of Psychology*, 46: 121–53; also, Goldberg and Huxley, *Common Mental Disorders*, op. cit.; and P. Tyrer (1990) 'The division of neurosis: a failed classification', *Journal of the Royal Society of Medicine*, 83: 614–16.

37. W. Eaton and C. Ritter (1988) 'Distinguishing anxiety from depression with field survey data', *Psychological Medicine*, 18: 155–66.

38. Goldberg and Huxley, *Common Mental Disorders*, op. cit.

39. J. Angst (1990) 'Depression and anxiety: a review of studies in the community and in primary care', in N. Sartorius, D. Goldberg, G. de Girolmano, J. Costa e Silva, Y. LeCrubier and H.-U. Wittchen (eds.), *Psychological Disorders in General Medical Settings*. Bern: Huber-Hogrefe.

40. Clark, Watson and Reynolds, 'Diagnosis and classification of psychopathology', op. cit.

41. D. Watson, L. A. Clark, K. Weber, J. S. Assenheimer, M. E. Strauss and R. A. McCormick (1995) 'Testing a tripartite model: II. Exploring the symptom structure of anxiety and depression in student, adult, and patient samples', *Journal of Abnormal Psychology*, 104: 15–25; and idem, (1995) 'Testing a tripartite model: I. Evaluating the convergent and discriminant validity of anxiety and depression symptom scales', *Journal of Abnormal Psychology*, 104: 3–14.

42. N. C. Andreasen (1989) 'Scale for the Assessment of Negative Symptoms (SANS)', *British Journal of Psychiatry*, 155 (Supplement 7), 53–8.

43. L. J. Chapman, J. P. Chapman and M. L. Raulin (1976) 'Scales for physical and social anhedonia', *Journal of Abnormal Psychology*, 85: 374–82.

44. J. K. Wing and G. W. Brown (1970) *Institutionalism and Schizophrenia*. London: Cambridge University Press.

45. P. Barham and R. Hayward (1990) 'Schizophrenia as a life process', in R. P. Bentall (ed.), *Reconstructing Schizophrenia*. London: Routledge.

46. R. Warner (1985) *Recovery from Schizophrenia: Psychiatry and Political Economy*. New York: Routledge & Kegan Paul.

47. E. C. Johnstone, D. G. C. Owens, A. Gold, T. Crow and J. F. MacMillan (1981) 'Institutionalization and the defects of schizophrenia', *British Journal of Psychiatry*, 139: 195–203.

48. T. Lewander (1994) 'Neuroleptics and the neuroleptic-induced deficit syndrome', *Acta Psychiatrica Scandinavica*, 89: 8–13; N. R. Schooler (1994) 'Deficit symptoms in schizophrenia: negative symptoms versus neuroleptic-induced deficits', *Acta Psychiatrica Scandinavica*, 89: 21–6.

49. M. Harrow, C. A. Yonan, J. R. Sands and J. Marengo (1994) 'Depression in schizophrenia: are neuroleptics, akinesia or anhedonia involved?' *Schizophrenia Bulletin*, 20: 327–38.

50. Norman and Malla, 'Dysphoric mood and symptomatology', op. cit.

51. S. R. Hirsch, A. G. Jolley, T. E. Barnes, P. F. Liddle, D. A. Curson, A. Patel, A. York, S. Bercu and M. Patel (1989) 'Dysphoric and depressive symptoms in schizophrenia', *Schizophrenia Research*, 2: 259–64.

52. M. F. Pogue-Geile and M. Harrow (1987) 'Negative symptoms in schizophrenia: longitudinal characteristics and etiological hypotheses', in P. D. Harvey and E. F. Walker (eds.), *Positive and Negative Symptoms of Psychosis: Description, Research and Future Directions*. Hillsdale, NJ: Erlbaum.

53. W. T. Carpenter, D. W. Heinrichs and A. M. I. Wagman (1988) 'Deficit and nondeficit forms of schizophrenia', *American Journal of Psychiatry*, 145: 578–83.

54. B. Kirkpatrick, R. W. Buchanan, P. D. McKenney, L. D. Alphs and W. T. Carpenter (1989) 'The Schedule for the Deficit Syndrome: an instrument for research in schizophrenia', *Psychiatry Research*, 30: 119–23.

55. J. K. Bouricius (1989) 'Negative symptoms and schizophrenia', *Schizophrenia Bulletin*, 15: 201–7.

56. H. Berenbaum and T. F. Oltmanns (1992) 'Emotional experience and expression in schizophrenia and depression', *Journal of Abnormal Psychology*, 101: 37–44.

57. A. M. Kring, S. L. Kerr, D. A. Smith and J. M. Neale (1993) 'Flat affect does not reflect diminished subjective experience of emotion', *Journal of Abnormal Psychology*, 102: 507–17.

58. I. Myin-Germeys, P. A. E. G. Delespaul and M. W. deVries (2000) 'Schizophrenia patients are more emotionally active than is assumed based on their behaviour', *Schizophrenia Bulletin*, 26: 847–53.

59. C. E. Sison, M. Alpert, R. Fudge and R. M. Stern (1996) 'Constricted expressiveness and psychological reactivity in schizophrenia', *Journal of Nervous and Mental Disease*, 184: 589–97.

60. M. Mayer, M. Alpert, P. Stastny, D. Perlick and M. Empfield (1985) 'Multiple contributions to clinical presentation of flat affect in schizophrenia', *Schizophrenia Bulletin*, 11: 420–6.

61. J. J. Blanchard, A. Kring, J. M. Neale (1994) 'Flat affect and deficits in affective expression in schizophrenia: a test of neuropsychological models', *Schizophrenia Bulletin*, 20: 311–25.

62. For a summary of this work, see H. Ellgring and S. Smith (1998) 'Affect regulation during psychosis', in F. W. Flack and D. J. Laird (eds.), *Emotions in Psychopathology: Theory and Research*. New York: Oxford University Press.

63. S. Rado (1956) *Psychoanalysis of Behaviour: Collected Papers* (2 vols). New York: Grune & Stratton.

64. P. Meehl (1962) 'Schizotaxia, schizotypia, schizophrenia', *American Psychologist*, 17: 827–38.

65. M. Harrow, R. R. Grinker, P. S. Holzman and L. Kayton (1977) 'Anhedonia and schizophrenia', *American Journal of Psychiatry*, 134: 794–7.

66. J. Katsanis, W. G. Iacono and M. Beiser (1990) 'Anhedonia and perceptual aberration in first-episode psychotic patients and their relatives', *Journal of Abnormal Psychology*, 99: 202–6.

67. J. J. Blanchard, A. S. Bellack and K. T. Mueser (1994) 'Affective and social correlates of physical and social anhedonia in schizophrenia', *Journal of Abnormal Psychology*, 103: 719–28.

68. J. Katsanis, W. G. Iacono, M. Beiser and L. Lacey (1992) 'Clinical correlates of anhedonia and perceptual aberration in first-episode patients with schizophrenia and affective disorders', *Journal of Abnormal Psychology*, 101: 184–91.

69. J. J. Blanchard, K. T. Mueser and A. S. Bellack (1998) 'Anhedonia, positive and negative affect and social functioning in schizophrenia', *Schizophrenia Bulletin*, 24: 413–24.

70. L. Ciompi (1988) *The Psyche and Schizophrenia: The Bond between Affect and Logic*. Cambridge, MA: Harvard University Press; L. Ciompi (1998) 'Is schizophrenia an affective disease?' in W. F. Flack and J. D. Laird (eds.), *Emotions in Psychopathology*, New York: Oxford University Press.

Chapter 10   Depression and the Pathology of Self

1. D. L. Rosenhan and M. E. P. Seligman (1989) *Abnormal Psychology* (2nd edn). New York: W. W. Norton.

2. A. Kleinman (1988) *Rethinking Psychiatry*. New York: Free Press.

3. R. A. Shweder (1991) *Thinking through Cultures: Expeditions in Cultural Psychology*. Cambridge, MA: Harvard University Press.

4. M. MacLachlan (1997) *Culture and Health*. London: Wiley.

5. P. Snaith (1995) 'Depression: a need for new directions in practice and research', *Journal of Psychosomatic Research*, 39: 943–7; D. Pilgrim and R. P. Bentall (1999) 'The medicalisation of misery: a critical realist analysis of the concept of depression', *Journal of Mental Health*, 8: 261–74.

6. H. Kuhs (1991) 'Depressive delusion', *Psychopathology*, 24: 106–14. E. Lattuada, A. Serretti, C. Cusin, M. Gasperini and E. Smeraldi (1999) 'Symptomatologic analysis of psychotic and non-psychotic depression', *Journal of Affective Dis-*

orders, 54: 183–7. See also M. Thakur, J. Hays, K. Krishnan and R. Rangar (1999) 'Clinical, demographic and social characteristics of psychotic depression', *Psychiatry Research*, 86: 99–106.

7. F. Benazzi (1999) 'Bipolar versus psychotic outpatient depression', *Journal of Affective Disorders*, 55: 63–6.

8. A. T. Beck (1976) *Cognitive Therapy and the Emotional Disorders*. New York: International Universities Press; A. T. Beck, A. J. Rush, B. F. Shaw and G. Emery (1979) *Cognitive Therapy of Depression*. New York: Guilford Press.

9. L. Y. Abramson, M. E. P. Seligman and J. D. Teasdale (1978) 'Learned helplessness in humans: critique and reformulation', *Journal of Abnormal Psychology*, 78: 40–74.

10. F. Heider (1958) *The Psychology of Interpersonal Relations*. New York: Wiley.

11. H. M. Zullow, G. Oettingen, C. Peterson and M. E. P. Seligman (1988) 'Pessimistic explanatory style in the historical record: CAVEing LBJ, Presidential candidates, and East versus West Berlin', *American Psychologist*, 43: 673–82.

12. For a recent discussion of these problems, see K. Reivich (1995) 'The measurement of explanatory style', in G. M. Buchanan and M. E. P. Seligman (eds.), *Explanatory Style*. Hillsdale, NJ: Lawrence Erlbaum.

13. C. Peterson, L. Luborsky and M. E. P. Seligman (1983) 'Attributions and depressive mood shifts: a case study using the symptom-context method', *Journal of Abnormal Psychology*, 92: 93–103.

14. H. M. Zullow (1995) 'Pessimistic rumination in American politics and society', in Buchanan and Seligman (eds.), *Explanatory Style*, op. cit.

15. Zullow et al., 'Pessimistic explanatory style in the historical record', op. cit.

16. P. Sweeny, K. Anderson and S. Bailey (1986) 'Attributional style and depression: a meta-analytic review', *Journal of Personality and Social Psychology*, 50: 774–91.

17. C. J. Robins and A. H. Hayes (1995) 'The role of causal attributions in the prediction of depression', in Buchanan and Seligman (eds.), *Explanatory Style*, op. cit.

18. H. Lyon, M. Startup and R. P. Bentall (1999) 'Social cognition and the manic defense', *Journal of Abnormal Psychology*, 108: 273–82.

19. W. K. Campbell and C. Sedikides (1999) 'Self-threat magnifies the self-serving bias: a meta-analytic integration', *Review of General Psychology*, 3: 23–43.

20. See S. E. Taylor (1988) *Positive Illusions*. New York: Basic Books.

21. S. Mineka, C. L. Pury and A. G. Luten (1995) 'Explanatory style in anxiety and depression', in Buchanan and Seligman (eds.), *Explanatory Style*, op. cit.

22. G. I. Metalsky, L. J. Halberstadt and L. Y. Abramson (1987) 'Vulnerability to depressive mood reactions: towards a more powerful test of the diathesis/stress and causal mediation components of the reformulated theory of depression', *Journal of Personality and Social Psychology*, 52: 386–93.

23. Robins and Hayes, 'The role of causal attributions', op. cit.

24. L. B. Alloy, L. Y. Abramson, W. G. Whitehouse, M. E. Hogan, N. A. Tashman, D. L. Steinberg, D. T. Rose and P. Donovan (1999) 'Depressogenic cognitive

styles: predictive validity, information processing and personality characteristics, and developmental origins', *Behaviour Research and Therapy*, 37: 503–31.

25. L. Y. Abramson, G. I. Metalsky and L. B. Alloy (1989) 'Hopelessness depression: a theory-based subtype of depression', *Psychological Review*, 96: 358–72.

26. A. T. Beck, R. A. Steer, M. Kovacs and B. Garrison (1985) 'Hopelessness and eventual suicide: a ten-year prospective study of patients hospitalized with suicidal ideation', *American Journal of Psychiatry*, 142: 559–63; M. E. Weishaar and A. T. Beck (1990) 'The suicidal patient: how should the therapist respond?', in K. Hawton and P. Cowen (eds.), *Dilemmas and Difficulties in the Management of Psychiatric Patients*. Oxford: Oxford University Press.

27. R. Drake and P. G. Cotton (1986) 'Depression, hopelessness and suicide in chronic schizophrenia', *British Journal of Psychiatry*, 148: 554–9.

28. H. Tennen and S. Herzenberger (1987) 'Depression, self-esteem and the absence of self-protective attributional biases', *Journal of Personality and Social Psychology*, 52: 72–80; H. Tennen, S. Herzenberger and H. F. Nelson (1987) 'Depressive attributional style: the role of self-esteem', *Journal of Personality*, 55: 631–60.

29. D. M. Romney (1994) 'Cross-validating a causal model relating attributional style, self-esteem, and depression: an heuristic study', *Psychological Reports*, 74: 203–7.

30. P. Robson (1989) 'Development of a new self-report measure of self-esteem', *Psychological Medicine*, 19: 513–18.

31. G. W. Brown, A. T. Bifulco and B. Andrews (1990) 'Self-esteem and depression: IV. Effect on course and recovery', *Social Psychiatry and Psychiatric Epidemiology*, 25: 244–9; G. W. Brown, A. T. Bifulco, H. O. Veiel and B. Andrews (1990) 'Self-esteem and depression: II. Social correlates of self-esteem', *Social Psychiatry and Psychiatric Epidemiology*, 25: 225–34.

32. J. D. Campbell (1990) 'Self-esteem and the clarity of the self-concept', *Journal of Personality and Social Psychology*, 59: 538–49.

33. J. Dent and J. D. Teasdale (1988) 'Negative cognition and the persistence of depression', *Journal of Abnormal Psychology*, 97: 29–34; C. Hammen, D. G. Dyke and D. J. Micklovitch (1986) 'Stability and severity parameters of depressive self-schema responding', *Journal of Social and Clinical Psychology*, 4: 23–45; C. Hammen, T. Marks, A. Mayall and R. de Mayo (1985) 'Depressive self-schemas, life stress and vulnerability to depression', *Journal of Abnormal Psychology*, 94: 308–19; J. M. G. Williams, D. Healy, J. D. Teasdale, W. White and E. S. Paykel (1990) 'Dysfunctional attitudes and vulnerability to persistent depression', *Psychological Medicine*, 20: 375–81.

34. Lyon, Startup, Bentall, 'Social cognition and the manic defense', op. cit.

35. K. D. Greenier, M. H. Kernis and S. B. Waschull (1995) 'Not all high (or low) self-esteem people are the same: theory and research on stability of self-esteem', in M. H. Kernis (ed.), *Efficacy, Agency, and Self-Esteem*. New York: Plenum; M. H. Kernis (1993) 'The role of stability and level of self-esteem in psychological functioning', in R. F. Baumeister (ed.), *Self-Esteem: The Puzzle of Low Self-Regard*. New York: Plenum; M. H. Kernis, D. P. Cornell, C. R. Sun, A. Berry and T. Harlow (1993) 'There's more to self-esteem than whether it is high or low: the importance of stability of self-esteem', *Journal of Personality and Social Psychology*, 65: 1190–204.

36. K. D. Greenier, M. H. Kernis, C. W. McNamara, S. B. Waschull, A. J. Berry, C. E. Herlocker and T. A. Abend (1999) 'Individual differences in reactivity to events: re-examining the roles of stability and level of self-esteem', *Journal of Personality*, 67: 185–208.

37. Beck, *Cognitive Therapy and the Emotional Disorders*, op. cit.

38. G. W. Lloyd and W. A. Lishman (1975) 'Effects of depression on the speed of recall of pleasant and unpleasant experiences', *Psychological Medicine*, 5: 173–80.

39. J. D. Teasdale and S. J. Fogarty (1979) 'Differential effects of induced mood on retrieval of pleasant and unpleasant events from episodic memory', *Journal of Abnormal Psychology*, 3: 248–57.

40. J. Glover (1999) *Humanity: A Moral History of the Twentieth Century*. London: Jonathan Cape.

41. E. T. Higgins (1987) 'Self-discrepancy: a theory relating self and affect', *Psychological Review*, 94: 319–40; E. T. Higgins, R. Bond, R. Klein and T. J. Strauman (1986) 'Self-discrepancies and emotional vulnerability: how magnitude, accessibility and type of discrepancy influence affect', *Journal of Personality and Social Psychology*, 41: 1–15.

42. T. J. Strauman (1989) 'Self-discrepancies in clinical depression and social phobia: cognitive structures that underline emotional disorders?' *Journal of Abnormal Psychology*, 98: 14–22.

43. For a detailed discussion of this issue, see J. Boldero and J. Francis (1999) 'Ideals, oughts, and self-regulation: are there qualitatively distinct self-guides?' *Asian Journal of Social Psychology*, 2: 343–55.

44. T. J. Strauman and E. T. Higgins (1987) 'Automatic activation of self-discrepancies and emotional syndromes: when cognitive structures influence affect', *Journal of Abnormal Psychology*, 98: 14–22; T. J. Strauman, A. M. Lemieux and C. L. Coe (1993) 'Self-discrepancy and natural killer cell activity: immunological consequences of negative self-evaluation', *Journal of Personality and Social Psychology*, 64: 1042–52.

45. R. P. Bentall, P. Kinderman and K. Manson (in submission) 'Self-discrepancies in bipolar-affective disorder'.

46. For an empirical demonstration that Higgins's self-guide and Beck's self-schema concepts are highly correlated, see N. Fairbrother and M. Moretti (1998) 'Sociotropy, autonomy and self-discrepancy: status in depressed, remitted depressed, and control participants', *Cognitive Therapy and Research*, 22: 279–96.

47. A. N. Weissman and A. T. Beck (1978) 'Development and validation of the Dysfunctional Attitude Scale', paper presented at the Annual Meeting of the Association for the Advancement of Behavior Therapy, Chicago. For a review of

the scale's advantages and disadvantages, see J. M. G. Williams (1992) *The Psychological Treatment of Depression* (2nd edn). London: Routledge.

48. Z. V. Segal and R. E. Ingram (1994) 'Mood priming and construct activation in tests of cognitive vulnerability to unipolar depression', *Clinical Psychology Review*, 14: 663–95.

49. Williams et al., 'Dysfunctional attitudes', op. cit.

50. Alloy et al., 'Depressogenic cognitive styles', op. cit.

51. A. T. Beck (1983) 'Cognitive therapy of depression: new perspectives', in P. J. Clayton and J. E. Barrett (eds.), *Treatment of Depression: Old Controversies and New Approaches*. New York: Raven Press.

52. S. J. Blatt, D. Quinlan, E. Chevron, C. McDonald and D. Zurroff (1982) 'Dependency and self-criticism: psychological dimensions of depression', *Journal of Consulting and Clinical Psychology*, 50: 113–24.

53. I. H. Gotlib and C. L. Hammen (1992) *Psychological Aspects of Depression: Towards a Cognitive-Interpersonal Integration*. Chichester: Wiley.

54. H. H. Kelley (1967) 'Attribution theory in social psychology', in D. Levine (ed.), *Nebraska Symposium on Motivation*, vol. 15. Lincoln: University of Nebraska Press, pp. 192–240.

55. Quoted in M. Gilbert (1996) *The Boys: Triumph over Adversity*. London: Weidenfeld & Nicolson.

56. G. L. Flett, P. Pliner and K. R. Blankstein (1995) 'Preattributional dimensions in self-esteem and depressive symptomatology', *Journal of Social Behavior and Personality*, 10: 101–22.

57. W. Ickes and M. A. Layden (1978) 'Attributional styles', in J. H. Harvey, W. Ickes and R. F. Kidd (eds.), *New Directions in Attribution Research*, vol. 2. Hillsdale, NJ: Lawrence Erlbaum, pp. 119–92.

58. R. P. Bentall, P. Kinderman and K. Bowen-Jones (1999) 'Response latencies for the causal attributions of depressed, paranoid and normal individuals: availability of self-representations', *Cognitive Neuropsychiatry*, 4: 107–18.

59. J. P. Forgas, G. H. Bower and S. J. Moylan (1990) 'Praise or blame? Affective influences on attributions for achievement', *Journal of Personality and Social Psychology*, 59: 809–19.

60. R. P. Bentall and S. Kaney (in submission) 'Attributional lability in depression and paranoia: psychopathology and the attribution–self-representation cycle'.

61. Zullow et al., 'Pessimistic explanatory style in the historical record', op. cit.

62. Peterson et al., 'Attributions and depressive mood shifts', op. cit.

63. Kernis, 'The role of stability and level of self-esteem', op. cit.

64. Taylor, *Positive Illusions*, op. cit.

65. Campbell and Sedikides, 'Self-threat magnifies the self-serving bias', op. cit.; S. E. Taylor, E. Neter and H. A. Wayment (1995) 'Self-evaluation processes', *Personality and Social Psychology Bulletin*, 21: 1278–87.

66. D. Dunning, A. Leuenberger and D. A. Sherman (1995) 'A new look at motivated inference: are self-serving theories of success a product of motivational forces?' *Journal of Personality and Social Psychology*, 69: 58–68.

67. C. Sedikides, W. K. Campbell, G. D. Reeder and A. J. Elliot (1998) 'The self-serving bias in relational context', *Journal of Personality and Social Psychology*, 74: 378–86.

68. S. Nolen-Hoeksema (1991) 'Responses to depression and their effects on the duration of depressed mood', *Journal of Abnormal Psychology*, 100: 569–82.

69. J. Scott, B. Stanton, A. Garland and N. Ferrier (2000) 'Cognitive vulnerability in patients with bipolar disorder', *Psychological Medicine*, 30: 467–72; J. A. Sweeney, J. A. Kmiec and D. J. Kupfer (2000) 'Neuropsychologic impairments in bipolar and unipolar mood disorders on the CANTAB neurocognitive battery', *Biological Psychiatry*, 48: 674–84.

70. S. Lyubomirsky, N. D. Caldwell and S. Nolen-Hoeksema (1998) 'Effects of ruminative and distracting responses to depressed mood on retrieval of autobiographical memories', *Journal of Personality and Social Psychology*, 75: 166–77.

71. S. Lyubomirsky and S. Nolen-Hoeksema (1995) 'Effects of self-focused rumination on negative thinking and interpersonal problem solving', *Journal of Personality and Social Psychology*, 69: 176–90.

72. S. Nolen-Hoeksema and J. Morrow (1991) 'A prospective study of depression and posttraumatic stress symptoms after a natural disaster: the 1989 Loma Prieta earthquake', *Journal of Personality and Social Psychology*, 61: 115–21.

73. N. Just and L. B. Alloy (1997) 'The response styles theory of depression: tests and an extension of the theory', *Journal of Abnormal Psychology*, 106: 221–9.

74. S. Nolen-Hoeksema, A. McBride and J. Larson (1997) 'Rumination and psychological distress among bereaved partners', *Journal of Personality and Social Psychology*, 72: 855–62.

75. S. Nolen-Hoeksema, L. E. Parker and J. Larson (1994) 'Ruminative coping with depressed mood following loss', *Journal of Personality and Social Psychology*, 67: 92–104.

76. C. L. Rusting and S. Nolen-Hoeksema (1998) 'Regulating responses to anger: effects of rumination and distraction on angry mood', *Journal of Personality and Social Psychology*, 74: 790–803.

77. S. Nolen-Hoeksema (2000) 'The role of rumination in depressive disorders and mixed anxiety/depressive symptoms', *Journal of Abnormal Psychology*, 109: 504–11.

78. R. J. Davidson (1999) 'Neuropsychological perspectives on affective styles and their cognitive consequences', in T. Dalgleish and M. Power (eds.), *Handbook of Cognition and Emotion*. London: Wiley, pp. 103–23.

79. Described in I. H. Gotlib and L. Y. Abramson (1999) 'Attributional theories of emotion', in Dalgleish and Power (eds.), *Handbook*, op. cit., pp. 615–36.

80. D. Healy (1987) 'Rhythm and blues: neurochemical, neuropharmacological and neuropsychological implications of a hypothesis of circadian rhythm dysfunction in the affective disorders', *Psychopharmacology*, 93: 271–85.

81. D. Healy (1997) *The Anti-Depressant Era*. Cambridge, MA: Harvard University Press.

82. T. H. Monk, D. J. Kupfer, E. Frank and A. Ritenour (1991) 'The social rhythm metric (SRM): measuring daily social rhythms over 12 weeks', *Psychiatry Research*, 36: 195–207; M. P. Szuba, A. Yager, B. Guze, E. Allen and L. R. Baxter (1992) 'Disruption of social circadian rhythms in major depression: a preliminary report', *Psychiatry Research*, 42: 221–30.

83. D. Healy and J. M. Waterhouse (1995) 'The circadian system and the therapeutics of affective disorders', *Pharmacology and Therapeutics*, 65: 241–63.

Chapter 11   A Colourful Malady

1. V. Woolf (1978) *The Letters of Virginia Woolf*, Vol. 4: *1929–1931*, ed. N. Nicholson and J. Trautmann. London: Hogarth Press.

2. K. R. Jamison (1996) *An Unquiet Mind*. London: Picador.

3. A. H. Weingartner, H. Miller and D. L. Murphy (1977) 'Mood-state-dependent retrieval of verbal associations', *Journal of Abnormal Psychology*, 86: 276–84.

4. J. M. G. Williams and H. Markar (1991) 'Money hidden and rediscovered in subsequent manic phases: a case of state-dependent re-enactment', *British Journal of Psychiatry*, 159: 579–81.

5. G. M. Davidson (1957) 'Manic-depressive psychosis: theory and practice', *Journal of Nervous and Mental Disease*, 125: 87–95.

6. F. K. Goodwin and K. R. Jamison (1990) *Manic-Depressive Illness*. Oxford: Oxford University Press.

7. S. L. McElroy, P. E. Keck, H. G. Pope, J. I. Hudson, G. L. Faedda and A. C. Swann (1992) 'Clinical and research implications of the diagnosis of dysphoric or mixed mania or hypomania', *American Journal of Psychiatry*, 149: 1633–44.

8. G. A. Carlson and F. K. Goodwin (1973) 'The stages of mania', *Archives of General Psychiatry*, 28: 221–8.

9. F. Cassidy, K. Forest, M. Murry and B. J. Carroll (1998) 'A factor analysis of the signs and symptoms of mania', *Archives of General Psychiatry*, 55: 27–32.

10. N. C. Andreasen (1979) 'Thought, language and communication disorders: diagnostic significance', *Archives of General Psychiatry*, 36: 1325–30.

11. E. Jones (1962) *The Life and Work of Sigmund Freud* (abridged edition). London: Hogarth Press.

12. K. Abraham (1911/1927) 'Notes on the psychoanalytic investigation and treatment of manic-depressive insanity and allied conditions', in E. Jones (ed.), *Selected Papers of Karl Abraham*. London: Hogarth.

13. S. Rado (1928) 'The problem of melancholia', *International Journal of Psychoanalysis*, 9: 420–38.

14. This position was taken, for example, by H. J. Eysenck in a series of books and papers published throughout his career, including H. J. Eysenck and G. D. Wilson (eds.) (1973) *The Experimental Study of Freudian Theories*. London: Methuen; and H. J. Eysenck (1985) *The Decline and Fall of the Freudian Empire*. Harmondsworth: Penguin.

15. J. M. Neale (1988) 'Defensive function of manic episodes', in T. F. Oltmanns and B. A. Maher (eds.), *Delusional Beliefs*. New York: Wiley.

16. D. Lam and G. Wong (1997) 'Prodromes, coping strategies, insight and social functioning in bipolar affective disorder', *Psychological Medicine*, 27: 1091–100; J. A. Smith and N. Tarrier (1992) 'Prodromal symptoms in manic depressive psychosis', *Social Psychiatry and Psychiatric Epidemiology*, 27: 245–8; G. Wong and D. Lam (1999) 'The development and validation of the coping inventory for prodromes of mania', *Journal of Affective Disorders*, 53: 57–65.

17. G. Fava (1999) 'Subclinical symptoms in mood disorders', *Psychological Medicine*, 29: 47–61; G. I. Keitner, D. A. Solomon, C. E. Ryan, I. W. Miller and A. Mallinger (1996) 'Prodromal and residual symptoms in bipolar I disorder', *Comprehensive Psychiatry*, 37: 362–7.

18. K. C. Winters and J. M. Neale (1985) 'Mania and low self-esteem', *Journal of Abnormal Psychology*, 94: 282–90.

19. D. P. Crowne and D. Marlowe (1960) 'A new scale of social desirability independent of psychopathology', *Journal of Consulting Psychology*, 24: 349–54.

20. J. Scott, B. Stanton, A. Garland and N. Ferrier (2000) 'Cognitive vulnerability in patients with bipolar disorder', *Psychological Medicine*, 30: 467–72.

21. J. R. Stroop (1935) 'Studies of interference in serial verbal reactions', *Journal of Experimental Psychology*, 18: 643–62.

22. I. H. Gotlib and C. D. McCann (1984) 'Construct accessibility and depression', *Journal of Personality and Social Psychology*, 47: 427–39; J. M. G. Williams and K. Broadbent (1986) 'Distraction by emotional stimuli: use of a Stroop task with suicide attempters', *British Journal of Clinical Psychology*, 25: 101–10.

23. S. Channon, D. R. Hemsley and P. de Silva (1988) 'Selective processing of food words in anorexia nervosa', *British Journal of Clinical Psychology*, 27: 259–60.

24. A. M. Mathews and C. MacLeod (1985) 'Selective processing of threat cues in anxiety states', *Behaviour Research and Therapy*, 23: 563–9.

25. R. P. Bentall and M. Thompson (1990) 'Emotional Stroop performance and the manic defence', *British Journal of Clinical Psychology*, 29: 235–7.

26. C. C. French, A. Richards and E. J. C. Scholfield (1996) 'Hypomania, anxiety and the emotional Stroop', *British Journal of Clinical Psychology*, 35: 617–26.

27. R. P. Bentall, J. Highfield and T. Woodnut (in preparation) 'Self-esteem fluctuations and vulnerability to bipolar symptoms'.

28. M. H. Kernis (1993) 'The role of stability and level of self-esteem in psychological functioning', in R. F. Baumeister (ed.), *Self-Esteem: The Puzzle of Low Self-Regard*. New York: Plenum, pp. 167–82.

29. N. A. Reilly-Harrington, L. B. Alloy, D. M. Fresco and W. G. Whitehouse (1999) 'Cognitive style and life events interact to predict bipolar and unipolar symptomatology', *Journal of Abnormal Psychology*, 108: 567–78.

30. S. L. Johnson, B. Meyer, C. Winett and J. Small (2000) 'Social support and self-esteem predict changes in bipolar depression but not mania', *Journal of Affective Disorders*, 58: 79–86.

31. Personal communication from J. Scott.

32. H. Lyon, M. Startup and R. P. Bentall (1999) 'Social cognition and the manic defense', *Journal of Abnormal Psychology*, 108: 273–82.

33. C. M. Ashworth, I. M. Blackburn and F. M. McPherson (1982) 'The performance of depressed and manic patients on some repertory grid measures', *British Journal of Medical Psychology*, 55: 247–55; S. E. Owen and B. Nurcombe (1970) 'The application of the Semantic Differential Test in a case of manic-depressive psychosis', *Australian and New Zealand Journal of Psychiatry*, 4: 148–54.

34. C. R. Hammen, T. Marks, A. Mayall and R. de Mayo (1985) 'Depressive self-schemas, life stress and vulnerability to depression', *Journal of Abnormal Psychology*, 94: 308–19; J. Dent and J. D. Teasdale (1988) 'Negative cognition and the persistence of depression', *Journal of Abnormal Psychology*, 97: 29–34; J. M. G. Williams, D. Healy, J. D. Teasdale, W. White and E. S. Paykel (1990) 'Dysfunctional attitudes and vulnerability to persistent depression', *Psychological Medicine*, 20: 375–81.

35. R. A. Depue, P. F. Collins and M. Luciana (1996) 'A model of neurobiology: environment interaction in developmental psychopathology', in M. F. Lenzenweger and J. J. Haugaard (eds.), *Frontiers of Developmental Psychopathology*. New York: Oxford University Press, pp. 44–76; R. A. Depue and W. G. Iacano (1989) 'Neurobehavioural aspects of affective disorders', *Annual Review of Psychology*, 40: 457–92.

36. J. Gray (1994) 'Three fundamental emotion systems', in P. Ekman and R. J. Davidson (eds.), *The Nature of Emotion: Fundamental Questions*. Oxford: Oxford University Press, pp. 243–7.

37. B. Meyer, S. Johnson and C. Carver (1999) 'Exploring behavioural activation and inhibition sensitivities among college students at-risk for mood disorders', *Journal of Psychopathology and Behavioral Assessment*, 21: 275–92.

38. S. L. Johnson, D. Sandow, B. Meyer, R. Winters, I. Miller, D. Solomon and G. Keitner (2000) 'Increases in manic symptoms after life events involving goal attainment', *Journal of Abnormal Psychology*, 109: 721–7.

39. D. Healy (1987) 'Rhythm and blues: neurochemical, neuropharmacological and neuropsychological implications of a hypothesis of circadian rhythm dysfunction in the affective disorders', *Psychopharmacology*, 93: 271–85. See also P. C. Whybrow (1998) *A Mood Apart: A Thinker's Guide to Emotion and its Disorder*. London: Picador.

40. C. L. Raison, H. M. Klein and M. Steckler (1999) 'The moon and madness reconsidered', *Journal of Affective Disorders*, 53: 99–106.

41. Goodwin and Jamison, *Manic-Depressive Illness*, op. cit.

42. T. Wehr, D. A. Sack and N. E. Rosenthal (1987) 'Sleep production as a final common pathway in the genesis of mania', *American Journal of Psychiatry*, 144: 201–4; T. A. Wehr (1991) 'Sleep-loss as a possible mediator of diverse causes of mania', *British Journal of Psychiatry*, 159: 576–8. See also J. B. Wright (1993) 'Mania following sleep deprivation', *British Journal of Psychiatry*, 163: 679–80.

43. J. I. Hudson, J. F. Lipinski, P. E. Keck, H. G. Aizley, S. E. Lukas, A. J. Rothschild, C. M. Waternaux and D. J. Kupfer (1992) 'Polysomnographic characteristics of

young manic patients: comparisons with unipolar depressed patients and normal control subjects', *Archives of General Psychiatry*, 49: 378–83.

44. B. Barbini, S. Bertelli, C. Colombo and E. Smeralsi (1996) 'Sleep loss as a possible factor in augmenting manic episodes', *Psychiatry Research*, 65: 121–5.

45. E. Leibenluft, P. S. Albert, N. E. Rosenthal and T. A. Wehr (1996) 'Relationship between sleep and mood in patients with rapid-cycling bipolar disorder', *Psychiatry Research*, 63: 161–8.

46. S. Malkoff-Schwartz, E. Frank, B. Anderson, J. T. Sherrill, L. Siegel, D. Patterson and D. J. Kupfer (1998) 'Stressful life events and social rhythm disruption in the onset of manic and depressive episodes of bipolar disorder', *Archives of General Psychiatry*, 55: 702–7; S. Malkoff-Schwartz, E. Frank, B. P. Anderson, S. A. Hlastala, J. F. Luther, J. T. Sherrill and D. J. Kupfer (2000) 'Social rhythm disruption and stressful life events in the onset of bipolar and unipolar episodes', *Psychological Medicine*, 30: 1005–16.

47. C. Colombo, F. Benedetti, B. Barbini, E. Campori and E. Smeraldi (1999) 'Rate of switch from depression to mania after therapeutic sleep deprivation in bipolar depression', *Psychiatry Research*, 86: 267–70.

48. S. Nolen-Hoeksema (1991) 'Responses to depression and their effects on the duration of depressed mood', *Journal of Abnormal Psychology*, 100: 569–82. See also the detailed discussion of Nolen-Hoeksema's work in the previous chapter.

49. J. Thomas and R. P. Bentall (2002) 'Hypomanic traits and response styles to depression', *British Journal of Clinical Psychology*, 41: 309–13.

50. Lam and Wong, 'Prodromes, coping strategies, insight and social functioning', op. cit.

Chapter 12   Abnormal Attitudes

1. D. Schreber (1903/1955) *Memoirs of my Nervous Illness* (trans. I. Macalpine and R. A. Hunter). London: Dawsons.

2. S. Freud (1911/1950) 'Psychoanalytic notes upon an autobiographical account of a case of paranoia (Dementia Paranoides)', *Collected Papers* (vol. III). London: Hogarth Press.

3. M. Stone (1997) *Healing the Mind: A History of Psychiatry from Antiquity to the Present*. New York: Norton.

4. Schreber, *Memoirs of my Nervous Illness*, op. cit.

5. I. Macalpine and R. A. Hunter (1955) 'Preface', in D. Schreber (1903/1955) *Memoirs*, op. cit.

6. Freud, 'Psychoanalytic notes', op. cit.

7. E. Bleuler (1911/1950) *Dementia Praecox or the Group of Schizophrenias* (trans. E. Zinkin). New York: International Universities Press.

8. K. Colby, S. Weber and F. D. Hilf (1971) 'Artificial paranoia', *Artificial Intelligence*, 2: 1–25; K. M. Colby (1977) 'Appraisal of four psychological theories of paranoid phenomena', *Journal of Abnormal Psychology*, 86: 54–9; K. M. Colby,

W. S. Faught and R. C. Parkinson (1979) 'Cognitive therapy of paranoid conditions: heuristic suggestions based on a computer simulation', *Cognitive Therapy and Research*, 3: 55–60.

9. M. Rokeach (1964) *The Three Christs of Ypsilanti: A Narrative Study of Three Lost Men*. New York: Vintage Books.

10. P. Jorgensen and J. Jensen (1994) 'Delusional beliefs in first admitters', *Psychopathology*, 27: 100–12.

11. P. Trower and P. Chadwick (1995) 'Pathways to defense of the self: a theory of two types of paranoia', *Clinical Psychology: Science and Practice*, 2: 263–78.

12. H. Haltenhof, H. Ulrich and W. Blanenburg (1999) 'Themes of delusion in 84 patients with unipolar depression', *Krankenhauspsychiatrie*, 10: 87–90; H. Kuhs (1991) 'Depressive delusion', *Psychopathology*, 24: 106–14.

13. J. P. Leff, M. Fisher and A. C. Bertelsen (1976) 'A cross-national epidemiological study of mania', *British Journal of Psychiatry*, 129: 428–42.

14. For good descriptive accounts of many of these types of delusions, see: M. D. Enoch and W. H. Trethowan (1979) *Uncommon Psychiatric Syndromes* (2nd edn). Bristol: Wright; and L. Franzini and J. M. Grossberg (1995) *Eccentric and Bizarre Behaviors*. New York: John Wiley.

15. P. K. Chadwick (1992) *Borderline: A Psychological Study of Paranoia and Delusional Thinking*. London: Routledge.

16. I. McGilchrist and J. Cutting (1995) 'Somatic delusions in schizophrenia and the affective psychoses', *British Journal of Psychiatry*, 167: 350–61.

17. M. Musalek, M. Bach, V. Passweg and S. Jaeger (1990) 'The position of delusional parasitosis in psychiatric nosology and classification', *Psychopathology*, 23: 115–24; M. Musalek, S. Zadro-Jaeger, O. M. Lesch and H. Walter (1992) 'Traumatic events and traumatizing life conditions in delusional parasitosis: the significance of social isolation and tactile sensations in the pathogenesis of delusional parasitosis', *Psychiatrica Fennica*, 23 (Supplement): 162–70.

18. J. H. Segal (1989) 'Erotomania revisited: from Kraepelin to DSM-III-R', *American Journal of Psychiatry*, 146: 1261–6.

19. D. Enoch (1991) 'Delusional jealousy and awareness of reality', *British Journal of Psychiatry*, 159 (Supplement 14): 52–6.

20. M. Hamilton (ed.) (1983) *Fish's Psychopathology*. Bristol: Wright.

21. A. Young and K. Leafhead (1996) 'Betwixt life and death: case studies of the Cotard delusion', in P. W. Halligan and J. C. Marshall (eds.), *Method in Madness: Case Studies in Cognitive Neuropsychiatry*. Hove: Psychology Press, pp. 147–71.

22. G. E. Berrios and R. Luque (1995) 'Cotard's syndrome: analysis of 100 cases', *Acta Psychiatrica Scandinavica*, 91: 185–8.

23. J. Capgras and J. Reboul-Lachaux (1923/1994) 'L'illusion des "sosies" dans un délire systématise chronique', *History of Psychiatry*, 5: 117–30.

24. P. Coubon and G. Fail (1927/1994) 'Syndrome d'illusion de Frégoli et schizophrénie', *History of Psychiatry*, 5: 134–8.

25. D. N. Anderson (1988) 'The delusion of inanimate doubles', *British Journal of Psychiatry*, 153: 694–9.

26. K. Schneider (1949/1974) 'The concept of delusion', in S. R. Hirsch and M. Shepherd (eds.), *Themes and Variations in European Psychiatry*. Bristol: John Wright & Sons, pp. 33–9.

27. P. A. Garety, B. S. Everitt and D. R. Hemsley (1988) 'The characteristics of delusions: a cluster analysis of deluded subjects', *European Archives of Psychiatry and Neurological Sciences*, 237: 112–14.

28. D. M. Ndetei and A. Vadher (1984) 'Frequency and clinical significance of delusions across cultures', *Acta Psychiatrica Scandinavica*, 70: 73–6. For a more recent study, comparing delusional themes in Austria and Pakistan, which found persecutory delusions to be the most common in both countries, see T. Stompe, A. Friedman, G. Ortwein, R. Strobl, H. R. Chaudhry, N. Najam and M. R. Chaudhry (1999) 'Comparisons of delusions among schizophrenics in Austria and Pakistan', *Psychopathology*, 32: 225–34.

29. M. F. Sendiony (1976) 'Cultural aspects of delusions: a psychiatric study of Egypt', *Australian and New Zealand Journal of Psychiatry*, 10: 201–7.

30. K. Kim, D. Li, Z. Jiang and X. Cui (1993) 'Schizophenic delusions among Koreans, Korean-Chinese and Chinese: a transcultural study', *International Journal of Social Psychiatry*, 39: 190–9.

31. J. Mitchell and A. D. Vierkant (1989) 'Delusions and hallucinations as a reflection of the subcultural milieu among psychotic patients of the 1930s and 1980s', *Journal of Psychology*, 123: 269–74.

32. American Psychiatric Association (1994) *Diagnostic and Statistical Manual for Mental Disorders* (4th edition). Washington, DC: APA.

33. D. J. Harper (1992) 'Defining delusions and the serving of professional interest: the case of "paranoia"', *British Journal of Medical Psychology*, 65: 357–69. See also D. Harper (1994) 'Histories of suspicion in a time of conspiracy: a reflection on Aubrey Lewis's history of paranoia', *History of the Human Sciences*, 7: 89–109.

34. See, for example, K. S. Kendler, W. Glazer and H. Morgenstern (1983) 'Dimensions of delusional experience', *American Journal of Psychiatry*, 140: 466–9; P. A. Garety and D. R. Hemsley (1987) 'The characteristics of delusional experience', *European Archives of Psychiatry and Neurological Sciences*, 236: 294–8.

35. M. Harrow, A. W. MacDonald, J. R. Sands and M. L. Silverstein (1995) 'Vulnerability to delusions over time in schizophrenia and affective disorders', *Schizophrenia Bulletin*, 21: 95–109; M. Harrow, F. Rattenbury and F. Stoll (1988) 'Schizophrenic delusions: an analysis of their persistence, of related premorbid ideas and three major dimensions', in T. F. Oltmanns and B. A. Maher (eds.), *Delusional Beliefs*. New York: John Wiley, pp. 184–211.

36. P. A. Garety (1985) 'Delusions: problems in definitions and measurement', *British Journal of Medical Psychology*, 58: 25–34.

37. G. E. Berrios (1991) 'Delusions as "wrong beliefs": a conceptual history', *British Journal of Psychiatry*, 159 (Supplement 14): 6–13.

38. I got this quote from *5,000 Gems of Wit and Wisdom*, by L. Peter, London: Treasure Press. My efforts to find the original source failed, but it was too good to pass up.

39. S. G. Brush (1974) 'Should the history of science be rated X?' *Science*, 183: 1164–72.

40. G. N. Gilbert and M. Mulkay (1984) *Opening Pandora's Box: A Sociological Analysis of Scientists' Discourse*. Cambridge: Cambridge University Press.

41. G. Kelly (1955) *The Psychology of Personal Constructs* (Vol. 1). New York: Norton.

42. R. P. Bentall (1990) 'The syndromes and symptoms of psychosis: or why you can't play 20 questions with the concept of schizophrenia and hope to win', in R. P. Bentall (ed.), *Reconstructing Schizophrenia*. London: Routledge, pp. 23–60.

43. K. Popper (1963) *Conjectures and Refutations: The Growth of Scientific Knowledge*. London: Routledge.

44. J. S. B. T. Evans (1989) *Bias in Human Reasoning: Causes and Consequences*. Hove: Erlbaum; R. S. Nickerson (1998) 'Confirmation bias: a ubiquitous phenomenon in many guises', *Review of General Psychology*, 2: 175–220.

45. K. Moser, V. Gadenne and J. Schroeder (1988) 'Under what conditions does confirmation seeking obstruct scientific progress?' *Psychological Review*, 95: 572–4.

46. S. Schneider (1998) 'Peace and paranoia', in J. H. Berke, S. Pierides, A. Sabbadini and S. Schneider (eds.), *Even Paranoids have Enemies: New Perspectives on Paranoia and Persecution*. London: Routledge, pp. 203–18.

47. D. Mayerhoff, D. Pelta, C. Valentino and M. Chakos (1991) 'Real-life basis for a patient's paranoia', *American Journal of Psychiatry*, 148: 682–3.

48. W. G. Niederland (1959) 'Schreber: father and son', *Psychoanalytic Quarterly*, 28: 151–69; and Niederland (1960) 'Schreber's father', *Journal of the American Psychoanalytic Association*, 8: 492–9. See also M. Schatzman (1973) *Soul Murder: Persecution in the Family*. London: Penguin Books.

49. Z. Lothane (1992) *In Defense of Schreber: Soul Murder and Psychiatry*. Hillsdale, NJ: Analytic Press.

50. J. Mirowsky and C. E. Ross (1983) 'Paranoia and the structure of powerlessness', *American Sociological Review*, 48: 228–39.

51. T. Harris (1987) 'Recent developments in the study of life events in relation to psychiatric and physical disorders', in B. Cooper (ed.), *Psychiatric Epidemiology: Progress and Prospects*, London: Croom Helm, pp. 81–102.

52. R. Day, J. A. Neilsen, A. Korten, G. Ernberg, K. C. Dube, J. Gebhart, A. Jablensky, C. Leon, A. Marsella, M. Olatawura, N. Sartorius, E. Stromgren, R. Takahashi, N. Wig and L. C. Wynne (1987) 'Stressful life events preceding the onset of acute schizophrenia: a cross-national study from the World Health Organization', *Culture, Medicine and Psychiatry*, 11: 123–206.

53. T. Fuchs (1999) 'Life events in late paraphrenia and depression', *Psychopathology*, 32: 60–9.

54. D. Bhugra, J. Leff, R. Mallett, G. Der, B. Corridan and S. Rudge (1997) 'Incidence and outcome of schizophrenia in Whites, African-Caribbeans and Asians in London', *Psychological Medicine*, 27: 791–8; G. Harrison, D. Owens, A. Holton, D. Neilsen and D. Boot (1988) 'A prospective study of severe mental disorder in Afro-Caribbean patients', *Psychological Medicine*, 18: 643–57.

55. B. A. Maher (1974) 'Delusional thinking and perceptual disorder', *Journal of Individual Psychology*, 30: 98–113; B. A. Maher (1988) 'Anomalous experience and delusional thinking: the logic of explanations', in Oltmanns and Maher (eds.), *Delusional Beliefs*, op. cit.; B. A. Maher (1992) 'Models and methods for the study of reasoning in delusions', *Revue Européenne de Psychologie Appliquée*, 42: 97–102.

56. B. A. Maher and J. S. Ross (1984) 'Delusions', in H. E. Adams and P. Suther (eds.), *Comprehensive Handbook of Psychopathology*. New York: Plenum.

57. A. F. Cooper and A. R. Curry (1976) 'The pathology of deafness in the paranoid and affective psychoses of later life', *Journal of Psychosomatic Medicine*, 20: 97–105; A. F. Cooper, R. F. Garside and D. W. Kay (1976) 'A comparison of deaf and non-deaf patients with paranoid and affective psychoses', *British Journal of Psychiatry*, 129: 532–8; D. W. Kay, A. F. Cooper, R. F. Garside and M. Roth (1976) 'The differentiation of paranoid from affective psychoses by patients' premorbid characteristics', *British Journal of Psychiatry*, 129: 207–15.

58. P. G. Zimbardo, S. M. Andersen and L. G. Kabat (1981) 'Induced hearing deficit generates experimental paranoia', *Science*, 212: 1529–31.

59. N. C. Moore (1981) 'Is paranoid illness associated with sensory defects in the elderly?' *Journal of Psychosomatic Research*, 25: 69–74; J. A. G. Watt (1985) 'Hearing and premorbid personality in paranoid states', *American Journal of Psychiatry*, 142: 1453–5.

60. Capgras and Reboul-Lachaux, 'L'illusion des "sosies"', op. cit .

61. See, for example, Enoch and Trethowan, *Uncommon Psychiatric Syndromes*, op. cit.

62. H. D. Ellis and K. W. Pauw (1994) 'The cognitive neuropsychiatric origins of the capgras delusion', in A. S. David and J. C. Cutting (eds.), *The Neuropsychology of Schizophrenia*. Hove: Erlbaum.

63. H. D. Ellis and A. W. Young (1990) 'Accounting for delusional misidentifications', *British Journal of Psychiatry*, 157: 239–48.

64. H. D. Ellis and M. B. Lewis (2001) 'Capgras delusion: a window on face recognition', *Trends in Cognitive Sciences*, 5: 149–56.

65. H. D. Ellis, A. W. Young, A. H. Quale and K. W. de Paul (1997) 'Reduced autonomic responses to faces in Capgras delusion', *Proceedings of the Royal Society of London*, 264: 1085–92. See, also, a more detailed study of face recognition in a single case of Capgras syndrome, reported in H. D. Ellis, M. B. Lewis, H. F. Moselhy, and A. W. Young (2000) 'Automatic without autonomic responses to familiar faces: differential components of covert face recognition in a case of Capgras delusion', *Cognitive Neuropsychiatry*, 5: 255–69. For an independent replication of this finding, see W. Hirstein and V. S. Ramachandran (1997) 'Capgras syndrome: a novel probe for understanding neural representation of identity and familiarity of persons', *Proceedings of the Royal Society of London*, 264: 437–44.

66. A. W. Young (1994) 'Recognition and reality', in E. M. R. Critchley (ed.), *The Neurological Boundaries of Reality*. London: Farrand Press.

67. L. LaRusso (1978) 'Sensitivity of paranoid patients to nonverbal cues', *Journal of Abnormal Psychology*, 87: 463–71.

68. P. J. Davis and M. G. Gibson (2000) 'Recognition of posed and genuine facial expressions of emotion in paranoid and nonparanoid schizophrenia', *Journal of Abnormal Psychology*, 109: 445–50.

69. W. G. Johnson, J. M. Ross and M. A. Mastria (1977) 'Delusional behavior: an attributional analysis of development and modification', *Journal of Abnormal Psychology*, 86: 421–6.

70. L. J. Chapman and J. P. Chapman (1988) 'The genesis of delusions', in Oltmanns and Maher (eds.), *Delusional Beliefs*, op. cit.

71. S. Escher, M. Romme, A. Buiks, P. Delespaul and J. van Os (2002) 'Formation of delusional ideation in adolescents hearing voices: a prospective study', *American Journal of Medical Genetics (Neuropsychiatric Genetics)*, 14: 913–20.

72. L. P. Ullmann and L. Krasner (1969) *A Psychological Approach to Abnormal Behavior*. Englewood Cliffs, NJ: Prentice-Hall.

73. R. P. Bentall and S. Kaney (1989) 'Content-specific information processing and persecutory delusions: an investigation using the emotional Stroop test', *British Journal of Medical Psychology*, 62: 355–64. For replications of this finding, see: C. F. Fear, H. Sharp and D. Healy (1996) 'Cognitive processes in delusional disorder', *British Journal of Psychiatry*, 168: 61–7; and P. Kinderman (1994) 'Attentional bias, persecutory delusions and the self concept', *British Journal of Medical Psychology*, 67: 53–66.

74. J. M. G. Williams, A. Mathews and C. MacLeod (1996) 'The emotional Stroop task and psychopathology', *Psychological Bulletin*, 120: 3–24.

75. K. M. Leafhead, A. W. Young and T. K. Szulecka (1996) 'Delusions demand attention', *Cognitive Neuropsychiatry*, 1: 5–16.

76. S. Kaney, M. Wolfenden, M. E. Dewey and R. P. Bentall (1992) 'Persecutory delusions and the recall of threatening and non-threatening propositions', *British Journal of Clinical Psychology*, 31: 85–7. See also R. P. Bentall, S. Kaney and K. Bowen-Jones (1995) 'Persecutory delusions and recall of threat-related, depression-related and neutral words', *Cognitive Therapy and Research*, 19: 331–43.

77. M. Phillips and A. S. David (1997) 'Abnormal visual scan paths: a psychophysiological marker of delusions in schizophrenia', *Schizophrenia Research*, 29: 235–54; M. Phillips and A. S. David (1997) 'Visual scan paths are abnormal in deluded schizophrenics', *Neuropsychologia*, 35: 99–105.

78. C. D. Frith (1994) 'Theory of mind in schizophrenia', in David and Cutting (eds.), *The Neuropsychology of Schizophrenia*, op. cit., pp. 147–61; C. D. Frith (1992) *The Cognitive Neuropsychology of Schizophrenia*. Hillsdale, NJ: Lawrence Erlbaum.

79. C. D. Frith and R. Corcoran (1996) 'Exploring "theory of mind" in people with schizophrenia', *Psychological Medicine*, 26: 521–30.

80. R. Corcoran, C. D. Frith and G. Mercer (1995) 'Schizophrenia, symptomatology and social inference: investigating "theory of mind" in people with schizophrenia', *Schizophrenia Research*, 17: 5–13. See also R. Corcoran, C. Cahill and

C. D. Frith (1997) 'The appreciation of visual jokes in people with schizophrenia: a study of "mentalizing" ability', *Schizophrenia Research*, 24: 319–27.

81. Y. Sarfati, M. C. Hardy-Bayle, C. Besche and D. Widlocher (1997) 'Attributions of intentions to others in people with schizophrenia: a non-verbal exploration with comic strips', *Schizophrenia Research*, 25: 199–209; Y. Sarfati, M. C. Hardy-Bayle, E. Brunet and D. Widlocher (1999) 'Investigating theory of mind in schizophrenia: influence of verbalization in disorganized and non-disorganized patients', *Schizophrenia Research*, 37: 183–90; Y. Sarfati, J. Nadel, J. F. Chevalier and D. Widlocher (1997) 'Attribution of mental states to others by schizophrenic patients', *Cognitive Neuropsychiatry*, 2: 1–17.

82. R. Langdon, P. Michie, P. B. Ward, N. McConaghy, S. V. Catts and M. Coltheart (1997) 'Defective self and/or other mentalising in schizophrenia: a cognitive neuropsychological approach', *Cognitive Neuropsychiatry*, 2: 167–93.

83. V. M. Drury, E. J. Robinson and M. Birchwood (1998) '"Theory of mind" skills during an acute episode of psychosis and following recovery', *Psychological Medicine*, 28: 1101–12.

84. D. Murphy (1998) 'Theory of mind in a sample of men with schizophrenia detained in a special hospital: its relationship to symptom profiles and neuropsychological tests', *Criminal Behaviour and Mental Health*, 8: 13–26; F. Walston, R. C. Blennerhassett and B. G. Charlton (2000) '"Theory of mind", persecutory delusions and the somatic marker hypothesis', *Cognitive Neuropsychiatry*, 5: 161–74.

85. N. Kerr, R. I. M. Dunbar and R. P. Bentall (2003) 'Theory of mind in bipolar affective disorder', *Journal of Affective Disorders*, 73: 253–9.

86. S. Kaney and R. P. Bentall (1989) 'Persecutory delusions and attributional style', *British Journal of Medical Psychology*, 62: 191–8.

87. Fear, Sharp and Healy, 'Cognitive processes', op. cit.

88. C. L. Candido and D. M. Romney (1990) 'Attributional style in paranoid vs depressed patients', *British Journal of Medical Psychology*, 63: 355–63.

89. H. Kristev, H. Jackson and D. Maude (1999) 'An investigation of attributional style in first-episode psychosis', *British Journal of Clinical Psychology*, 88: 181–94.

90. H. J. Lee and H. T. Won (1998) 'The self-concepts, the other-concepts, and attributional style in paranoia and depression', *Korean Journal of Clinical Psychology*, 17: 105–25; H. T. Won and H. J. Lee (1997) 'The self-concept and attributional style in a paranoid group', *Korean Journal of Clinical Psychology*, 16: 173–82.

91. H. M. Sharp, C. F. Fear and D. Healy (1997) 'Attributional style and delusions: an investigation based on delusional content', *European Psychiatry*, 12: 1–7.

92. S. Kaney and R. P. Bentall (1992) 'Persecutory delusions and the self-serving bias', *Journal of Nervous and Mental Disease*, 180: 773–80.

93. P. A. White (1991) 'Ambiguity in the internal/external distinction in causal attribution', *Journal of Experimental Social Psychology*, 27: 259–70.

94. See, for example, K. Reivich (1995) 'The measurement of explanatory style',

in G. M. Buchanan and M. E. P. Seligman (eds.), *Explanatory Style*. Hillsdale, NJ: Lawrence Erlbaum. In general, studies have shown that the Attributional Style Questionnaire has extremely poor psychometric properties and, in particular, that scores on individual items show poor consistency. It has continued to be the most widely used attributional measure mainly because of the lack of a viable alternative.

95. P. Kinderman and R. P. Bentall (1996) 'The development of a novel measure of causal attributions: the Internal Personal and Situational Attributions Questionnaire', *Personality and Individual Differences*, 20: 261–4. See also L. Day and J. Maltby (2000) 'Can Kinderman and Bentall's suggestion for a personal and situational attributions questionnaire be used to examine all aspects of attributional style?' *Personality and Individual Differences*, 29: 1047–55.

96. D. R. Hemsley and P. A. Garety (1986) 'The formation and maintenance of delusions: a Bayesian analysis', *British Journal of Psychiatry*, 149: 51–6.

97. S. F. Huq, P. A. Garety and D. R. Hemsley (1988) 'Probabilistic judgements in deluded and nondeluded subjects', *Quarterly Journal of Experimental Psychology*, 40A: 801–12.

98. P. A. Garety, D. R. Hemsley and S. Wessely (1991) 'Reasoning in deluded schizophrenic and paranoid patients', *Journal of Nervous and Mental Disease*, 179: 194–201.

99. Y. Linney, E. Peters and P. Ayton (1998) 'Reasoning biases in delusion-prone individuals', *British Journal of Clinical Psychology*, 37: 285–302.

100. C. H. John and G. Dodgson (1994) 'Inductive reasoning in delusional thought', *Journal of Mental Health*, 3: 31–49; see also H. F. Young and R. P. Bentall (1995) 'Hypothesis testing in patients with persecutory delusions: comparison with depressed and normal subjects', *British Journal of Clinical Psychology*, 34: 353–69.

101. R. E. J. Dudley, C. H. John, A. W. Young and D. E. Over (1997) 'The effect of self-referent material on the reasoning of people with delusions', *British Journal of Clinical Psychology*, 36: 575–84.

102. H. F. Young and R. P. Bentall (1997) 'Probabilistic reasoning in deluded, depressed and normal subjects: effects of task difficulty and meaningful versus nonmeaningful materials', *Psychological Medicine*, 27: 455–65.

103. K. Salzinger (1984) 'The immediacy hypothesis in a theory of schizophrenia', in D. Spaulding and J. K. Cole (eds.), *Theories of Schizophrenia and Psychosis: Nebraska Symposium on Motivation*. Lincoln: University of Nebraska Press.

104. R. E. J. Dudley, C. H. John, A. W. Young and D. E. Over (1997) 'Normal and abnormal reasoning in people with delusions', *British Journal of Clinical Psychology*, 36: 243–58.

105. Young and Bentall, 'Probabilistic reasoning', op. cit.

106. Popper, *Conjectures and Refutations*, op. cit.

107. H. H. Farris and R. Revlin (1989) 'Sensible reasoning in two tasks: rule discovery and hypothesis evaluation', *Memory and Cognition*, 17: 221–32; J. E. Tschirgi (1980) 'Sensible reasoning: a hypothesis about hypotheses', *Child Development*, 51: 1–10.

108. R. P. Bentall and H. F. Young (1996) 'Sensible-hypothesis-testing in deluded, depressed and normal subjects', *British Journal of Psychiatry*, 168: 372–5.

109. A. W. Kruglanski and D. M. Webster (1996) 'Motivated closing of the mind: "seizing" and "freezing"', *Psychological Review*, 103: 263–83.

110. G. Roberts (1991) 'Delusional belief systems and meaning in life: a preferred reality?' *British Journal of Psychiatry*, 159 (Supplement 14): 19–28.

111. R. P. Bentall and R. Swarbrick (in press) 'The best laid schemas of paranoid patients', *Psychology and Psychotherapy: Theory, Research and Practice*

112. S. M. Colbert and E. R. Peters (2002) 'Need for closure and jumping-to-conclusions in delusion-prone individuals', *Journal of Nervous and Mental Disease*, 190: 27–31.

113. A. P. Morrison (1998) 'Cognitive behaviour therapy for psychotic symptoms of schizophrenia', in N. Tarrier, A. Wells and G. Haddock (eds.), *Treating Complex Cases: The Cognitive Behavioural Therapy Approach*. London: Wiley, pp. 195–216.

114. D. Freeman, P. A. Garety and E. Kuipers (2001) 'Persecutory delusions: developing the understanding of belief maintenance and emotional distress', *Psychological Medicine*, 31: 1293–306.

115. J. C. Rosen (1995) 'The nature of body dysmorphobic disorder and treatment with cognitive behavior therapy', *Cognitive and Behavioral Practice*, 2: 143–66.

Chapter 13   On the Paranoid World View

1. Quoted in J. Ronson (2001) *Them: Adventures with Extremists*. London: Picador.

2. Andrew Grove, Chief Executive Officer of the Intel Corporation, quoted in the *New York Times*, 18 December 1994.

3. For a full account, see R. P. Bentall, R. Corcoran, R. Howard, R. Blackwood and P. Kinderman (2001) 'Persecutory delusions: a review and theoretical integration', *Clinical Psychology Review*, 21: 1143–92.

4. Readers of a particularly obsessional bent will find these earlier versions (models 1.1, 2.1 and 3.1 respectively) described in the following publications: R. P. Bentall (1994) 'Cognitive biases and abnormal beliefs: towards a model of persecutory delusions', in A. S. David and J. Cutting (eds.), *The Neuropsychology of Schizophrenia*. Hove: Lawrence Erlbaum, pp. 337–60; R. P. Bentall, P. Kinderman and S. Kaney (1994) 'The self, attributional processes and abnormal beliefs: towards a model of persecutory delusions', *Behaviour Research and Therapy*, 32: 331–41; R. P. Bentall and P. Kinderman (1998) 'Psychological processes and delusional beliefs: implications for the treatment of paranoid states', in S. Lewis, N. Tarrier and T. Wykes (eds.), *Outcome and Innovation in the Psychological Treatment of Schizophrenia*. Chichester: Wiley, pp. 119–44.

5. The assumption that delusions reflect attempts to explain troubling experiences is apparent, for example, in Brendan Maher's anomalous perception theory, in

Chris Frith and Rhiannon Corcoran's ideas about the role of theory-of-mind deficits in persecutory delusions, in the work that Sue Kaney, Peter Kinderman and I have conducted on paranoia, and also in Philippa Garety and David Hemsley's studies of the way in which deluded patients reason about hypotheses.

6. K. M. Colby, S. Weber and F. D. Hilf (1971) 'Artificial paranoia', *Artificial Intelligence*, 2: 1–25; K. M. Colby (1977) 'Appraisal of four psychological theories of paranoid phenomena', *Journal of Abnormal Psychology*, 86: 54–9; K. M. Colby, W. S. Faught and R. C. Parkinson (1979) 'Cognitive therapy of paranoid conditions: heuristic suggestions based on a computer simulation', *Cognitive Therapy and Research*, 3: 55–60.

7. D. Freeman, P. Garety, D. Fowler, E. Kuipers, G. Dunn, P. Bebbington and C. Hadley (1998) 'The London–East Anglia randomized controlled trial of cognitive-behaviour therapy for psychosis. IV: Self-esteem and persecutory delusions', *British Journal of Clinical Psychology*, 37: 415–30.

8. B. Bowins and G. Shugar (1998) 'Delusions and self-esteem', *Canadian Journal of Psychiatry*, 43: 154–8.

9. C. Barrowclough, N. Tarrier, L. Humphreys, J. Ward, L. Gregg and B. Andrews (in press) 'Self-esteem in schizophrenia: the relationship between self-evaluation, family attitudes and symptomatology', *Journal of Consulting and Clinical Psychology*.

10. C. L. Candido and D. M. Romney (1990) 'Attributional style in paranoid vs depressed patients', *British Journal of Medical Psychology*, 63: 355–63.

11. H. M. Lyon, S. Kaney and R. P. Bentall (1994) 'The defensive function of persecutory delusions: evidence from attribution tasks', *British Journal of Psychiatry*, 164: 637–46.

12. T. E. Oxman, S. D. Rosenberg, P. P. Schnurr and G. Tucker (1988) 'Somatization, paranoia and language', *Journal of Communication Disorders*, 21: 33–50.

13. P. Kinderman and R. P. Bentall (1996) 'Self-discrepancies and persecutory delusions: evidence for a defensive model of paranoid ideation', *Journal of Abnormal Psychology*, 105: 106–14.

14. P. Kinderman (1994) 'Attentional bias, persecutory delusions and the self concept', *British Journal of Medical Psychology*, 67: 53–66.

15. H. J. Lee (2000) 'Attentional bias, memory bias and the self-concept in paranoia', *Psychological Science*, 9: 77–99.

16. Lyon, Kaney and Bentall, 'The defensive function of persecutory delusions', op. cit.

17. R. P. Bentall and S. Kaney (1996) 'Abnormalities of self-representation and persecutory delusions', *Psychological Medicine*, 26: 1231–7. Another type of implicit self-measure, based on the self-referent encoding effect, was used in this study but produced more equivocal results. For simplicity, I have not described it in the main text.

18. C. F. Fear, H. Sharp and D. Healy (1996) 'Cognitive processes in delusional disorder', *British Journal of Psychiatry*, 168: 61–7.

19. P. Kinderman and R. P. Bentall (2000) 'Self-discrepancies and causal attri-

butions: studies of hypothesized relationships', *British Journal of Clinical Psychology*, 39: 255–73.

20. P. Trower and P. Chadwick (1995) 'Pathways to defense of the self: a theory of two types of paranoia', *Clinical Psychology: Science and Practice*, 2: 263–78.

21. J. Gleick (1988) *Chaos: Making a New Science*. London: Heinemann.

22. R. P. Bentall and S. Kaney (1989) 'Content-specific information processing and persecutory delusions: an investigation using the emotional Stroop test', *British Journal of Medical Psychology*, 62: 355–64; Fear, Sharp and Healy, 'Cognitive processes in delusional disorder', op. cit.

23. R. P. Bentall, S. Kaney and K. Bowen-Jones (1995) 'Persecutory delusions and recall of threat-related, depression-related and neutral words', *Cognitive Therapy and Research*, 19: 331–43; S. Kaney, M. Wolfenden, M. E. Dewey and R. P. Bentall (1992) 'Persecutory delusions and the recall of threatening and non-threatening propositions', *British Journal of Clinical Psychology*, 31: 85–7.

24. P. J. Davis and M. G. Gibson (2000) 'Recognition of posed and genuine facial expressions of emotion in paranoid and nonparanoid schizophrenia', *Journal of Abnormal Psychology*, 109: 445–50; L. LaRusso (1978) 'Sensitivity of paranoid patients to nonverbal cues', *Journal of Abnormal Psychology*, 87: 463–71.

25. E. Bodner and M. Mikulincer (1998) 'Learned helplessness and the occurrence of depressive-like and paranoid-like responses: the role of attentional focus', *Journal of Personality and Social Psychology*, 74: 1010–23.

26. D. T. Gilbert, B. W. Pelham and D. S. Krull (1988) 'On cognitive busyness: when person perceivers meet persons perceived', *Journal of Personality and Social Psychology*, 54: 733–40; D. T. Gilbert (1991) 'How mental systems believe', *American Psychologist*, 46: 107–19; D. T. Gilbert, S. E. McNutty, T. A. Giuliano and J. E. Benson (1992) 'Blurry words and fuzzy deeds: the attribution of obscure behavior', *Journal of Personality and Social Psychology*, 62: 18–25.

27. C. Frith (1994) 'Theory of mind in schizophrenia', in David and Cutting (eds.), *The Neuropsychology of Schizophrenia*, op. cit., pp. 147–61; C. D. Frith (1992) *The Cognitive Neuropsychology of Schizophrenia*. Hillsdale, NJ: Lawrence Erlbaum.

28. P. Kinderman, R. I. M. Dunbar and R. P. Bentall (1998) 'Theory of mind deficits and causal attributions', *British Journal of Psychology*, 71: 339–49.

29. J. Taylor and P. Kinderman (2002) 'An analogue study of attributional complexity, theory of mind deficits and paranoia', *British Journal of Psychology*, 93: 137–40.

30. O. Sabri, R. Erkwoh, M. Schreckenberger, A. Owega, H. Sass and U. Buell (1997) 'Correlation of positive symptoms exclusively to hyperperfusion or hypoperfusion of cerebral cortex in never-treated schizophrenics', *Lancet*, 349: 1735–9.

31. K. P. Ebmeir, D. H. R. Blackwood, C. Murray, V. Souza, M. Walker, N. Dougall, A. P. R. Moffoot, R. E. O'Carroll and G. M. Goodwin (1993) 'Single photon emission computed tomography with 99mTc-Exametazine in unmedicated schizophrenic patients', *Biological Psychiatry*, 33: 487–95; R. D. Kaplan, H. Szechtman, S. Franco, B. Szechtman, C. Nahmias, E. S. Garnett, S. List and J. M.

Cleghorn (1993) '3 clinical syndromes of schizophrenia in untreated subjects: relation to brain glucose activity measured by PET', *Schizophrenia Research*, 11: 47–54; P. F. Liddle, K. J. Friston, C. D. Frith, S. R. Hirsch, T. Jones and R. S. Frackowiak (1992) 'Patterns of cerebral blood flow in schizophrenia', *British Journal of Psychiatry*, 160: 179–86.

32. N. Blackwood, R. J. Howard, D. H. ffytche, A. Simmons, R. P. Bentall and R. M. Murray (2000) 'Imaging attentional and attributional biases: an fMRI approach to paranoid delusions', *Psychological Medicine*, 30: 873–83.

33. B. Kirkpatrick and X. F. Amador (1995) 'The study of paranoia and suspiciousness', *Biological Psychiatry*, 38: 496–7.

34. W. Maier, D. Lichtermann, J. Minges and R. Heun (1993) 'Personality disorders among the relatives of schizophrenia patients', *Schizophrenia Bulletin*, 20: 481–93; E. Squires-Wheeler, A. E. Skodol, A. Bassett and L. Erlenmeyer-Kimling (1989) 'DSM-III-R schizotypal personality traits in offspring of schizophrenic disorder, affective disorder, and normal control parents', *Journal of Psychiatric Research*, 23: 229–39.

35. H. Schanda, P. Berner, E. Gabriel, M. L. Kronberger and B. Kufferle (1983) 'The genetics of delusional psychoses', *Schizophrenia Bulletin*, 9: 563–70.

36. E. Zigler and M. Glick (1988) 'Is paranoid schizophrenia really camouflaged depression?', *American Psychologist*, 43: 284–90.

Chapter 14   The Illusion of Reality

1. Brian's case is described in more detail in my earlier book with Peter Slade (P. D. Slade and R. P. Bentall (1988) *Sensory Deception: A Scientific Analysis of Hallucination*. London: Croom-Helm).

2. G. E. Berrios (1996) *The History of Mental Symptoms: Descriptive Psychopathology since the Nineteenth Century*. Cambridge: Cambridge University Press.

3. J. Jaynes (1979) *The Origins of Consciousness in the Breakdown of the Bicameral Mind*. London: Penguin.

4. I. Leudar and P. Thomas (2000) *Voices of Reason, Voices of Insanity: Studies of Verbal Hallucinations*. London: Routledge.

5. J. Preuss (1975) 'Mental disorders in the Bible and Talmud', *Israeli Annals of Psychiatry and Related Disciplines*, 13: 221–38.

6. T. R. Sarbin and J. B. Juhasz (1967) 'The historical background of the concept of hallucination', *Journal of the History of the Behavioral Sciences*, 5: 339–58.

7. J.-E. D. Esquirol (1832) 'Sur les illusions des sens chez aliénés', *Archives Générales de Médecine*, 2: 5–23.

8. American Psychiatric Association (1994) *Diagnostic and Statistical Manual for Mental Disorders* (4th edn). Washington, DC: APA.

9. Slade and Bentall, *Sensory Deception*, op. cit.

10. K. Jaspers (1913/1963) *General Psychopathology* (trans. J. Hoenig and M. W. Hamilton). Manchester: Manchester University Press.

11. C. H. Mellor (1970) 'First-rank symptoms of schizophrenia', *British Journal of Psychiatry*, 117: 15–23.

12. P. M. Salkovskis (1985) 'Obsessional-compulsive problems: a cognitive behavioural analysis', *Behaviour Research and Therapy*, 23: 571–83.

13. K. Schneider (1959) *Clinical Psychopathology*. New York: Grune & Stratton.

14. N. Sartorius, R. Shapiro and A. Jablensky (1974) 'The international pilot study of schizophrenia', *Schizophrenia Bulletin*, 1: 21–5.

15. G. Asaad and B. Shapiro (1986) 'Hallucinations: theoretical and clinical overview', *American Journal of Psychiatry*, 143: 1088–97.

16. L. J. Miller, E. O'Connor and T. DiPasquale (1993) 'Patients' attitudes to hallucinations', *American Journal of Psychiatry*, 150: 584–8.

17. I. Al-Issa (1978) 'Sociocultural factors in hallucinations', *International Journal of Social Psychiatry*, 24: 167–76; I. Al-Issa (1995) 'The illusion of reality or the reality of an illusion: hallucinations and culture', *British Journal of Psychiatry*, 166: 368–73; A. Jablensky, N. Sartorius, G. Ernberg, M. Anker, A. Korten, J. E. Cooper, R. Day and A. Bertelsen (1992) 'Schizophrenia: manifestations, incidence and course in different cultures', *Psychological Medicine* (Supplement 20): 1–97.

18. W. Pryse-Phillips (1971) 'An olfactory reference syndrome', *Acta Psychiatrica Scandinavica*, 47: 484–509.

19. J. S. Strauss (1969) 'Hallucinations and delusions as points on continua function: rating scale evidence', *Archives of General Psychiatry*, 21: 581–6.

20. M. Romme and S. Escher (eds.) (1993) *Accepting Voices*. London: MIND Publications.

21. For reviews of the medical evidence, see Asaad and Shapiro, 'Hallucinations', op. cit., and Slade and Bentall, *Sensory Deception*, op. cit.

22. R. K. Siegel and M. E. Jarvick (1975) 'Drug-induced hallucinations in animals and man', in R. K. Siegel and L. J. West (eds.), *Hallucinations: Behavior, Experience and Theory*. New York: Wiley.

23. E. C. Johnstone, J. F. MacMillan and T. J. Crow (1987) 'The occurrence of organic disease of possible or probable aetiological significance in a population of 268 cases of first episode schizophrenia', *Psychological Medicine*, 17: 371–9.

24. J. R. Cornelius, J. Mezzich, H. Fabrega, M. D. Cornelius, J. Myers and R. F. Ulrich (1991) 'Characterizing organic hallucinosis', *Comprehensive Psychiatry*, 32: 338–44.

25. M. Pennings and M. Romme (1996) 'Stemmen horen bij schizofrenie patienten, patienten met een dissociatieve stoornis en bij niet patienten', in M. de Hert, E. Thijs, I. Peuskens, D. Petri and B. van Raay (eds.), *Zin in waanzin: De wereld van schizofrenie*. Antwerp: EPO, pp. 137–50.

26. I. Leudar, P. Thomas, D. McNally and A. Glinsky (1997) 'What voices can do with words: pragmatics of verbal hallucinations', *Psychological Medicine*, 27: 885–98.

27. P. Chadwick and M. Birchwood (1994) 'The omnipotence of voices: a cognitive approach to auditory hallucinations', *British Journal of Psychiatry*, 164: 190–201; P. Chadwick and M. Birchwood (1995) 'The omnipotence of voices II: The beliefs about voices questionnaire (BAVQ)', *British Journal of Psychiatry*, 166: 773–6.

28. M. Birchwood, A. Meaden, P. Trower, P. Gilbert and J. Plaistow (2000) 'The power and omnipotence of voices: subordination and entrapment by voices and significant others', *Psychological Medicine*, 30: 337–44.

29. A. P. Morrison (2001) 'The interpretation of intrusions in psychosis: an integrative cognitive approach to hallucinations and delusions', *Behavioural and Cognitive Psychotherapy*, 29: 257–76. See also A. P. Morrison, A. Wells and S. Nothard (2000) 'Cognitive factors in predisposition to auditory and visual hallucinations', *British Journal of Clinical Psychology*, 39: 67–78.

30. A. P. Morrison and A. Wells (in press) 'A comparison of metacognitions in patients with hallucinations, delusions, panic disorder, and non-patient controls', *Behaviour Research and Therapy*.

31. Al-Issa, 'The illusion of reality or the reality of an illusion?', op. cit.

32. Jablensky et al., 'Schizophrenia', op. cit.

33. H. L. Lenz (1964) *Verleichende Psychiatrie: Ein Studie über die Beziehung von Kultur, Sociologie und Psychopathologie*. Vienna: Wilhelm Mandrich.

34. J. Kroll and B. Bachrach (1982) 'Visions and psychopathology in the Middle Ages', *Journal of Nervous and Mental Disease*, 170: 41–9.

35. T. X. Barber and D. S. Calverley (1964) 'An experimental study of "hypnotic" (auditory and visual) hallucinations', *Journal of Abnormal and Social Psychology*, 63: 13–20.

36. S. Mintz and M. Alpert (1972) 'Imagery vividness, reality testing and schizophrenic hallucinations', *Journal of Abnormal and Social Psychology*, 19: 310–16.

37. H. F. Young, R. P. Bentall, P. D. Slade and M. E. Dewey (1987) 'The role of brief instructions and suggestibility in the elicitation of hallucinations in normal and psychiatric subjects', *Journal of Nervous and Mental Disease*, 175: 41–8. For a more complex experiment demonstrating that hallucinating patients are excessively suggestible in the auditory modality, see G. Haddock, P. D. Slade and R. P. Bentall (1995) 'Auditory hallucinations and the verbal transformation effect: the role of suggestions', *Personality and Individual Differences*, 19: 301–6.

38. A. Margo, D. R. Hemsley and P. D. Slade (1981) 'The effects of varying auditory input on schizophrenic hallucinations', *British Journal of Psychiatry*, 139: 122–7.

39. A. G. Gallagher, T. G. Dinin and L. V. J. Baker (1994) 'The effects of varying auditory input on schizophrenic hallucinations: a replication', *British Journal of Medical Psychology*, 67: 67–76.

40. G. L. Belenky (1979) 'Unusual visual experiences reported by subjects in the British Army study of sustained operations, Exercise Early Call', *Military Medicine*, 144: 695–6.

41. N. L. Comer, L. Madow and J. J. Dixon (1967) 'Observations of sensory deprivation in a life-threatening situation', *American Journal of Psychiatry*, 124: 164–9.

42. R. K. Siegel (1984) 'Hostage hallucinations: visual imagery induced by isolation and life-threatening stress', *Journal of Nervous and Mental Disease*, 172: 264–72.

43. W. D. Reese (1971) 'The hallucinations of widowhood', *British Medical Journal*, 210: 37–41.

44. A. Grimby (1993) 'Bereavement among elderly people: grief reactions, post-bereavement hallucinations and quality of life', *Acta Psychiatrica Scandinavica*, 87: 72–80.

45. A. Grimby (1998) 'Hallucinations following the loss of a spouse: common and normal events among the elderly', *Journal of Clinical Geropsychology*, 4: 65–74.

46. R. Lange, J. Houran, T. M. Harte and R. A. Haves (1996) 'Contextual mediation of perceptions in hauntings and poltergeist-like experiences', *Perceptual and Motor Skills*, 82: 755–62.

47. B. K. Toone, E. Cooke and M. H. Lader (1981) 'Electrodermal activity in the affective disorders and schizophrenia', *Psychological Medicine*, 11: 497–508.

48. R. Cooklin, D. Sturgeon and J. P. Leff (1983) 'The relationship between auditory hallucinations and spontaneous fluctuations of skin conductance in schizophrenia', *British Journal of Psychiatry*, 142: 47–52.

49. Leudar et al., 'What voices can do with words', op. cit.

50. L. N. Gould (1948) 'Verbal hallucinations and activity of vocal musculature', *American Journal of Psychiatry*, 105: 367–72; L. N. Gould (1950) 'Verbal hallucinations and automatic speech', *American Journal of Psychiatry*, 107: 110–19.

51. T. Inouye and A. Shimizu (1970) 'The electromyographic study of verbal hallucination', *Journal of Nervous and Mental Disease*, 151: 415–22.

For other demonstrations of subvocalization in patients suffering from auditory hallucinations, see: F. J. McGuigan (1966) 'Covert oral behavior and auditory hallucinations', *Psychophysiology*, 3: 73–80; and M. F. Green and M. Kinsbourne (1990) 'Subvocal activity and auditory hallucinations: clues for behavioral treatments', *Schizophrenia Bulletin*, 16: 617–25.

52. L. N. Gould (1949) 'Auditory hallucinations and subvocal speech', *Journal of Nervous and Mental Disease*, 109: 418–27.

53. P. Green and M. Preston (1981) 'Reinforcement of vocal correlates of auditory hallucinations by auditory feedback: a case study', *British Journal of Psychiatry*, 139: 204–8.

54. J. R. Stevens and A. Livermore (1982) 'Telemetered EEG in schizophrenia: spectral analysis during abnormal behaviour episodes', *Journal of Neurology, Neurosurgery and Psychiatry*, 45: 385–95.

55. P. K. McGuire, G. M. Shah and R. M. Murray (1993) 'Increased blood flow in Broca's area during auditory hallucinations', *Lancet*, 342: 703–6.

56. D. A. Silbersweig, E. Stern, C. Frith, C. Cahill, A. Holmes, S. Grootoonk, J. Seaward, P. McKenna, S. E. Chua, L. Schnorr, T. Jones and R. S. J. Frackowiak (1995) 'A functional neuroanatomy of hallucinations in schizophrenia', *Nature*, 378: 176–9.

57. R. E. Hoffman (1986) 'Verbal hallucinations and language production processes in schizophrenia', *Behavioral and Brain Sciences*, 9: 503–48.

58. K. Akins and D. Dennett (1986) 'Who may I say is calling?' *Behavioral and Brain Sciences*, 9: 517–18.

59. G. L. Stephens and G. Graham (2000) *When Self-Consciousness Breaks: Alien Voices and Inserted Thoughts*. Cambridge, MA: MIT Press.

60. M. K. Johnson, S. Hashtroudi and D. S. Lindsay (1993) 'Source monitoring', *Psychological Bulletin*, 114 (1): 3–28; M. K. Johnson and C. L. Raye (1981) 'Reality monitoring', *Psychological Review*, 88: 67–85.

61. B. Miles (1998) *Paul McCartney: Many Years from Now*. London: Vintage.

62. A. B. Heilbrun (1980) 'Impaired recognition of self-expressed thought in patients with auditory hallucinations', *Journal of Abnormal Psychology*, 89: 728–36.

63. A. B. Heilbrun, N. A. Blum and M. Haas (1983) 'Cognitive vulnerability to auditory hallucinations: preferred imagery mode and spatial location of sounds', *British Journal of Psychiatry*, 143: 294–9; R. P. Bentall, G. A. Baker and S. Havers (1991) 'Reality monitoring and psychotic hallucinations', *British Journal of Clinical Psychology*, 30: 213–22.

64. P. Rankin and P. O'Carrol (1995) 'Reality monitoring and signal detection in individuals prone to hallucinations', *British Journal of Clinical Psychology*, 34: 517–28.

65. Bentall et al., 'Reality monitoring', op. cit.

66. M. L. Seal, S. F. Crowe and P. Cheung (1997) 'Deficits in source monitoring in subjects with auditory hallucinations may be due to differences in verbal intelligence and verbal memory', *Cognitive Neuropsychiatry*, 2: 273–90.

67. G. Brebion, X. Amador, A. David, D. Malaspina and Z. Sharif (2000) 'Positive symptomatology and source monitoring failure in schizophrenia: an analysis of symptom-specific effects', *Psychiatry Research*, 95: 119–31. For a slightly different kind of source-monitoring experiment which produced results that are consistent with the argument I am making in this chapter, see N. Franck, P. Rouby, E. Daprati, J. Dalery, M. Marie-Cardine and N. Georgieff (2000) 'Confusion between silent and overt reading in schizophrenia', *Schizophrenia Research*, 41: 357–68.

68. R. P. Bentall and P. D. Slade (1985) 'Reality testing and auditory hallucinations: a signal-detection analysis', *British Journal of Clinical Psychology*, 24: 159–69.

69. Rankin and O'Carrol, 'Reality monitoring and signal detection', op. cit.

70. G. Brebion, M. J. Smith, X. Amador, D. Malaspina and J. M. Gorman (1998) 'Word recognition, discrimination accuracy, and decision bias in schizophrenia: association with positive symptomatology and depressive symptomatology', *Journal of Nervous and Mental Disease*, 186: 604–9.

71. C. A. Baker and A. P. Morrison (1998) 'Cognitive processes in auditory hallucinations: attributional biases and metacognition', *Psychological Medicine*, 28: 1199–208; A. P. Morrison and G. Haddock (1997) 'Cognitive factors in source monitoring and auditory hallucinations', *Psychological Medicine*, 27: 669–79.

72. I. Ensum and A. P. Morrison (in press) 'The effects of focus of attention on attributional bias in patients experiencing auditory hallucinations', *Behaviour Research and Therapy*.

73. L. C. Johns and P. K. McGuire (1999) 'Verbal self-monitoring and auditory hallucinations in schizophrenia', *Lancet*, 353: 469–70; L. C. Johns, S. Rossell, C.

Frith, F. Ahmad, D. Hemsley, E. Kuipers and P. K. McGuire (2001) 'Verbal self-monitoring and auditory hallucinations in people with schizophrenia', *Psychological Medicine*, 31: 705–15.

74. H. Szechtman, E. Woody, K. S. Bowers and C. Nahmias (1998) 'Where the imaginal appears real: a positron emission tomography study of auditory hallucinations', *Proceedings of the National Academy of Sciences, USA*, 95: 1956–60.

75. Leudar and Thomas, *Voices of Reason, Voices of Insanity*, op. cit.

76. G. L. Stephens and G. Graham (2000) *When Self-Consciousness Breaks*, op. cit.

77. A. P. Morrison and C. A. Baker (2000) 'Intrusive thoughts and auditory hallucinations: a comparative study of intrusions in psychosis', *Behaviour Research and Therapy*, 38: 1097–106.

78. A. P. Morrison (2001) 'The interpretation of intrusions in psychosis: an integrative cognitive approach to hallucinations and delusions', *Behavioural and Cognitive Psychotherapy*, 29: 257–76.

79. D. M. Wegner (1994) *White Bears and Other Unwanted Thoughts: Suppression, Obsession and the Psychology of Mental Control*. New York: Guilford.

80. L. Sass (1992) *Madness and Modernism: Insanity in the Light of Modern Art, Literature, and Thought*. New York: Basic Books.

Chapter 15   The Language of Madness

1. Source unknown.

2. E. Kraepelin (1905) *Lectures in Clinical Psychiatry* (revised 2nd edn). London: Baillière, Tindall and Cox.

3. ibid. The quotation is as given in R. D. Laing's *The Divided Self* (London: Tavistock Press, 1960) with Laing's italics.

4. E. Bleuler (1911/1950) *Dementia Praecox or the Group of Schizophrenias* (trans. E. Zinkin). New York: International Universities Press.

5. E. von Domarus (1944) 'The specific laws of logic in schizophrenia', in J. S. Kasanin (ed.), *Language and Thought in Schizophrenia*. New York: Norton.

6. L. S. Vygotsky (1934) 'Thought in schizophrenia', *Archives of Neurological Psychiatry*, 31: 1063–77.

7. K. Goldstein (1944) 'Methodological approach to the study of schizophrenic thought disorder', in Kasanin (ed.), *Language and Thought*, op. cit.

8. N. Cameron (1944) 'Experimental analysis of schizophrenic thinking', in Kasanin (ed.), *Language and Thought*, op. cit.

9. N. Cameron (1947) *The Psychology of Behavior Disorders*. Boston: Houghton Mifflin. For a detailed account of Cameron's work, see L. J. Chapman and J. P. Chapman (1973). *Disordered Thought in Schizophrenia*. Englewood Cliffs, NJ: Prentice-Hall.

10. Chapman and Chapman, *Disordered Thought*, op. cit.

11. S. Rochester and J. R. Martin (1979) *Crazy Talk: A Study of the Discourse of Psychotic Speakers*. New York: Plenum.

12. N. C. Andreasen (1982) 'Should the term "thought disorder" be revised?' *Comprehensive Psychiatry*, 23: 291–9.

13. N. C. Andreasen (1979) 'The clinical assessment of thought, language and communication disorders', *Archives of General Psychiatry*, 36: 1315–21.

14. N. C. Andreasen (1979) 'Thought, language and communication disorders: diagnostic significance', *Archives of General Psychiatry*, 36: 1325–30.

15. For replications of this finding, see: P. D. Harvey, E. A. Earle-Boyer and M. S. Wielgus (1984). 'The consistency of thought disorder in mania and schizophrenia: an assessment of acute psychotics', *Journal of Nervous and Mental Disease*, 172: 458–63; and L. S. Grossman and M. Harrow (1991) 'Thought disorder and cognitive processes in mania', in P. A. Magaro (ed.), *Annual Review of Psychopathology*, Newbury Park, CA: Sage.

16. R. D. Laing (1960) *The Divided Self*. London: Tavistock Press.

17. M. Harrow and M. Prosen (1978) 'Intermingling and the disordered logic as influences on schizophrenic thought', *Archives of General Psychiatry*, 35: 1213–18; M. Harrow and M. Prosen (1979) 'Schizophrenic thought disorders: bizarre associations and intermingling', *American Journal of Psychiatry*, 136: 293–6.

18. For a review, see Chapter 11 of Chapman and Chapman, *Disordered Thought in Schizophrenia*, op cit.

19. L. J. Chapman and J. P. Chapman (1974) 'Schizophrenic response to affectivity in word definition', *Journal of Abnormal Psychology*, 83: 616–22.

20. A. Shimkunas (1972) 'Demand for intimate self-disclosure and pathological verbalizations in schizophrenia', *Journal of Abnormal Psychology*, 80: 197–205.

21. G. Haddock, M. Wolfenden, I. Lowens, N. Tarrier and R. P. Bentall (1995) 'The effect of emotional salience on the thought disorder of patients with a diagnosis of schizophrenia', *British Journal of Psychiatry*, 167: 618–20.

22. N. M. Docherty, I. M. Evans, W. H. Sledge, J. P. Seibyl and J. H. Krystal (1994) 'Affective reactivity of language in schizophrenia', *Journal of Nervous and Mental Disease*, 182: 98–102; N. M. Docherty and A. S. Hebert (1997) 'Comparative affective reactivity of different types of communication disturbances in schizophrenia', *Journal of Abnormal Psychology*, 106: 325–30.

23. S. Tai, G. Haddock and R. P. Bentall (in submission) 'The effects of emotional salience on thought disorder in patients with bipolar affective disorder'.

24. W. M. Grove and N. C. Andreasen (1985) 'Language and thinking in psychosis', *Archives of General Psychiatry*, 42: 26–32.

25. M. Harrow and J. G. Miller (1980) 'Schizophrenic thought disorders and impaired perspective', *Journal of Abnormal Psychology*, 89: 717–27.

26. Rochester and Martin, *Crazy Talk*, op. cit.

27. B. A. Maher, K. O. McKean and B. McLaughlin (1966) 'Studies in psychotic language', in P. J. Stone, R. F. Bales, Z. Namenworth and D. M. Ogilvie (eds.), *The General Inquirer: A Computer Approach to Content Analysis*. Cambridge, MA: MIT Press.

28. Quoted in Rochester and Martin, *Crazy Talk*, op. cit.

29. P. D. Harvey and J. M. Neale (1983) 'The specificity of thought disorder to schizophrenia: research methods in their historical perspective', in B. A. Maher and W. B. Maher (eds.), *Progress in Experimental Personality Research*. New York: Academic Press.

30. T. Wykes and J. Leff (1982) 'Disordered speech: differences between manics and schizophrenics', *Brain and Language*, 15: 117–24.

31. P. D. Harvey (1983) 'Speech competence in manic and schizophrenic psychosis: the association between clinically rated thought disorder and cohesion and reference performance', *Journal of Abnormal Psychology*, 92: 368–77. For similar findings, see: A. B. Ragin and T. F. Oltmanns (1986) 'Lexical cohesion and formal thought disorder during and after psychotic episodes', *Journal of Abnormal Psychology*, 95: 181–3.

32. Elaine Chaika of Providence College in Rhode Island (*Understanding Psychotic Speech: Beyond Freud and Chomsky*. Springfield, IL: Charles C. Thomas, 1990; see also 'On analysing psychotic speech: what model should we use?', in A. Sims (ed.) (1995) *Speech and Language Disorders in Psychiatry*. London: Gaskell) has questioned aspects of Halliday and Hasan's theory of cohesion, arguing that some speech can have ample cohesive ties but still remain incoherent. An example of such speech from a schizophrenia patient she studied was as follows:

Her parents that she's so proud of she goes out, leaves the ice cream and eats it and on the way and we don't know what happens the fact. You can interpolate and say that she ate the ice cream and brought it home.

In her own research, Chaika asked schizophrenia patients and ordinary people to watch and then talk about a short film, 'The Ice Cream Stories', concerning a young girl who is refused cash for ice cream from her mother but who manages to persuade her father to supply the necessary money. Using an analysis similar to that employed by Rochester and Martin, she found no evidence of abnormal cohesive ties, although there was evidence of excessive exophoria.

Chaika's findings certainly did not imply that the speech of thought-disordered patients is normal. They often had difficulty constructing narratives that followed the temporal ordering of the events in the story. When the normal participants misperceived some aspect of the story, their misperception generally fitted in with the story line (for example, they mistook the flavour of the ice cream bought by the girl) whereas the misperceptions of the schizophrenia patients sometimes deviated from the story line significantly (for example, one patient reported that the girl in the story moved a shop counter rather than leaned against it). Sometimes the schizophrenia patients veered off the story line and never returned to it.

33. N. M. Docherty, M. DeRosa and N. C. Andreasen (1996) 'Communication disturbances in schizophrenia and mania', *Archives of General Psychiatry*, 53: 358–64.

34. Docherty and Hebert, 'Comparative affective reactivity', op. cit.

35. R. E. Hoffman, L. Kirstein, S. Stopek and D. V. Cicchetti (1982) 'Apprehending schizophrenic discourse: a structural analysis of the listener's task', *Brain and Language*, 15: 207–33.

36. R. E. Hoffman, S. Stopek and N. C. Andreasen (1986) 'A comparative study of manic vs schizophrenic speech disorganization', *Archives of General Psychiatry*, 43: 831–5.

37. A. W. Beveridge and K. Brown (1985) 'A critique of Hoffman's analysis of schizophrenic speech', *Brain and Language*, 24: 174–81.

38. D. M. Barch and H. Berenbaum (1996) 'Language production and thought disorder in schizophrenia', *Journal of Abnormal Psychology*, 105: 81–8.

39. Chaika, 'On analysing psychotic speech', op. cit.

40. P. D. Harvey (1985) 'Reality monitoring in mania and schizophrenia: the association between thought disorder and performance', *Journal of Abnormal Psychology*, 92: 368–77; P. D. Harvey (1988) 'Cognitive deficits and thought disorder: a retest study', *Schizophrenia Bulletin*, 14: 57–66; P. D. Harvey and M. Serper (1990) 'Linguistic and cognitive failures in schizophrenia: a multivariate analysis', *Journal of Nervous and Mental Disease*, 178: 487–94.

41. Y. Sarfati, M. C. Hardy-Bayle, C. Besche and D. Widlocher (1997) 'Attributions of intentions to others in people with schizophrenia: a non-verbal exploration with comic strips', *Schizophrenia Research*, 25: 199–209; Y. Sarfati and M. C. Hardy-Bayle (1999) 'How do people with schizophrenia explain the behaviour of others? A study of theory of mind and its relationship to thought and speech disorganization in schizophrenia', *Psychological Medicine*, 29: 613–20; Y. Sarfati, M. C. Hardy-Bayle, E. Brunet and D. Widlocher (1999) 'Investigating theory of mind in schizophrenia: influence of verbalization in disorganized and non-disorganized patients', *Schizophrenia Research*, 37: 183–90; Y. Sarfati, C. Passerieux and M. C. Hardy-Bayle (2000) 'Can verbalization remedy the theory of mind deficit in schizophrenia?' *Psychopathology*, 33: 246–51; Y. H. B. Sarfati, J. Nadel, J. F. Chevalier and D. Widlocher (1997) 'Attribution of mental states to others by schizophrenic patients,' *Cognitive Neuropsychiatry*, 2: 1–17.

42. T. F. Oltmanns and J. M. Neale (1978) 'Distractability in relation to other aspects of schizophrenic disorder', in S. Schwartz (ed.), *Language and Cognition in Schizophrenia*. Hillsdale, NJ. Erlbaum.

43. See, for example, P. D. Harvey, E. A. Earle-Boyer and J. C. Levinson (1986) 'Distractability and discourse failure: their association in mania and schizophrenia', *Journal of Nervous and Mental Disease*, 174: 274–9.

44. D. Barch and H. Berenbaum (1994) 'The relationship between information processing and language production', *Journal of Abnormal Psychology*, 103: 241–50.

45. C. M. Adler, T. E. Goldberg, A. K. Malhotra, D. Pickar and A. Breier (1998) 'Effects of ketamine on thought disorder, working memory, and semantic memory in healthy volunteers', *Biological Psychiatry*, 43: 811–16.

46. T. E. Goldberg and D. R. Weinberger (2000) 'Thought disorder in schizophrenia: a reappraisal of older formulations and an overview of some recent studies', *Cognitive Neuropsychiatry*, 5: 1–19.

47. For a discussion of these effects and their relevance to psychiatric disorders, see: E. Chen, P. McKenna and A. Wilkins (1995) 'Semantic processing and categorisation in schizophrenia', in A. Sims (ed.), *Speech and Language Disorders in Psychiatry*. London: Gaskell; and M. Spitzer (1997) 'A cognitive neuroscience view of schizophrenic thought disorder', *Schizophrenia Bulletin*, 23: 29–50.

48. See, for example: L. Clare, P. J. McKenna, A. M. Mortimer and A. D. Baddeley (1993) 'Memory in schizophrenia: what is impaired and what is preserved?' *Neuropsychologia*, 31: 1225–41; and P. J. McKenna, A. M. Mortimer and J. R. Hodges (1994) 'Semantic memory and schizophrenia', in A. S. David and J. C. Cutting (eds.), *The Neuropsychology of Schizophrenia*. Hove: Erlbaum.

49. Spitzer, 'A cognitive neuroscience view', op. cit.

50. T. E. Goldberg, M. Aloia, M. L. Gourovitch, D. Missar, D. Pickar and D. R. Weinberger (1998) 'Cognitive substrates of thought disorder, I: The semantic system', *American Journal of Psychiatry*, 155: 1671–6.

51. Goldberg and Weinberger, 'Thought disorder in schizophrenia', op. cit.

52. B. A. Maher, T. C. Manschreck, T. M. Hoover and C. C. Weisstein (1987) 'Thought disorder and measured features of language production in schizophrenia', in P. D. Harvey and E. Walker (eds.), *Positive and Negative Symptoms in Psychosis: Description, Research and Future Directions*. Hillsdale, NJ: Erlbaum; T. C. Manschreck, B. A. Maher, J. J. Milavetz, D. Ames, C. C. Weisstein and M. L. Schneyer (1988) 'Semantic priming in thought disordered schizophrenic patients', *Schizophrenia Research*, 1: 61–6.

53. Spitzer, 'A cognitive neuroscience view', op. cit.

54. M. Spitzer, U. Braun, L. Hermie and S. Maier (1993) 'Associative semantic network dysfunction in thought disordered schizophrenic patients', *Biological Psychiatry*, 34: 864–77.

55. M. Aloia, M. L. Gourovitch, D. Missar, D. Pickar, D. R. Weinberger and T. E. Goldberg (1998) 'Cognitive substrates of thought disorder, II: specifying a candidate cognitive mechanism', *American Journal of Psychiatry*, 155: 1677–84. See also D. M. Barch, J. D. Cohen, D. Servan-Schreiber, S. Steingard, S. Steinhauer and D. P. van Kammen (1996) 'Semantic priming in schizophrenia: an examination of spreading activation using word pronounciation and multiple SOAs', *Journal of Abnormal Psychology*, 105: 592–601.

56. D. M. Barch and H. Berenbaum (1996) 'Language production and thought disorder in schizophrenia', *Journal of Abnormal Psychology*, 105: 81–8.

57. Grossman and Harrow, 'Thought disorder and cognitive processes in mania', op. cit.

Chapter 16 Things are Much More Complex than they Seem

1. J. B. S. Haldane (1923) *Daedalus, or Science and the Future*. London: Kegan Paul.

2. R. Mojtabai and R. O. Rieder (1998) 'Limitations of the symptom-orientated approach to psychiatric research', *British Journal of Psychiatry*, 173: 198–202.

3. See, for example, his comments about delusions in G. E. Berrios (1991) 'Delusions as "wrong beliefs": a conceptual history', *British Journal of Psychiatry*, 159: 6–13.

4. T. Honderich (1993) *How Free are You?: The Determinism Problem*. Oxford: Oxford University Press.

5. R. Warner (1985) *Recovery from Schizophrenia: Psychiatry and Political Economy*. New York: Routledge & Kegan Paul.

6. P. Sturmey (1996) *Functional Analysis in Clinical Psychology*. Chichester: Wiley.

7. B. A. Maher (1974) 'Delusional thinking and perceptual disorder', *Journal of Individual Psychology*, 30: 98–113.

8. S. Escher, M. Romme, A. Buiks, P. Delespaul and J. van Os (2002) 'Formation of delusional ideation in adolescents hearing voices: a prospective study', *American Journal of Medical Genetics (Neuropsychiatric Genetics)*, 114: 913–20.

9. G. Haddock, P. D. Slade and R. P. Bentall (1995) 'Auditory hallucinations and the verbal transformation effect: the role of suggestions', *Personality and Individual Differences*, 19: 301–6; S. Mintz and M. Alpert (1972) 'Imagery vividness, reality testing and schizophrenic hallucinations', *Journal of Abnormal and Social Psychology*, 19: 310–16; H. F. Young, R. P. Bentall, P. D. Slade and M. E. Dewey (1987) 'The role of brief instructions and suggestibility in the elicitation of hallucinations in normal and psychiatric subjects', *Journal of Nervous and Mental Disease*, 175: 41–8.

10. M. Birchwood, Z. Iqbal, P. Chadwick and P. Trower (2000) 'Cognitive approach to depression and suicidal thinking in psychosis: 1. Ontogeny of post-psychotic depression', *British Journal of Psychiatry*, 177: 516–21.

11. Z. Iqbal, M. Birchwood, P. Chadwick and P. Trower (2000) 'Cognitive approach to depression and suicidal thinking in psychosis: 2. Testing the validity of a social rank model', *British Journal of Psychiatry*, 177: 522–8.

12. D. H. Erickson, M. Beiser and W. G. Iacono (1998) 'Social support predicts 5-year outcome in first-episode schizophrenia', *Journal of Abnormal Psychology*, 107: 681–5.

13. P. Meehl (1962) 'Schizotaxia, schizotypia, schizophrenia', *American Psychologist*, 17: 827–38. See Chapter 5 of this book for more details.

14. G. S. Claridge (1990) 'Can a disease model of schizophrenia survive?', in R. P. Bentall (ed.), *Reconstructing Schizophrenia*. London: Routledge.

15. K. H. Nuechterlein and K. L. Subotnik (1998) 'The cognitive origins of schizo-

phrenia and prospects for intervention', in T. Wykes, N. Tarrier and S. Lewis (eds.), *Outcome and Innovation in Psychological Treatment of Schizophrenia*. Chichester: Wiley.

16. L. Y. Abramson, G. I. Metalsky and L. B. Alloy (1989) 'Hopelessness depression: a theory-based subtype of depression', *Psychological Review*, 96: 358–72; L. Y. Abramson, M. E. P. Seligman and J. D. Teasdale (1978) 'Learned helplessness in humans: critique and reformulation', *Journal of Abnormal Psychology*, 78: 40–74.

17. M. H. Kernis (1993) 'The role of stability and level of self-esteem in psychological functioning', in R. F. Baumeister (ed.), *Self-Esteem: The Puzzle of Low Self-Regard*. New York: Plenum, pp. 167–82; M. H. Kernis, D. P. Cornell, C. R. Sun, A. Berry and T. Harlow (1993) 'There's more to self-esteem than whether it is high or low: the importance of stability of self-esteem', *Journal of Personality and Social Psychology*, 65: 1190–204.

18. K. D. Greenier, M. H. Kernis, C. W. McNamara, S. B. Waschull, A. J. Berry, C. E. Herlocker and T. A. Abend (1999) 'Individual differences in reactivity to events: re-examining the roles of stability and level of self-esteem', *Journal of Personality*, 67: 185–208.

19. A. Gottschalk, M. S. Bauer and P. C. Whybrow (1995) 'Evidence of chaotic mood variation in bipolar disorder', *Archives of General Psychiatry*, 52: 947–59.

20. J. Gleick (1988) *Chaos: Making a New Science*. London: Heinemann.

21. I. Myin-Germeys, J. van Os, J. E. Schwartz, A. Stone and P. Delespaul (2001) 'Emotional reactivity to daily stress in psychosis', *Archives of General Psychiatry*, 58: 1137–44.

22. I. Myin-Germeys, L. Krabbendam, J. Jolles, P. A. E. G. Delespaul and J. van Os (2002) 'Are cognitive impairments associated with sensitivity to stress in schizophrenia? An experience sampling study', *American Journal of Psychiatry*, 159: 443–9.

23. W. Tschacher (1996) 'The dynamics of psychosocial crises: time courses and causal models', *Journal of Nervous and Mental Disease*, 184: 172–9. See also W. Tschacher, C. Scheier and Y. Hashimoto (1997) 'Dynamical analysis of schizophrenia courses', *Biological Psychiatry*, 41: 428–37.

24. A. Gumley, C. A. White and K. Power (1999) 'An interacting cognitive subsystems model of relapse and the course of psychosis', *Clinical Psychology and Psychotherapy*, 6: 261–78.

25. J. A. Smith and N. Tarrier (1992) 'Prodromal symptoms in manic depressive psychosis', *Social Psychiatry and Psychiatric Epidemiology*, 27: 245–8.

26. M. Birchwood (1996) 'Early intervention in psychotic relapse: cognitive approaches to detection and management', in G. Haddock and P. D. Slade (eds.), *Cognitive-Behavioural Interventions with Psychotic Disorders*. London: Routledge, pp. 171–211.

27. G. W. Brown (1984) 'The discovery of expressed emotion: induction or deduction?', in J. Leff and C. Vaughn (eds.) *Expressed Emotion in Families: Its Significance for Mental Health*. New York: Guilford, pp. 7–25.

28. G. W. Brown, M. Carstairs and G. Topping (1958) 'Post-hospital adjustment of chronic mental patients', *Lancet*, ii: 685–9.

29. G. W. Brown, E. M. Monck, G. M. Carstairs and J. K. Wing (1962) 'Influence of family life on the course of schizophrenia disorders', *British Journal of Preventative and Social Medicine*, 16: 55–68.

30. G. W. Brown and M. Rutter (1966) 'The measurement of family activities and relationships: a methodological study', *Human Relations*, 19: 241–63.

31. The only widely used alternative to the Camberwell Family Interview is the Five Minute Speech Sample, which (as the name suggests) is based on the analysis of five minutes of speech in which the relative talks about the patient. See A. B. Magana, M. J. Goldstein, M. Karno, D. J. Miklowitz, J. Jenkins and I. R. H. Falloon (1986) 'A brief method of assessing expressed emotion in relatives of psychiatric patients', *Psychiatry Research*, 17: 203–12.

32. P. E. Bebbington and E. Kuipers (1994) 'The predictive utility of expressed emotion in schizophrenia', *Psychological Medicine*, 24: 707–18. For a more recent meta-analysis that reached essentially the same conclusions, see R. L. Butzlaff and J. M. Hooley (1998) 'Expressed emotion and psychiatric relapse', *Archives of General Psychiatry*, 55: 547–52.

33. C. E. Vaughn and J. Leff (1976) 'The influence of family and social factors on the course of psychiatric illness: a comparison of schizophrenic and depressed neurotic patients', *British Journal of Psychiatry*, 129: 125–37.

34. J. P. Leff and C. Vaughn (1980) 'The interaction of life-events and relatives' expressed emotion in schizophrenia and depressive neurosis', *British Journal of Psychiatry*, 136: 146–53.

35. J. M. Hooley, J. Orley and J. D. Teasdale (1989) 'Predictors of relapse in unipolar depressives: expressed emotion, marital distress and perceived criticism', *Journal of Abnormal Psychology*, 98: 229–37.

36. D. J. Miklowitz, M. J. Goldstein, K. H. Nuechterlein, K. S. Snyder and J. Mintz (1988) 'Family factors and the course of bipolar affective disorder', *Archives of General Psychiatry*, 45: 225–31.

37. N. Tarrier and G. Turpin (1992) 'Psychosocial factors, arousal and schizophrenic relapse: the physiological data', *British Journal of Psychiatry*, 161: 3–11.

38. M. Goldstein, I. Rosenfarb, S. Woo and K. Nuechterlein (1994) 'Intrafamilial relationships and the course of schizophrenia', *Acta Psychiatrica Scandinavica*, 90 (Supplement 384): 60–6.

39. C. Barrowclough, N. Tarrier, L. Humphreys, J. Ward, L. Gregg and B. Andrews (in press) 'Self-esteem in schizophrenia: the relationship between self-evaluation, family attitudes and symptomatology', *Journal of Consulting and Clinical Psychology*.

40. D. J. Miklowitz, M. J. Goldstein, I. R. Falloon and J. A. Doane (1984) 'Interactional correlates of expressed emotion in the families of schizophrenics', *British Journal of Psychiatry*, 144: 482–7.

41. D. J. Miklowitz (1994) 'Family risk indicators in schizophrenia', *Schizophrenia Bulletin*, 20: 137–49.

42. C. R. Brewin, B. MacCarthy, K. Duda and C. E. Vaughn (1991) 'Attribution and expressed emotion in the relatives of patients with schizophrenia', *Journal of Abnormal Psychology*, 100: 546–54.

43. C. Barrowclough, M. Johnston and N. Tarrier (1994) 'Attributions, expressed emotion and patient relapse: an attributional model of relatives' response to schizophrenic illness', *Behavior Therapy*, 25: 67–88.

44. G. Fadden, P. E. Bebbington and L. Kuipers (1987) 'The impact of functional psychiatric illness on the patient's family', *British Journal of Psychiatry*, 150: 285–92.

45. E. Kuipers and D. Raune (2000) 'The early development of expressed emotion and burden in the families of first-onset psychosis', in M. Birchwood, D. Fowler and C. Jackson (eds.), *Early Intervention in Psychosis*. London: Wiley, pp. 128–40.

46. D. Diamond and J. Doane (1994) 'Disturbed attachment and negative affective style: an intergenerational spiral', *British Journal of Psychiatry*, 164: 770–81.

47. G. Paley, D. A. Shapiro and A. Worrall-Davies (2000) 'Familial origins of expressed emotion in relatives of people with schizophrenia', *Journal of Mental Health*, 9: 655–63.

48. E. Kuipers and E. Moore (1995) 'Expressed emotion and staff–client relationships: implications for community care of the severely mentally ill', *International Journal of Mental Health*, 24: 13–26; E. Moore, R. A. Ball and L. Kuipers (1992) 'Expressed emotion in staff working with the long-term adult mentally ill', *British Journal of Psychiatry*, 161: 802–8; E. Moore and E. Kuipers (1999) 'The measurement of expressed emotion in relationships between staff and service users: the use of short speech samples', *British Journal of Clinical Psychology*, 38: 345–56; N. Oliver and E. Kuipers (1996) 'Stress and its relationship to expressed emotion in community mental health workers', *International Journal of Social Psychiatry*, 42: 150–9.

49. R. A. Ball, E. Moore and L. Kuipers (1992) 'Expressed emotion in community care staff: a comparison of patient outcome in a nine month follow-up of two hostels', *Social Psychiatry and Psychiatric Epidemiology*, 27: 35–9.

50. K. S. Snyder, C. J. Wallace, K. Moe and R. P. Liberman (1994) 'Expressed emotion by residential care workers and residents' symptoms and quality of life', *Hospital and Community Psychiatry*, 45: 1141–3.

51. P. E. Bebbington, J. Bowen, S. R. Hirsch and E. A. Kuipers (1995) 'Schizophrenia and psychosocial stresses', in S. R. Hirsch and D. R. Weinberger (eds.), *Schizophrenia*. Oxford: Blackwell, pp. 587–604.

52. G. W. Brown and T. Harris (1978) *Social Origins of Depression*. New York: Free Press.

53. G. W. Brown and P. Moran (1998) 'Emotion and the etiology of depressive disorders', in W. F. Flack and J. D. Laird (eds.), *Emotions in Psychopathology: Theory and Research*. New York: Oxford University Press, pp. 171–84.

54. G. W. Brown and R. Prudo (1981) 'Psychiatric disorders in a rural and an urban population: 1. Aetiology of depression', *Psychological Medicine*, 11: 581–99.

55. G. W. Brown and J. L. T. Birley (1968) 'Crises and life changes and the onset of schizophrenia', *Journal of Health and Social Behaviour*, 9: 203–14.

56. Bebbington et al., 'Schizophrenia and psychosocial stresses', op. cit.

57. S. Hirsch, J. Bowen, J. Emami, P. Cramer, A. Jolley, C. Haw and M. Dickinson (1996) 'A one year prospective study of the effect of life events and medication in the aetiology of schizophrenic relapse', *British Journal of Psychiatry*, 168: 49–56.

58. S. L. Johnson and J. E. Roberts (1995) 'Life events and bipolar disorder: implications from biological theories', *Psychological Bulletin*, 117: 434–49.

59. S. L. Johnson and I. Miller (1997) 'Negative life events and time to recovery from episodes of bipolar disorder', *Journal of Abnormal Psychology*, 106: 449–57.

60. R. Finlay-Jones and G. W. Brown (1981) 'Types of stressful life events and the onset of anxiety and depressive disorders', *Psychological Medicine*, 11: 803–15.

61. Brown and Moran, 'Emotion and the etiology of depressive disorders', op. cit.

62. T. Harris (1987) 'Recent developments in the study of life events in relation to psychiatric and physical disorders', in B. Cooper (ed.), *Psychiatric Epidemiology: Progress and Prospects*. London: Croom Helm, pp. 81–102.

63. R. Day, J. A. Neilsen, A. Korten, G. Ernberg, K. C. Dube, J. Gebhart, A. Jablensky, C. Leon, A. Marsella, M. Olatawura, N. Sartorius, E. Stromgren, R. Takahashi, N. Wig and L. C. Wynne (1987) 'Stressful life events preceding the onset of acute schizophrenia: a cross-national study from the World Health Organization', *Culture, Medicine and Psychiatry*, 11: 123–206; T. Fuchs (1999) 'Life events in late paraphrenia and depression', *Psychopathology*, 32: 60–9.

64. S. Malkoff-Schwartz, E. Frank, B. Anderson, J. T. Sherrill, L. Siegel, D. Patterson and D. J. Kupfer (1998) 'Stressful life events and social rhythm disruption in the onset of manic and depressive episodes of bipolar disorder', *Archives of General Psychiatry*, 55: 702–7.

65. S. L. Johnson, D. Sandow, B. Meyer, R. Winters, I. Miller, D. Solomon and G. Keitner (2000) 'Increases in manic symptoms after life events involving goal attainment', *Journal of Abnormal Psychology*, 109: 721–7.

66. Bebbington et al., 'Schizophrenia and psychosocial stresses', op. cit.

67. M. Bowers, N. Boutros, D. C. D'Souza and S. Madonick (2001) 'Substance abuse as a risk factor for schizophrenia and related disorders', *International Journal of Mental Health*, 30: 33–57; A. Johns (2001) 'Psychiatric effects of cannabis', *British Journal of Psychiatry*, 178: 116–22.

68. S. M. Stakowski, M. P. DelBello, D. E. Fleck and S. Arndt (2000) 'The impact of substance abuse on the course of bipolar disorder', *Biological Psychiatry*, 48: 477–85.

69. E. S. Brown, T. Suppes, B. Adinoff and N. R. Thomas (2001) 'Drug abuse and bipolar disorder: comorbidity or misdiagnosis?' *Journal of Affective Disorders*, 65: 105–15; K. T. Mueser, P. R. Yarnold, S. D. Rosenberg, C. Swett and K. M. Miles (2000) 'Substance use in hospitalized severely mentally ill psychiatric patients: prevalence, correlates and subgroups', *Schizophrenia Bulletin*, 26: 179–92; I. L. Fowler, V. J. Carr, N. T. Carter and T. J. Lewin (1998) 'Patterns of current and lifetime substance use in schizophrenia', *Schizophrenia Bulletin*, 24: 433–55.

70. K. H. Nuechterlein, M. E. Dawson, M. Giltin, J. Ventura, M. J. Goldstein, K. S. Snyder, C. M. Yee and J. Mintz (1992) 'Developmental processes in schizophrenic disorders: longitudinal studies of vulnerability and stress', *Schizophrenia Bulletin*, 18: 387–425.

Chapter 17   From the Cradle to the Clinic

1. J. Milton (1671) *Paradise Regained*.
2. S. Lewis, N. Tarrier, G. Haddock, R. P. Bentall, P. Kinderman, D. Kingdon, R. Siddle, R. Drake, J. Everitt, K. Leadley, A. Benn, K. Grazebrook, C. Haley, S. Akhtar, L. Davies, S. Palmer, B. Faragher and G. Dunn (2002) 'Randomised, controlled trial of cognitive-behaviour therapy in early schizophrenia: acute phase outcomes', *British Journal of Psychiatry*, 181 (Supplement 43): s91–s97. See also R. J. Drake, C. J. Haley, S. Akhtar and S. W. Lewis (2000) 'Causes of duration of untreated psychosis in schizophrenia', *British Journal of Psychiatry*, 177: 511–15.
3. H. Hafner, K. Maurer, W. Loffler and A. Riecher-Rossler (1993) 'The influence of age and sex on the onset and early course of schizophrenia', *British Journal of Psychiatry*, 162: 80–6.
4. F. K. Goodwin and K. R. Jamison (1990) *Manic-Depressive Illness*. Oxford: Oxford University Press.
5. E. Leibenluft (1996) 'Women with bipolar illness: clinical and research issues', *American Journal of Psychiatry*, 153: 163–73.
6. A. M. Vicente and J. L. Kennedy (1997) 'The genetics of neurodevelopment and schizophrenia', in M. S. Keshavan and R. M. Murray (eds.), *Neurodevelopment and Adult Psychopathology*. Cambridge: Cambridge University Press.
7. I. Feinberg (1982) 'Schizophrenia and late maturational brain changes in man', *Psychopharmocology Bulletin*, 18: 29–31.
8. E. T. Bullmore, P. O'Connell, S. Frangou and R. M. Murray (1997) 'Schizophrenia as a developmental disorder of neural network integrity: the dysplastic net hypothesis', in Keshavan and Murray (eds.), *Neurodevelopment and Adult Psychopathology*, op. cit.
9. H. Hafner, W. an der Heiden, S. Behrens, W. F. Gattaz, M. Hambrecht, W. Loffler, K. Maurer, P. Munk-Jorgensen, B. Nowotny, A. Riecher-Rossler and A. Stein (1998) 'Causes and consequences of the gender difference in age at onset of schizophrenia', *Schizophrenia Bulletin*, 24: 99–113.
10. Quoted in A. Jablensky (1999) 'The conflict of the nosologists: views on schizophrenia and manic-depressive illness in the early part of the 20th century', *Schizophrenia Research*, 39: 95–100.
11. R. Lewontin (2000) *The Triple Helix: Gene, Organism and Environment*. Cambridge, MA: Harvard University Press.
12. W. T. Dickins and J. R. Flynn (2001) 'Heritability estimates versus large environmental effects: the IQ paradox resolved', *Psychological Review*, 108: 346–69.

13. A. E. Farmer (1996) 'The genetics of depressive disorders', *International Review of Psychiatry*, 8: 369–72.

14. R. Mojtabai and R. O. Rieder (1998) 'Limitations of the symptom-orientated approach to psychiatric research', *British Journal of Psychiatry*, 173: 198–202.

15. H. Berenbaum, T. F. Oltmanns and I. I. Gottesman (1987) 'A twin study perspective on positive and negative symptoms of schizophrenia', in P. D. Harvey and E. F. Walker (eds.), *Positive and Negative Symptoms of Psychosis: Description, Research and Future Directions*. Hillsdale, NJ: Erlbaum.

16. K. Kendler, L. Karkowski-Shuman, F. A. O'Neill, R. E. Straub, C. J. MacLean and D. Walsh (1997) 'Resemblance of psychotic symptoms and syndromes in affected sibling pairs from the Irish study of high-density schizophrenia families: evidence for possible etiologic heterogeneity', *American Journal of Psychiatry*, 154: 191–8.

17. M. T. Singer and L. C. Wynne (1965) 'Thought disorder and family relations of schizophrenics. III. Methodology using projective techniques', *Archives of General Psychiatry*, 12: 187–200; M. T. Singer and L. C. Wynne (1965) 'Thought disorder and family relations of schizophrenics. IV. Results and implications', *Archives of General Psychiatry*, 12: 201–12.

18. 'Projective' rather than standardized tests were employed. In these kinds of tests, for example the familiar Rorschach test in which the participant is asked to describe a series of ink blots, the person being assessed is asked to generate imaginative responses which are then analysed for their meaning. Most projective tests were designed by psychoanalysts or psychologists inspired by Freud's theory, and they have tended to fall into disuse, largely because the interpretation of the participant's responses is highly subjective, and scores are often unreliable. However, Singer and Wynne used a very detailed scoring protocol in order to avoid this criticism.

19. An apparent exception, which seems to have knocked British research into communication deviance stone dead, was a study reported in S. R. Hirsch and J. P. Leff (1971) 'Parental abnormalities of verbal communication in the transmission of schizophrenia', *Psychological Medicine*, 1: 118–27. In fact, differences between the parents of schizophrenia patients and the parents of psychiatric controls were observed in this study, although only a minority of the parents of the schizophrenia patients showed evidence of communication deviance.

20. N. M. Docherty, J. P. Rhinewine, R. P. Labhart and S. W. Gordinier (1998) 'Communication disturbance and family psychiatric history in parents of schizophrenic patients', *Journal of Nervous and Mental Disease*, 186: 761–8.

21. N. M. Docherty, M. J. Hall and S. W. Gordinier (1998) 'Affective reactivity of speech in schizophrenia patients and their nonschizophrenic relatives', *Journal of Abnormal Psychology*, 107: 461–7.

22. M. A. Nugter, P. M. A. J. Dingemans, D. H. Linszen and A. J. W. van der Does (1997) 'The relationships between expressed emotion, affective style and communication deviance in recent-onset schizophrenia', *Acta Psychiatrica Scandinavica*, 96: 445–51.

23. O. Gambini, A. Campana, F. Macciardi and S. Scarone (1997) 'A preliminary report of a strong genetic component for thought disorder in normals', *Neuropsychobiology*, 36: 13–18.

24. D. K. Kinney, P. S. Holzman, B. Jacobsen, L. Jansson, B. Faber, W. Hildebrand, E. Kasell and M. E. Zimbalist (1997) 'Thought disorder in schizophrenic and control adoptees and their relatives', *Archives of General Psychiatry*, 54: 475–9.

25. K.-E. Wahlberg, L. C. Wynne, H. Oja, P. Keskitalo, L. Pykalainen, L. Lahti, J. Moring, M. Naarala, A. Sorri, M. Seitamaa, K. Laksy, J. Kolassa and P. Tienari (1997) 'Gene–environment interaction in vulnerability to schizophrenia: findings from the Finnish Adoptive Family Study of Schizophrenia', *American Journal of Psychiatry*, 154: 355–62; K.-E. Wahlberg, L. C. Wynne, H. Oja, P. Keskitalo, H. Anais-Tanner, P. Koistinen, T. Tarvainen, H. Hakko, J. Moring, M. Naarala, A. Sorri and P. Tienari (2000) 'Thought disorder index of Finnish adoptees and communication deviance of their adoptive parents', *Psychological Medicine*, 30: 127–36.

26. F. L. Coolidge, L. L. Thede and K. L. Jang (2001) 'Heritability of personality disorders in childhood: a preliminary investigation', *Journal of Personality Disorders*, 15: 33–40; A. A. Dahl (1993) 'The personality disorders: a critical review of family, twin and adoption studies', *Journal of Personality Disorders* (Supplement 1): 86–99; S. Torgersen, S. Lygren, P. A. Oien, I. Skre, S. Onstad, J. Edvardsen, K. Tambs and E. Kringlen (2000) 'A twin study of personality disorders', *Comprehensive Psychiatry*, 41: 416–25.

27. K. S. Kendler, A. M. Gruenberg and J. S. Strauss (1981) 'An independent analysis of the Copenhagen sample of the Danish Adoption Study of Schizophrenia: III. The relationship between paranoid psychosis (delusional disorder) and the schizophrenia spectrum disorders', *Archives of General Psychiatry*, 38: 985–7; K. S. Kendler and P. Hays (1981) 'Paranoid psychosis (delusional disorder) and schizophrenia: a family history study', *Archives of General Psychiatry*, 38: 547–51; K. S. Kendler, C. C. Masterson and K. L. Davis (1985) 'Psychiatric illness in first-degree relatives of patients with paranoid psychosis, schizophrenia and medical illness', *British Journal of Psychiatry*, 147: 524–31.

28. R. H. Dworkin, M. F. Lenzenweger, S. O. Moldin, G. F. Skillings and S. E. Levick (1988) 'A multidimensional approach to the genetics of schizophrenia', *American Journal of Psychiatry*, 145: 1077–83; A. Jorgensen, T. W. Teasdale, J. Parnas, F. Schulsinger, H. Shulsinger and S. A. Mednick (1987) 'The Copenhagen High-Risk Project: the diagnosis of maternal schizophrenia and its relation to offspring diagnosis', *British Journal of Psychiatry*, 151: 753–7; S. Onstad, I. Skre, S. Torgersen and E. Kringlen (1991) 'Subtypes of schizophrenia: evidence from a twin-family study', *Acta Psychiatrica Scandinavica*, 84: 203–6.

29. R. C. Lewontin (1993) *The Doctrine of DNA: Biology as Ideology*. London: Penguin.

30. S. H. Barondes (1998) *Mood Genes: Hunting for the Origins of Mania and Depression*. Oxford: Oxford University Press.

31. Vicente and Kennedy, 'The genetics of neurodevelopment and schizophrenia', op. cit.

32. J.-P. Changeux and S. Dehaene (1989) 'Neuronal models of cognitive functions', *Cognition*, 33: 63–109.

33. W. T. Greenough, J. E. Black and C. S. Wallace (1987) 'Experience and brain development', *Child Development*, 58: 539–59; W. T. Greenough (1993) 'Brain adaption to experience: an update', in M. H. Johnson (ed.), *Brain Development and Cognition: A Reader*. Oxford: Blackwell.

34. J. L. Elman, E. A. Bates, M. H. Johnson, A. Karmiloff-Smith, D. Parisi and K. Plunkett (1999) *Rethinking Innateness: A Connectionist Perspective on Development*. Cambridge, MA: MIT Press.

35. For an excellently accessible description of these new techniques, see Barondes, *Mood Genes*, op. cit.

36. D. F. Levinson, M. Mahtani, D. J. Nancarrow, D. M. Brown, L. Kruglyak, A. Kirby, N. K. Hayward, R. R. Crowe, N. C. Andreasen, D. W. Black, J. M. Silverman, J. Endicott, L. Sharpe, R. C. Mohs, L. J. Siever, M. K. Walters, D. P. Lennon, H. L. Jones, D. A. Nertney, M. J. Daly, M. Gladis and B. J. Mowry (1998) 'Genome scan of schizophrenia', *American Journal of Psychiatry*, 155: 741–50; L. E. DeLisi, S. H. Shaw, T. J. Crow, G. Shields, A. B. Smith, V. W. Larach, N. Wellman, J. Loftus, B. Nanthakumar, K. Razi, J. Stewart, M. Comazzi, A. Vita, T. Heffner and R. Sherrington (2002) 'A genome-wide scan for linkage to chromosomal regions in 382 sibling pairs with schizophrenia or schizoaffective disorder', *American Journal of Psychiatry*, 159: 803–12.

37. J. A. Egeland, D. S. Gerhard, D. L. Pauls, J. N. Sussex, K. K. Kidd, C. R. Allen, A. M. Hostetter and D. E. Housman (1987). 'Bipolar affective disorder linked to DNA markers on chromosome 11', *Nature*, 325: 783–7.

38. J. R. Kelsoe, E. I. Ginns, J. A. Egeland, D. S. Gerhard, A. M. Goldstein, S. J. Bale, D. L. Pauls, R. T. Long, K. K. Kidd, G. Conte, D. E. Housman and S. M. Paul (1989) 'Re-evaluation of the linkage relationship between chromosome 11p loci and the gene for bipolar affective disorder in the Old Order Amish', *Nature*, 342: 238–43.

39. C. Barr (1998) 'Why two findings which were eventually refuted have been seminal for the field of psychiatric genetics', *Journal of Psychosomatic Research*, 44: 625–6.

40. D. Hill (1988) 'Psychiatric delusions', *New Statesman*, 12 September.

41. R. Sherrington, J. Brynjolfsson, H. Pertursson, M. Potter, K. Dudleston, B. Barraclough, J. Wasmuth, M. Dobbs and H. G. Gurling (1988) 'Localization of a susceptibility locus for schizophrenia on chromosome 5', *Nature*, 336: 164–7.

42. J. L. Kennedy, L. A. Giuffra, H. W. Moises, L. I. Cavalli-Sforza, A. J. Pakstis, J. R. Kidd, C. M. Castiglione, L. Wetterberg and K. K. Kidd (1988) 'Evidence against linkage of schizophrenia to markers on chromosome 5 in a northern Swedish pedigree', *Nature*, 336: 167–70.

43. D. St Clair, D. Blackwood, W. Muir, D. Baillie, A. Hubbard, A. Wright and J. Evans (1989) 'No linkage of chromosome 5q11–q13 markers to schizophrenia in Scottish families', *Nature*, 339: 305–9.

44. S. D. Detera-Wadleigh, L. R. Goldin, R. Sherrington et al. (1989) 'Exclusion of

linkage to 5q11–13 in families with schizophrenia and other psychiatric disorders', *Nature*, 340: 391–3.

45. G. Turecki, G. A. Rouleau, J. J. Mari and K. Morgan (1996) 'A systematic evaluation of linkage studies in bipolar disorder', *Acta Psychiatrica Scandinavica*, 93: 317–26; S. G. Simpson and J. R. DePaulo (1998) 'Genetics', in P. J. Goodnick (ed.), *Mania: Clinical and Research Perspectives*. Washington, DC: American Psychiatric Association.

46. The dopamine hypothesis, discussed in Chapter 4, was proposed when it was discovered that anti-psychotic drugs block dopamine receptors. There are five known types of dopamine receptor, and the genes for all five types are known. Reviewing the molecular evidence, Petter Portin and Y. O. Alanen of the University of Turku in Finland ('A critical review of genetic studies of schizophrenia. II: Molecular genetic studies', *Acta Psychiatrica Scandinavica*, 95: 73–80, 1997) have concluded that, 'On the whole, it seems that molecular genetic studies lend only minor support to the dopamine theory of schizophrenia.'

47. D. B. Wildenauer, S. G. Schwab, W. Maier and S. D. Detera-Wadleigh (1999) 'Do schizophrenia and affective disorder share susceptibility genes?' *Schizophrenia Research*, 39: 107–11.

48. T. J. Crow (1997) 'Current status of linkage for schizophrenia: polygenes of vanishingly small effect or multiple false positives?' *American Journal of Medical Genetics (Neuropsychiatric Genetics)*, 74: 99–103; Portin and Alanen, 'A critical review of genetic studies of schizophrenia, II, op. cit.

49. Crow, 'Current status of linkage for schizophrenia', op. cit.

50. Schizophrenia Linkage Collaborative Group for Chromosomes 3 and 6a (1996) 'Additional support for schizophrenia linkage on chromosomes 6 and 8: a multicenter study', *American Journal of Medical Genetics (Neuropsychiatric Genetics)*, 67: 580–94.

51. L. E. DeLisi, S. H. Shaw, T. J. Crow, G. Shields, A. B. Smith, V. W. Larach, N. Wellman, J. Loftus, B. Nanthakumar, K. Razi, J. Stewart, M. Comazzi, A. Vita, T. Heffner and R. Sherrington (2002) 'A genome-wide scan for linkage to chromosomal regions in 382 sibling pairs with schizophrenia or schizoaffective disorder', *American Journal of Psychiatry*, 159: 803–12.

52. S. O. Moldin (1997) 'The maddening hunt for madness genes', *Nature Genetics*, 17: 127–9.

53. K. K. Kidd (1997) 'Can we find genes for schizophrenia?' *American Journal of Medical Genetics (Neuropsychiatric Genetics)*, 74: 104–11; E. Rall (1998) 'Commentary: where are the genes specifying mental illness?' *Journal of Nervous and Mental Disease*, 186: 722–3.

54. A. Serretti, F. Macciardi, M. Catalano, L. Bellodi and E. Smeraldi (1999) 'Genetic variants of dopamine receptor D4 and psychopathology', *Schizophrenia Bulletin*, 25: 609–18.

55. M. Boyle (1990) *Schizophrenia: A Scientific Delusion*. London: Routledge; R. Marshall (1990) 'The genetics of schizophrenia: axiom or hypothesis?' in R. P. Bentall (ed.), *Reconstructing Schizophrenia*. London: Routledge; S. Rose, L. J.

Kamin and R. C. Lewontin (1985) *Not in our Genes*. Harmondsworth: Penguin.

56. Consistent with this conclusion, a recent study of Irish families with a 'high density' of schizophrenia found six chromosomal regions associated with psychosis, but found that very few families were 'positive' with respect to more than one region. See R. E. Straub, C. J. MacLean, Y. Ma, B. T. Webb, M. V. Myakishev, C. Harris-Kerr, B. Wormley, H. Sadek, B. Kadambi, F. A. O'Neill, D. Walsh and K. S. Kendler (2002) 'Genome-wide scans of three independent sets of 90 Irish multiplex schizophrenia families and follow-up of selected regions in all families provides evidence for multiple susceptibility genes', *Molecular Psychiatry*, 7: 542–59.

57. I. Feinberg (1997) 'Schizophrenia as an emergent disorder of late brain maturation', in Keshavan and Murray (eds.), *Neurodevelopment and Adult Psychopathology*, op. cit.

58. P. R. Huttenlocher (1979) 'Synaptic density in human frontal cortex – developmental changes and effects of aging', *Brain Research*, 163: 195–205; P. R. Huttenlocher (1990) 'Morphometric study of human cerebral cortex development', *Neuropsychologia*, 517–27.

59. G. Edelman (1989) *Neural Darwinism: The Theory of Neuronal Group Selection*. Oxford: Oxford University Press.

60. N. Davies, A. Russell, P. Jones and R. M. Murray (1998) 'Which characteristics of schizophrenia predate psychosis?' *Journal of Psychiatric Research*, 32: 121–31.

61. Feinberg, 'Schizophrenia and late maturational brain changes', op. cit.; R. E. Hoffman and T. H. McGlashan (1993) 'Parallel distributed processing and the emergence of schizophrenic symptoms', *Schizophrenia Bulletin*, 19: 257–61.

62. M. Davidson, A. Reichenberg, J. Rabinowitz, M. Weiser, Z. Kaplan and M. Mark (1999) 'Behavioral and intellectual markers for schizophrenia in apparently healthy male adolescents', *American Journal of Psychiatry*, 156: 1328–35.

63. E. F. Walker (1994) 'Neurodevelopmental precursors of schizophrenia', in A. S. David and J. C. Cutting (eds.), *The Neuropsychology of Schizophrenia*. Hove: Erlbaum.

64. E. F. Walker, K. E. Grimes, D. M. Davis and A. J. Smith (1993) 'Childhood precursors of schizophrenia: facial expressions of emotion', *American Journal of Psychiatry*, 150: 1654–60.

65. M. F. Pogue-Geile and M. Harrow (1987) 'Negative symptoms in schizophrenia: longitudinal characteristics and etiological hypotheses', in P. D. Harvey and E. F. Walker (eds.), *Positive and Negative Symptoms of Psychosis: Description, Research and Future Directions*. Hillsdale, NJ: Erlbaum.

66. M. Cannon, E. Walsh, C. Hollis, M. Kargin, E. Taylor, R. M. Murray and P. B. Jones (2001) 'Predictors of later schizophrenia and affective psychosis among attendees at a child psychiatry department', *British Journal of Psychiatry*, 178: 420–6.

67. S. A. Mednick and F. Schulsinger (1965) 'A longitudinal study of children with a high risk for schizophrenia: a preliminary report', in S. Vandenberg (ed.), *Methods and Goals in Human Behavior Genetics*. New York: Academic Press.

68. L. Erlenmeyer-Kimling and B. Cornblatt (1987) 'The New York High-Risk Project: a follow-up report', *Schizophrenia Bulletin*, 13: 451–63.

69. J. Marcus, S. L. Hans, S. Nagler, J. G. Aurbach, A. F. Mirsky and A. Aubrey (1987) 'Review of the NIMH Israeli Kibbutz–City Study and the Jerusalem Infant Development Study', *Schizophrenia Bulletin*, 13: 425–39.

70. P. H. Venables (1990) 'Longitudinal research on schizophrenia', in Bentall (ed.), *Reconstructing Schizophrenia*, op. cit.

71. T. D. Cannon, S. A. Mednick and J. Parnas (1990) 'Two pathways to schizophrenia in children at risk', in L. Robins and M. Rutter (eds.), *Straight and Devious Pathways from Childhood to Adulthood*. Cambridge: Cambridge University Press.

72. L. Erlenmeyer-Kimling, B. Cornblatt, A. S. Bassett, S. O. Moldin, U. Hilldoff-Adamo and S. Roberts (1990) 'High-risk children in adolescence and young adulthood: course of global adjustment', in Robins and Rutter (eds.), *Straight and Devious Pathways*, op. cit.

73. L. Erlenmeyer-Kimling, U. H. Adamo, D. Rock, S. A. Roberts, A. S. Bassett, E. Squires-Wheeler, B. A. Cornblatt, J. Endicott, S. Pape and I. I. Gottesman (1997) 'The New York High-Risk Project: prevalence and comorbidity of axis-I disorders in offspring of schizophrenic parents at 25-year follow-up', *Archives of General Psychiatry*, 54: 1096–102.

74. J. R. Asarnow (1988) 'Children at risk for schizophrenia: converging lines of evidence', *Schizophrenia Bulletin*, 14: 613–31.

75. C. Hollis and E. Taylor (1997) 'Schizophrenia: a critique from the developmental psychopathology perspective', in Keshavan and Murray (eds.), *Neurodevelopment and Adult Psychopathology*, op. cit.

76. Cannon, Mednick and Parnas, 'Two pathways to schizophrenia', op. cit.

77. R. H. Dworkin, B. A. Cornblatt, R. Friedmann, L. M. Kaplansky, J. A. Lewis, A. Rinalsi, C. Shilliday and L. Erlenmeyer-Kimling (1993) 'Childhood precursors of affective vs social deficits in adolescents at risk for schizophrenia', *Schizophrenia Bulletin*, 19: 563–76; L. R. Freedman, D. Rock, S. A. Roberts, B. A. Cornblatt and L. Erlenmeyer-Kimling (1998) 'The New York High-Risk Project: attention, anhedonia and social outcome', *Schizophrenia Research*, 30: 1–9.

78. P. B. Jones and D. J. Done (1997) 'From birth to onset: a developmental perspective of schizophrenia in two national birth cohorts', in Keshavan and Murray (eds.), *Neurodevelopment and Adult Psychopathology*, op. cit.

79. E. Frenkel, S. Kugelmass, M. Nathan and L. J. Ingraham (1995) 'Locus of control and mental health in adolescence and adulthood', *Schizophrenia Bulletin*, 21: 219–26.

80. S. A. Mednick (1970) 'Breakdown in individuals at high risk of schizophrenia: possible predisposing perinatal factors', *Mental Hygiene*, 54: 50–63.

81. S. W. Lewis, M. J. Owen and R. M. Murray (1989) 'Obstetric complications and schizophrenia: methodology and mechanisms', in S. C. Schulz and C. A. Tamming (eds.), *Schizophrenia: A Scientific Focus*. New York: Oxford University Press; S. L. Buka, M. T. Tsuang and L. P. Lipsitt (1993) 'Pregnancy/delivery complications and psychiatric diagnosis: a prospective study', *Archives of General Psychiatry*, 50: 151–6.

82. D. J. Done, E. C. Johnstone, C. D. Frith, J. Golding, P. M. Shepard and T. J. Crow (1991) 'Complications of pregnancy and delivery in relation to psychosis in adult life: data from the British Perinatal Mortality Survey', *British Medical Journal*, 302: 1576–80.

83. E. O'Callaghan, T. Gibson, H. A. Colohan, P. Buckley, D. G. Walshe, C. Larkin and J. L. Waddington (1992) 'Risk of schizophrenia in adults born after obstetric complications and their association with early onset of illness: a controlled study', *British Medical Journal*, 305: 1256–9.

84. D. Cotter, C. Larkin, J. L. Waddington and E. O'Callaghan (1996) 'Season of birth in schizophrenia: clue or cul-de-sac?', in J. L. Waddington and P. F. Buckley (eds.), *The Neurodevelopmental Basis for Schizophrenia*. New York: Chapman Hall, pp. 17–30; E. F. Torrey, J. Miller, R. Rawlings and R. H. Yolken (1997) 'Seasonality of births in schizophrenia and bipolar disorder: a review of the literature', *Schizophrenia Research*, 28: 1–38.

85. E. F. Torrey and R. H. Yolken (1995) 'Could schizophrenia be a viral zoonosis transmitted from house cats?' *Schizophrenia Bulletin*, 21: 167–77.

86. S. Mednick, R. A. Machon, M. O. Huttenen and D. Bonnett (1988) 'Adult schizophrenia following prenatal exposure to an influenza epidemic', *Archives of General Psychiatry*, 45: 188–92; P. C. Sham, E. O'Callaghan, N. Takei, G. K. Murray, E. H. Hare and R. M. Murray (1992) 'Increased risk of schizophrenia following prenatal exposure to influenza', *British Journal of Psychiatry*, 160: 461–6.

87. T. J. Crow and D. J. Done (1992) 'Prenatal exposure to influenza does not cause schizophrenia', *British Journal of Psychiatry*, 161: 390–5; L. Erlenmeyer-Kimling, Z. Folnegovic, V. Hrabak-Zerjavic, B. Borcic, V. Folnegovic-Smale and E. Susser (1994) 'Schizophrenia and prenatal exposure to the 1957 A2 influenza epidemic', *American Journal of Psychiatry*, 151: 1496–8; J.-P. C. J. Selten and J. P. J. Slaets (1994) 'Second trimester exposure to 1957 A2 influenza epidemic is not a risk factor for schizophrenia', *Schizophrenia Research*, 11: 95; E. Susser, S. P. Lin, A. S. Brown, L. H. Lumey and L. Erlenmeyer-Kimling (1994) 'No relation between risk of schizophrenia and prenatal exposure to influenza in Holland', *American Journal of Psychiatry*, 151: 922–4.

88. N. Takei, P. C. Sham, E. O'Callaghan, G. Glover and R. M. Murray (1995) 'Schizophrenia: increased risk associated with winter and city birth: a case-control study in 12 regions within England and Wales', *Journal of Epidemiology and Community Health*, 49: 106–7; H. Verdoux, N. Takei, R. Cassou de Saint Mathurin, R. M. Murray and M. L. Bourgeois (1997) 'Seasonality of birth in schizophrenia: the effect of regional population density', *Schizophrenia Research*, 23: 175–80.

89. E. O'Callaghan, D. Cotter, K. Colgan and C. Larkin (1995) 'Confinement of winter birth excess in schizophrenia to the urban-born and its gender specificity', *British Journal of Psychiatry*, 166: 51–4.

90. P. B. Mortensen, C. B. Pedersen, T. Westergaard, J. Wohlfahrt, H. Ewald, O. Mors, P. K. Andersen and M. Melbye (1999) 'Effects of family history and place and season of birth on the risk of schizophrenia', *New England Journal of Medicine*, 340: 603–8.

91. Cotter et al., 'Season of birth in schizophrenia', op. cit.

92. E. S. Susser and S. P. Lin (1992) 'Schizophrenia after prenatal exposure to the Dutch hunger winter of 1944–1945', *Archives of General Psychiatry*, 49: 983–8.

93. J. McGrath and R. Murray (1995) 'Risk factors for schizophrenia: from conception to birth', in S. R. Hirsch and D. R. Weinberger (eds.), *Schizophrenia*. Oxford: Blackwell, pp. 187–205.

94. ibid.

95. C. M. Hultman, P. Sparen, N. Takei, R. M. Murray and S. Cnattingius (1999) 'Prenatal and perinatal risk factors for schizophrenia, affective psychosis, and reactive psychosis of early onset: case control study', *British Medical Journal*, 318: 421–6.

96. J. B. Lohr and H. S. Bracha (1989) 'Can schizophrenia be related to prenatal exposure to alcohol? Some speculations', *Schizophrenia Bulletin*, 15: 595–603.

97. H. A. Nasrallah (1997) 'Neurodevelopment and affective disorders', in Keshavan and Murray (eds.), *Neurodevelopment and Adult Psychopathology*, op. cit.

98. J. Worland, R. Edenhart-Pepe, D. G. Weeks and P. M. Koren (1984) 'Cognitive evaluation of children at risk: IQ, differentiation and egocentricity', in N. F. Watt, E. J. Anthony, L. C. Wynne and J. E. Rolf (eds.), *Children at Risk of Schizophrenia: A Longitudinal Perspective*. Cambridge: Cambridge University Press.

99. J. J. van Os, P. Jones, G. Lewis, M. Wadsworth and R. M. Murray (1996) 'Evidence for similar developmental precursors of chronic affective illness and schizophrenia in a general population birth cohort', *Archives of General Psychiatry*, 54: 625–31.

100. M. Cannon, P. Jones, C. Gilvarry, L. Rifkin, K. McKenzie, A. Foerster and R. M. Murray (1997) 'Premorbid social functioning in schizophrenia and bipolar disorder: similarities and differences', *American Journal of Psychiatry*, 154: 1544–50.

101. Torrey et al., 'Seasonality of births in schizophrenia and bipolar disorder', op. cit.

102. Nasrallah, 'Neurodevelopment and affective disorders', op. cit.

103. A. S. Brown, J. van Os, C. Driessens, H. W. Hoek and E. S. Susser (2000) 'Further evidence of relation between prenatal famine and major affective disorder', *American Journal of Psychiatry*, 157: 190–5.

Chapter 18 The Trials of Life

1. A. Camus (1955) *The Myth of Sisyphus*. London: Hamish Hamilton.

2. P. Larkin (1988) 'This be the verse', *Collected Poems*. London: Faber & Faber.

3. L. Johnstone (1999) 'Do families cause "schizophrenia"?: Revisiting a taboo subject', *Changes*, 17: 77–90.

4. L. Kuipers, M. Birchwood and R. D. McCreadie (1992) 'Psychosocial family intervention in schizophrenia: a review of empirical studies', *British Journal of Psychiatry*, 160: 272–5.

5. G. Bateson, D. D. Jackson, J. Haley and J. Weakland (1956) 'Towards a theory of schizophrenia', *Behavioral Science*, 1: 251–64.

6. R. D. Laing and A. Esterson (1964) *Sanity, Madness and the Family: Families of Schizophrenics*. London: Tavistock.

7. P. Sedgwick (1982) *Psychopolitics*. London: Pluto Press.

8. J. Bowlby (1965) *Child Care and the Growth of Love* (2nd edn). Harmondsworth: Penguin.

9. S. J. Suomi (1997) 'Long-term effects of different early rearing experiences on social, emotional, and physiological development in nonhuman primates', in M. S. Keshavan and R. M. Murray (eds.), *Neurodevelopment and Adult Psychopathology*. Cambridge: Cambridge University Press, pp. 104–16.

10. For a review of evidence on the social and cognitive consequences of insecure attachment, see E. Meins (1997) *Security of Attachment and the Social Development of Cognition*. Hove: Psychology Press.

11. M. Main (1991) 'Metacognitive knowledge, metacognitive monitoring, and singular (coherent) vs. multiple model of attachment: findings and future directions for research', in C. M. Parkes, J. Stevenson-Hinde and P. Marris (eds.), *Attachment across the Life Cycle*. London: Routledge, pp. 127–59.

12. P. Fonagy, S. Redfern and A. Charman (1997) 'The relationship between belief-desire reasoning and a projective measure of attachment security (SAT)', *British Journal of Developmental Psychology*, 15: 51–63.

13. Meins, *Security of Attachment*, op. cit.; E. Meins, C. Fernyhough, J. A. Russell and D. Clark-Carter (1998) 'Security of attachment as a predictor of symbolic and mentalizing abilities: a longitudinal study', *Social Development*, 7: 1–24.

14. A. Myhrman, P. Rantakallio, M. Isohanni, P. Jones and U. Partanen (1996) 'Unwantedness of pregnancy and schizophrenia in the child', *British Journal of Psychiatry*, 169: 637–40.

15. For readable accounts of attachment theory, see J. Holmes (1993) *John Bowlby and Attachment Theory*. London: Routledge; and Parkes, Stevenson-Hinde and Marris (eds.), *Attachment across the Life Cycle*, op. cit.

16. M. Dozier, A. L. Stevenson, S. W. Lee and D. I. Velligan (1991) 'Attachment organization and familial overinvolvement for adults with serious psychopathological disorders', *Development and Psychopathology*, 3: 475–89.

17. M. Dozier and S. W. Lee (1995) 'Discrepancies between self and other-report

of psychiatric symptomatology: effects of dismissing attachment strategies', *Development and Psychopathology*, 7: 217–26.

18. K. D. Mickelson, R. C. Kessler and P. R. Shaver (1997) 'Adult attachment in a nationally representative sample', *Journal of Personality and Social Psychology*, 73: 1092–106.

19. M. L. Cooper, P. R. Shaver and N. L. Collins (1998) 'Attachment style, emotion regulation, and adjustment in adolescence', *Journal of Personality and Social Psychology*, 74: 1380–97. For a study of disturbed adolescents that found a relationship between paranoid personality characteristics and the dismissing-avoidant attachment style, see also D. S. Rosenstein and H. A. Horowitz (1996) 'Adolescent attachment and psychopathology', *Journal of Consulting and Clinical Psychology*, 64: 244–53.

20. P. Rankin, R. P. Bentall, J. Hill and P. Kinderman (submitted) 'Parental relationships and paranoid delusions: comparisons of currently ill, remitted and normal people'.

21. J. Schiffman, J. LaBrie, J. Carter, C. Tyrone, F. Schulsinger, J. Parnas and S. Mednick (2002) 'Perception of parent–child relationships in high-risk families, and adult schizophrenia outcome of offspring', *Journal of Psychiatric Research*, 36: 41–7.

22. K.-E. Wahlberg, L. C. Wynne, H. Oja, P. Keskitalo, L. Pykalainen, I. Lahti, J. Moring, N. Naarala, A. Sorri, M. Seitamaa, K. Laksy, J. Kolassa and P. Tienari (1997) 'Gene–environment interaction in vulnerability to schizophrenia: findings from the Finnish Adoptive Family Study of Schizophrenia', *American Journal of Psychiatry*, 154: 355–62.

23. E. Kuipers and D. Raune (2000) 'The early development of expressed emotion and burden in the families of first-onset psychosis', in M. Birchwood, D. Fowler and C. Jackson (eds.), *Early Intervention in Psychosis*. London: Wiley, pp. 128–40.

24. N. J. Goldstein (1987) 'The UCLA high-risk project', *Schizophrenia Bulletin*, 13: 505–14.

25. M. J. Goldstein (1998) 'Adolescent behavioral and intrafamilial precursors of schizophrenia spectrum disorders', *International Clinical Psychopharmacology*, 13 (Supplement 1): 101.

26. M. E. Seligman, C. Peterson, N. J. Kaslow, R. L. Tanenbaum, L. B. Alloy and L. Y. Abramson (1984) 'Attributional style and depressive symptoms among children', *Journal of Abnormal Psychology*, 93: 235–8.

27. K. Durkin (1995) *Developmental Social Psychology*. Oxford: Blackwell; F. D. Fincham and K. M. Cain (1986) 'Learned helplessness in humans: a developmental analysis', *Developmental Review*, 6: 301–33; E. Turk and B. Bry (1992) 'Adolescents' and parents' explanatory styles and parents' causal explanations about their adolescents', *Cognitive Therapy and Research*, 16: 349–57.

28. J. Garber and C. Flynn (2001) 'Predictors of depressive cognitions in young adolescents: negative interpersonal context leads to personal vulnerability', *Cognitive Therapy and Research*, 25: 353–76.

29. C. Hammen (1991) *Depression Runs in Families: The Social Context of Risk and Resilience in Children of Depressed Mothers.* London: Springer-Verlag.

30. L. B. Alloy, L. Y. Abramson, W. G. Whitehouse, M. E. Hogan, N. A. Tashman, D. L. Steinberg, D. T. Rose and P. Donovan (1999) 'Depressogenic cognitive styles: predictive validity, information processing and personality characteristics, and developmental origins', *Behaviour Research and Therapy*, 37: 503–31.

31. L. B. Alloy, L. Y. Abramson, N. A. Tashman, D. S. Berrebbi, M. E. Hogan, W. G. Whitehouse, A. G. Crossfield and A. Morocco (2001) 'Developmental origins of cognitive vulnerability to depression: parenting, cognitive and inferential feedback styles of the parents of individuals at high and low cognitive risk for depression', *Cognitive Therapy and Research*, 25: 397–423. For an earlier relevant study from the same research group, see: D. T. Rose, L. Y. Abramson, C. J. Hodulik, L. Halberstadt and G. Leff (1994) 'Heterogeneity of cognitive style among depressed inpatients', *Journal of Abnormal Psychology*, 103: 419–29.

32. D. Diamond and J. Doane (1994) 'Disturbed attachment and negative affective style: an intergenerational spiral', *British Journal of Psychiatry*, 164: 770–81; G. Paley, D. A. Shapiro and A. Worrall-Davies (2000) 'Familial origins of expressed emotion in relatives of people with schizophrenia', *Journal of Mental Health*, 9: 655–63.

33. G. Harrison, D. Owens, A. Holton, D. Neilson and D. Boot (1988) 'A prospective study of severe mental disorder in Afro-Caribbean patients', *Psychological Medicine*, 18: 643–57.

34. D. Bhugra, M. Hilwig, B. Hossein, H. Marceau, J. Neehall, J. P. Leff, R. Mallett and G. Der (1996) 'First contact incidence rates of schizophrenia in Trinidad and one-year follow-up', *British Journal of Psychiatry*, 169: 587–92; F. W. Hickling (1995) 'The incidence of first-contact schizophrenia in Jamaica', *British Journal of Psychiatry*, 167: 193–6.

35. G. Hutchinson, N. Takei, T. A. Fahy, D. Bhugra, C. Gilvarry, O. Moran, R. Mallett, P. Sham, J. Leff and R. M. Murray (1996) 'Morbid risk of schizophrenia in first-degree relatives of white and Afro-Caribbean patients with psychosis', *British Journal of Psychiatry*, 171: 776–80; P. A. Sugarman and D. Crawford (1994) 'Schizophrenia in the Afro-Caribbean community', *British Journal of Psychiatry*, 164: 474–80.

36. J.-P. Selten, N. Veen, W. Feller, J. D. Blom, D. Schols, W. Camoenie, J. Oolders, M. van der Velden, H. W. Hoek, V. M. Rivero, Y. van der Graaf and R. Kahn (2001) 'Incidence of psychotic disorders in immigrant groups to The Netherlands', *British Journal of Psychiatry*, 178: 367–72.

37. K. Zolkowska, G. E. Cantor and T. F. McNeil (2001) 'Increased rates of psychosis amongst immigrants to Sweden: is migration a risk factor for psychosis?' *Psychological Medicine*, 31: 669–78.

38. C. Haasen, M. Lambert, R. Mass and M. Kraesz (1998) 'Impact of ethnicity on the prevalence of psychiatric disorders among migrants in Germany', *Ethnicity and Health*, 3: 159–65.

39. F. W. Hickling (1991) 'Double jeopardy: psychopathology of Black mentally ill returned to Jamaica', *International Journal of Social Psychiatry*, 37: 80–9.

40. J. Boydell, J. van Os, J. McKenzie, J. Allardyce, R. Goel, R. G. McCreadie and R. M. Murray (2001) 'Incidence of schizophrenia in ethnic minorities in London: ecological study into interactions with environment', *British Medical Journal*, 323: 1–4.

41. D. Bhugra, J. Leff, R. Mallett, G. Der, B. Corridan and S. Rudge (1997) 'Incidence and outcome of schizophrenia in Whites, African-Caribbeans and Asians in London', *Psychological Medicine*, 27: 791–8.

42. M. MacLachlan (1997) *Culture and Health*. London: Wiley.

43. J. Berry (1988) 'Acculturation and mental health', in Pierre Dasen, John Berry and Norman Sartorius (eds.), *Health and Cross-Cultural Psychology: Towards Applications*. Thousand Oaks, CA: Sage.

44. R. E. L. Faris and H. W. Dunham (1939) *Mental Disorders in Urban Areas*. Chicago: Chicago University Press.

45. D. L. Gerald and L. G. Houston (1953) 'Family setting and the ecology of schizophrenia', *Psychiatric Quarterly*, 27: 90–101.

46. A. S. McNaught, S. E. Jeffries, C. A. Harvey and A. S. Quale (1997) 'The Hampstead Schizophrenia Survey 1991: incidence and migration in inner London', *British Journal of Psychiatry*, 170: 307–11.

47. C. B. Pedersen and P. B. Mortensen (2001) 'Evidence of a dose–response relationship between urbanicity during upbringing and schizophrenia risk', *Archives of General Psychiatry*, 58: 1039–46.

48. V. K. Varma, N. N. Wig, H. R. Phookun, A. K. Misra, C. B. Khare, B. M. Tripathi, P. B. Behere, E. S. Yoo and E. S. Susser (1997) 'First-onset schizophrenia in the community: relationship of urbanization with onset, early manifestations and typology', *Acta Psychiatrica Scandinavica*, 96: 431–8.

49. American Psychiatric Association (1994) *Diagnostic and Statistical Manual for Mental Disorders* (4th edition). Washington, DC: APA.

50. L. A. Goodman, S. D. Rosenberg, K. T. Mueser and R. E. Drake (1997) 'Physical and sexual assault history in women with serious mental illness: prevalence, correlates, treatment, and future research directions', *Schizophrenia Bulletin*, 23: 685–96.

51. K. T. Mueser, L. A. Goodman, S. L. Trumbetta, S. D. Rosenberg, F. C. Osher, R. Vidaver, P. Auciello and D. W. Foy (1998) 'Trauma and posttraumatic stress disorder in severe mental illness', *Journal of Consulting and Clinical Psychology*, 66: 493–9.

52. M. Hyun, S. D. Friedman and D. L. Dunner (2000) 'Relationship of childhood physical and sexual abuse to adult bipolar disorder', *Bipolar Disorder*, 2: 121–35; R. D. Levitan, S. V. Parikh, A. D. Lesage, K. M. Hegadoren, M. Adams, S. H. Kennedy and P. N. Goering (1998) 'Major depression in individuals with a history of childhood physical or sexual abuse: relationship to neurovegetative features, mania, and gender', *American Journal of Psychiatry*, 155: 1746–52.

53. B. M. Cohen and M. Z. Cooper (1954) 'A follow-up study of World War II prisoners of war', Veterans Administration Medical Monograph. Washington: US Government Printing Office; G. W. Beebe (1975) 'Follow-up studies of World War II and Korean War prisoners', *American Journal of Epidemiology*, 101: 400–2.

54. R. E. Eberly and B. E. Engdahl (1991) 'Prevalence of somatic and psychiatric disorders among former prisoners of war', *Hospital and Community Psychiatry*, 42: 807–13.

55. R. W. Butler, K. T. Mueser, J. Sprock and D. L. Braff (1996) 'Positive symptoms of psychosis in posttraumatic stress disorder', *Biological Psychiatry*, 39: 839–44; K. T. Mueser and R. W. Butler (1987) 'Auditory hallucinations in combat-related chronic posttraumatic stress disorder', *American Journal of Psychiatry*, 144: 299–302.

56. L. Eitinger (1967) 'Schizophrenia among concentration camp survivors', *International Journal of Psychiatry*, 5: 403–8.

57. J. D. Kinzie and J. J. Boehnlein (1989) 'Post-traumatic psychosis among Cambodian refugees', *Journal of Traumatic Stress*, 2: 185–98.

58. Y. Neria, E. J. Bromet, S. Sievers, J. Lavelle and L. J. Fochtmann (2002) 'Trauma exposure and posttraumatic stress disorder in psychosis: findings from a first-admission cohort', *Journal of Consulting and Clinical Psychology*, 70: 246–51.

59. J. E. D. Esquirol (1843/1965) *Mental Maladies: A Treatise on Insanity*. New York: Hafner.

60. R. E. Kendell, J. C. Chalmers and C. Platz (1986) 'Epidemiology of puerperal psychoses', *British Journal of Psychiatry*, 150: 662–73.

61. I. F. Brockington, K. F. Cernik, E. M. Schofield, A. R. Downing, A. F. Francis and C. Keelan (1981) 'Puerperal psychosis: phenomena and diagnosis', *Archives of General Psychiatry*, 38: 829–33.

62. I. Brockington (1996) *Motherhood and Mental Health*. Oxford: Oxford University Press.

63. J. W. Ellason and C. A. Ross (1997) 'Childhood trauma and psychiatric symptoms', *Psychological Reports*, 80: 447–50; C. A. Ross, G. Anderson and P. Clark (1994) 'Childhood abuse and the positive symptoms of schizophrenia', *Hospital and Community Psychiatry*, 42: 489–91.

64. J. Read and N. Argyle (1999) 'Hallucinations, delusions and thought disorder among adult psychiatric inpatients with a history of child abuse', *Psychiatric Services*, 51: 534–5.

65. P. Hammersley, A. Dias, G. Todd, K. Bowen-Jones, B. Reilly and R. P. Bentall (in press) 'Childhood trauma and hallucinations in bipolar affective disorder: a preliminary investigation', *British Journal of Psychiatry*.

66. The specific association between trauma and hallucinations has also been reported in studies of women who have been abused. Bernadine Ensink (*Confusing Realities: A Study of Child Sexual Abuse and Psychiatric Symptoms*. Amsterdam: VU University Press, 1992), a psychologist working at the University of Amsterdam, interviewed 100 women who had sought psychological help for problems

relating to sexual abuse. Thirty-four per cent reported hallucinatory flashbacks of their experiences, 42 per cent reported visual hallucinations, and 43 per cent reported hearing voices. In general, the women who experienced auditory hallucinations had been victims of the most severe forms of sexual abuse.

67. C. Fernyhough and J. Russell (1997) 'Distinguishing one's own voice from those of others: a function for private speech?' *International Journal of Behavioral Development*, 20: 651–65.

68. A. Honig, M. A. J. Romme, B. J. Ensink, S. Escher, M. H. A. Pennings and M. W. DeVries (1998) 'Auditory hallucinations: a comparison between patients and nonpatients', *Journal of Nervous and Mental Disease*, 186: 646–51.

69. J. Read, B. D. Perry, A. Moskowitz and J. Connolly (2001) 'The contribution of early traumatic events to schizophrenia in some patients: a traumagenic neurodevelopmental model', *Psychiatry: Interpersonal and Biological Processes*, 64: 319–45.

70. R. W. Heinrichs (2001) *In Search of Madness: Schizophrenia and Neuroscience*. Oxford: Oxford University Press.

71. For example, see the study by Butler et al. cited earlier in this chapter.

72. E. Bleuler (1911/1950) *Dementia Praecox or the Group of Schizophrenias* (trans. E. Zinkin). New York: International Universities Press.

73. M. F. Green (1998) *Schizophrenia from a Neurocognitive Perspective: Probing the Impenetrable Darkness*. Boston: Allyn & Bacon.

74. G. S. Hall (1916) *Adolescence*. New York: Appleton.

75. R. E. Muus (1996) *Theories of Adolescence*. New York: McGraw-Hill; J. C. Coleman and L. B. Hendry (1999) *The Nature of Adolescence* (3rd edn). London: Routledge.

76. E. H. Erikson (1950) *Childhood and Society*. New York: Norton.

77. C. Harrop and P. Trower (2001) 'Why does schizophrenia develop at late adolescence?', *Clinical Psychology Review*, 21: 241–66.

78. P. D. McGorry, C. McFarlane, G. C. Patton, R. Bell, M. E. Hibbert, H. J. Jackson and G. Bowes (1995) 'The prevalence of prodromal features of schizophrenia in adolescence: a preliminary survey', *Acta Psychiatrica Scandinavica*, 92: 241–9.

79. B. A. Cornblatt, M. F. Lenzenweger, R. H. Dworkin and L. Erlenmeyer-Kimling (1992) 'Childhood attentional dysfunctions predict social deficits in unaffected adults at risk for schizophrenia', *British Journal of Psychiatry*, 161 (Supplement 18): 59–64.

80. A. P. Morrison (2001) 'The interpretation of intrusions in psychosis: an integrative cognitive approach to hallucinations and delusions', *Behavioural and Cognitive Psychotherapy*, 29: 257–76.

81. K. Popper (1961) *The Poverty of Historicism*. London: Routledge.

Chapter 19   Madness and Society

1. Quoted in N. Zierold (1991) *The Moguls*. New York: Silman-James.

2. E. Kraepelin (1899/1990) *Psychiatry: A Textbook for Students and Physicians*, Vol. 1: *General Psychiatry*. Canton, MA: Watson Publishing International.

3. W. Mayer-Gross, E. Slater and M. Roth (1975) *Clinical Psychiatry*. London: Cassell.

4. A. Lewis (1934) 'The psychopathology of insight', *British Journal of Medical Psychology*, 14: 332–48.

5. X. F. Amador and H. Kronengold (1998) 'The description and meaning of insight in psychosis', in X. F. Amador and A. S. David (eds.), *Insight and Psychosis*. Oxford: Oxford University Press, pp. 15–32.

6. World Health Organization (1973) *International Pilot Study of Schizophrenia*. Geneva: WHO; X. F. Amador, M. Flaum, N. C. Andreasen, D. H. Strauss, S. A. Yale, S. C. Clark and J. M. Gorman (1994) 'Awareness of illness in schizophrenia and schizoaffective and mood disorders', *Archives of General Psychiatry*, 51: 826–36; M. A. Weiler, M. H. Fleisher and D. McArthur-Campbell (2000) 'Insight and symptom change in schizophrenia', *Schizophrenia Research*, 45: 29–36.

7. A. S. David (1998) 'The clinical importance of insight', in Amador and David (eds.), *Insight and Psychosis*, op. cit., pp. 332–51; A. S. David (1999) ' "To see ourselves as others see us" ', *British Journal of Psychiatry*, 175: 210–16.

8. For a study of recent historical trends in the use of coercion in Britain see M. Hotopf, S. Wall, A. Buchanan, S. Wessely and R. Churchill (2000) 'Changing patterns in the use of the Mental Health Act 1983 in England, 1984–1996', *British Journal of Psychiatry*, 176: 479–84.

For evidence from Finland, see H. R. Kaltiala, J. Korkeila, C. Tuohimaeki, T. Tuori and V. Lehtinen (2000) 'Coercion and restrictions in psychiatric inpatient treatment', *European Psychiatry*, 15: 213–19.

For evidence from the USA, see S. K. Hoge, C. W. Lidz, M. Eisenberg and W. Gardner (1997) 'Perceptions of coercion in the admission of voluntary and involuntary psychiatric patients', *International Journal of Law and Psychiatry*, 20: 167–81.

For evidence from New Zealand, see B. G. McKenna, A. I. F. Simpson and T. M. Laidlaw (1999) 'Patient perception of coercion on admission to acute psychiatric services: the New Zealand experience', *International Journal of Law and Psychiatry*, 22: 143–53.

Finally, for evidence that patients' perceptions that they are being coerced are often accurate, see C. W. Lidz, E. P. Mulvey, S. K. Hoge, B. L. Kirsch, J. Monahan, M. Eisenberg, W. Gardner and L. H. Roth (1998) 'Factual sources of psychiatric patients' perceptions of coercion in the hospital admission process', *American Journal of Psychiatry*, 155: 1254–60.

9. V. W. Swayze (1995) 'Frontal leukotomy and related psychosurgical procedures

chotics (1935–1954): a historical overview', *American*
52: 505–15.

oxic Psychiatry. London: Fontana.

'The fate of the mentally ill in Germany during the Third
Medicine, 18: 575–81.

)88) *Racial Hygiene: Medicine under the Nazis*. Cambridge,
ersity Press.

13. J. Le ra. 99) *The Rise and Fall of Modern Medicine*. London: Little,
Brown & Co.

14. See, for example, recent systematic reviews published electronically (and avail-
able at academic libraries) by the international 'Cochrane' collaborative network
of researchers, which provides evidence on the effectiveness of treatments for the
British National Health Service and other health care providers: B. Thornley, C. E.
Adams and G. Award (2001) 'Chlorpromazine versus placebo for schizophrenia
(*Cochrane Review*)', *The Cochrane Library*, 3. Oxford: Update Software; C. B.
Joy, C. E. Adams and S. M. Lawrie (2001) 'Haloperidol versus placebo for
schizophrenia (*Cochrane Review*)', *The Cochrane Library*, 3. Oxford: Update
Software.

15. R. Warner (1985) *Recovery from Schizophrenia: Psychiatry and Political
Economy*. New York: Routledge & Kegan Paul.

16. W. A. Brown and L. R. Herz (1989) 'Response to neuroleptic drugs as a device
for classifying schizophrenia', *Schizophrenia Bulletin*, 15: 123–8.

17. B. J. Kinon, J. M. Kane, C. Johns, R. Perovich, M. Ismi, A. Koreen and P.
Weiden (1993) 'Treatment of neuroleptic resistant relapse', *Psychopharmacology
Bulletin*, 29: 309–14.

18. P. F. Kennedy, H. I. Hershon and R. J. McGuire (1971) 'Extrapyramidal
disorders after prolonged phenothiazine therapy', *British Journal of Psychiatry*,
118: 509–18.

19. G. Sullivan and D. Lukoff (1990) 'Sexual side effects of antipsychotic medication: evaluation and interventions', *Hospital and Community Psychiatry*, 41:
1238–41.

20. J. Day, P. Kinderman and R. P. Bentall (1997) 'Discordant views of neuroleptic
side effects: a potential source of conflict between patients and professionals', *Acta
Psychiatrica Scandinavica*, 97: 93–7.

21. R. Robinson, P. McHugh and M. Follstein (1975) 'Measurement of appetite
disturbance in severe psychiatric disorders', *Journal of Psychiatric Research*, 12:
59–68.

22. D. B. Allison, J. L. Mentore, M. Heo, L. P. Chandler, J. C. Cappelleri, M. C.
Infante and P. Weiden (1999) 'Antipsychotic-induced weight gain: a comprehensive research synthesis', *American Journal of Psychiatry*, 156: 1686–96.

23. T. van Putten and P. R. May (1978) 'Subjective response as a predictor of
outcome in pharmacotherapy', *Archives of General Psychiatry*, 35: 477–80; T.
van Putten, P. R. May, S. R. Marder and L. A. Wittman (1981) 'Subjective response
to antipsychotic drugs', *Archives of General Psychiatry*, 38: 187–90.

24. M. Harrow, C. A. Yonan, J. R. Sands and J. Marengo (1994) 'Depression in schizophrenia: are neuroleptics, akinesia or anhedonia involved?', *Schizophrenia Bulletin*, 20: 327–38.

25. T. Lewander (1994) 'Neuroleptics and the neuroleptic-induced deficit syndrome', *Acta Psychiatrica Scandinavica*, 89: 8–13; N. R. Schooler (1994) 'Deficit symptoms in schizophrenia: negative symptoms versus neuroleptic-induced deficits', *Acta Psychiatrica Scandinavica*, 89: 21–6.

26. T. J. Crow, J. F. MacMillan, A. L. Johnson and E. C. Johnstone (1986) 'The Northwick Park study of first episodes of schizophrenia. II: A randomised controlled trial of prophylactic neuroleptic treatment', *British Journal of Psychiatry*, 148: 120–7.

27. N. Thorogood, P. Cowen, J. Mann, M. Murphy and M. Vessey (1992) 'Fatal myocardial infarction and use of psychotropic drugs in young women', *Lancet*, 340: 1067–8; W. A. Ray, S. Meredith, P. B. Thapa, K. G. Meador, K. Hall and K. T. Murray (2001) 'Antipsychotics and the risk of sudden death', *Archives of General Psychiatry*, 58: 1161–7; W. A. Ray and K. G. Meador (2002) 'Antipsychotics and sudden death: is thoridazine the only bad actor?', *British Journal of Psychiatry*, 180: 483–4.

28. S. N. Caroff (1980) 'The neuroleptic malignant syndrome', *Journal of Clinical Psychiatry*, 41: 79–83.

29. M. N. G. Dukes (ed.) (1992) *Meyler's Side Effects of Drugs*. Amsterdam: Elsevier.

30. I am grateful to Professor Simon Wessely of the Institute of Psychiatry in London, who first drew my attention to this risk associated with neuroleptics.

31. E. C. Atbasoglu, S. K. Schultz and N. C. Andreasen (2001) 'The relationship of akathisia with suicidality and depersonalization among patients with schizophrenia', *Journal of Neuropsychiatry and Clinical Neurosciences*, 13: 336–41; H. Lars (2001) 'A critical review of akathisia and its possible association with suicidal behaviour', *Human Psychopharmacology: Clinical and Experimental*, 16: 495–505; M. Z. Azhar and S. L. Varama (1992) 'Akathisia-induced suicidal behaviour', *European Psychiatry*, 7: 239–41; J. L. Schulte (1985) 'Homicide and suicide associated with akathisia and haloperidol', *American Journal of Forensic Psychiatry*, 6: 3–7.

32. T. van Putten, S. R. Marder and J. Mintz (1990) 'A controlled dose comparison of haloperidol in newly admitted schizophrenic patients', *Archives of General Psychiatry*, 47: 754–8; J. P. McEvoy, G. E. Hogarty and S. Steingard (1991) 'Optimal dose of neuroleptic in acute schizophrenia: a controlled study of the neuroleptic threshold and higher haloperidol dose', *Archives of General Psychiatry*, 48: 739–45; A. Rifkind, S. Doddi, B. Karagigi, M. Bornstein and M. Wachspress (1991) 'Dosage of haloperidol for schizophrenia', *Archives of General Psychiatry*, 48: 166–70.

33. P. Bollini, S. Pampallona, M. J. Orza, M. E. Adams and T. C. Chalmers (1994) 'Antipsychotic drugs: is more worse? A meta analysis of the published randomized controlled trials', *Psychological Medicine*, 24: 307–16.

34. Royal College of Psychiatrists (1993) *Consensus Statement on the Use of High Dose Antipsychotic Medication* (CR 26). Royal College of Psychiatrists.

35. A. F. Lehman, D. M. Steinwachs, L. B. Dixon, H. H. Goldman, F. Osher, L. Postrado, J. E. Scott, J. W. Thompson, M. Fahey, P. Fisher, J. A. Kasper, A. Lyles, E. A. Skinner, R. Buchanan, W. T. Carpenter, J. Levine, E. A. McGlynn, R. Rosenheck and J. Zito (1998) 'Translating research into practice: the Schizophrenia Patient Outcomes Research Team (PORT) treatment recommendations', *Schizophrenia Bulletin*, 24: 1–10.

36. L. M. Flynn (1998) 'Patterns of usual care for schizophrenia: initial results from the Schizophrenia Patient Outcomes Research Team (PORT) Client Survey', *Schizophrenia Bulletin*, 24: 30–2; D. Cohen (1997) 'A critique of the use of neuroleptic drugs in psychiatry', in S. Fisher and R. P. Greenberg (eds.), *From Placebo to Panacea: Putting Psychiatric Drugs to the Test*. New York: Wiley, pp. 173–228.

In an as yet unpublished study carried out by myself and Jennie Day, in which we collected data on neuroleptic treatment from 212 patients on psychiatric wards in the North West of England and North Wales between 1995 and 1998, we found that the median dose of medication received by the patients was equivalent to 600 milligrams of chlorpromazine a day and approximately a quarter of the patients were on doses equivalent to 1 gram of chlorpromazine or more.

37. H. Hippius and D. Healy (1996) 'The founding of the CNIP and the discovery of clozapine (interview)', in D. Healy (ed.), *The Psychopharmacologists*. London: Chapman & Hall, pp. 187–213.

38. J. Kane, G. Honigfeld, J. Singer and H. Meltzer (1988) 'Clozapine for the treatment-resistant schizophrenic', *Archives of General Psychiatry*, 45: 789–96.

39. H. Meltzer and D. Healy (1996) 'A career in biological psychiatry (interview)', in Healy (ed.), *The Psychopharmacologists*, op. cit., pp. 483–507.

40. T. Van Putten, B. D. Marshall, R. Liberman and J. Mintz (1993) 'Systematic dosage reduction in treatment-resistant schizophrenic patients', *Psychopharmacology Bulletin*, 29: 315–20.

41. J. Geddes, N. Freemantle, P. Harrison and P. Bebbington (2000) 'Atypical antipsychotics in the treatment of schizophrenia: systematic overview and meta-regression analysis', *British Medical Journal*, 321: 1371–6.

42. American psychiatrist Peter Breggin takes this kind of position. See Breggin, *Toxic Psychiatry*, op. cit.

43. L. R. Mosher and A. Z. Menn (1978) 'Community residential treatment for schizophrenia: two-year follow-up', *Hospital and Community Psychiatry*, 29: 715–23; L. R. Mosher, R. Vallone and A. Menn (1995) 'The treatment of acute psychosis without neuroleptics: six-week psychopathology outcome data from the Soteria project', *International Journal of Social Psychiatry*, 41: 157–73.

44. H. S. Sullivan (1962) *Schizophrenia as a Human Process*. New York: Norton.

45. F. B. Evans (1996) *Harry Stack Sullivan: Interpersonal Theory and Psychotherapy*. London: Routledge.

46. K. T. Mueser and H. Berenbaum (1990) 'Psychodynamic treatment of schizophrenia: is there a future?', *Psychological Medicine*, 20: 253–62.

47. A. H. Stanton, J. G. Gunderson, P. H. Knapp, A. F. Frank, M. L. Vannicelli, R. Schnitzer and R. Rosenthal (1984) 'Effects of psychotherapy in schizophrenia: I. Design and implementation of a controlled study', *Schizophrenia Bulletin*, 10: 520–63; J. G. Gunderson, A. F. Frank, H. M. Katz, M. L. Vannicelli, J. P. Frosch and P. H. Knapp (1984) 'Effects of psychotherapy in schizophrenia: II. Comparative outcome of two forms of treatment', *Schizophrenia Bulletin*, 10: 564–98.

48. T. H. McGlashan (1984) 'The Chestnut Lodge follow-up study I: Follow-up methodology and study sample', *Archives of General Psychiatry*, 41: 575–85; T. H. McGlashan (1984) 'The Chestnut Lodge follow-up study II: Long-term outcome of schizophrenia and affective disorders', *Archives of General Psychiatry*, 41: 586–601; M. H. Stone (1986) 'Exploratory psychotherapy in schizophrenia-spectrum patients', *Bulletin of the Menninger Clinic*, 50: 287–306.

49. J. P. Leff, L. Kuipers, R. Berkowitz, R. Eberlein-Fries and D. Sturgeon (1982) 'A controlled trial of intervention with families of schizophrenic patients', *British Journal of Psychiatry*, 141: 121–34.

50. J. P. Leff, L. Kuipers, R. Berkowitz and D. Sturgeon (1985) 'A controlled trial of social intervention in the families of schizophrenic patients', *British Journal of Psychiatry*, 146: 594–600.

51. I. R. H. Falloon, J. L. Boyd, C. W. McGill, M. Williamson, J. Razani, H. B. Moss, A. M. Gilderman and G. M. Simpson (1985) 'Family management in the prevention of morbidity of schizophrenia: clinical outcome of a two-year longitudinal study', *Archives of General Psychiatry*, 42: 887–96.

52. G. E. Hogarty, C. M. Anderson, D. J. Reiss, S. J. Kornblith, D. P. Greenwald, R. F. Ulrich and M. Carter (1991) 'Family psychoeducation, social skills training and maintenance chemotherapy in the aftercare treatment of schizophrenia. II: Two year effects of a controlled study on relapse and adjustment', *Archives of General Psychiatry*, 48: 340–7.

53. N. Tarrier, C. Barrowclough, C. E. Vaughn, J. S. Bamrah, K. Porceddu, S. Watts and H. Freeman (1988) 'The community management of schizophrenia: a controlled trial of a behavioural intervention with families to reduce relapse', *British Journal of Psychiatry*, 153: 532–42; N. Tarrier, C. Barrowclough, C. E. Vaughn, J. S. Bamrah, K. Porceddu, S. Watts and H. Freeman (1989) 'The community management of schizophrenia: a controlled trial of a behavioural intervention with families to reduce relapse: a two-year follow-up', *British Journal of Psychiatry*, 154: 625–8.

54. W. G. Pitschel, S. Leucht, J. Baeumil, W. Kissling and R. R. Engel (2001) 'The effects of family interventions on relapse and rehospitalisation in schizophrenia: a meta-analysis', *Schizophrenia Bulletin*, 27: 73–92.

55. N. Tarrier, C. Barrowclough, K. Porceddu and E. Fitzpatrick (1994) 'The Salford family intervention project: relapse rates of schizophrenia at five and eight years', *British Journal of Psychiatry*, 165: 829–32.

56. D. J. Miklowitz, T. L. Simoneau, E. L. George, J. A. Richards, A. Kalbag, N. Sachs-Ericsson and R. Suddath (2000) 'Family focused treatment of bipolar

disorder: 1-year effects of a psychoeducational program in conjunction with pharmacotherapy', *Biological Psychiatry*, 48: 582–92.

57. A. T. Beck, A. J. Rush, B. F. Shaw and G. Emery (1979) *Cognitive Therapy of Depression*. New York: Guilford.

58. P. Chadwick and C. F. Lowe (1990) 'The measurement and modification of delusional beliefs', *Journal of Consulting and Clinical Psychology*, 58: 225–32.

59. G. Haddock, R. P. Bentall and P. D. Slade (1993) 'Psychological treatment of chronic auditory hallucinations: two case studies', *Behavioural and Cognitive Psychotherapy*, 21: 335–46.

60. P. Chadwick and M. Birchwood (1994) 'The omnipotence of voices: a cognitive approach to auditory hallucinations', *British Journal of Psychiatry*, 164: 190–201.

61. D. G. Kingdon and D. Turkington (1994) *Cognitive-Behavioural Therapy of Schizophrenia*. Hove: Lawrence Erlbaum.

62. L. Yusupoff and N. Tarrier (1996) 'Coping strategy enhancement for persistent hallucinations and delusions', in G. Haddock and P. D. Slade (eds.), *Cognitive-Behavioural Interventions with Psychotic Disorders*. London: Routledge, pp. 71–85.

63. N. Tarrier, R. Beckett, S. Harwood, A. Baker, L. Yusupoff and I. Ugarteburu (1993) 'A trial of two cognitive-behavioural methods of treating drug-resistant residual psychotic symptoms in schizophrenic patients. I: Outcome', *British Journal of Psychiatry*, 162: 524–32.

64. P. A. Garety, L. Kuipers, D. Fowler, F. Chamberlain and G. Dunn (1994) 'Cognitive behavioural therapy for drug-resistant psychosis', *British Journal of Medical Psychology*, 67: 259–71.

65. T. Sensky, D. Turkington, D. Kingdon, J. L. Scott, J. Scott, R. Siddle, M. O'Carrol and T. R. E. Barnes (2000) 'A randomized controlled trial of cognitive-behaviour therapy for persistent symptoms in schizophrenia resistant to medication', *Archives of General Psychiatry*, 57: 165–72.

66. E. Kuipers, P. Garety, D. Fowler, G. Dunn, P. Bebbington, D. Freeman and C. Hadley (1997) 'The London–East Anglia randomised controlled trial of cognitive-behavioural therapy for psychosis. I: Effects of the treatment phase', *British Journal of Psychiatry*, 171: 319–27; E. Kuipers, D. Fowler, P. Garety, D. Chizholm, D. Freeman, G. Dunn, P. Bebbington and C. Hadley (1998) 'London–East Anglia randomised controlled trial of cognitive-behavioural therapy for psychosis. III: Follow-up and economic considerations', *British Journal of Psychiatry*, 173: 61–8.

67. N. Tarrier, L. Yusupoff, C. Kinner, E. McCarthy, A. Gladhill, G. Haddock and J. Morris (1998) 'A randomized controlled trial of intense cognitive behaviour therapy for chronic schizophrenia', *British Medical Journal*, 317: 303–7.

68. The trial design is described in S. Lewis, N. Tarrier, G. Haddock, R. P. Bentall, P. Kinderman, D. Kingdon, R. Siddle, R. Drake, J. Everitt, K. Leadley, A. Benn, K. Grazebrook, C. Haley, S. Akhtar, L. Davies, S. Palmer, B. Faragher and G. Dunn (2002) 'Randomised, controlled trial of cognitive-behaviour therapy in early schizophrenia: acute phase outcomes', *British Journal of Psychiatry*, 181

(Supplement 43): s91–s97. The 18-month outcome report is in preparation for publication at the time of writing.

69. A. Gumley, K. Power, M. O'Grady, L. Mcnay, J. Reilly, K. Athanasios, A. Tait, Z. Chouliara and C. White (in press) 'A randomised controlled trial of targeted cognitive behaviour therapy: effects on relapse at 12 months', *Psychological Medicine*.

70. D. H. Lam, J. Bright, S. Jones, P. Hayward, N. Schuck, D. Chisholm and P. Sham (2000) 'Cognitive therapy for bipolar illness: a pilot study of relapse prevention', *Cognitive Therapy and Research*, 24: 503–20; A. Perry, N. Tarrier, R. Morriss, E. McCarthy and K. Limb (1999) 'Randomised controlled trial of efficacy of teaching patients with bipolar disorder to identify early symptoms of relapse and obtain treatment', *British Medical Journal*, 318: 149–53; J. Scott, A. Garland and S. Moorhead (2001) 'A pilot study of cognitive therapy in bipolar disorder', *Psychological Medicine*, 31: 459–67.

71. R. J. Wyatt (1995) 'Early intervention in schizophrenia: can the course of illness be altered?', *Biological Psychiatry*, 38: 1–3.

72. R. J. Drake, C. J. Haley, S. Akhtar and S. W. Lewis (2000) 'Causes of duration of untreated psychosis in schizophrenia', *British Journal of Psychiatry*, 177: 511–15.

73. A. R. Yung, L. J. Phillips, P. D. McGorry, C. A. McFarlane, S. Francey, S. Harrigan, G. C. Patton and H. J. Jackson (1998) 'Prediction of psychosis: a step towards indicated prevention of psychosis', *British Journal of Psychiatry*, 172 (Supplement 33): 14–20.

74. P. D. McGorry, L. J. Phillips, A. R. Yung, S. Francey, D. Germano, J. Bravin, A. MacDonald, N. Hearn, P. Amminger and L. O'Dwyer (2000) 'A randomized controlled trial of interventions in the pre-psychotic phase of psychotic disorders', *Schizophrenia Research*, 41: 9; P. D. McGowry, A. R. Yung, L. J. Phillips, H. P. Yen, S. Francey, E. M. Cosgrave, D. Germano, J. Bravin, T. McDonald, A. Blair, S. Adlard and H. J. Jackson (2002) 'Randomized controlled trial of interventions designed to reduce the risk of progression to first-episode psychosis in a clinical sample with subthreshold symptoms', *Archives of General Psychiatry*, 59: 921–8.

75. J. L. Rosen, S. W. Woods, J. Miller-Tandy and T. H. McGlashan (2002) 'Prospective observations of emerging psychosis', *Journal of Nervous and Mental Disease*, 190: 133–41.

76. R. P. Bentall and A. P. Morrison (2002) 'More harm than good: the case against using antipsychotic drugs to prevent severe mental illness', *Journal of Mental Health*, 11: 351–6.

77. A. P. Morrison, R. P. Bentall, P. French, L. Walford, A. Kilcommons, A. Knight, M. Kreutz and S. W. Lewis (2002) 'A randomised controlled trial of early detection and cognitive therapy for preventing transition to psychosis in high risk individuals: study design and interim analysis of transition rate and psychological risk factors', *British Journal of Psychiatry*, 181 (Supplement 43): s78–s84.

78. R. P. Bentall (1992) 'A proposal to classify happiness as a psychiatric disorder', *Journal of Medical Ethics*, 18: 94–8; K. W. M. Fulford (2002) 'Values in psychiatric diagnosis: executive summary of a report to the chair of the ICD-12/DSM-VI

coordination taskforce (dateline 2010)', *Psychopathology*, 35: 132–8; P. Sedgwick (1982) *Psychopolitics*. London: Pluto Press.

79. Of course, for many people, this is a big if. However, the popular perception, fostered by the mass media, that psychosis very often leads to dangerous behaviour, is ill founded. For recent discussions of the evidence, see: A. O'Kane and R. P. Bentall (2000) 'Psychosis and offending', in J. McGuire, T. Mason and A. O'Kane (eds.), *Behaviour, Crime and Legal Processes: A Guide for Forensic Practitioners*. London: Wiley, pp. 161–76; P. Taylor and P. J. Gunn (1999) 'Homicides by people with mental illness: myth and reality', *British Journal of Psychiatry*, 174: 9–14.

Index